Breath Analysis
for Clinical Diagnosis and Therapeutic Monitoring

Breath Analysis
for Clinical Diagnosis and Therapeutic Monitoring

editors

Anton Amann
Innsbruck Medical University and ETH-Zürich

David Smith
Keele University, UK

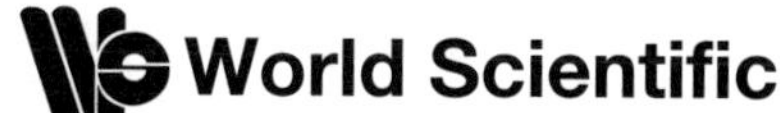

World Scientific

NEW JERSEY • LONDON • SINGAPORE • BEIJING • SHANGHAI • HONG KONG • TAIPEI • CHENNAI

Published by

World Scientific Publishing Co. Pte. Ltd.

5 Toh Tuck Link, Singapore 596224

USA office: 27 Warren Street, Suite 401-402, Hackensack, NJ 07601

UK office: 57 Shelton Street, Covent Garden, London WC2H 9HE

British Library Cataloguing-in-Publication Data
A catalogue record for this book is available from the British Library.

BREATH ANALYSIS FOR CLINICAL DIAGNOSIS AND THERAPEUTIC MONITORING (With CD-ROM)

ISBN 981-256-284-2

Printed in Singapore by World Scientific Printers (S) Pte Ltd

CONTENTS

FOREWORD

This book is a compilation of review papers and original research papers written by authorities in the field of breath analysis that are based on their presentations at the conference "Breath Gas Analysis for Medical Diagnostics" held at the University of Applied Sciences in Dornbirn, Austria, during September 23rd to 26th, 2004, organised by Anton Amann and Marco Freek with support from Oskar Müller and Karl Unterkofler. Included in this book are descriptions of the instrumentation developed for breath analysis, breath sampling methodologies and pilot case studies. It is intended as a treatise on the present state of development and the application of breath analysis to medicine and physiology. A primary purpose is to stimulate the entry of new workers into this exciting and potentially important field.

It has been known for centuries that the odour or smell of an individual is in some cases an indicator or a symptom of disease, even though the nature of the disease was not always understood. The classic case of this is the sweet smell of a person suffering from diabetes resulting from the excessive amount of acetone emitted in the breath and through the skin. The concentrations of compounds generated within the body reflect normal biochemistry and abnormalities due to pathophysiological processes. This, of course, is now an essential part of clinical diagnosis. Blood analysis is a routine part of clinical investigations, but usually it is the non-volatile compounds such as proteins and ions measured in blood that are the check for abnormalities. Nevertheless, volatile compounds must also carry information concerning the biochemical status of the individual.

Following the developments in analytical techniques after the Second World War period, in particular the development of gas chromatography mass spectrometry, GC-MS,[1] serious experiments were carried out to measure the metabolites present in exhaled breath in several diseased states. A most valuable review of the results of these early experiments was published in 1983.[2] This paper stimulated much of the subsequent work that

---

[1] reviewed by Gohlke RS and McLafferty FW, *J Am Soc Mass Spectrom* 1993; **4**: 367

[2] Manolis A, *Clin Chem* 1983; **29**: 5

has led to the clearer understanding that we have today of the potential of breath analysis for clinical diagnosis and therapeutic monitoring. Thus, it is known that a large number of volatile compounds appear at the trace level in the breath of even healthy individuals, and other compounds appear in the breath of diseased individuals. It is also the case that certain of the normally-occurring compounds are greatly elevated during disease; acetone and diabetes have already been mentioned, but to these can be added ammonia in renal disease, nitric oxide in asthma and small hydrocarbons (ethane and pentane) during oxidative stress, to mention just a few. The informative review by Manolis includes several more examples. However, a major problem has been the inability to reproduce many of the observations, which cast a cloud over the use of breath analysis in medicine. Undoubtedly, this is due to the inadequacies of the analytical methods and sampling methodologies and it is these topics that are now being successfully addressed, as reported in this book.

It has been said that as many as 300 and even 3000 trace gases are present in breath. Such has been indicated by experiments that have combined trapping techniques (such as solid phase microextraction, SPME) with GC-MS analyses. Even if it is accepted that many of these compounds are exogenous, it is reasonable to expect that many others are endogenously produced. Some of these compounds must play a significant role in the biochemistry occurring in the body and potentially they could be used diagnostically. However, many of these compounds are at such low levels in the blood/breath that they cannot yet be quantified sufficiently accurately with current techniques. A number of these volatile compounds can be identified and quantified sufficiently accurately in breath to allow meaningful physiological and clinical measurements to be made. Some of them are known disease markers (ammonia, acetone) and some are real candidates as markers of disease (formaldehyde, acetaldehyde, isoprene, ethane, pentane, etc.). It is the further detailed studies of these readily identifiable and quantifiable compounds that offer to place breath analysis on a firm foundation in medicine and biology, whilst progressing towards the more challenging analysis of lower level compounds that must be present and which are the repository of valuable clinical information.

Hence, a major challenge is to develop analytical techniques that allow these volatile compounds to be identified and quantified to sufficient accuracy to be useful in diagnosis. So what are the instrumental requirements for breath analysis to become a reliable tool for medical diagnostics and therapy? Ideally, a wide range of diverse volatile organic and inorganic compounds must be unambiguously identified and accurately quantified in exhaled breath in real time, obviating sample collection into bags or onto traps, because this can compromise the sample by selectively favouring certain compounds (*e.g.* because of differential adsorption rates, etc.) and also introduce exogenous impurities. This is a real analytical challenge made even more demanding by the fact that most of the metabolites will be present at the parts-per-billion (ppb) level or lower, although in the diseased state some will be present at the parts-per-million level (ppm) and much greater, so a wide dynamic range of sensitivity is also desirable. The compounds known to be present in exhaled breath range from the simple diatomic inorganic molecules, nitric oxide, NO, and carbon monoxide, CO, the small hydrocarbon molecule ethane, C_2H_6, carbonyl sulfide, OCS, dimethylsulfide, $(CH_3)_2S$, and ammonia, NH_3, to polyatomic molecules such as alcohols, including ethanol, C_2H_5OH, aldehydes such as acetaldehyde, CH_3CHO, ketones, including acetone, CH_3COCH_3, and higher-order alcohols, aldehydes and ketones, such as heptanone. In this mix there are also high-order hydrocarbons and other types of organic compounds.

Given the widely different physical properties of these compounds, it is now understood that no single analytical method can be used to detect and quantify all of them. Laser optical spectroscopy is very specific and can be made accurately quantitative, but it is only useful for some specific (low molecular weight) compounds, such as NO, CO and C_2H_6. GC-MS can separate and analyse the components of multi-component mixtures like breath, and the use of this technique has provided the majority of the data available to date on breath analysis. However, using GC-MS it is difficult to analyse low molecular weight polar organic compounds such as formaldehyde and sticky compounds like amines. Furthermore, each gas chromatographic column must be calibrated for all compounds, as must the ion source/analytical mass spectrometer. The latest developments in analytical techniques, especially selected ion flow tube mass spectrometry, SIFT MS, and proton transfer reaction mass spectrometry, PTR-MS, which both use mass spectrometry coupled with chemical ionisation and flow tube technology, are very valuable tools for real time accurate quantitative breath analysis of a wide variety of compounds, as is indicated in some chapters in this book. The benefits derived by the patients and clinicians from reliable real time breath analysis are clear in that no trauma is involved and the results are immediately available to the clinician, thus allowing rapid diagnosis and early treatment. Hence the reason for the growing research base for this subject.

What are the achievements so far using the available techniques? The chapters in this book provide some answers to this question. Notable are the SIFT-MS longitudinal studies of the major breath metabolites carried out to establish the concentration distributions for a few healthy individuals. These are required if abnormal breath levels are to be recognised. Such studies have indicated, for example, that in renal failure breath ammonia can be massively greater than normal, in some cases as much as 100 times greater, and breath acetone can be massively elevated in diabetes. The level of breath isoprene (2-methyl-1,3-butadiene) is relatively low in healthy individuals, but there is clear evidence that its level in breath is elevated following haemodialysis, probably the result of the peroxidation of lipids by free radicals produced at the dialysis membrane. Breath isoprene levels also vary during sleeping, as shown by recent PTR-MS measurements.

Some of these breath analyses have been carried out on-line and in real time. A further good example of such are the PTR-MS breath analyses carried out in the sleep laboratory using a mask or a catheter to collect the breath samples, as reported in a chapter in this book. No blood- or urine-based invasive procedures can achieve what these non-invasive breath analyses can achieve. The data flow using these on-line methods can be very large and this allows very accurate measurements of the time variations in breath concentrations to be made from which additional insights into lung physiology, other physiological processes (including metabolic rates) and pharmacokinetics can be obtained. This has been well demonstrated by studying ethanol metabolism using SIFT-MS, as is reported in a chapter in this book. Further to these aspects, it has been demonstrated how several metabolites can be quantified simultaneously in only single breath exhalations. This is potentially important since diagnosis may be clearer and co-morbidity recognised when several metabolites can be monitored simultaneously. For example, analysis of the breath of patients with renal failure (elevated ammonia) also indicates those patients who are diabetic (elevated acetone) and also shows if the patients have been smoking cigarettes (presence of acetonitrile). Another such example is the decrease in breath acetone following feeding with a protein meal after a fasting period and the associated increase in breath ammonia due to protein metabolism. These are but a few examples of what is possible when exhaled breath can be reliably analysed, especially on-line.

To further exploit the diagnostic potential of breath analysis, not only analytical problems but also basic methodological issues have to be addressed. In practice, this means that it is essential to differentiate between the levels of particular endogenous compounds in the healthy and diseased states and, crucially, to recognise exogenous compounds, *i.e.* those that have been inhaled from ambient air via the lungs or absorbed through the skin. This is now possible due to the remarkable developments in gas analysis and in sampling methodology during the last few decades, which are briefly referred to below and described in some detail in this book.

Exogenous compounds introduced into inhaled air, such as anaesthetic gases, readily flow across the lung interface into the blood. Similarly, truly endogenous compounds such as ammonia, acetone, etc., readily flow to the lungs via the blood stream and appear in exhaled breath. Clearly, the blood concentrations and the volatilities of the compounds will be first-order parameters in determining their concentrations in the exhaled breath. The liquid phase/gas phase partition coefficients for many of the compounds that are now known to be generated in the body have been determined by experiment and so breath concentrations can readily be converted to blood concentrations and vice versa (unless the pH of the blood has an influence, as it does for ammonia).

An important yet underappreciated aspect of breath analysis and its interpretation concerns the different blood-gas kinetics of the various compounds present in exhaled breath and where they are produced in the body. Some of them, such as NO and CO, are not only transported to the lungs by the blood stream, but are also produced in the airways and/or in the paranasal sinuses. Modelling of the influence of haemodynamics and lung mechanics on the concentration patterns of trace compounds in exhaled breath can provide additional information about the production and elimination rates of these compounds. This is of particular concern for very volatile compounds such as methane, ethane, pentane and isoprene, the concentrations of which in exhaled breath significantly depend on the heart rate and the breathing rate, as well as the breath volume. A more detailed knowledge of the behaviour of other marker compounds such as lipophilic hydrocarbons under different haemodynamic and respiratory conditions is surely important. The use of concentration patterns of such compounds for cancer screening, for example, must be complemented by information on their variability with heart rate and breath volume.

Further to this, breath compounds such as isoprene could provide estimates of the ventilation–perfusion ratios and their variations within the lungs. At present, such estimates can only be obtained by injecting inert gases with different physicochemical properties (*e.g.* different solubilities in water and lipophilic compartments) into the blood stream and measuring their concentrations in exhaled breath. The multiple inert gas elimination technique, MIGET,[3] provides detailed information on the variation of ventilation–perfusion ratios, but this technique is not easily translated to clinical practice, especially in intensive care units. It is possible that endogenously-produced or ubiquitous exogenous compounds could be used to obtain some of the information supplied by MIGET technology. Hence, the scope for using volatile compounds in these investigations might be much broader than previously envisaged.

Real progress has been made in understanding the biochemical pathways to some of the volatile breath metabolites, especially NO, but much more needs to be done in parallel with further reliable breath analyses. A very good example of the combination of basic biochemical knowledge and advanced analytical techniques can be seen in the diagnostic application of NO. The discovery by Murad, Furchgott and Ignarro that this small inorganic molecule is endogenously produced and exerts multiple physiological functions[4] has led to the realization that endogenously-derived gases can participate in the regulation of physiological processes. Similarly, CO can be produced endogenously and although it is toxic in "high" concentrations, it is now known to have various cytoprotective effects in the body, as is reported in a chapter in this book. So, these small molecules can be important metabolites, messenger molecules, and antibacterial or cytoprotective agents. That this was not realised earlier is mainly due to sampling and detection difficulties due to the relatively low concentrations of these diatomic molecules in exhaled breath. The development of new methods to quantify NO in breath, especially the small hand-held devices that have recently been developed, allows and encourages their use in the clinical environment, for example, to study asthma. Important as NO and CO are as biomarkers, they are just two species amongst many other breath metabolites.

So, how has the detection of the many trace gas species in exhaled breath (including NO and CO) supported clinical diagnosis to date? Recent research in this area has largely proceeded via several uncoordinated programmes in various laboratories in Europe and the United States, which have been concerned principally with the development of sampling methodology, analytical techniques and pilot experiments. The major objective of this book is to review and report this work. Many laboratories have

---

[3]Roca J, Wagner PD, *Thorax* 1994; **49**: 815
[4]Barnes PJ, *Ann Med* 1995; **27**: 389

adopted GC-MS as the well-established analytical method. The use of the newer techniques (SIFT-MS, PTR-MS, laser spectroscopy, ion mobility spectrometry) will allow both the previous, mostly GC-MS, finding to be checked in more laboratories and hospitals and encourage the development of acceptable sampling methodologies. The exploitation of the fast flow tube techniques (SIFT-MS, PTR-MS) is particularly promising for real time breath analysis (*i.e.* avoiding sample collection). Close collaboration between researchers using the various analytical techniques will surely assist the identification of breath markers of particular diseases. In this way, breath composition will become a valuable research tool for detecting and identifying volatile metabolites with ready-to-use, on-line databases to assist clinical diagnosis.

So, to summarise, the real key to the advancement of breath analysis as a clinical tool resides in reliable identification and quantification of the trace gases present and a proper understanding of the basic biochemical mechanisms that generate these trace gases. Ideally, the analytical methods should satisfy the needs outlined previously — on-line, real time analysis avoiding sample collection into bags or onto traps; simultaneous accurate analyses of several metabolites over a wide concentration range (down to the parts-per-billion, ppb, level and below) without the need for constant re-calibration; results immediately available to assist rapid diagnosis; high sample rate and hence rapid time response for analysis of single exhalations; can be used when the patient is sleeping or comatose (*e.g.* in the intensive care unit). Whilst the SIFT-MS and PTR-MS analytical techniques fulfil many of these requirements, their lower limits of detection are currently limited to about 0.1 ppb, and they are rather large instruments unsuitable for use in restricted spaces like intensive care units. However, these detection limits are constantly being lowered by further research and development and smaller instruments are currently under construction so that restricted space will no longer be an issue.

These exciting developments point the way towards the routine exploitation of breath analysis for diagnosis and therapy. Just imagine the value of a reliable breath test that indicates the presence of tumours in the body! There is some evidence from trapping/GC-MS measurements that high-order hydrocarbons are present in the breath of cancer patients, but at such low levels that, as yet, this has not been confirmed by other techniques. It has also been demonstrated that urine from cancer patients contains formaldehyde (at levels undetectable in the urine of healthy volunteers), so it seems likely that this compound is also present in their breath. But will it be present at levels that it can be accurately quantified using the available analytical methods? It is important questions such as this that are driving this new area of science and which are revealing the need for more basic research and new instrument development.

In conclusion, the contents of this book represent the current status of the methods used for breath analysis and how they have been exploited to date in clinical diagnosis, therapeutic monitoring and for physiological measurements. Some glances into the future are also given in the book, especially in instrument development, and the future prospects for breath analysis in medicine are discussed. The work reported in this book has only revealed the great potential of breath analysis. Further research will surely establish it as a valuable addition to the armoury of the clinical practitioner.

We are indebted to all the authors of the chapters in this book without whose interest and skill the book could not have been produced. We are especially grateful for the wise advice and critical comments of Jochen Schubert, Patrik Španěl and Wolfram Miekisch, and for the technical support of Pierre Funck, Venelin Chernogorov, and especially Marco Freek, in the production and presentation of this book.

Finally, we thank the Government of Vorarlberg and the Bernhard Lang Research Association (Austria) for their financial support in the production of this book.

<table>
<tr><td>Anton Amann</td><td style="text-align:right">Innsbruck and Keele</td></tr>
<tr><td>David Smith</td><td style="text-align:right">31 January, 2005</td></tr>
</table>

PART A

NEW ANALYTICAL TECHNIQUES

SELECTED ION FLOW TUBE MASS SPECTROMETRY, SIFT-MS, FOR ON-LINE TRACE GAS ANALYSIS OF BREATH

D. SMITH

Institute of Science and Technology in Medicine,
Medical School, Keele University,
Thornburrow Drive, Hartshill, Stoke-on-Trent, ST4 7QB, UK

P. ŠPANĚL

V. Čermák Laboratory, J. Heyrovský Institute of Physical Chemistry,
Academy of Sciences of the Czech Republic,
Dolejškova 3, CZ-182 23 Prague 8, Czech Republic

1. Introduction

The objective of this short review paper is to describe the principles of the novel selected ion flow tube mass spectrometry, SIFT-MS, analytical technique and how it can be utilised for real time, on line analysis of the trace gases in ambient air and especially exhaled breath. Real-time detection and quantification of the wide variety of trace gases that are present in atmospheric air and exhaled breath are especially challenging using electron ionisation mass spectrometry, because the gas loading of the ion source by N_2 and O_2 (as well as water vapour) can be excessive. To circumvent this problem, various forms of membrane have been used that allow the passage of particular (polar) trace gas/vapour species into the ion source whilst blocking the major air gases.[1] However, these membranes also inhibit the passage of other trace gases (notably hydrocarbons) and so careful calibration of the membrane transmission for each trace gas is essential if meaningful quantification is to be achieved. Alternatively, to avoid the simultaneous ionisation of different compounds, separation of the multiple components in a mixture and their identification can be achieved using gas chromatography mass spectrometry, GC-MS.[2] Although GC-MS has been used to effect for trace gas analysis of air and breath at the parts per billion (ppb) level, and apparently at the parts per trillion (ppt) level, collection of the trace gases from relatively large volumes of air and breath samples is usually required either onto cryogenic traps or adsorption traps[3] and this is obviously not real-time monitoring. Also, GC-MS is not a practical technique for the separation and detection of some low molecular weight compounds such as ammonia and formaldehyde.[3,4]

In order to realise a real-time analytical method that does not suffer from the above deficiencies, but which supplements GC-MS and the other analytical methods more suitable for analyses of prepared samples, we have developed SIFT-MS.[5] As we will show, this is a quantitative mass spectrometric method that exploits chemical ionisation using judiciously-selected precursor positive ions that react during a defined (short) reaction time with the trace gases in air and breath samples that are introduced into a helium stream in a flow tube. This powerful combination of the fast flow tube technique, chemical ionisation and quantitative mass spectrometry allows accurate quantitative analyses of several trace gases simultaneously in air and exhaled breath down to the ppb regime of concentration on time scales of seconds. Thus, for example, several metabolites in single breath exhalations can be quantified on-line and in real time. The facility to choose precursor ions for the analysis of particular media illustrates the versatility of SIFT-MS and demonstrates its advantage over most other analytical methods.

In this paper, we briefly describe the SIFT-MS analytical method and the physics and the ion chemistry on which it is based followed by some examples of its use, principally for breath analysis.

2. Selected Ion Flow Tube Mass Spectrometry, SIFT-MS

SIFT-MS was realised from our familiarity with the selected ion flow tube, SIFT, technique that was conceived and developed almost thirty years ago[6] for the study of ion-neutral reactions at thermal interaction energies.[7] Initially, SIFT was developed to satisfy the need for the great deal of kinetic data on gas phase ion-neutral reactions that are required to describe the production of the molecule observed in cold interstellar clouds.[8,9] However, we now use the SIFT technique to develop the kinetics database that is required for SIFT-MS.

2.1. *Principle of SIFT-MS*

The principle of the SIFT-MS technique is simply explained with reference to the line diagram shown in Figure 1. Positive ions are created in an ion source and from the mixture of ion species that are inevitably present a current of ions of a given mass-to-charge ratio is selected using a quadrupole mass filter.[7,10,11] These ions (variously called the precursor ions or reagent ions) are injected into a fast-flowing inert carrier gas (usually pure helium at a pressure of ca. 100 Pa, ca. 1 Torr) through a Venturi-type orifice (diameter typically 1 mm). They are convected along a flow tube (typically 30 to 100 cm long) as a cold ion swarm possessing a Maxwellian velocity distribution appropriate to the temperature of the carrier gas (usually 300 K). The ions are sampled from the flowing swarm via a pinhole orifice (ca. 3 mm diameter) located at the downstream end of the flow tube and pass into a differentially-pumped quadrupole mass spectrometer where they are mass analysed and detected by a channeltron multiplier/pulse counting system.

A sample of ambient air, exhaled breath or the headspace of a liquid (*e.g.* urine) is then introduced into the helium carrier gas/precursor ion swarm at a known flow rate via a heated calibrated capillary (as depicted in Figure 1). If the precursor ions are chosen judiciously they react rapidly with the trace gases in the sample but not with the major air components (N_2, O_2, H_2O, CO_2, Ar). It turns out that only H_3O^+, NO^+, and O_2^+ precursor ions are suitable and it is these ions that are routinely used for SIFT-MS

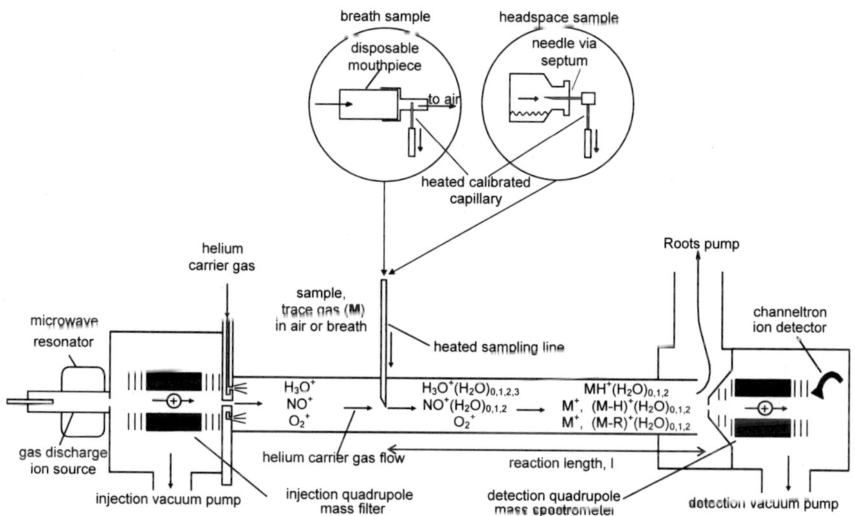

Fig. 1. A schematic of the selected ion flow tube mass spectrometer, SIFT-MS, instrument. The ions listed in the flow tube are the precursor ions (upstream) and examples of the product ions (downstream). The sampling methods are indicated in the large circles; see the text.

analyses. The ion-molecule reactions result in characteristic product ions for each of the trace gas species that are present in the air/breath sample and these product ions also are detected and counted by the downstream mass spectrometer detection system (Figure 1). The quantification of the trace gases (*i.e.* determination of their partial pressures in ppb or ppm) is well illustrated using, for example, the reaction of H_3O^+ with trace gas species M:

$$H_3O^+ + M \longrightarrow MH^+ + H_2O \tag{1}$$

Clearly, the loss of the precursor H_3O^+ ions, and hence the production of the MH^+ ions, is dependent on the number density of M molecules in the carrier gas, [M]. It can be shown from a consideration of the kinetics of the reaction involved (*i.e.* the rate coefficient k) and the flow dynamics (*i.e.* flow velocities and reaction time t) that the count rates of the H_3O^+ ions, $[H_3O^+]$, and the MH^+ ions, $[MH^+]$, at the downstream detection system are given by the relation:

$$[MH^+]_t = [H_3O^+]\, k\, [M]\, t \tag{2}$$

Thus, [M] is readily determined and if the k values and the product ions of the reactions of several species of M in the sample can be identified then the number densities (partial pressures) of each M species can be determined simultaneously. The rate coefficients for hundreds of reactions of the three precursor ions H_3O^+, NO^+, and O_2^+ have been determined with several types of organic molecules;[12-34] see also the compilation of rate coefficients.[35] The kinetic data obtained is used to construct the database for SIFT-MS, as described below.

It must be noted that whilst relation (2) properly demonstrates the principle of SIFT-MS analysis it is oversimplified for accurate analysis and certain conditions apply, notably that the fractional loss of the precursor ions must not be large (in practice less than about 10 %). Also, when the mass-to-charge ratio, m/z, value of the product ion that is used for the analysis of a particular compound is greatly different than the m/z of the precursor ion, then differential diffusion of these ions to the walls of the flow tube must be accounted for in the analysis. Also, mass discrimination against larger m/z ions in the analytical quadrupole mass spectrometer can play a role. It is fortunate that differential diffusion enhances the count rates of the heavier ions and mass discrimination diminishes their count rates. These two opposing phenomena tend to cancel each other, but for accurate analyses their combined effect must be considered. We have carried out a thorough experimental study of this, which has led to improvements in the SIFT-MS analytical software[36] and allows these phenomena to be properly accounted for in the analyses. This has been discussed in detail in a recent paper.[37] Further, when humid air or breath is analysed, cluster ions of the kind $H_3O^+(H_2O)_{1,2,3}$ and $NO^+(H_2O)_{1,2,3}$ usually form in the carrier gas and these can react with M molecules to form ions like $MH^+(H_2O)_{1,2}$. The ion chemistry involved in these reactions is well understood and has been discussed in detail in our previous papers.[24,38,39] However, for accurate SIFT-MS analyses, it is required that all the product ions originating from M are included in the quantification of M.[39] This careful approach to all aspects of SIFT-MS analyses has ensured that this technique is quite accurate for the quantitative analysis of the trace gases in humid air and even single exhalations of breath.

2.2. *Detection Limit, Accuracy, and Precision*

The detection limit of a SIFT-MS instrument can be assessed using typical values of the parameters that determine the product ion count rates, viz. the helium carrier gas pressure, typically 95 Pa (0.7 Torr) and its temperature, usually 300 K, the reaction time, typically 3 ms, and the sample gas to carrier gas flow rate ratio, which is typically 0.04 in our current instruments, and the precursor ion count rate. For a typical count rate of H_3O^+ precursor ions of 10^5 s^{-1} and a typical reaction rate coefficient k of 3×10^{-9} cm^3 s^{-1} (see Refs. 13, 35, and 40), a concentration of about 10 ppb of acetone in the air corresponds to a product ion count rate of about 10 counts per second (c/s), as derived using relation (2). Thus, the detection limit of a typical SIFT-MS instrument for any compound that reacts with precursor ions at a rate close to the above k value is 1 ppb for an integration time of 1 s at a product ion count rate of 1 c/s. Clearly, for longer counting times and higher precursor ion count rates the detection sensitivity is proportionally increased and trace gases present at sub-ppb concentrations can be measured. The precision (reproducibility) of the measurement is largely determined by the counting statistics. The standard error of each individual measurement is determined from the square root of the total number of the product ions counted by the detection system and is routinely displayed with the calculated ppb value.[30] Typical values of the standard error for the measurements of common breath metabolites (ammonia, acetone) from single exhalations range from $\pm5\,\%$ to ±20 %. The precision improves by a factor 1.7 for values obtained from three consecutive exhalations ($\pm3\,\%$ to $\pm12\,\%$).

2.3. *Modes of Operation*

SIFT-MS instruments can be operated in two modes. Using the full-scan
(FS) mode a complete mass spectrum is obtained by sweeping the detection
quadrupole over a selected mass-charge ratio, m/z, range for a chosen time
whilst a sample of air or breath is introduced into the carrier gas at a steady
flow rate (see Figure 2). The *count rates* of the ions are then calculated
from the numbers of counts and the total sampling time for each ion. The
mass spectra are interpreted by relating the product ion peaks to the trace
gases present in the sample from a detailed knowledge of the ion chemistry
and the in-built database. Using the multiple ion monitoring (MIM) mode,
only the count rates of the precursor ions and those of selected product ions

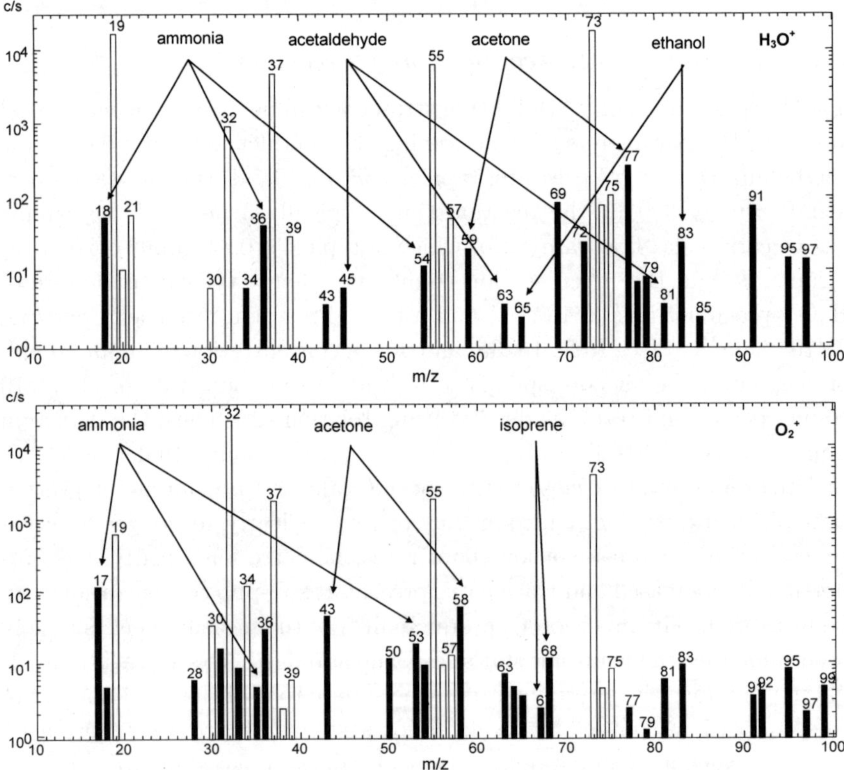

Fig. 2.   SIFT-MS spectra of a breath sample obtained using H_3O^+ and O_2^+ precursor
ions, clearly indicating the common breath metabolites. Reproduced from Ref. 67 with
permission from IOP publishing, copyright 2003.

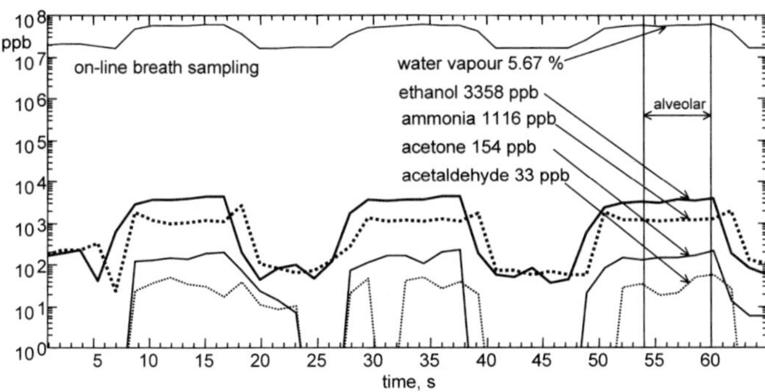

Fig. 3.   The concentrations of water vapour and the breath metabolites indicated in three sequential breath exhalations obtained simultaneously using the MIM mode of SIFT-MS analysis. Note the very wide concentration range from that of water vapour down to acetaldehyde. The known breath water vapour concentration acts as a very valuable internal calibration for the analyses. Reproduced from Ref. 70 with permission from IOP publishing, copyright 2002.

are monitored as air or breath displaces the ambient air at the entrance to the sample entry port (see Figure 1). This is achieved by rapidly switching the downstream mass spectrometer between the masses of all the primary ions and the selected product ions and dwelling on each of these masses for a predetermined short time interval (see Figure 3). This real-time monitoring is possible because of the fast time response of SIFT-MS, largely determined by the fast flow rates of the carrier gas along the flow tube and the sample gas along the inlet tube. The response time is about 20 ms. There is no fundamental limit to the number of different ion masses that can be recorded simultaneously using this technique. However, with the values of the precursor ion count rates currently available in SIFT-MS instruments, the practical limit is about fourteen ions at trace gas concentrations in the ppb regime. If larger numbers of ions need to be monitored it is much more convenient to sequentially record several full scan spectra in the time allowed by the sample volume and construct a table of count rates of all ions within the m/z range.[36]

2.4. Sampling Procedures

SIFT-MS analysis of ambient air is achieved by simply opening the sampling port to allow the air to enter the carrier gas (via the calibrated capillary; see Figure 1) whilst the detection mass spectrometer is operated in the FS or the MIM mode. Sample results obtained using both modes are given in Figures 2 and 3 and also later. Analysis of exhaled breath can be achieved by obtaining FS and MIM mode spectra while a breath sample collected into a bag or a glass vessel flows into the sampling port; this can be extended until the sample is exhausted; the longer the sampling time the greater the sensitivity. But sample collection into vessels has its problems, especially for water-soluble compounds like ammonia and those compounds that readily adsorb onto vessel surfaces. SIFT-MS is unique in that these problems can be avoided, since on line, real time analysis is allowed and single breath exhalations can be analysed for several metabolites simultaneously (as shown in Figure 3) as the breath displaces ambient air at the entrance to the sampling port. The MIM mode is now used almost exclusively for such breath analysis. For the breath donor this is a painless procedure that even frail patients can complete. In practice, several exhalation and inhalation cycles are easily delivered which allows a breath-by-breath consistency check to be made. An additional unique feature of SIFT-MS is that the humidity of an air and breath sample can be obtained routinely (from the distribution of the hydrated hydronium ions in the helium[41]). Since the humidity of exhaled breath is known (6 % at normal body temperature) it serves as a valuable internal validation of the sample flow rate and the other physical parameters involved in the quantification.[41] SIFT-MS can also be used to great effect to analyse volatile compounds emitted by aqueous solutions such as urine,[41] slurries,[42] food products[44] (solid and liquid) and cell cultures.[45,46] The sampling procedures have been described in previous paper.[47] To derive liquid phase concentrations from headspace (vapour phase) concentrations (also blood concentrations from breath levels), Henry's Law constants need to be known and several of these have been obtained using SIFT-MS to analyse the headspace of standard solutions of common breath metabolite compounds in water.[47]

2.5. *A Note on the Ion Chemistry Underpinning SIFT-MS*

As previously stated, the application of SIFT-MS to the analysis of complex media such as exhaled breath, in which a wide variety of trace gas species may be present, requires an extensive kinetics database that includes the reactions of H_3O^+, NO^+, and O_2^+ with each of the compounds present. This database has been constructed to include hundreds of compounds by many SIFT studies.[12−29,31] It is inappropriate to discuss the details of this ion chemistry in this short review; rather the reader is referred to the published papers and a longer review.[48] It is worthy of note that when the reactions of the many compounds with each of the three precursor ions, and indeed with the cluster ions that may be present, are fully understood, these three ions can be used simultaneously to analyse breath samples. This minimises the chance of wrong compound identifications and improves quantification.[24] It turns out that H_3O^+ and NO^+ are valuable reagent ions for many classes of organic compounds[48,49] and O_2^+ is more valuable for the analysis of small inorganic species such as NO, NO_2 (see Ref. 22) and NH_3 (see Refs. 50 and 51). There are a few organic compounds that have required special kinetic studies, including H_2CO (Ref. 52), H_2S (Ref. 52), and HCN (Ref. 53), and these can know be analysed with confidence in moist air samples, including exhaled breath. Following these exhaustive studies, SIFT-MS is now a reliable, accurate and versatile method for the analysis of trace gases in air and breath. The facility to rapidly switch between three precursor ions adds a new dimension to real-time gas analysis. Finally, a vital point to recognise is that for meaningful clinical diagnosis by breath analysis, the metabolites need to be quantified to better than a factor of two accuracy. This disqualifies most breath analysis techniques, but SIFT-MS is well capable of achieving the required accuracy without the need for regular re-calibration.[37,39,54,55]

2.6. *Validation of the Quantitative Accuracy of SIFT-MS*

It is, of course, important to provide experimental evidence that SIFT-MS is an accurate and absolute analytical technique, especially because it has been stressed that conventional calibration of these instruments is unnecessary. The first approach to providing such evidence was to investigate its precision and accuracy for the analysis of trace gases in dry air when potential complications due to the presence of water vapour (as discussed previously) are avoided. Thus, we have established the validity of SIFT-MS for the analyses of several organic vapours in dry air, including ethanol, benzene, acetone and trichloroethylene, over a wide range of partial pressures by preparing standard atmospheres by both the syringe injection technique and the permeation tube method.[54,55] This established that the accuracy of SIFT-MS measurements is better than 10 % over the 10 ppb to 20 ppm range of partial pressures of these compounds.

Since ambient air is humid (1 2 % relative humidity) and exhaled breath is very humid (6 % relative humidity) it is obviously important to account for the effect of water vapour on SIFT-MS analyses. Thus, we have carried out detailed studies (involving several classes of compounds) of the kinetics of the complex reactions that occur as the water vapour concentration in the helium carrier gas of the SIFT-MS instrument is varied.[24,38,39] This has led to the development of a refined analytical procedure that accounts for the presence of water vapour[39] and which, very significantly, also provides a measurement of the humidity of the sample, as mentioned previously.[41] This study has shown that when the overall ion chemistry and the kinetics are understood and properly accounted for, the quantification of trace gases in humid air and exhaled breath is not distorted by the water vapour in the sample (*i.e.* the quantification is not dependent on the humidity of the sample). This unique feature of SIFT-MS also allows the accurate quantification of volatile trace compounds in the headspace of aqueous liquids such as urine, which is valuable for clinical diagnosis.[52,56]

2.7. *SIFT-MS Instrumentation*

The TransSIFT 400 instrument is now commercially available. TransSIFT 400 has a mass of some 200 kg and requires only a single-phase mains power supply capable of supplying 4 kWatts of power. The ion source for this instrument, which provides a stable source of the required H_3O^+, NO^+, and O_2^+ precursor ions, is a microwave discharge through (moist) laboratory air at a pressure of typically 0.5 Torr that dissipates just a few Watts of power. Hence, special ion source gases are not required. We have designed a new monolithic rectangular resonator that forms a robust microwave plasma ion source.[57] TransSIFT 400 has an integral computer that performs instrument control and all data analysis. This versatile instrument is manufactured by Trans Spectra Ltd, Newcastle-under-Lyme, Staffs, UK. The detection quadrupole mass spectrometer in current instruments can be scanned up to m/z values of 250. Smaller benchtop instruments operating on SIFT-MS principles are also being developed by Trans Spectra Ltd (see `www.transspectra.com`).

3. SIFT-MS Case Studies

In this section, we show, using previously published work, that SIFT-MS is a valuable addition to the available trace gas analytical techniques. Its unique features have already been alluded to and include accurate, on line, real time analyses of ambient air, of single breath exhalations and the headspace above liquids such as urine and *in vitro* cell cultures. Thus, it has applications in many areas including environmental[58,59] and agriculture sciences,[60–62] health and safety practice,[54,55] medical,[51,63] and veterinary[43] sciences and in food and flavour research.[44] However, in this paper we focus on breath analysis with the occasional mention of urine and cell/bacterial headspace analyses. To date, we have carried out few in-depth SIFT-MS studies, so the main purpose of the following sections is to illustrate the unique contribution that SIFT-MS makes to breath analysis and not to present detailed results.

3.1. *Physiological Breath Composition*

Much of the excitement in the development of SIFT-MS lies in its potential for on-line and real time non-invasive breath analysis and urine headspace analysis for clinical diagnosis, therapeutic monitoring and physiology studies. For these studies SIFT-MS is currently uniquely versatile. Its wide-ranging applications have been alluded to previously, but the newness of the technique has not yet allowed many of these applications to be thoroughly investigated. Even so, we have explored some interesting areas to demonstrate its potential and some of these we now briefly describe beginning with studies involving healthy volunteers.

3.1.1. *Common breath metabolites*

Figure 2 shows FS spectra obtained using H_3O^+ and O_2^+ precursor ions when a breath sample from the same individual input directly into the sampling port is analysed. It shows the breath metabolites common to all individuals, the most abundant being ammonia, acetone, ethanol and isoprene.[64–67] The concentrations are given in parts per billion, ppb, and they fall within the typical range for healthy people. However, the concentrations of the various metabolites are subject somewhat to diurnal and nocturnal variations and diet, and vary for different individual. A limited SIFT-MS study of the concentrations of ammonia, acetone, isoprene, ethanol and acetaldehyde in the breath of five volunteers over a period of 30 days has been carried out in order to explore these variations and thus to establish "baselines" for each individual.[67] Breath samples were analysed in the early morning on arrival at the SIFT-MS laboratory. Real time analyses of three consecutive breath exhalations were carried out for each individual using the MIM mode (see Figure 3). The precision achieved, calculated from the counting statistics (see Section 2) for the individual compounds, was typically $\pm 5\,\%$ for ammonia, $\pm 7\,\%$ for acetone and $\pm 30\,\%$ for isoprene, and ethanol. Sufficient data were acquired over the 30 days to allow concentration distributions to be obtained for ammonia, acetone, isoprene and ethanol (see the distributions for ammonia and acetone in Figure 4). These showed that the ammonia, acetone and isoprene concentrations exhibited

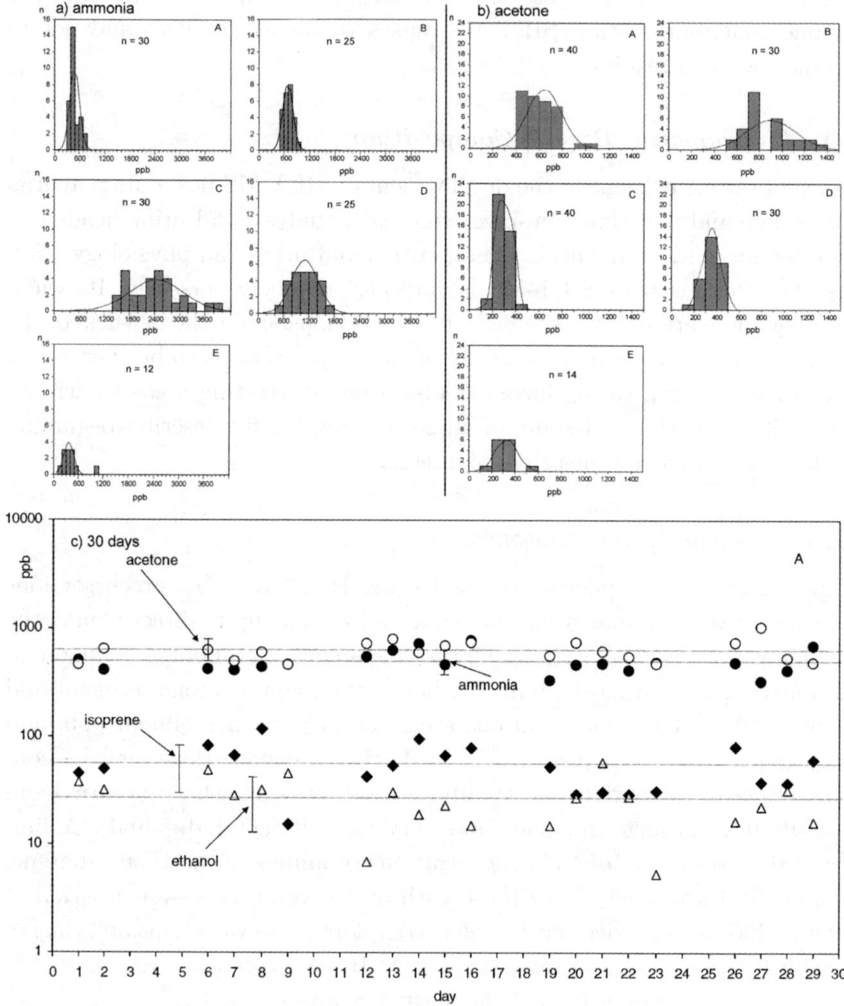

Fig. 4.   *Above:* Histograms of breath ammonia and acetone for five subjects obtained over a 30 day period. *Below:* The day-by-day variations in the concentrations in ppb of breath acetone, ammonia, isoprene and ethanol for one individual. The horizontal lines represent the mean values for each metabolite over the period of observation and the bars represent the standard deviations. Reproduced from Ref. 67 with permission from IOP publishing, copyright 2003.

sensibly normal distributions, with coefficients of variation of typically 0.3. Obvious and statistically significant differences are apparent in the mean concentrations of these metabolites between the five individuals except for acetaldehyde, the concentrations of which were relatively low and close to the instrument detection limit, such that meaningful distributions could not be obtained. The spreads in the mean concentrations in ppb of each metabolite amongst the five subjects are as follows: ammonia, 422–2389; acetone, 293–870; isoprene, 55–121; ethanol, 27–153; acetaldehyde, 2–5. There are no obvious patterns in the distributions of these five metabolites for these individuals, except that the ammonia levels were greatest in the breath of the two oldest subjects. Details are given in the published paper Ref. 67. Note in Figure 4c the variations of the metabolite concentrations for subject A over the 30 day period. Although this study is very preliminary and many more studies need to be performed for many more individuals at different times of day, after meals, etc, and over longer periods, the study does suggest that the patterns of the different breath metabolites may represent crude "fingerprints" for each individual. What is quite certain is that the concentrations of some of these metabolites are greatly elevated in the breath of those suffering from particular diseases (ammonia – renal failure; acetone – diabetes), well beyond the normal variations for healthy individuals, demonstrating the potential of breath analysis for clinical diagnosis (see later and Refs. 66 and 68).

3.1.2. *Influence of food*

The question that is always asked when discussing the value of breath analysis for clinical diagnosis is "what is the influence of food ingestion?" To investigate the influence of food intake (and starvation) on the levels of breath metabolites, we carried out a study of selected metabolites in the exhaled breath of six healthy volunteers following the ingestion of a liquid protein meal[66] and subsequently of a liquid carbohydrate meal.[69] Alveolar breath levels of ammonia, acetone, ethanol and isoprene were taken from single exhalations (using the MIM mode) in the morning following overnight fasting and then for several hours after ingestion of the meals. Prior to feeding, the acetone levels were relatively high and the corresponding ammonia levels were relatively low in the breath of all six volunteers. Following feeding, the acetone levels all decreased as the body was nourished (Figure 4). Initially, the ammonia levels all reduced towards a minimum value near to 200 ppb about 30 minutes after feeding by both the protein and the carbohydrate meals and then began to increase in the breath of all six volunteers. For the (nitrogen-containing) protein meal the ammonia increased to values obviously greater than their respective initial values, as shown in Figure 5a, whereas for the carbohydrate meal it asymptotically approached the initial values prior to feeding. Actually, it is the mean of the levels of breath ammonia and acetone from the six volunteers that are shown as functions of time in Figure 5, although the curves for each individual show the same forms. We hypothesise that the initial "dip" in the ammonia level is the result of an increase in portal blood flow as the stomach is loaded with the meal.[66,68] This initially lowers the blood ammonia level before it returns to normal in the case of the carbohydrate meal and actually increases beyond this as the protein is metabolised. It is relevant to note that a similar decrease in the breath ammonia was observed when the stomach was loaded with a volume (about 500 mL) of water,[70] again supporting the above hypothesis. There were unexpected increases in the breath ethanol levels following the ingestion of both the protein and carbohydrate meals, which we traced to the presence of traces of ethanol in the liquid meals.

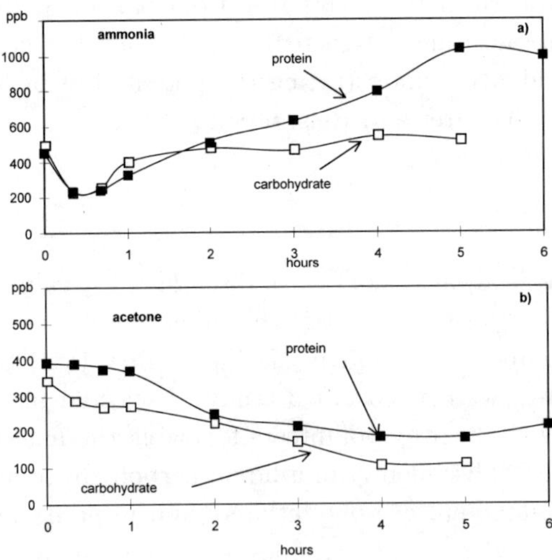

Fig. 5.   The time variation of a) breath ammonia and b) breath acetone concentrations (in ppb) following the ingestion of liquid protein and carbohydrate meals, as indicated. The individual points are the mean values of the concentrations of these metabolites for six healthy individuals, but it must be stated that the forms of these curves are similar for all six individuals. The concentrations were obtained from single breath exhalations using the MIM mode. The interesting features of these data are discussed in the text, see also Refs. 66 and 69.

These studies well demonstrate the capability of SIFT-MS to follow changes in breath trace gas levels on short (single exhalations – seconds) and long (hour) time scales, as is further demonstrated below.

Throughout the several hours duration of the above meal studies, the isoprene levels in the breath of each volunteer did not change significantly. Isoprene is the most abundant hydrocarbon present in breath. It is formed in the later stages of cholesterol synthesis and its blood/breath concentration is influenced by the rate of cholesterol synthesis in the body.[68,71] In principle, it can be quantified in breath by SIFT-MS using H_3O^+, NO^+, and O_2^+ precursor ions, although the presence of methanol can cause problems when using H_3O^+.[72] In a separate study we quantified isoprene in the breath of 29 healthy volunteers over a period of about six months and at various times of the day.[73] These observations were originally initiated following suggestions in the literature that breath isoprene levels may be indicators of psychological stress.[65] These measurements indicate that the normal levels of breath isoprene are 83 ppb (SD ±45 ppb).[73] Interestingly, in another study we observed that the breath isoprene levels of some patients suffering from end-stage renal failure following haemodialysis actually increase (see Ref. 63 and Sec. 3.3.2 below).

3.1.3. *Ethanol metabolism*

A very simple but graphic further demonstration of SIFT-MS in physiological studies is our observation of ethanol metabolism via breath analysis. This study shows the rapidity and accuracy of breath analysis and how the concentrations of metabolites can be followed over much longer periods with good time resolution. Thus, following the ingestion of small amounts of ethanol dissolved in 500 mL of water by two individuals, the concentrations of ethanol, acetaldehyde, ammonia, acetone and water vapour were measured simultaneously in single breath exhalations using the MIM mode as shown in Figure 3.[70] In this way, the concentrations of these compounds were tracked in real time obviating sample collection into bags or onto traps. The data obtained for the variation of breath ethanol and acetaldehyde levels with time are shown in Figure 6. The apparent breath ethanol levels are initially high due to mouth contamination, but they reduce as it is cleared from the mouth, fall to minimum levels, rise as ethanol passes into the blood stream (and hence the breath), reach maximum levels and finally decay. This study and another SIFT-MS study[74] show that for moderate doses of ethanol, its decay quickly exhibits first-order kinetics (a single exponential

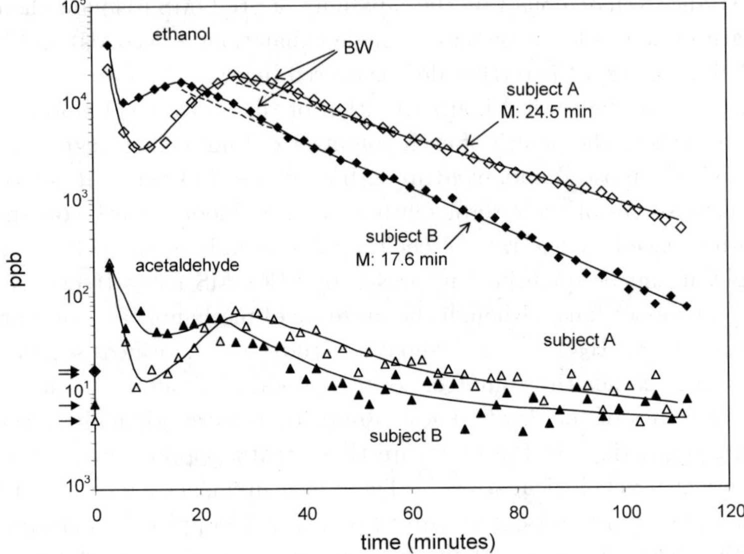

Fig. 6.   The variation with time (minutes) of the breath concentrations of ethanol and acetaldehyde (in ppb) in two healthy subjects following the ingestion of 500 mL water/ 7.5 mL ethanol mixtures. The initial decline from high values is due to mouth emissions. The subsequent increases to peak values are due to the passage of ethanol into the blood stream.   The decays of ethanol are due to both dispersal into body water (BW) and metabolism (M), the latter partially producing the observed acetaldehyde.   The small arrows on the y-axis indicate pre-dose values. Reproduced from Ref. 70 with permission from IOP publishing, copyright 2002.

decay), whereas for relatively large ethanol doses, the initial decay is slow, indicating saturation kinetics. The ethanol levels reach concentrations that are only approximately consistent with its dilution in blood and body water (the latter can be determined using our FA-MS technique[75,76], which is described on page 439 in this volume). For smaller ethanol doses, and following a meal, the breath ethanol increases only slightly indicating that under these circumstances the ethanol is largely metabolised in the stomach. We have suggested that the time delay (following ethanol ingestion) before the breath ethanol begins to increase (see Figure 5b) is an indicator of the gastric emptying rate. The appearance of breath acetaldehyde correlates well with the ethanol, indicating that it is mostly formed from the metabolism of the ethanol. Note that the acetaldehyde levels are about three orders-of-magnitude lower than those of the ethanol and that they are obtained from single breath exhalations simultaneously. As emphasised previously, the water vapour partial pressure is routinely measured in all SIFT-MS analyses (see Figure 3) and since it is known in exhaled breath (about 6 %), this measurement acts as an internal calibration of the precision and accuracy of the breath analyses. Further details of this study are reported in a previous paper.[70]

3.2. *Exposure to Exogenous Toxic Substances*

This is an important area of public concern.[77] The limited objective here is to show how SIFT-MS can contribute to the monitoring of exposure. Our efforts to date have been limited to studies of the breath and urine headspace of smokers and the controlled exposure to one organic solvent.

The dangers of smoking, and to a less extent passive smoking, have been well documented and publicised. It was discovered a few years ago[72,78] that amongst the many toxic compounds contained in cigarette smoke is acetonitrile and that this cyanide is retained in the body and appears in exhaled breath. It is present in the exhaled breath of smokers at measurable concentrations several days after cessation of smoking. But does this compound also appear in the urine of smokers? To investigate this, a SIFT-MS study has been carried out of acetonitrile both in the exhaled breath and the headspace of urine of several cigarette smokers and of several non-smokers as controls.[79] The results of this study show that acetonitrile is readily detected by SIFT-MS in breath (Figure 7) and urinary headspace[79] of the smokers at levels dependent on the cigarette consumption, but is practically absent from the breath and urine headspace of non-smokers. Further to these experiments, we have determined the Henry's Law partition coefficients for dilute aqueous solutions of acetonitrile,[79] which allow the deter-

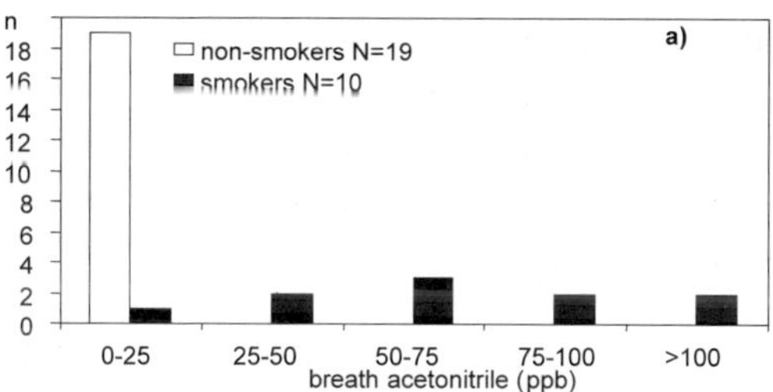

Fig. 7.   Concentration distributions for breath (vapour phase) acetonitrile concentration (*n* is the number of samples within 40 ppb concentration intervals) for non-smokers and smokers, as indicated. The *N* values are the total numbers of individuals in each category. Data from Ref. 79 with permission from Elsevier, copyright 2003.

mination of liquid phase urinary acetonitrile concentrations from headspace concentrations. The results of this study show that acetonitrile concentrations in the breath of smokers are within the range 17–124 ppb (mean value 69 ppb), which are in close agreement with previous studies.[78,80] The urinary acetonitrile concentrations for the same cohort of smokers are within the range 0–150 μg/L (mean value 57 μg/L), which are close to the typical concentrations determined previously in the blood of smokers.[81] These combined data imply that the acetonitrile is equilibrated amongst the body fluids (blood, total body water and urine) and that excretion occurs via both exhaled breath and urine. So both media can be analysed for acetonitrile to detect exposure to cigarette smoke. We have detected acetonitrile in the breath of non-smokers regularly exposed to cigarette smoke (spouses), but at a much reduced level that is close to the current detection limit of SIFT-MS. However, this detection limit is continuously being lowered and soon more extended SIFT-MS studies of passive smoking can be initiated. SIFT-MS has been used by others to monitor isoprene, acetone, ammonia and ethanol in breath before and after cigarette smoking.[82]

A great deal of work has been carried out by several health and safety agencies to monitor the exposure of workers to volatile compounds, principally using blood analysis. Less effort has been given to the exploitation of breath analysis, which had been considered to be less reliable. However, we now know that SIFT-MS can be used for accurate breath analysis,[55] both quickly and non-invasively, for example at the entrance and exit to factories. This now provides the means for efficiently screening workers for exposure. To demonstrate this, we have carried out some pilot experiments in collaboration with experienced health and safety scientists. This study showed that following several hours of exposure to a controlled atmosphere of perchloroethylene, C_2Cl_4, this chlorocarbon is easily detected in the breath some 16 hours later at a level of about 1 ppm. After a brief period of exercise, the C_2Cl_4 level had reduced by about an order of magnitude. The value of such work in factory health and safety monitoring is clear. In New Zealand SIFT-MS has been used for *in situ* analysis of solvents in breath and blood.[83]

On a related theme, we have carried out pilot studies of anaesthetic gases halothane, isoflurane and sevoflurane in breath. Before this was possible, the kinetics database must be extended to include these compounds in order to identify monitor ions for SIFT-MS analyses.[27] The data in Figure 8 show how these gases can be detected in exhaled breath and how they decay with time, as shown by the single breath exhalations. SIFT-MS can now be used

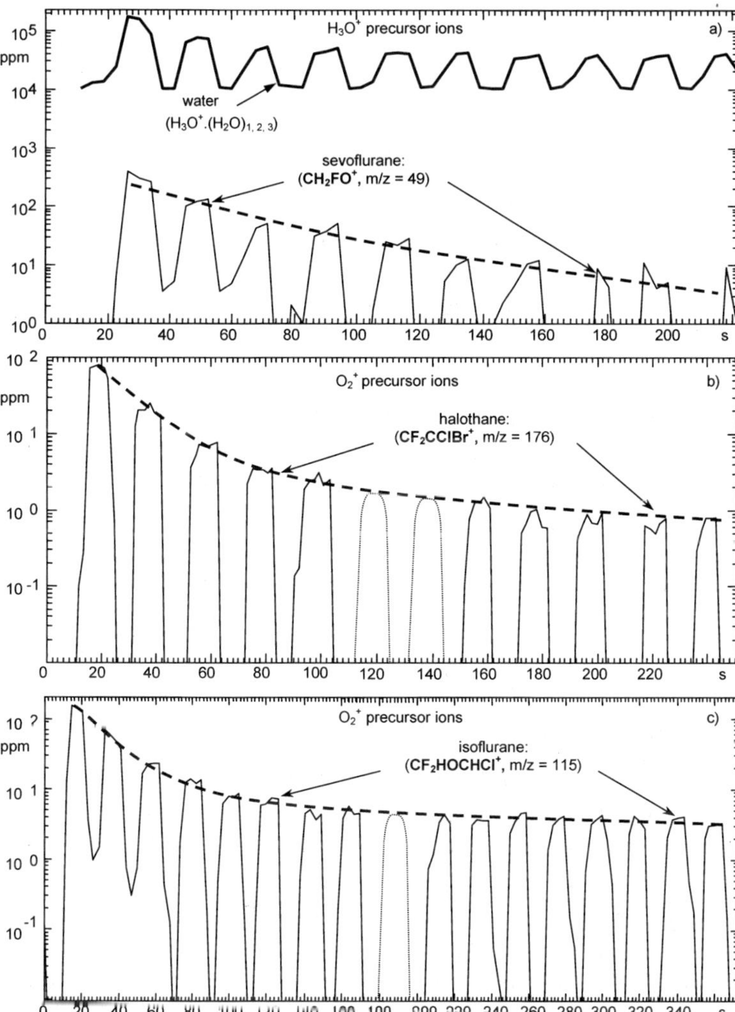

Fig. 8.   The decay with time (seconds) of anaesthetic gases in breath (concentrations in parts per million, ppm) following brief exposure to these gases. **a)** CH_2FO^+ ions produced by H_3O^+ precursor ions monitoring sevoflurane. Note the apparent increase in breath water level when sevoflurane is in the breath, which shows that the H_3O^+/ sevoflurane ion chemistry catalyses the production of H_3O^+ hydrates. **b)** CF_2CClBr^+ ions produced by O_2^+ precursor ions monitoring halothane. **c)** $CF_2HOCHCl^+$ ions produced by O_2^+ as precursor ions monitoring isoflurane. Reproduced from Ref. 27 with permission from Wiley, copyright 2002.

to check for potentially dangerous levels of these compounds in the breath of operating theatre staff and also to monitor the post-operative loss of these anaesthetic gases from the body of patients.

3.3. *Clinical Studies, Disease Related*

A major motivation for the development of SIFT-MS is for the detection of diseases in their early stages, non-invasively and painlessly, via exhaled breath and urine headspace analysis. Clearly, to achieve this, reliable markers of diseases have to be recognisable in these biological media and hence our initial studies have followed the obvious pathway of studying patients with known diseases. The choice of which diseases to investigate to date has been influenced, in part, by the medical specialties of local clinicians and biologists. Hence, to date, our studies have mostly involved nephrologists, urologists, oncologists and cell biologists, but with specialists in gynaecology, psychiatry and respiratory medicine now becoming involved. Many pilot experiments are currently underway, the results of which will be reported in due course. Here we summarise the results of some partially completed pilot studies involving both breath analysis and urinary headspace analysis.

3.3.1. *Helicobacter pylori infection*

The ability of SIFT-MS to quantify ammonia accurately in exhaled breath[50] has an important application in the screening for colonisation of the gastrointestinal tract with the urea-splitting organism *Helicobacter pylori*.[84] The standard test to detect the presence of this bacterium is to give an oral dose of carbon-13-labelled urea ($^{13}CO(NH_2)_2$) and to observe an increase of the carbon-13 component of the breath carbon dioxide ($^{13}CO_2$) using conventional isotope ratio mass spectrometry.[84] The biochemistry involved implies that ammonia should also be emitted following ingestion of the urea, and this we recognised very early in our SIFT-MS pilot studies. Thus, using SIFT-MS we observed a significant increase (4 ppm) of breath level of ammonia 20 to 40 minutes after an oral dose of 2 grams of normal urea ($^{12}CO(NH_2)_2$) in a volunteer known to be infected with *H. pylori*.[85] Also, when a person who is not infected swallowed the same dose of urea solution, no significant enhancement of breath ammonia was observed at about 30 minutes. Corresponding increases of breath ammonia have been confirmed in later studies of mouth and breath ammonia levels measured using other techniques.[84] Recent follow-up SIFT-MS studies on another *H. pylori* positive volunteer are in substantial agreement with our above observations (see the paper by C. Penault *et al.*[86] on page 393 of this book). Thus, breath analysis of ammonia has the potential to become a cheap, rapid and effective way of diagnosing *H. pylori* infection.

On a related topic, we have been investigating the molecular emissions from bacterial cultures, especially *Pseudomonas aeruginosa* (PA). The rationale is look for a molecular marker of PA and thus to investigate if the level of colonisation by PA of the lungs of children with cystic fibrosis can be assessed. The remarkable result from our initial study is that PA cultures emit copious amounts of hydrogen cyanide into the gas phase.[53,87] It therefore seems likely that we will be able to detect hydrogen cyanide in the breath of these patients with all its ramifications for treatment and improving the quality of life.

3.3.2. *Renal failure*

It is to be expected that the breath of patients suffering from kidney and/or liver disease will be rich in metabolites compared to that of healthy individuals and our SIFT-MS studies show that this is indeed the case. Figure 9a shows an FS spectrum obtained using H_3O^+ precursor ions for a bag sample of breath obtained from a patient suffering from end-stage renal failure prior to haemodialysis treatment. As can be seen, the normal breath metabolites are present, but it is obvious that some of them, especially ammonia and acetone, are at much greater levels than normal (compare Figure 9a with Figure 2a). From these SIFT-MS studies it is now clear that increased breath ammonia is characteristic of end-stage renal failure.[51] The elevated breath ammonia levels correlate well with high blood levels of urea in these patients. The levels of these breath metabolites are reduced to normal by haemodialysis treatment, as is graphically illustrated in Figure 9b where the breath ammonia levels are followed during the course of the haemodialysis session. The elevated breath acetone is simply explained by the fact this patient is also diabetic (see Ref. 65 for further discussion). These studies also showed that abnormally high levels of breath ethanol and isoprene occur in some of these patients.[85]

Subsequent SIFT-MS breath analyses for a renal patient cohort involved the location of the SIFT-MS instrument in the dialysis unit of the local hospital to allow on-line, real time breath analyses to be performed. The exhaled breath of some 20 patients was sampled on line before their dialysis sessions. Simultaneous single breath concentration profiles of ammonia, acetone and isoprene were obtained for each patient and also for several healthy controls using the MIM mode of data collection. These measurements were repeated for the patients immediately after about three hours of dialysis when it was seen that the abnormally high breath concentrations

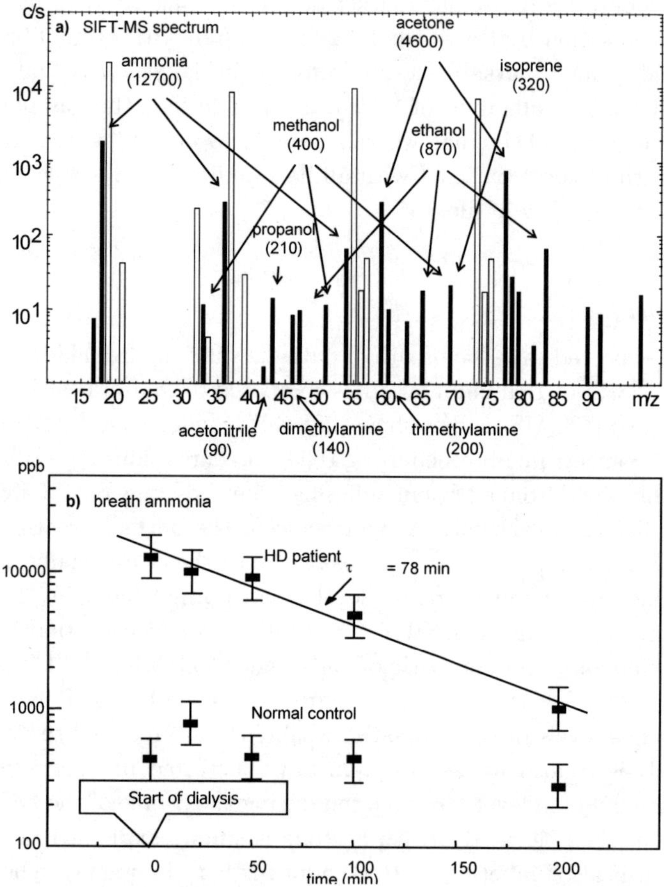

Fig. 9. **a)** SIFT-MS spectra of exhaled breath of a patient suffering from end-stage renal failure showing the major breath metabolites and their concentrations in ppb in parentheses. By comparing this spectrum with that for a healthy individual shown in Figure 2a it is obvious that the breath ammonia and acetone are greatly increased, indicating that the patient is both uraemic and diabetic. The presence of acetonitrile indicates that the patient is a smoker. **b)** Reduction of breath ammonia for the same individual during a haemodialysis session together with the breath ammonia for a control in the same environment. See also Ref. 51 for detailed discussion.

of most metabolites reduce towards normal levels.[51,63] Very obvious again was the dramatic reduction in the breath ammonia. It is worth mentioning that even the frail patients involved in these studies had no difficulty in providing direct breath samples for SIFT-MS analysis.

In this same study it was observed that the isoprene level actually increased in the breath of some of the patients following the haemodialysis treatment.[63] Prior to dialysis, the patients' mean breath isoprene concentrations (113 ppb, SD ±50 ppb) were significantly greater than those for the healthy controls (89 ppb, SD ±36 ppb), and immediately following the dialysis treatment breath isoprene had increased significantly (147 ppb, SD ±75 ppb). Some of the patients were also clearly distressed following the treatment. As yet, it is not clear if the increased breath isoprene is due to psychological stress or biochemical stress resulting from acute tissue injury, perhaps reflecting the bio-incompatibility of blood with dialysis membranes. The intriguing possibility is that breath isoprene may be an indicator of psychological stress and may be a useful, non-invasive tool to monitor complications associated with end-stage renal failure and its treatment. This study is ongoing.

3.3.3. *Substance abuse*

Checking for solvent and drug abuse is now becoming another valuable application of SIFT-MS, its real time feature being especially useful for this. We have recently used SIFT-MS to quantify CS_2 in breath following a dose of Antabuse (disulfiram) commonly used to inhibit alcohol ingestion by abusers. The CS_2 appears in the exhaled breath several hours after the ingestion of the Antabuse, and surprisingly the breath acetone is greatly elevated from normal! This has not previously been recognised and requires further investigation, because the Antabuse may be having an adverse influence on metabolism. Recently, we have initiated a study of SIFT-MS detection of volatile compounds in exhaled breath of cannabis smokers and those ingesting other illegal substances, including γ hydroxybutyrate (see the paper by R. Bloor *et al.*[88] on page 409 in this volume).

3.3.4. *Urine analysis; infection and cancer*

Urine analysis is commonly used for clinical diagnosis, but analysis using "wet chemistry" and dipsticks is the common practice. We have begun to investigate the potential value of urine headspace analysis by SIFT-MS for the detection of clinical disease and obtained some potentially important results.[56] In analysing liquid headspace it should be recognised that some compounds are partitioned between the liquid and vapour phases according to the pH of the urine, notably ammonia and fatty acids. However, the pH does not markedly influence the concentrations of most VOCs in urine headspace,[42,56] so compounds such as acetone and ethanol, that are always present in urine, can be quantified with confidence.

Our initial experiments involved the analysis of volatile compounds in the headspace of urine taken from healthy normal controls and patients suffering from prostate and bladder cancer. When some acidified samples were analysed using O_2^+ precursor ions, large signals at $m/z = 30$ were observed. We now understand that HNO_2 and both NO and NO_2 are present in the headspace of the acidified urine, the last two species resulting from the partial dissociation of the HNO_2.[89] Further investigations showed that the urine samples the headspace of which contained elevated levels of the nitrogen oxides were bacterially infected. Thus, it is now understood that the bacteria reduces the nitrates, naturally present in the urine, to nitrites which in acidic solution produce nitrous acid, which partially breaks down to NO, NO_2 and H_2O.[90] The concentrations of these oxides of nitrogen in the headspace of bacterially infected urine are typically several ppm rising to tens of ppm. Such large levels are always obvious and easily quantified. Thus, SIFT-MS offers a rapid, non-invasive check for urinary infection.[56]

A more exciting discovery from these experiments was of formaldehyde in the urinary headspace,[52] most especially in those samples given by the bladder cancer patients, but not in those from the healthy controls. Formaldehyde analysis by SIFT-MS is not so simple as for most other VOCs, but it can be achieved with care.[52] This important observation points the way to a non-invasive check on the presence of these tumours in the body. We are currently pursuing this line of research with urgency, for obvious reasons, by investigating urine from patients suffering from colorectal cancer and breast cancer (see the mention in Ref. 79). It seems certain that other molecular markers of tumours will be present at detectable levels, as other studies have suggested.[91,92]. So our short SIFT-MS study, which is currently being extended to include breath analysis, merely represents a beginning to this important topic.

In support of the above studies we have initiated studies of the molecular emissions from cancer cell lines *in vitro*. In a recent paper[45] we have reported the discovery that acetaldehyde is released by the lung cancer cell lines SK-MES and CALU-1 *in vitro*. The acetaldehyde concentration in the headspace of the medium/cell culture was found to be proportional to the number of cancer cells in the medium (typically 10^8). From these data, the acetaldehyde production rates of the SK-MES cells and the CALU-1 cells were determined to be 1×10^6 and 1.5 to 3×10^6 molecules/cell/minute respectively. Assuming that similar production rates of acetaldehyde pertain to lung cancer cells *in vivo*, the size of tumours that may be detectable using SIFT-MS breath analysis can be estimated. Thus, it does seem feasible that lung tumours may be detectable via breath analysis. The potential value of this approach to the early diagnosis of cancer and to industrial cell biotechnology is briefly discussed in a recent paper.[45]

4. Summary, Some Concluding Remarks and Future Prospects for SIFT-MS

We have described the unique features of selected ion flow tube mass spectrometry, SIFT-MS, for accurate, real-time analysis of trace gases in air, exhaled breath and liquid headspace. Sample collection into bags or onto traps, which can compromise the sample, is unnecessary. This new analytical method can be used to detect most gases in dry or moist air down to parts per billion levels in times of seconds, including most permanent gases and the vapours of organic liquids and solids. Areas of application that have only been briefly explored to date include environmental and soil sciences, biological monitoring and food science. In this paper we have given special attention to breath analysis and highlighted its potential for clinical diagnosis and therapeutic monitoring, when the unique capability of SIFT-MS for analysing single breath exhalations on-line and in real time provides the clinician with immediate results and presents the most fragile patients with minimal stress. We have also shown the potential of SIFT-MS for the analysis of urinary headspace and how it can be used to detect urinary tract infection and even the presence of body tumours. Molecular emissions from cancer cell lines *in vitro* are being explored to support this exciting and potentially important topic. Thus, the potential of SIFT-MS for non invasive diagnosis of and therapeutic monitoring via breath analysis is unparalleled. However, SIFT-MS is in its early stages of development and with more users its value to medical and biological sciences and other areas will be further revealed.

Commercial SIFT-MS instruments (and also FA-MS instruments; see the article by Španěl and Smith[76] on page 439 of this volume) are now available from Trans Spectra Limited, Newcastle-under-Lyme, UK, the authors of this review being co-founders and directors of this company.

Acknowledgements

We are grateful for the help and support of all the co-authors of our cited papers without which some of the SIFT-MS work in medicine and cell biology, animal husbandry and health and safety practice would not have been possible. We especially acknowledge our co-workers in the SIFT-MS core team Dr. Tianshu Wang, Dr. Ann Diskin, and Edward Hall.

References

1. Campbell L, Jones AH, Wilson HK. Evaluation of occupational exposure to carbon disulphide by blood, exhaled air, and urine analysis. *Am J Ind Med* 1985; **8**: 143–153.
2. Karasek F, Clement R. *Basic Gas Chromatography–Mass Spectrometry.* Amsterdam: Elsevier,1988.
3. Phillips M, Greenberg J. Ion-trap detection of volatile organic compounds in alveolar breath. *Clin Chem* 1992; **38**: 60–65.
4. Sanchez JM, Sacks RD. GC analysis of human breath with a series-coupled column ensemble and a multibed sorption trap. *Anal Chem* 2003; **75**: 2231–2236.
5. Španěl P, Smith D. Selected ion flow tube: a technique for quantitative trace gas analysis of air and breath. *Med Biol Eng Comput* 1996; **34**: 409–419.
6. Adams N, Smith D. The selected ion flow tube (SIFT): a technique for studying thermal energy ion–neutral reactions. *Int J Mass Spectrom Ion Physics* 1976; **21**: 349–359.
7. Smith D, Adams N. The selected ion flow tube (SIFT): studies of ion-neutral reactions. *Adv Atom Mol Phys* 1987; **24**: 1–49.
8. Smith D. The ion chemistry of interstellar clouds. *Chemical Reviews* 1992; **92**: 1473–1485.
9. Smith D, Španěl P. Ions in the terrestrial atmosphere and in interstellar clouds. *Mass Spectrom Rev* 1996; **14**: 255–278.
10. Smith D, Španěl P. Swarm techniques. In: Dunning F, ed. *Experimental Methods in the Physical Sciences: Atomic, Molecular, and Optical Physics: Charged Particles,* New York: Academic Press, 1995.
11. Smith D, Španěl P. SIFT applications in mass spectrometry. In: Lindon J, Tranter G, Holmes J, eds. Encyclopaedia of Spectroscopy and Spectrometry., London: Academic Press, 1999: 2092–2105.
12. Španěl P, Smith D. SIFT studies of the reactions of H_3O^+, NO^+ and O_2^+ with a series of alcohols. *Int J Mass Spectrom Ion Processes* 1997; **167/168**: 375–388.
13. Španěl P, Ji Y, Smith D. SIFT studies of the reactions of H_3O^+, NO^+ and O_2^+ with a series of aldehydes and ketones. *Int J Mass Spectrom Ion Processes* 1997; **165/166**: 25–37.
14. Španěl P, Smith D. SIFT studies of the reactions of H_3O^+, NO^+ and O_2^+ with a series of volatile carboxylic acids and esthers. *Int J Mass Spectrom Ion Processes* 1998; **172**: 137–147.

15. Španěl P, Smith D. SIFT studies of the reactions of H_3O^+, NO^+ and O_2^+ with several ethers. *Int J Mass Spectrom Ion Processes* 1998; **172**: 239–247.

16. Španěl P, Smith D. SIFT studies of the reactions of H_3O^+, NO^+ and O_2^+ with several amines and other nitrogen containing molecules. *Int J Mass Spectrom* 1998; **176**: 203–211.

17. Španěl P, Smith D. SIFT studies of the reactions of H_3O^+, NO^+ and O_2^+ with some organosulphur molecules. *Int J Mass Spectrom* 1998; **176**: 167–176.

18. Španěl P, Smith D. SIFT studies of the reactions of H_3O^+, NO^+ and O_2^+ with several aliphatic and aromatic hydrocarbons. *Int J Mass Spectrom* 1998; **181**: 1–10.

19. Španěl P, Smith D. SIFT studies of the reactions of H_3O^+, NO^+ and O_2^+ with several amine isomers of $C_5H_{13}N$. *Int J Mass Spectrom* 1999; **185/186/187**: 139–147.

20. Španěl P, Smith D. SIFT studies of the reactions of H_3O^+, NO^+ and O_2^+ with some chloroalkanes and chloroalkenes. *Int J Mass Spectrom* 1999; **184**: 157–181.

21. Španěl P, Smith D. SIFT studies of the reactions of H_3O^+, NO^+ and O_2^+ with several aromatic and aliphatic monosubstituted hydrocarbons. *Int J Mass Spectrom* 1999; **189**: 213–223.

22. Španěl P, Smith D. An investigation of the reactions of H_3O^+ and O_2^+ with NO, NO_2, N_2O and HNO_2 in support of selected ion flow tube mass spectrometry. *Rapid Commun Mass Spectrom* 2000; **14**: 646–651.

23. Španěl P, Smith D. Quantification of hydrogen sulphide in humid air by selected ion flow tube mass spectrometry SIFT-MS. *Rapid Commun Mass Spectrom* 2000; **14**: 1136–1140.

24. Smith D, Diskin A, Ji Y, Španěl P. Concurrent use of H_3O^+, NO^+ and O_2^+ precursor ions for the detection and quantification of diverse trace gases in the presence of air and breath by selected ion flow tube mass spectrometry. *Int J Mass Spectrom* 2001; **209**: 81–97.

25. Španěl P, Van Doren J, Smith D. A selected ion flow tube study of the reactions of H_3O^+, NO^+ and O_2^+ with saturated and unsaturated aldehydes and subsequent hydration of the product ions. *Int J Mass Spectrom* 2002; **213**: 163–176.

26. Španěl P, Wang TS, Smith D. A selected ion flow tube, SIFT, study of the reactions of H_3O^+, NO^+ and O_2^+ ions with a series of diols. *Int J Mass Spectrom* 2002; **218**: 227–236.

27. Wang TS, Smith D, Španěl P. Selected ion flow tube studies of the reactions of H_3O^+, NO^+ and O_2^+ with the anaesthetic gases halothane, isoflurane and sevoflurane. *Rapid Commun Mass Spectrom* 2002; **16**: 1860–1870.

28. Španěl P, Diskin A, Wang TS, Smith D. A SIFT study of the reactions of H_3O^+, NO^+ and O_2^+ with hydrogen peroxide and peroxyacetic acid. *Int J Mass Spectrom* 2003; **228**: 269–283.

29. Wang TS, Španěl P, Smith D. A selected ion flow tube study of the reactions of H_3O^+, NO^+ and O_2^+ with some phenols, phenyl alcohols and cyclic carbonyl compounds in support of SIFT-MS and PTR-MS. *Int J Mass Spectrom* 2004; **239**: 139–146.

30. Diskin A, Wang TS, Smith D, Španěl P. A selected ion flow tube (SIFT) study of the reactions of H_3O^+, NO^+ and O_2^+ ions with a series of alkenes in support of SIFT-MS. *Int J Mass Spectrom* 2002; **218**: 87–101.

31. Smith D, Wang TS, Španěl P. Analysis of ketones by selected ion flow tube mass spectrometry. *Rapid Commun Mass Spectrom* 2003; **17**: 2655–2660.

32. Smith D, Wang TS, Španěl P. A SIFT study of the reactions of H_2ONO^+ ions with several types of organic molecules. *Int J Mass Spectrom* 2003; **230**: 1–9.

33. Wang TS, Španěl P, Smith D. Selected Ion Flow Tube, SIFT, studies of the reactions of H_3O^+, NO^+ and O_2^+ with eleven $C_{10}H^{16}$ monoterpenes. *Int J Mass Spectrom* 2003; **228**: 117–126.

34. Dryahina K, Polasek M, Španěl P. A selected ion flow tube, SIFT, study of the reactions of H_3O^+, NO^+ and O_2^+ ions with several nitroalkenes in the presence of water vapour. *Int J Mass Spectrom* 2004; **239**: 57–65.

35. Anicich V. *An Index of the Literature for Bimolecular Gas Phase Cation-Molecule Reaction Kinetics*. JPL Publication 03-19. Pasadena: NASA, 2003.

36. Španěl P. *TransSIFT Software*. Newcastle-under-Lyme: Trans Spectra Limited, 2003.

37. Španěl P, Smith D. Quantitative selected ion flow tube mass spectrometry: the influence of ionic diffusion and mass discrimination. *J Am Mass Spectrom Soc* 2001; **12**: 863–872.

38. Španěl P, Smith D. Reactions of hydrated hydronium ions and hydrated hydroxide ions with some hydrocarbons and oxygen-bearing organic molecules. *J Phys Chem* 1995; **99**: 15551–15556.

39. Španěl P, Smith D. Influence of water vapour on selected ion flow tube mass spectrometric analyses of trace gases in humid air and breath. *Rapid Commun Mass Spectrom* 2000; **14**: 1898–1906.

40. Ikezoe Y, Matsuoka S, Takebe M, Viggiano A. *Gas Phase Reaction Rate Constants through 1986*. Tokyo: Maruzen, 1987.

41. Španěl P, Smith D. On-line measurement of the absolute humidity of air, breath and liquid headspace samples by selected ion flow tube mass spectrometry. *Rapid Commun Mass Spectrom* 2001; **15**: 563–569.

42. Diskin AM, Španěl P, Smith D. Increase of acetone and ammonia in urine headspace and breath during ovulation quantified using selected ion flow tube mass spectrometry. *Physiol Meas* 2003; **24**: 191–199.

43. Smith D, Španěl P, Jones J. Analysis of volatile emissions from porcine faeces and urine using selected ion flow tube mass spectrometry. *Bioresource Technology* 2000; **75**: 27–33.

44. Španěl P, Smith D. Selected ion flow tube–mass spectrometry: detection and real-time monitoring of flavours released by food products. *Rapid Commun Mass Spectrom* 1999; **13**: 585–597.

45. Smith D, Wang TS, Sule-Suso J, Španěl P, Haj AE. Quantification of acetaldehyde released by lung cancer cells in vitro using selected ion flow tube mass spectrometry. *Rapid Commun Mass Spectrom* 2003; **17**: 845–850.

46. Smith D, Wang TS, Španěl P. Kinetics and isotope patterns of ethanol and acetaldehyde emissions from yeast fermentations of glucose and

glucose-6,6-d2 using selected ion flow tube mass spectrometry: a case study. *Rapid Commun Mass Spectrom* 2002; **16**: 69–76.

47. Španěl P, Diskin A, Abbott S, Wang TS, Smith D. Quantification of volatile compounds in the headspace of aqueous liquids using selected ion flow tube mass spectrometry. *Rapid Commun Mass Spectrom* 2002; **16**: 2184–2153.

48. Smith D, Španěl P. Selected ion flow tube mass spectrometry (SIFT-MS) for on-line trace gas analysis. *Mass Spectrom Rev* 2005; Published on-line 2004: dx.doi.org/2010.1002/mas.20033.

49. Španěl P, Smith D. A selected ion flow tube study of the reactions of NO^+ and O_2^+ ions with some organic molecules: The potential for trace gas analysis of air. *J Chem Phys* 1996; **104**: 1893–1899.

50. Španěl P, Davies S, Smith D. Quantification of ammonia in human breath by the selected ion flow tube analytical method using H_3O^+ and O_2^+ precursor ions. *Rapid Commun Mass Spectrom* 1998; **12**: 763–766.

51. Davies S, Španěl P, Smith D. Quantitative analysis of ammonia on the breath of patients in end-stage renal failure. *Kidney Int* 1997; **52**: 223–228.

52. Španěl P, Smith D, Holland TA, Al Singary W, Elder JB. Analysis of formaldehyde in the headspace of urine from bladder and prostate cancer patients using selected ion flow tube mass spectrometry. *Rapid Commun Mass Spectrom* 1999; **13**: 1354–1359.

53. Španěl P, Wang TS, Smith D. Quantification of hydrogen cyanide in humid air by selected ion flow tube mass spectrometry. *Rapid Commun Mass Spectrom* 2004; **18**: 1869–1873.

54. Smith D, Španěl P, Thompson J, Rajan B, Cocker J, Rolfe P. The selected ion flow tube method for workplace analyses of trace gases in air and breath: its scope, validation, and applications. *Appl Occup Environ Hygiene* 1998; **13**: 817–825.

55. Španěl P, Cocker J, Rajan B, Smith D. Validation of the SIFT technique for trace gas analysis of breath using the syringe injection method. *Ann Occup Hyg* 1997; **41**: 373–378.

56. Smith D, Španěl P, Holland TA, al Singari W, Elder JB. Selected ion flow tube mass spectrometry of urine headspace. *Rapid Commun Mass Spectrom* 1999; **13**: 724–729.

57. Španěl P, Hall E, Workman C, Smith D. A directly coupled monolithic rectangular resonator forming a robust microwave plasma ion source for SIFT-MS *Plasma Sources Science and Technology* 2004; **13**: 282–284.

58. Smith D, Cheng P, Španěl P. Analysis of petrol and diesel vapour and vehicle engine exhaust gases using selected ion flow tube mass spectrometry (SIFT-MS). *Rapid Commun Mass Spectrom* 2002; **16**: 1124–1134.

59. Smith D, Španěl P, Dabill D, Cocker J, Rajan B. On-line analysis of diesel engine exhaust gases by selected ion flow tube mass spectrometry. *Rapid Commun Mass Spectrom* 2004; **18**: 2830–2838.

60. Clough T, Sherlock R, Mautner M, Milligan D, Wilson P, Freeman C, McEwan M. Emission of nitrogen oxides and ammonia from varying rates of applied synthetic urine and correlations with soil chemistry. *Austr J Soil Res* 2003; **41**: 421–438.

61. Milligan D, Wilson P, Mautner M, Freeman C, McEwan M, Clough T, Sherlock R. Real-time, high-resolution quantitative measurement of multiple soil gas emissions: Selected ion flow tube mass spectrometry. *J Environ Qual* 2002; **31**: 515–524.

62. Dewhurst R, Evans R, Mottram T, Španěl P, Smith D. Assessment of rumen processes using selected ion flow tube mass spectrometric analysis of rumen gases. *Dairy Science* 2001; **84**: 1438–1444.

63. Davies S, Španěl P, Smith D. A new 'online' method to measure increased exhaled isoprene in end-stage renal failure. *Nephrol Dial Transplant* 2001; **16**: 836–839.

64. Gelmont D, Stein RA, Mead JF. Isoprene — the main hydrocarbon in human breath. *Biochem Biophys Res Commun* 1981; **99**: 1456–1460.

65. Manolis A. The diagnostic potential of breath analysis. *Clin Chem* 1983; **29**: 5–15.

66. Smith D, Španěl P, Davies S. Trace gases in breath of healthy volunteers when fasting and after a protein-calorie meal: a preliminary study. *J Appl Physiol* 1999; **87**: 1584–1588.

67. Diskin AM, Španěl P, Smith D. Time variation of ammonia, acetone, isoprene and ethanol in breath: a quantitative SIFT-MS study over 30 days. *Physiol Meas* 2003; **24**: 107–119.

68. Miekisch W, Schubert JK, Noeldge-Schomburg GF. Diagnostic potential of breath analysis — focus on volatile organic compounds. *Clin Chim Acta* 2004; **347**: 25–39.

69. Španěl P, Davies S, Smith D. Breath ammonia dips after feeding independently of the protein content of the meal. *The FASEB Journal* 2000; **14**: A490.

70. Smith D, Wang TS, Španěl P. On-line, simultaneous quantification of ethanol, some metabolites and water vapour in breath following the ingestion of alcohol. *Physiol Meas* 2002; **23**: 477–489.

71. Hyspler R, Crhova S, Gasparic J, Zadak Z, Cizkova M, Balasova V. Determination of isoprene in human expired breath using solid-phase microextraction and gas chromatography-mass spectrometry. *J Chromatography B* 2000; **739**: 183–190.

72. Smith D, Španěl P. Application of Ion Chemistry and the SIFT Technique to the Quantitative Analysis of Trace Gases in Air and on Breath. *Int Rev Phys Chem* 1996; **15**: 231–271.

73. Španěl P, Davies S, Smith D. Quantification of breath isoprene using the selected ion flow tube mass spectrometric analytical method. *Rapid Commun Mass Spectrom* 1999; **13**: 1733–1738.

74. Wilson PF, Freeman CG, McEwan MJ, Milligan DB, Allardyce RA, Shaw GM. Alcohol in breath and blood: a selected ion flow tube mass spectrometric study. *Rapid Commun Mass Spectrom* 2001; **15**: 413–417.

75. Smith D, Španěl P. On-line determination of the deuterium abundance in breath water vapour by flowing afterglow mass spectrometry with applications to measurements of total body water. *Rapid Commun Mass Spectrom* 2001; **15**: 25–32.

76. Španěl P, Smith D. Flowing afterglow mass spectrometry (FA-MS) for the determination of the deuterium abundance in breath water vapour and aqueous liquid headspace. In: Amann A, Smith D, eds. *Breath Analysis for Clinical Diagnosis and Therapeutic Monitoring,* Singapore: World Scientific, 2005.

77. Španěl P, Rolfe P, Rajan B, Smith D. The selected ion flow tube (SIFT) — a novel technique for biological monitoring. *Ann Occup Hyg* 1996; **40**: 615–626.

78. Hansel A, Jordan A, Holzinger R, Prazeller P, Vogel W, Lindinger W. Proton-transfer reaction mass-spectrometry — online trace gas-analysis at the ppb level. *Int J Mass Spectrom Ion Processes* 1995; **149/150**: 609.

79. Abbott S, Elder J, Španěl P, Smith D. Quantification of acetonitrile in exhaled breath and urinary headspace using selected ion flow tube mass spectrometry. *Int J Mass Spectrom* 2003; **228**: 655–665.

80. Prazeller P, Karl T, Jordan A, Holzinger R, Hansel A, Lindinger W. Quantification of passive smoking using proton-transfer-reaction mass spectrometry. *Int J Mass Spectrom* 1998; **178**: L1–L4.

81. Houeto P, Hoffman JR, Got P, Dang Vu B, Baud FJ. Acetonitrile as a possible marker of current cigarette smoking. *Hum Exp Toxicol* 1997; **16**: 658–661.

82. Senthilmohan ST, McEwan MJ, Wilson PF, Milligan DB, Freeman CG. Real time analysis of breath volatiles using SIFT-MS in cigarette smoking. *Redox Rep* 2001; **6**: 185–187.

83. Wilson PF, Freeman CG, McEwan MJ, Milligan DB, Allardyce RA, Shaw GM. In situ analysis of solvents on breath and blood: a selected ion flow tube mass spectrometric study. *Rapid Commun Mass Spectrom* 2002; **16**: 427–432.

84. Vaira D, Holton J, Ricci C, Basset C, Gatta L, Perna F, Tampieri A, Miglioli M. Review article: Helicobacter pylori infection from pathogenesis to treatment — a critical reappraisal. *Aliment Pharmacol Ther* 2002; **16 Suppl 4**: 105–113.

85. Smith D, Španěl P. The novel selected-ion flow tube approach to trace gas analysis of air and breath. *Rapid Commun Mass Spectrom* 1996; **10**: 1183–1198.

86. Penault C, Španěl P, Smith D. Detection of *H. pylori* infection by breath ammonia following urea ingestion. In: Amann A, Smith D, eds. *Breath Analysis for Clinical Diagnosis and Therapeutic Monitoring,* Singapore: World Scientific, 2005.

87. Carroll W, Wang TS, Španěl P, Alcock A, Lenney W, Smith D. A Study of the volatile compounds emitted by Pseudomonas bacteria in vitro using selected ion flow tube mass spectrometry, SIFT-MS. *Pediatric Pulmonolog* 2005: in press.

88. Bloor R, Wang TS, Španěl P Smith D. Applications of selected ion flow tube mass spectrometry, SIFT-MS, in addiction research. In: Amann A, Smith D, eds. *Breath Analysis for Clinical Diagnosis and Therapeutic Monitoring,* Singapore: World Scientific, 2005.

89. Waldorf D, Babb A. Vapor-phase equilibrium of NO, NO_2, H_2O, and HNO_2. *J Chem Phys* 1963; **39**: 432–435.

90. Lundberg JO, Carlsson S, Engstrand L, Morcos E, Wiklund NP, Weitzberg E. Urinary nitrite: more than a marker of infection. *Urology* 1997; **50**: 189–191.
91. Kato S, Post GC, Bierbaum VM, Koch TH. Chemical ionization mass spectrometric determination of acrolein in human breast cancer cells. *Anal Biochem* 2002; **305**: 251–259.
92. Phillips M, Gleeson K, Hughes JM, Greenberg J, Cataneo RN, Baker L, McVay WP. Volatile organic compounds in breath as markers of lung cancer: a cross-sectional study. *Lancet* 1999; **353**: 1930–1933.

OCCUPATIONAL EXPOSURE ASSESSMENT THROUGH ANALYSIS OF HUMAN BREATH AND AMBIENT AIR USING IMR–MASS SPECTROMETRY

J. VILLINGER, S. PRAUN, J. RÖSSLER-GRAF, AND A. DORNAUER

V & F medical development GmbH,
A-6067 Absam, Austria

H. NEUMAYER AND E. BAUMGARTNER

Arbeitsmedizinisches Zentrum Hall,
A-6060 Hall i. T., Austria

1. Introduction

Non-invasive diagnosis has been of great interest to the medical industry since the times of Hippocrates. *Airsense*, a multi-component gas analyzer (see below), is a valuable tool for the analysis of organic and inorganic compounds in exhaled breath to monitor occupational exposure. This monitoring technique has been used for over 18 years in the analysis of gases from internal combustion engines (exhaust gases), gases from fuel cells and in catalytic converter research, as well as in environmental analysis and in the food industry, and is constantly being refined for medical diagnostic applications.

2. Methods

2.1. Technology

Airsense is a mass spectrometer, which is based on the use of ion–molecule reactions (IMR) coupled with quadrupole mass spectrometry (QMS), and provides a highly-sensitive method for on-line and off-line sampling of organic and inorganic compounds in exhaled breath.[1][5] Because low-energetic primary ions are used there is a soft charge exchange with the molecules of the exhaled breath introduced into the instrument; this largely suppresses the formation of molecular fragments, which is known to result from elec-

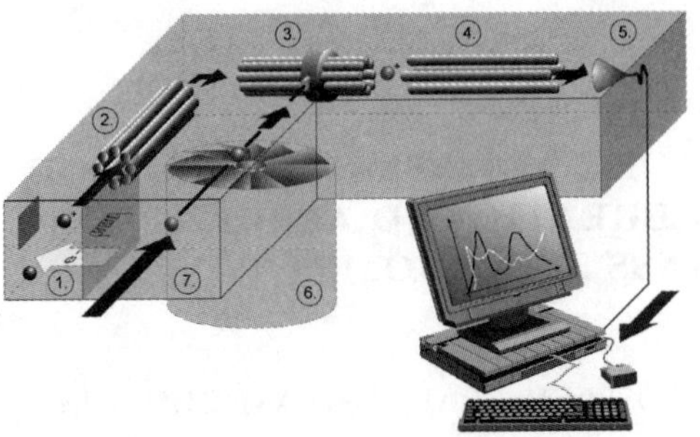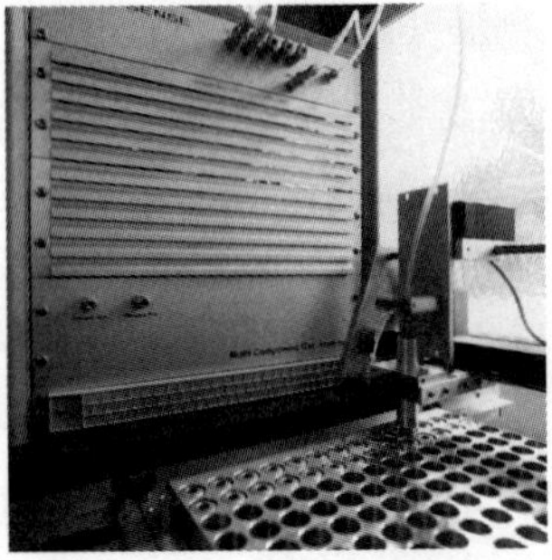

Fig. 1.   Setup of the *Airsense* instrument and the *V&F-autosampler*. 1: Primary ion source; 2: Octopole separation device; 3: Charge exchange cell; 4: Quadrupole–mass filter; 5: Particle detector; 6: Vacuum system; 7: Gas inlet system

tron impact ionization. A schematic diagram and a photograph of the *Airsense* instrument is shown in Figure 1.

Gaseous compounds and compounds dissolved in exhaled breath, *e.g.* aliphatics, aromatics, alcohols, aldehydes, ketones, carboxylic acids, amines, inorganic acids and bases are detected directly. At the same time, the major components of exhaled breath in volume percent levels can be monitored (carbon dioxide, oxygen, water and nitrogen), as well as the trace components (*e.g.* methane, isoprene, ammonia, nitrogen monoxide, acetaldehyde, acetone, acetonitrile, ethanol, propanol, butadiene, benzene, diethyl ether, toluene, dimethylformamide etc.) that are present in the parts-per-billion, ppb, to the parts-per-million, ppm, range. Analysis times for each species depend on the application, but range from a few milliseconds to seconds.

2.2. *Sampling Methods*

For an on-line breath analysis, the subject breathes into a heated transfer capillary of the breath-by-breath gas analyzer either a few centimetres in front of the transfer capillary or directly connected with a mask (see Figure 2). This method also allows the real-time monitoring of ambient air. For an off-line breath analysis, the subject breathes through a straw into a vial (see Figure 2), which is then air-sealed and analyzed with an autosampler-IMR-MS (see Figure 1).

By placing vials at different positions in a room, ambient air can be sampled at the same time. Thus, off-line sampling also allows the concentrations of compounds in exhaled breath to be compared with those in the

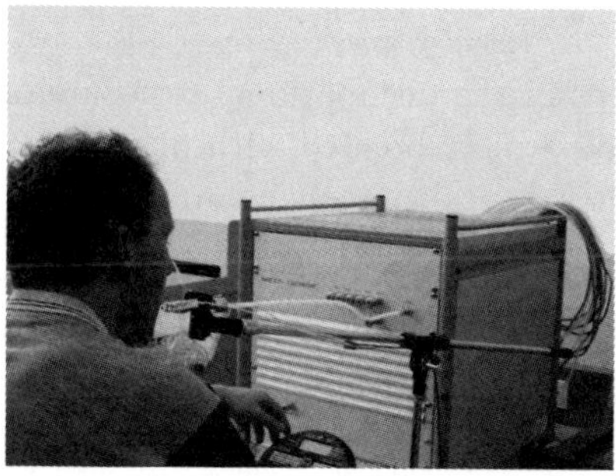 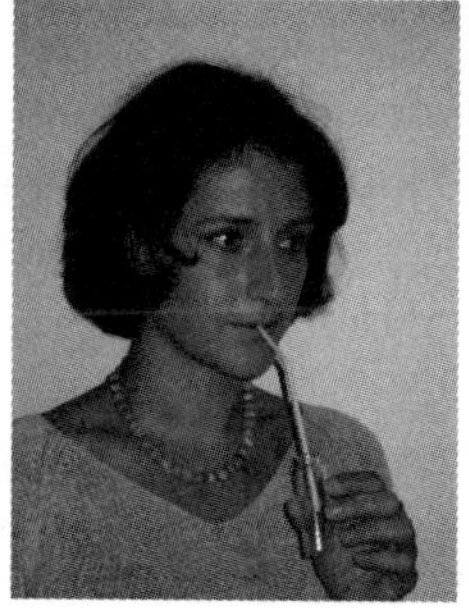

Fig. 2.　On-line and off-line sampling

ambient air. Neither on-line nor off-line sampling requires further concentration steps, such as adsorption onto stationary phases, for instance. Thus, sample preparations such as thermal desorption or elution is unnecessary.

3. Results

3.1. *Online*

3.1.1. *Gas clearance monitoring*

Figure 3 shows the clearance from the breath of propene, butadiene, benzene, and toluene, following the inhalation of a gas-mixture containing 5 ppm of these compounds.[6] The concentrations peaked at 1.1 ppm before reaching the initial concentration again after about three to six minutes.

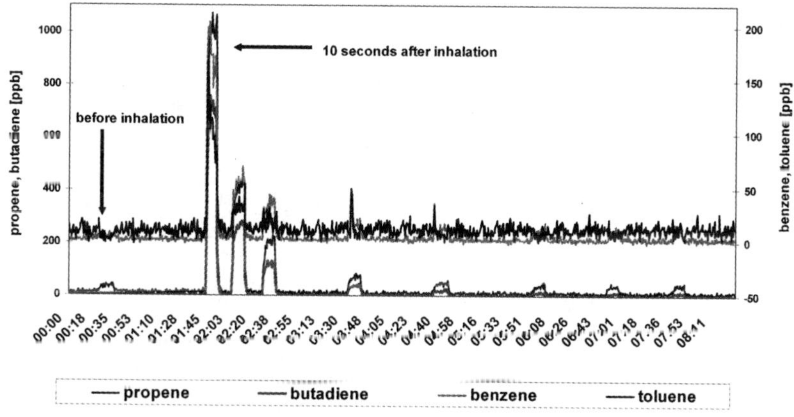

Fig. 3.　Gas clearance monitoring after inhalation of 5 ppm of propene, butadiene, benzene, toluene

3.1.2. *Emission from grinding discs*

Figure 4 shows selective differences in the occupational exposure of workers where different makes of grinding discs bonded with phenol resin were used. Benzene, formaldehyde, phenol, and polycyclic aromatic hydrocarbons (PAHs) were detected in real time.

3.1.3. *Monitoring of "Hoffmann analytes" in cigarette smoke*

Another example of on-line measurement is the "puff-per-puff" Hoffmann analysis of cigarette smoke. Four different kinds of cigarettes of a common brand are smoked by a "smoking machine". The concentration profiles of acetaldehyde are shown in Fig. 5.

3.2. *Offline*

3.2.1. *Pharmaceutical industry: dimethylformamide (DMF) in clean room ambient air and in exhaled breath*

DMF is a solvent used in the manufacture of drugs. When working with DMF, different concentrations of this solvent can be detected in different positions in the clean room and the decontamination room. The concentrations of DMF in the exhaled breath of a laboratory worker increased during exposure and decreased during the lunch break (see Figure 6).[7,8] There is

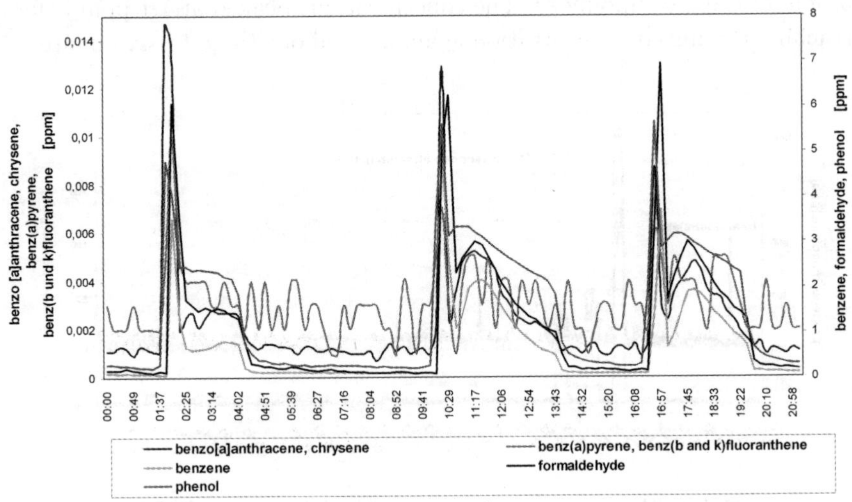

Fig. 4.   Emission from grinding discs bonded with phenol resin; 3 different makes

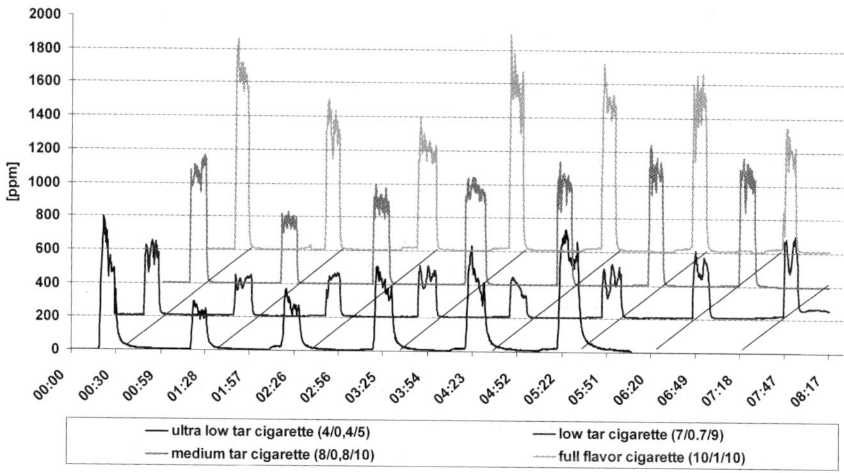

Fig. 5. Puff-per-puff analysis of different kinds of cigarettes of a common brand; acetaldehyde

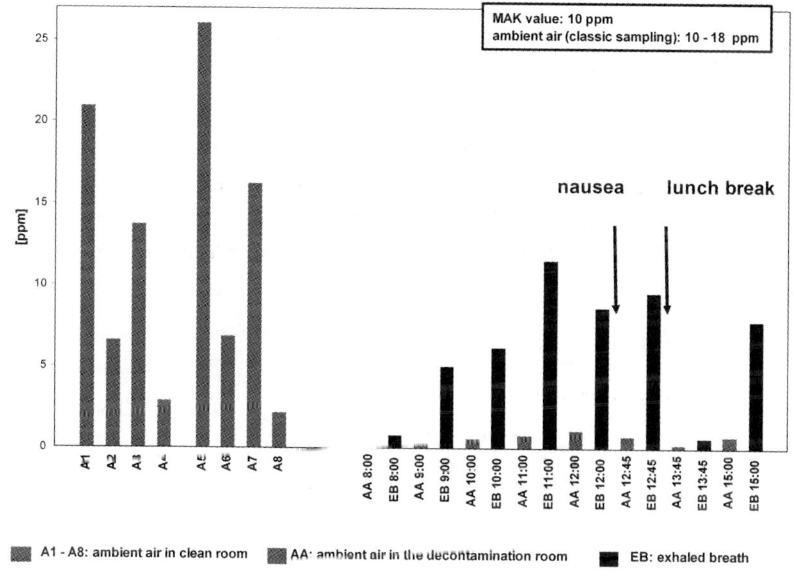

Fig. 6. Concentration profiles of dimethylformamide in ambient air and exhaled breath

a high correlation between the levels of DMF in the ambient air measured with glass vials (see 2.2) and its level in ambient air measured by the classic method (adsorption of DMF from the air onto silica gel; desorption with methanol; detection by gas chromatography). The concentrations at different places in the clean room varied from 3–26 ppm measured by IMR-MS compared to 10–18 ppm measured with gas chromatography.

3.2.2. *Glass manufacturing industry: diethyl ether, acetone; levels in exhaled breath (off-line) and in ambient air (on-line)*

Acetone and diethyl ether are used to clean lenses and prisms in the production of binoculars.[9] During the morning, the concentrations of these solvents in exhaled breath increase up to a level of 15 ppm. These levels decrease during the lunch break and increase again during the afternoon (see Figure 7). This again demonstrates the positive effect of (lunch) breaks in reducing occupational exposure.

As can be seen in Figure 8, the ambient air levels (on-line) in the production area vary widely in concentrations up to a maximum of 600 ppm.

3.2.3. *Spray painting: toluene; comparison of levels in blood and in exhaled breath*

Breath samples were collected every hour from four subjects in a spray painting plant where toluene is used as a solvent. These samples were then compared with blood samples taken before and after work.[10,11] Table 1 shows the parameters recorded (blood, breath and ambient air levels of toluene) and Figure 9 shows the concentration profile as recorded during working hours.

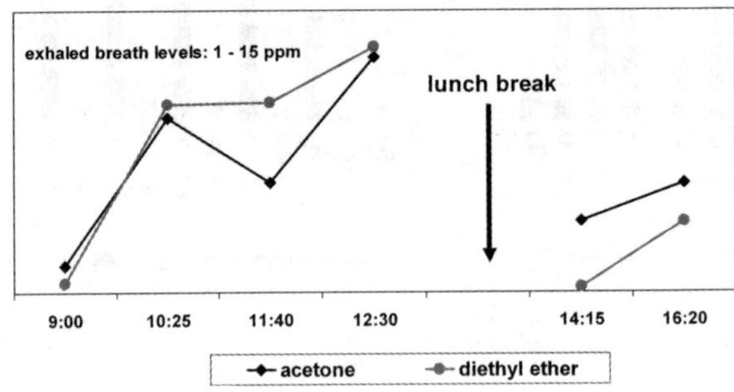

Fig. 7.   Time-dependent concentration profile of acetone and diethyl ether in exhaled breath (average of 6 persons)

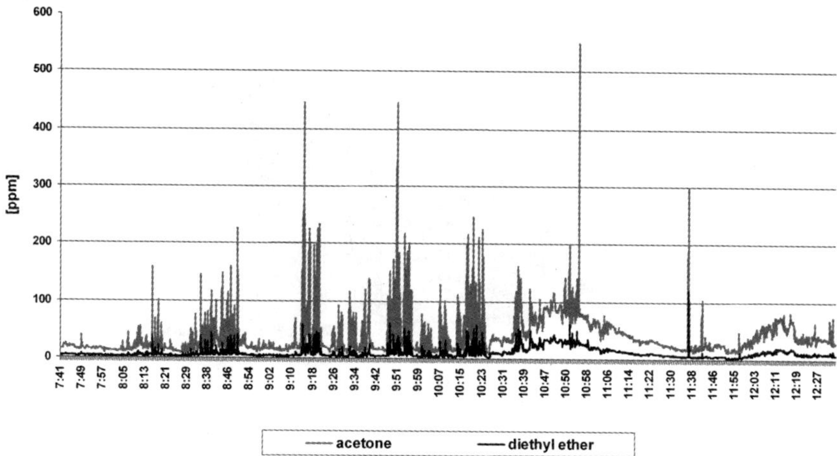

Fig. 8. Online ambient air measurement; acetone and diethyl ether

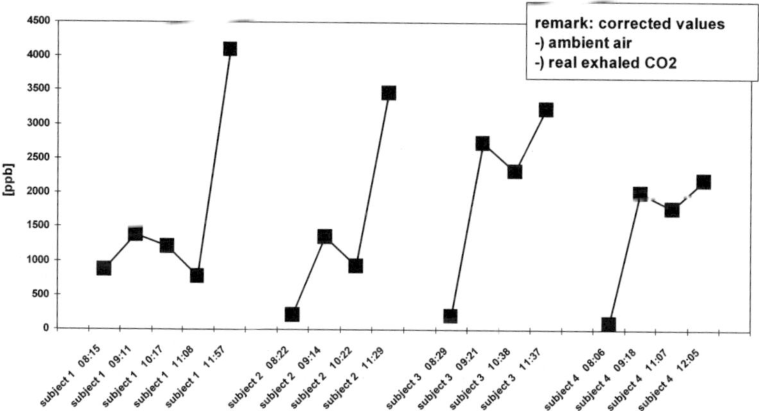

Fig. 9. Time-dependent concentration of toluene in exhaled breath of workers in a spray painting plant

Table 1. Sampling data recorded at the spray painting plant

	Before work	After work
Blood	0.478–2.16 μg/dL	8.00–14.31 μg/dL
Exhaled breath	66–232 ppb	372–3119 ppb
Ambient air	36 ppb	54 ppb
Ambient air in spray painting line	0.854–12.082 ppm	

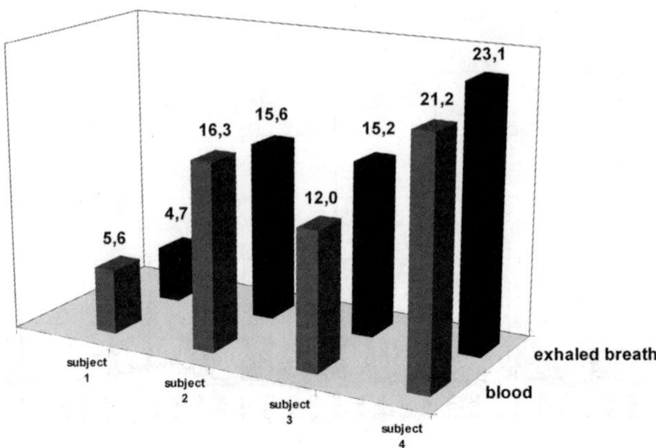

Fig. 10.   Comparison of toluene levels in blood and exhaled breath (ratio of post-exposure by pre-exposure)

Due to the individual sequences of operation, the initial concentration levels in subjects 1 and 2 were low. By contrast, the concentration levels in subjects 3 and 4 had peaked one hour after they had started to work and remained constant until the end of the working day. *Remark:* In order to record the actual breath toluene concentrations, the concentrations in the test room were subtracted from the exhaled breath levels, and normalized to the exhaled carbon dioxide concentrations.

Figure 10 shows the ratio of pre-exposure to post-exposure toluene levels. After only four hours of exposure the toluene levels in the breath of the subjects were 4.7 to 23.1 times higher than the initial (pre-exposure) levels. Despite high variations amongst the individuals, the toluene concentrations in blood correlated well with breath levels, and reached $98.6\% \pm 17.2\%$ on average.

4. Conclusions

Breath analysis offers a non-invasive method to monitor occupational exposure levels. Using *Airsense*, a multi-component gas mixture, comprising organic and inorganic compounds, can be analysed simultaneously without the need for time-consuming sample preparations. The on-line (real time) and off-line (passive) analysis of exhaled breath and ambient air both offer a simple method to assess occupational exposure as the organic constituents of exhaled human breath are representative of blood-borne concentrations through gas exchange in the blood/breath interface in the lungs. In contrast to blood samples, which have to be taken to the lab, on-site breath samples allow the evaluation of concentration profiles within the working hours, thus allowing more precise and rapid conclusions to be drawn regarding the assessment of occupational exposure.

References

1. Villinger J, Federer W, Resch R, Lubich M, Sejkora W, Dornauer A. SIMS 500 — Rapid Low Energy Secondary Ion Mass Spectrometer for In-Line Analysis of Gaseous Compounds — Technology and Applications in Automotive Testing. In: *SAE Technical Paper Series 932017*. Warrendale, PA, USA: SAE Technical Paper Series 932017, 1993.
2. Portincasa P, Praun S, Berardino M, Moschetta A, Pistoia G, Montelli R, Scaccianoce G, Villinger J, Palasciano G. Novel soft ionization mass spectrometry (SIMS) monitors several components in human breath: studies in the fasting and fed period in healthy subjects. *Gastroenterology* 2004; **126** (Suppl 2): S1479.
3. Balint B, Donnelly LE, Hanazawa T, Kharitonov SA, Barnes PJ. Increased nitric oxide metabolites in exhaled breath condensate after exposure to tobacco smoke. *Thorax* 2001; **56**: 456–461.
4. Teranishi R, Mon TR, Robinson AB, Cary P, Pauling L. Gas chromatography of volatiles from breath and urine. *Anal Chem* 1972; **44**: 18–20.
5. Phillips M. Breath tests in medicine. *Sci Am* 1992; **267**: 74–79.
6. Ljungkvist G, Olin A, Torén K, Lärstad M. Simultaneous single-breath measurement of pentane, isoprene and nitric oxide using mass spectrometry. In: *ERS 13th Annual Congress, Vienna*, 2003: P577.
7. Brugnone F, Perbellini L, Gaffuri E, Turri P. Monitoring of industrial exposure to dimethylformamide by analysis of alveolar air. *G Ital Med Lav* 1984; **6**: 139–141.
8. Brugnone F, Perbellini L, Gaffuri E. *N-N*-dimethylformamide concentration in environmental and alveolar air in an artificial leather factory. *Br J Ind Med* 1980; **37**: 185–188.
9. Brugnone F, Perbellini L, Gaffuri E, Apostoli P. Biomonitoring of industrial solvent exposures in workers' alveolar air. *Int Arch Occup Environ Health* 1980; **47**: 245–261.
10. Chen ML, Chen SH, Guo BR, Mao IF. Relationship between environmental exposure to toluene, xylene and ethylbenzene and the expired breath concentrations for gasoline service workers. *J Environ Monit* 2002; **4**: 562–566.
11. Astrand I, Ehrner-Samuel H, Kilbom A, Ovrum P. Toluene exposure. I. Concentration in alveolar air and blood at rest and during exercise. *Work environ Health* 1972; **9**: 119–130.

PROTON TRANSFER REACTION TIME-OF-FLIGHT MASS SPECTROMETRY: A GOOD PROSPECT FOR DIAGNOSTIC BREATH ANALYSIS?

R. S. BLAKE, C. WHYTE, P. S. MONKS, AND A. M. ELLIS

Department of Chemistry,
University of Leicester,
Leicester, LE1 7RH, UK

1. Introduction

Although conceived little more than ten years ago, proton transfer reaction mass spectrometry (PTR-MS) has already seen widespread application as a tool for measuring trace amounts of volatile organic compounds (VOCs) in air.[1–3] In our own laboratory, we have a research programme underway in which PTR-MS is employed in studies of atmospheric chemistry, particularly as a mobile instrument for field campaigns. In order to gain as complete a picture as possible of the role of organic compounds in tropospheric chemistry, it is important to be able to monitor a wide range of VOCs in a relatively short period of time. Unfortunately, conventional PTR-MS instruments, in which a quadrupole filter is used for mass selection, are not the most efficient tools for carrying out such studies. The accumulation of an ion signal at a chosen mass-charge-ratio, m/z, necessarily results in rejection of all other ions. Consequently, acquisition of a full mass spectrum requires a lengthy scanning procedure in which each mass channel is sampled for a given period of time before stepping to the next m/z position.

In our work we have been exploring the use of time-of-flight mass spectrometry (TOF-MS) in place of a quadrupole filter in PTR-MS. The resulting PTR-TOF-MS technique offers great promise for rapidly monitoring a wide variety of species because of the multichannel detection capability of TOF-MS. Although our primary research targets are in atmospheric science, we feel that PTR-TOF-MS may also find important applications in medical diagnosis through the analysis of human breath. In particular, the ability to rapidly detect a wide range of VOCs may be suitable for 'fingerprinting' certain medical conditions.

In this article we describe the key design features and capabilities of our current PTR-TOF-MS instrument. In addition, we will outline a second-generation instrument, based on Hadamard transform time-of-flight mass spectrometry, which is currently under construction and which will potentially provide much higher detection sensitivity.

2. Experimental Details

A schematic illustration of the PTR-TOF-MS instrument is shown in Fig. 1. It consists of a small ion source and drift tube coupled to a time-of-flight mass spectrometer by an ion transfer region. H_3O^+ ions are generated in the ion source region either by a hollow cathode discharge through water vapour or by using a radioactive source. The former yields higher currents but the work reported here focuses on the radioactive source, a ^{241}Am alpha source.

Whichever source is used, the H_3O^+ ions are mixed with a continuously flowing air sample at the top of a drift tube and proton transfer occurs as the gas sample traverses the drift tube. Only those molecules with proton affinities greater than that of H_3O^+ will accept a proton, limiting the observable species to trace VOCs. Most VOCs, with the exception of

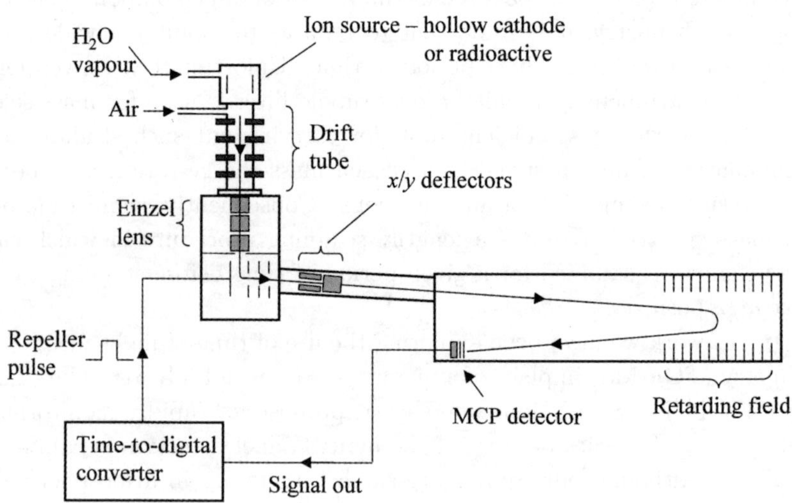

Fig. 1.   Block diagram of the PTR-TOF-MS instrument

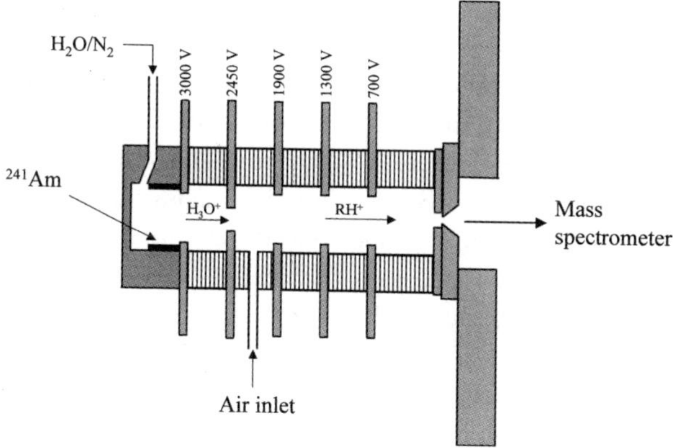

Fig. 2.   Expanded view of the ion source and drift tube. The ion source shown is a radioactive source based on alpha particle emission from ^{241}Am. Water vapour from a de-ionised water reservoir is carried into the ion source region by continuously flowing N_2.

mainly the lighter alkanes, will readily accept a proton from H_3O^+. Figure 2 shows a schematic of the ion source and drift tube: the design is similar to that reported by Hansen and co-workers.[4] Ions leave the drift tube through a small aperture and pass through a differential pumping region (not shown in Fig. 1) before encountering an ion transfer lens. The ion lens is a standard three-element einzel lens, which focuses the ion beam into the extraction region of a reflectron time-of-flight mass spectrometer. An extraction voltage is applied to drive a bunch of ions from the incoming continuous ion stream into the drift region of the TOF-MS. Ions reaching the detector, which in this instrument is a dual microchannel plate (MCP) detector, generate an output current which is amplified and fed into a pulse counting system consisting of a time-to-digital converter coupled to a computer. The TOF-MS and its data acquisition system were custom-built by Kore Technology (Ely, Cambridgeshire, UK). A more detailed account of the PTR-TOF-MS instrument can be found in a recent publication.[5]

3. Performance of the PTR-TOF-MS Instrument

The PTR-TOF MS instrument has been characterised with a number of standard calibration mixtures. As an illustration, Fig. 3 shows part of the mass spectrum from a 30-component VOC secondary gas standard produced by the National Physical Laboratory (Teddington, Middlesex, UK). This contains a variety of alkanes, alkenes and alkynes, including aromatics, all at the 1–10 ppbv level. The alkanes in the mixture cannot be detected by PTR-MS using H_3O^+ as the ionisation agent, but most of the unsaturated hydrocarbons can be detected.[6] Some of the prominent components of the mixture have been labeled in the spectrum.

Figure 3 also serves to demonstrate the mass resolution we can currently attain. Although the TOF-MS has a nominal mass resolution ($m/\Delta m$) of 3000, we find under our operating conditions that it is generally closer to 1000. With this resolution, ions that differ in mass by approximately one dalton are easily separated. However, ions from different compounds that are nominally isobaric, but in practice have slightly different masses, cannot be distinguished with our current instrument (a resolution in excess of 3000 would be required before this approach could begin to be useful).

Tests with various mixtures have shown that the instrument shows an excellent linear response over a wide concentration range. With the radioactive source, the detection sensitivity is such that individual VOCs at the ppbv level can be confidently detected (registering a few counts) in about 1–2 minutes. Figure 3 provides a good illustration of this, since it was accumulated over a 20 minute period and, for example, the benzene concentration in the gas standard is known to be 5.5 ppbv. The sensitivity we attain for a single species is well below that reported for current PTR-MS using instruments based on quadrupole MS.[1] However, it is im-

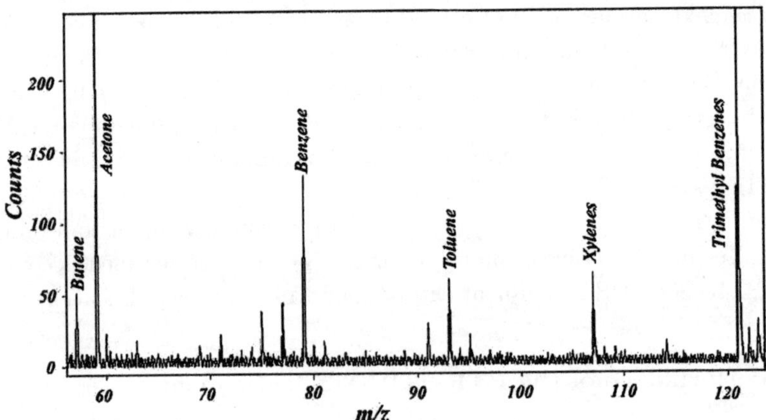

Fig. 3.   Section of the PTR-TOF-MS mass spectrum for a 30-component hydrocarbon mixture containing aromatics at concentrations less than 10 ppbv. This spectrum was accumulated over a 20 minute period. The large acetone and trimethylbenzene signals are due to contaminants (source unknown) inside the instrument, since these peaks remain intense after the calibration mixture is closed off.

portant to emphasise that this sensitivity is achieved over the whole mass range simultaneously, so benefit may accrue if the number of species being monitored is large.

There are three factors that play a role in limiting the detection sensitivity of the PTR-TOF-MS, which we specifically identify. First, our present radioactive ion source does not produce a particularly large H_3O^+ current. The alternative, the hollow cathode discharge source, yields roughly five times more ion current. However, there have been problems with the stability of this source and it needs more development work before we employ it as standard on our instrument. A second limiting factor may be that, with our current experimental arrangement, the ions leaving the drift tube are not sampled efficiently into the extraction region of the TOF-MS. Ion trajectory simulations using SIMION seem to confirm this and we are therefore currently exploring ways of improving the ion transfer optics to extract more ions into the TOF-MS. Finally, even if the above factors are addressed, a serious limitation is the duty cycle of the TOF-MS. Only a small proportion of the ion beam entering the mass spectrometer extraction region actually gets injected into the flight tube. We estimate that under our current operating conditions the duty cycle is in the region of 2–3 %. Thus 97–98 % of the ion signal is lost to the instrument. This is a serious limitation and if some or the entire missing signal could be collected the sensitivity of the instrument would be increased dramatically. The next section describes a potential solution, the use of Hadamard transform TOF-MS.

4. Solving the Duty Cycle Problem: Hadamard Transform TOF-MS

The limited duty cycle of standard orthogonal acceleration TOF-MS arises because, when a bunch of ions is injected into the flight tube, no further ions can be injected until the entire previous bunch has reached the detector. Although the duty cycle can be improved to some extent by lengthening the extractor/repeller region of the TOF-MS, and also by slowing down the incoming ion beam, it is difficult to recover more than a few percent of the missing signal through this means.

An alternative and highly effective solution has recently been demonstrated by Zare and co-workers,[7–9] the use of Hadamard transform TOF-MS. Instead of orthogonal acceleration of an ion beam into the flight tube, the ion beam is input in-line with the flight tube. This beam is then rapidly modulated using an in-line deflector, a Bradley–Nielson (BN) gate.[10] A BN gate is a fast-switching beam deflection device which can be set either to transmit ions undeflected, in which case the ions reach the detector, or can deflect the ions out of the path of the detector. In other words the BN gate has a binary (on or off) status depending on the level of an external voltage applied to it. If a pseudo-random sequence of on/off voltage pulses is applied continuously to the gate, the output from the MCP detector will show no apparent pattern when ions counts versus time is plotted. However, this raw data can be used to extract the time-of-flight spectrum, and hence the mass spectrum, if it is cross-correlated with the pseudo-random pulse sequence. This cross-correlation is a straightforward mathematical transformation known as a *Hadamard transformation.*

The key point about this approach is that it automatically achieves a 50 % duty cycle, and in fact a scheme has been developed which attains a 100 % duty cycle.[11] We are in the final stages of constructing the first PTR-TOF-MS instrument based on the Hadamard transform approach. When complete, and when in combination with the improved hollow-cathode discharge ion source, we anticipate that the gain in sensitivity will be dramatic and should allow individual VOCs to be detected at the 1 ppbv level in roughly one second. Again, we emphasise that this sensitivity will be available in *all* mass channels simultaneously, and when applied to breath analysis it should be practical to obtain a comprehensive VOC status report from a single human breath in just a few seconds of data accumulation. Such detailed information is potentially suitable for analysis by pattern recognition techniques, and we speculate that it may be possible to use pattern recognition to correlate certain medical conditions with specific mass spectral patterns. If this speculation has any validity, then PTR-HT-TOF-MS may find a role in rapid medical diagnosis through breath analysis.

5. Conclusions

A proton transfer reaction mass spectrometer based on time-of-flight mass spectrometry has been developed. The present version is capable of achieving a detection limit of 1 ppbv in all mass channels simultaneously in about one minute of data accumulation. A faster version of the instrument is currently being developed which, when fully operational, offers particularly exciting prospects for breath analysis. This new instrument should achieve detection at the 1 ppbv level in about one second and will enable the rapid capture of comprehensive VOC data. In combination with pattern recognition techniques, we speculate that this may provide information for the diagnosis of certain medical conditions, although of course much detailed clinical research would be required to establish if this claim has any validity.

Acknowledgements

The authors would like to acknowledge important contributions from a number of people, particularly Ceri Hughes, Keith Wilkinson and Gerry Butler.

References

1. Lindinger W, Hansel A, Jordan A. On-line monitoring of volatile organic compounds at pptv levels by means of proton-transfer-reaction mass spectrometry (PTR-MS): medical applications, food control, and environmental research. *Int J Mass Spectrom Ion Processes* 1998; **173**: 191–241.
2. Lindinger W, Hansel A, Jordan A. Proton-transfer-reaction mass spectrometry (PTR-MS): on-line monitoring of volatile organic compunds at pptv levels. *Chem Soc Rev* 1998; **27**: 347–354.
3. Hewitt C, Hayward S, Tani A. The application of proton transfer reaction-mass spectrometry (PTR-MS) to the monitoring and analysis of volatile organic compounds in the atmosphere. *J Environ Monitoring* 2003; **5**: 1–7.
4. Hanson D, Greenberg J, Henry B, Kosciuch E. Proton transfer reaction mass spectrometry at high drift tube pressure. *Int J Mass Spectrom Ion Processes* 2003; **223-224**: 507–518.
5. Blake R, Whyte C, Hughes C, Ellis A, Monks P. Demonstration of proton transfer reaction time-of-flight mass spectrometry for real-time analysis of trace volatile organic compounds. *Anal Chem* 2004; **76**: 3841–3845.
6. Španěl P, Smith D. SIFT studies of the reactions of H_3O^+, NO^+ and O_2^+ with several aliphatic and aromatic hydrocarbons. *Int J Mass Spectrom* 1998; **181**: 1–10.
7. Brock A, Rodriguez N, Zare R. Characterization of a Hadamard transform time-of-flight mass spectrometer. *Rev Sci Instrum* 2000; **71**: 1306–1318.
8. Fernandez F, Rodriguez N, Vadillo J, Wetterhall M, K M, Engelke F, Kimmel J, Zare R. Effect of sequence length, sequence frequency, and data acquisition rate on the performance of a Hadamard transform time-of-flight mass spectrometer. *J Am Soc Mass Spec* 2001; **12**: 1302–1311.
9. Zare R, Kimmel J, Fernández F. Hadamard transform time-of-flight mass spectrometry: more signal, more of the time. *Angewandte Chemie* 2003; **42**: 30–35.
10. Kimmel J, Engelke F, Zare R. Novel method for the production of finely spaced Bradbury–Nielson gates. *Rev Sci Instru* 2001; **72**: 4354–4357.
11. Trapp O, Kimmel J, Yoon O, Zuleta I, Fernandez F, Zare R. Continuous two-channel time-of-flight mass spectrometric detection of electrosprayed ions. *Angew Chemie* 2004; **43**: 6541–6544.

METABOLITES IN HUMAN BREATH:
ION MOBILITY SPECTROMETERS
AS DIAGNOSTIC TOOLS FOR LUNG DISEASES

J. I. BAUMBACH, W. VAUTZ, AND V. RUZSANYI

ISAS — Institute for Analytical Sciences,
Department of Metabolomics,
Bunsen–Kirchhoff-Straße 11, D-44139 Dortmund, Germany

L. FREITAG

Lung Hospital Hemer,
Theo-Funccius-Straße 1, D-58675 Hemer, Germany

1. Introduction

The aim of this chapter is to establish a quick and low-cost device for human breath analysis, in addition to investigations of blood and urine, as a non-invasive standard method in hospitals and for medical applications. This procedure is based on miniaturised ion mobility spectrometers supported by mass spectrometric validations. The full procedure, including sampling, pre-separation and identification of metabolites in human exhaled air, will be developed and implemented with a view to future use in hospitals. Metabolic profiling of the breath of healthy individuals and those suffering from different diseases, in particular lung cancer, will be considered at various lung hospitals and point-of-care centres.

It is well recognised in the medical community that people exhale volatile compounds that may carry important information about the health of the individuals. Thus, a successful detection of the products of different metabolic processes is attractive, especially if the detection limits of the spectrometric methods used are sufficiently low and the instruments are available at moderate price levels so that they can be used as standard methods in hospitals. The vision of the authors is to contribute to the development of breath analysis as a diagnostic method for disease in support of blood and urine analysis.

Human breath contains numerous volatile substances derived both from endogenous metabolism and exposure to ambient vapours and gases and their metabolites. Approximately 200 different compounds have been detected in human breath; some are correlated with various common disorders like diabetes, heart disease and possibly lung cancer.[1-20] Generally, the composition of different constituents in expired air is representative for blood concentrations resulting from gas exchange at the blood/breath interface in the lungs.[21] Thus, the presence and concentrations of specific volatile organic compounds, VOCs, in expired air are directly linked to their presence in the blood, which is in contact with diseased tissues and organs. Furthermore, metabolites derived from local bacterial infections in the airways can be also detected directly in breath. Pulmonary infections carry a significant risk for people with week immune systems, especially for long term and post-operative patients.

Different techniques are used for breath analysis. A popular sampling method is the use of Tedlar bags to collect human breath. The components of the exhaled breath sample are collected using a sorbent-trap or a cryo-trap followed by desorption into an analytical instrument such as the often used gas chromatograph with an analytical mass spectrometer, GC-MS.[22] This is a rather time consuming process with numerous steps that may lead to loss of analytes,[2,23] since different analytes may adsorb on the surface of the bag,[24] which is especially troublesome at trace gas levels. The number of compounds detected in exhaled air and their concentrations vary according to the sampling procedure and the analytical method used. The major VOCs found in the breath of healthy persons (with their typical concentrations in parts-per-billion by volume, ppbv) are isoprene (10–600), acetone (1–2000), ethanol (10–1000), methanol (150–200 ppbv). All are products of the standard metabolic processes.[9]

The high moisture of exhaled breath samples is a major problem for most analytical methods, except for SIFT-MS (see the article by Smith and Španěl[25] on page 3 of this book). It can seriously compromise GC-MS analyses and so the water vapour should be removed using a cryo-trap for GC-MS to be used effectively. Because these laboratory instruments are usually large and expensive and require an analysis time of nearly one to two hours, depending on the sample preparation steps necessary, there is a need for instruments that can perform on-line, real time breath analysis.

If the number of sample handling steps could be minimised and no additional carrier gases of high purity are required (like nitrogen or helium, as used in GC-MS), then on-line methods for effective breath analysis procedures become attractive for point-of-care applications. Then breath testing could be carried out in hospitals by regular hospital personnel. SIFT-MS is used in hospitals, but currently it is a relatively large instrument.

In recent years, ion mobility spectrometers, IMS, have been developed as comparatively small and effective devices to determine trace quantities of VOCs down to the low ppbv range, especially in air.[26] The major advantages of IMS devices are that no vacuum systems are required for their operation and ambient air can be used as a carrier gas. Worldwide, more than 70,000 units are in service, especially to detect chemical warfare agents, narcotics and explosives. The IMS instruments available on the market are also handheld.[27,28] Environmental pollutants like benzene, toluene and xylene (collectively known as BTX) or methyl-*tert*-butyl ether (MTBE) can be analyzed using different IMS at concentrations down to the ng/L level in air.[29–32]

2. Material and Methods: Ion Mobility Spectrometry

For the measurements described below, a custom designed IMS equipped with a ^{63}Ni β-ionization source was used.[29,32] The operating principle of the IMS and the operational details are summarized in Ref. 28. Therefore, only a brief description will be given here. The term ion mobility spectrometry refers to the method of characterising analytes in gases by their gas phase ion mobilities. The drift times of ion swarms formed using suitable ionisation sources and electrical shutters are normally measured. The product ions formed in defined chemical reactions of neutral analyte molecules with reactant ions are characteristic of the analyte molecules, so the mobility of these product ions may be used to identify the analyte molecules. The drift velocity v of the ions is related to the electric field strength E by the mobility k: one has $v = kE$. Therefore, the mobility is inversely proportional to the drift time, which is usually measured at a fixed drift length. Theoretical considerations show that the mobility is related to the collision rate of the ions with the gas molecules in which they are drifting (the reduced mass), the temperature, the dimensions of the ion (structural dependencies) and the collision integral. The collision integral, and therefore the mobility, is influenced by the size of the ions and molecules, their structures and polarisabilities. Therefore, a dependence of ion mobility on mass and structure is commonly observed. Thus, it is clear that isomeric forms of ions should be distinguishable.

Ion mobility spectrometry was originally developed for the detection of trace compounds in a gas, for example gaseous pollutants in air for military applications. It combines both high sensitivity and relatively low technical expenditure with a high speed data acquisition. The time to acquire a single spectrum is in the range of 10 ms to 50 ms. Thus, an IMS is an instrument suitable for process control, but due to the occurrence of ion-molecule reactions and relatively poor mass resolution of the ionic species formed, it is generally not good for identification of unknown compounds. The working principle is based on the drift of ions in a buffer gas at ambient pressure under the influence of a weak applied electric field. Unlike conventional low pressure mass spectrometry, the mean free path of the ions in the buffer gas is smaller than the dimensions of the instrument. Therefore, the different ion species that comprises an ion swarm drifting under such conditions separate in space according to their drift velocities, which are related to their different masses and geometrical structures. Collection of these ions by a Faraday cup results in a time-dependent signal corresponding to the mobility of the separated ions. Such an ion mobility spectrum contains information on the nature of the different trace compounds present in the sample gas from which the ions were formed. For the generation of ion swarms some additional components are required, including an ionisation source (normally ^{63}Ni β-radiation sources, UV-lamps or discharges), an ion shutter grid and a high voltage supply that delivers voltages between some 100 to 10,000 Volts to establish the electric field in the drift tube. The ions formed in the ionisation/reaction region (see below) drift under the influence of the static electric field of strength between 100 and about 1,000 V/cm counter to the buffer/carrier gas flow direction. The shutter control circuit drives the ion gate. The shutter opening time is normally fixed between some 10 μs and about 1 ms. Generally speaking, digital signal processing provides a better readability of the spectra obtained. Under ideal circumstances the final spectrum consists of clearly separated peaks. The amplification realised with different types of preamplifiers is between of 1 V/nA and 100 V/nA. The current measured lies in the range of some nano-ampères, sometimes as low as pico-ampères, and is converted into a signal voltage converted by commercial AD-cards into digital signals for further processing. It is necessary to shield the IMS against external electromagnetic disturbances. The gas flow rates must be controlled (normally in the range of some mL/min) as well as the temperature in the ionisation and drift regions.

The most important sections of the instrument are the ionisation and reaction regions and the drift region. The external homogenous electric field is established in the drift tube using several drift rings for uniformity. The carrier gas retains sample molecules within the ionisation region. There, direct ionisation can occur using UV-lamps or by chemical ionisation by collisions of the analyte with ionised carrier gas molecules formed by radioactive ionisation sources, and fragmentation in the case of discharges. The so-called drift gas flows from the Faraday plate/cup towards the ionisation region. Normally, if the shutter is closed, no ions can reach the drift region. The drift gas will protect the drift region and no neutral analyte molecules should enter the drift region. If the shutter is held closed all analyte molecules, neutrals and ions will pass through the gas outlet. During the shutter open time, some ions will enter the drift region. During several collisions with the surrounding gas molecules a steady drift velocity will be reached. If no chemical reactions occur, total spatial separation of the various ionic species will be reached at the Faraday-plate. Because of the influence of moving particles influencing the current to the metal plate, the Faraday cup is shielded by using a so-called aperture grid. Thus, only ions moving through the aperture grid are collected and directly converted into a current and later, using a preamplifier, into a voltage. The time-dependent voltage or current plotted against the time interval referenced to the shutter opening pulse, is called the ion mobility spectrum. The kind of product ions produced will differ depending on the method of ionisation. Frequently used are radioactive sources (alpha- and beta-radiation), UV-lamps with different photon energies between 8.6 eV and 11.7 eV, lasers, different kinds of discharges (including corona or so-called partial discharges) and electrospray (for further details see Ref. 28). Using nitrogen or air as the carrier gas, the carrier gas molecules are normally ionised directly by the β-particles. Positive carrier gas ions and free electrons will also be formed. These primary positive ions (called reaction or reactant ions) will undergo different chemical reactions with the analyte molecules to form so-called product ions by: proton transfer, nucleophilic attachment, hydride abstraction and other processes. The electrons may attach to sample molecules to form negative ions (electrophilic attachment, resonant attachment, dissociative attachment). Also, charge transfer and proton abstraction may occur. Often both positive and negative ions are formed. The formation of reactant ions depends on the activity of the ionisation source. However, the number of reactant ions produced is largely independent of the design of the reaction region.

All parts of the IMS that are in contact with the analytes are made from inert materials. Teflon was used for the ionization chamber and the drift tube. The shutter grid was built from parallel nickel wires and is closed by an electric field. All conducting surfaces and drift rings were constructed from brass. The rings are outside the drift tube and therefore are not in contact to the analytes. The drift tube was designed by Baumbach *et al.*[33] by modelling the homogeneity of the electric field. The electric field in the drift tube is established by using a high-voltage supply with a voltage divider connected to the drift rings placed at equal distance. The parameters of the IMS are summarised in Table 1.

Table 1.   Main parameters of the ^{63}Ni-IMS

Ionization source	^{63}Ni β-radiation source, 510 MBq
Length of the drift region	12 cm
Electric field strength	326 V/cm
Drift Volthage	4 kV
Shutter opening time	300 μs
Drift and sample gas	Synthetic air
Drift gas flow	100 mL/min
Sample gas flow	150 mL/min (optimised for breath analysis)
Temperature	25 °C (ambient)
Pressure	101 kPa (ambient)

To realize effective pre-separation of a rather complex exhaled air mixture, a 17 cm long polar multi-capillary chromatographic column (MCC, OV-5, Sibertech, LTD, Novosibirsk, Russia) was used made by combining approximately 1000 capillaries each with an inner diameter of 40 μm and a film thickness of 0.2 μm. This was coupled to the ^{63}Ni source IMS. The total column diameter of 3 mm allows operation with a carrier gas flow up to 150 mL/min, which is the optimum flow rate for the IMS. The heating of the column is essential to obtain reproducible results. To achieve rather comparable retention times, the MCC was held at 30 °C during the breath analysis procedure. To realize isothermal separation, a simple heating construction is needed, but it is only necessary to hold the temperature constant.

In the breath sampling process, the subject blows through a mouthpiece coupled to a brass adapter (designed by ISAS) via a Teflon tube ($\frac{1}{4}''$, Bohlender GmbH, Lauda, Germany), which is connected to a 10 mL stainless steel sample loop of an electric six-port valve (Nalco, Macherey-Nagel, Düren, Germany). By switching the six-port valve, breath is trans-

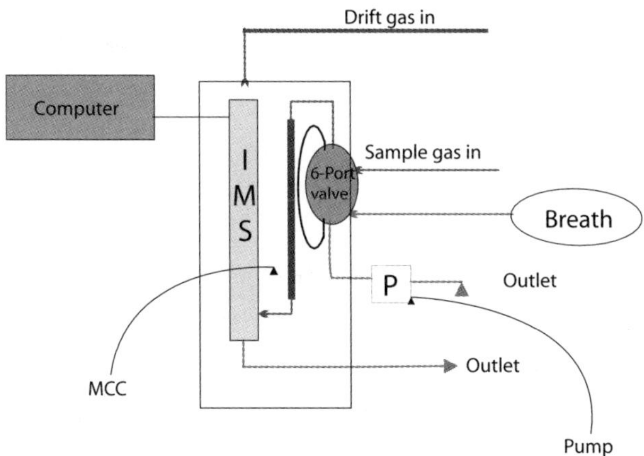

Fig. 1. Diagram of the breath sampling and analysis systems using MCC-Ni-IMS

ported by the carrier gas from the sample loop into the MCC. The separated compounds can be directly analysed by IMS. Therefore, the results can be achieved within 600 s depending on the separation time of the compounds. This construction enables a direct and rapid sampling at a known breath volume. The schematic drawing of the sampling and detection systems for breath analysis using MCC-^{63}Ni-IMS is shown in Fig. 1.

The loss of any molecules of the analyte on all parts of the analytical system must be avoided, especially when considering the detection of traces of analytes. The effective separation of water vapour is one major advantage of the MCC. Using other techniques like humidity sorbents or membrane separation units, some of the original analytes may be lost.

3. Results and Discussion

Two typical spectra obtained for a sample of acetone in air at concentrations of 100 and 500 ng/L are shown in Fig. 2. The two ion peaks observed arise from air (RIP· reactant ion peak) at 17.69 ms and the analyte acetone at 19.59 ms. The ionisation of acetone is realised by charge transfer between the air ions and the acetone molecule. Thus, it is clear that with higher concentration of the analyte in air, the RIP will decrease and the acetone-related peak will increase. In general, the peak position is relevant to identification and the peak area is related to the concentration of the analyte. Peak areas are often calculated using Gaussian-Curve-Analysis procedures. Furthermore, it is shown that concentrations much greater

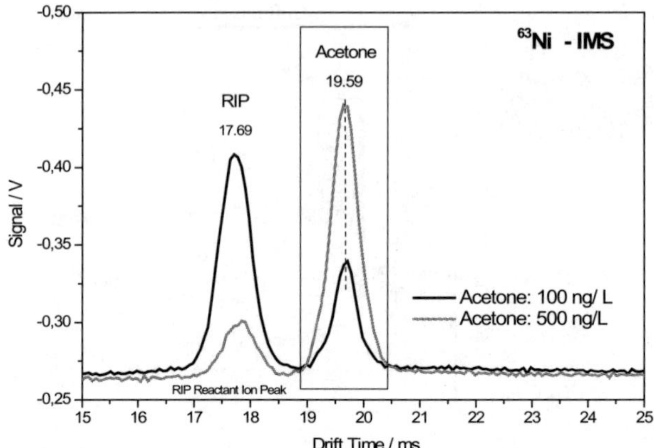

Fig. 2.   Ion mobility spectra of acetone in air (at concentrations of 100 and 500 ng/L)

than 500 ng/L of the analyte (acetone) in air will not be effectively ionised, because not enough reactant ions are available. Therefore, it should be noted that IMS is most suitable for *trace* gas analysis.

The combination of a chromatographic column with the IMS enables multidimensional data analysis and allows peak identification from both retention times and by using specific ion mobility data (arrival time at the Faraday plate) of the ions formed from the analytes. Therefore, retention times of the compounds separated by the MCC and drift times of the analytes are shown in so-called IMS-chromatograms. The MCC reduces the number of interactions in the ionisation region of the IMS, thus reducing cluster ion formation and avoids concurrent charge transfer due to the time-delayed entrance of the analytes. Hence, the effective ionisation of nearly all analytes in a given sample is achieved by proper selection of the GC and effective temperature programming of the chromatographic column.

Figure 3 shows the results of investigations of human exhaled breath. Ammonia, acetone and ethanol peaks and also the reactant ion peak (RIP) are seen as major signals. Smaller peaks will not be considered here. In addition, the K_0 values (see Ref. 28) are included in the inlet, showing a single spectrum at a fixed retention time. It is also clear in Fig. 3 that the water vapour, which is at really high values in exhaled air, is separated effectively using the MCC. Only during the first 20 s do large amounts of water vapour enter the ionisation region of the IMS. For other molecules, which have low proton affinities or result in unstable ions, the sensitivity of IMS can be seriously affected by water. In general, the MCC will reduce

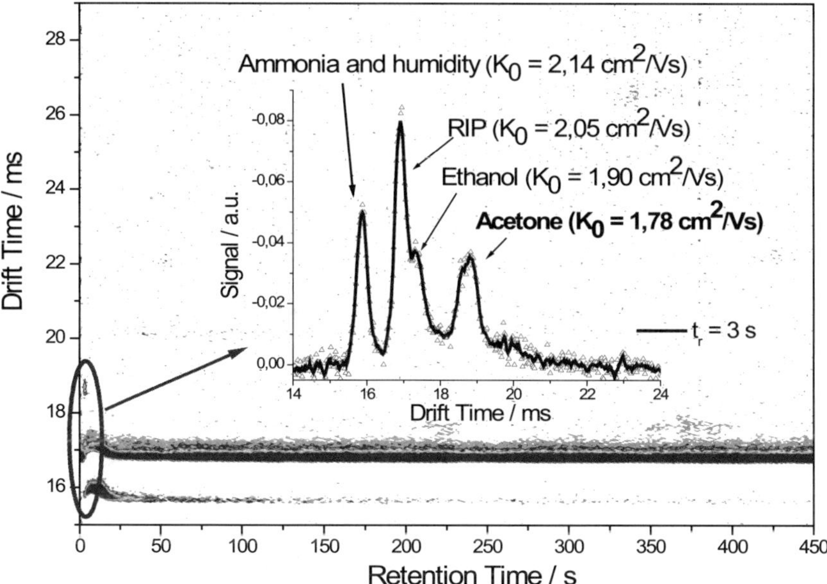

Fig. 3. IMS-chromatogram of human exhaled breath. *Inlet:* single spectrum at a fixed retention time of 3 s showing signals of the major constitutions, ammonia, ethanol and acetone

the influence of humidity. On the other hand, the main influence will be at higher drift times than about 17 ms at all retention times.

In cooperation with the lung hospital in Hemer, on-site measurements were carried out on the breath of 40 subjects, including 22 patients suffering from various pulmonary infections. Also, breath samples from 18 healthy persons were analysed on-line using the MCC-^{63}Ni-IMS. The full analysis was always carried out in the same room, where room air was analysed before each of the breath measurements. To reduce the risk of cross contaminations due to other physiological processes, the subjects had not ingested solids or liquids and not smoked for at least two hours before the breath measurements.

IMS-chromatograms for samples of the exhaled breath of a healthy person and a patient suffering from bacterial lung infection are shown in Figs. 4 and 5, respectively. The ambient air values have been subtracted from both sets of data. The colours refer to different peak heights like a peak-height diagram. The identified peaks are labelled with the corresponding mobility values, K_0, calculated from the drift time of the ions derived from

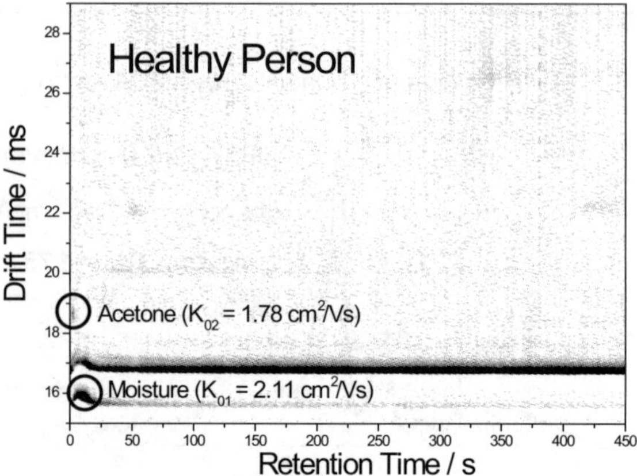

Fig. 4. IMS-chromatogram for a breath sample from a healthy person

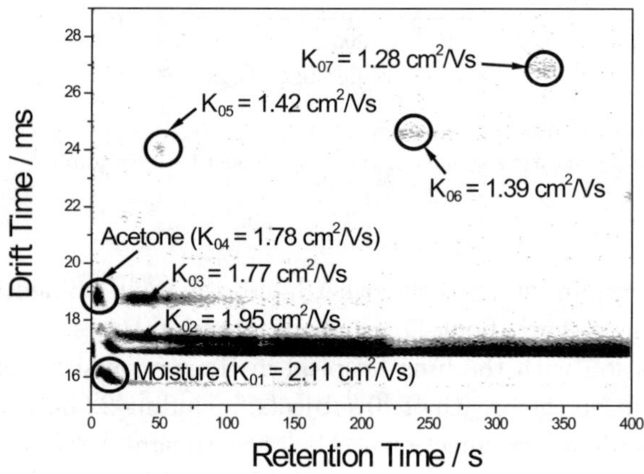

Fig. 5. IMS-chromatogram for a breath sample from a patient with lung infection

the analytes, taking into account the values of the electric field strength in the drift tube and the carrier gas pressure and temperature during the experiment (for further details see Ref. 28).

As mentioned above, the formation of so-called reactant ions (arising from the carrier gas air) and product ions (formed by the analytes) in IMS can be altered by the presence of water vapour. Therefore, the separation of water molecules is very important when analysing breath samples. Figs. 4 and 5 show that the water vapour in breath samples (mobility values $K_{01} = 2.11$ cm^2/Vs) could be effectively separated using the MCC.

The signals correlated to water vapour always appear at the beginning of the IMS-chromatogram. Thus, water vapour has no disturbing effect for peaks appearing at longer retention times. In the topographic plot of the exhaled breath of the healthy person, acetone (see Fig. 4) was identified based on its reduced mobility value ($K_{04} = 1.78$ cm^2/Vs). Acetone has a retention time similar to water, but the proton affinity of the acetone molecule is greater than that of the water molecule. So, proton transfer from protonated water molecules (reactant ions) to acetone molecules can produce protonated acetone molecules (product ions).

The two IMS-chromatograms in Figs. 4 and 5 are conspicuously different. In Fig. 5 the 2D-plot exhibits additional peaks occurring at retention times of 28 s ($K_{02} = 1.95$ cm^2/Vs) and 36 s ($K_{03} = 1.77$ cm^2/Vs). Both are probably due to the presence in the breath of degradation products of antibiotics or other drugs, because they were also found in the breath of several persons who had taken similar antibiotics. The peak at 50 s and $K_{05} = 1.42$ cm^2/Vs was also seen in the exhaled breath of patients suffering from *Pneumonia*. Two other larger analytes with lower mobilities ($K_{06} = 1.39$ cm^2/Vs and $K_{07} = 1.28$ cm^2/Vs) and longer retention times ($t_{\mathrm{ret6}} = 244$ s, $t_{\mathrm{ret7}} = 330$ s) were often detected in the breath of patients with bacterial infection and airway inflammation.

To identify the characteristic peaks, further measurements will be needed, and larger cohorts of patients and healthy persons will need to be investigated. Data will be processed using statistical methods to clearly correlate the characteristic pattern of the IMS-topographic plots with specific diseases. In the near future, different mass spectrometric methods (QMS, LTQ-FT and TOF) will be used to identify some of the metabolites detected by ion mobility spectrometry.

4. Conclusions

By coupling an ion mobility spectrometer and a multi-capillary column for pre-separation, investigations have been carried out to directly detect volatile metabolites in human exhaled breath. The total analysis was accomplished within time intervals of less than 500 s. The system constructed has sufficient sensitivity to detect the metabolites directly and provides characteristic IMS-Chromatograms (peak-height diagrams). The breath is introduced directly onto the MCC using a sample loop. The results of investigations on the breath of patients suffering from *Pneumonia* show the presence of different metabolites compared to the breath of healthy persons.

Further investigations using mass spectrometric methods should identify some of the metabolites found by ion mobility spectrometry. The opportunity for on-site and short-time analyses using air as the carrier gas at ambient pressure is the most important benefit of this MCC-IMS technique. To use MCC-IMS directly in the clinical setting allows results to be obtained within minutes, provides additional information to influence therapeutic strategy and facilitates the building of databases for several illnesses. The general aim of these studies is to include breath analysis as a method for early recognition of selected diseases on the basis of ion mobility spectrometry data.

Acknowledgements

The financial support of the Bundesministerium für Bildung und Forschung and the Ministerium für Wissenschaft und Forschung des Landes Nordrhein-Westfalen and the funding of the common project by G.A.S. Gesellschaft für Analytische Sensorensysteme mbH are gratefully acknowledged. The opportunity to work in the Lung Hospital in Hemer and the help of the assistants and doctors should be mentioned with thanks. The authors wish to express their special thanks to Mrs. Oberdrifter for laboratory support and Dr. Litterst and Dr. Westhoff for helpful discussions and for organising the clinical measurements (all in the Lung Cancer Hospital Hemer) and Mrs. S. Güssgen and L. Seifert (both ISAS Dortmund) for the support in operation of the ion mobility spectrometer and preparation of the data handling.

References

1. Phillips M. Method for the collection and assay of volatile organic compounds in breath. *Anal Biochem* 1997; **247**: 272–278.
2. Phillips M, Gleeson K, Hughes JM, Greenberg J, Cataneo RN, Baker L, McVay WP. Volatile organic compounds in breath as markers of lung cancer: a cross-sectional study. *Lancet* 1999; **353**: 1930–1933.
3. Phillips M, Greenberg J. Ion-trap detection of volatile organic compounds in alveolar breath. *Clin Chem* 1992; **38**: 60–65.
4. Rooth G, Ostenson S. Acetone in alveolar air, and the control of diabetes. *Lancet* 1966; **2**: 1102–1105.
5. Benolt FM, Davidson WR, Lovett AM, Nacson S, Ngo A. Breath analysis by atmospheric pressure ionization mass spectrometry. *Anal Chem* 1983; **55**: 805–807.

6. Bischoff R, Moenke-Wedler T, Bischoff G. On-line detection of volatile compounds in human breath., In: *4th European Congress of Oto-Rhino-Laryngology, Head and Neck Surgery*, 2000.

7. Cheng WH, Lee WJ. Technology development in breath microanalysis for clinical diagnosis. *J Lab Clin Med* 1999; **133**: 218–228.

8. Ehrmann S, Juengst J, Goschnick J, Everhard D. application of a gas sensor microarray to human breath analysis. *Sens & Actuators B* 1999; **3075**: 1–3.

9. Fenske JD, Paulson SE. Human breath emissions of VOCs. *J Air Waste Manag Assoc* 1999; **49**: 594–598.

10. Grote C, Pawliszyn J. Solid-phase microextraction for the analysis of human breath. *Anal Chem* 1997; **69**: 587–596.

11. Hansel A, Jordan A, Holzinger R, Prazeller P, Vogel W, Lindinger W. Proton transfer reaction mass spectrometry: on-line trace gas analysis at the ppb level. *Int J Mass Spectrom Ion Processes* 1995; **149/150**: 609–619.

12. Jansson BO, Larsson BT. Analysis of organic compounds in human breath by gas chromatography-mass spectrometry. *J Lab Clin Med* 1969; **74**: 961–966.

13. Jones AW, Lagesson V, Tagesson C. Origins of breath isoprene. *J Clin Pathol* 1995; **48**: 979–980.

14. Karl T, Prazeller P, Mayr D, Jordan A, Rieder J, Fall R, Lindinger W. Human breath isoprene and its relation to blood cholesterol levels: new measurements and modeling. *J Appl Physiol* 2001; **91**: 762–770.

15. Lindinger W, Hansel A, Jordan A. On-line monitoring of volatile organic compounds at pptv levels by means of proton-transfer-reaction mass spectrometry (PTR-MS) medical applications, food control and environmental research. *Int J Mass Spectrom Ion Processes* 1998; **173**: 191–241.

16. Manolis A. The diagnostic potential of breath analysis. *Clin Chem* 1983; **29**. 5–15.

17. Mendis S, Sobotka PA, Euler DE. Pentane and isoprene in expired air from humans: gas-chromatographic analysis of single breath. *Clin Chem* 1994; **40**: 1485–1488.

18. Phillips M, Erickson GA, Sabas M, Smith JP, Greenberg J. Volatile organic compounds in the breath of patients with schizophrenia. *J Clin Pathol* 1995; **48**: 466–469.

19. Ruzsanyi V, Sielemann S, Baumbach J. Determination of VOCs in human breath using IMS. *Int J Ion Mobility Spectrometry* 2002; **5**: 45–48.

20. Stein VB, Narang RS, Wilson L, Aldous KM. A simple, reliable method for the determination of chlorinated volatile organics in human breath and air using glass sampling tubes. *J Anal Toxicol* 1996; **20**: 145–150.

21. Pleil JD Lindstrom AB. Exhaled human breath measurement method for assessing exposure to halogenated volatile organic compounds. *Clin Chem* 1997; **43**: 723–730.

22. Gordon SM, Szidon JP, Krotoszynski BK, Gibbons RD, O'Neill HJ. Volatile organic compounds in exhaled air from patients with lung cancer. *Clin Chem* 1985, **31**. 1278–1282.

23. Pleil JD Lindstrom AB. Collection of a single alveolar exhaled breath for volatile organic compounds analysis. *Am J Ind Med* 1995; **28**: 109–121.

24. Wilson HK. Breath analysis. Physiological basis and sampling techniques. *Scand J Work Environ Health* 1986; **12**: 174–192.

25. Smith D, Španěl P. Selected ion flow tube mass spectrometry, SIFT-MS, for on-line trace gas analysis of breath., In: Amann A, Smith D, eds. *Breath Analysis for Clinical Diagnosis and Therapeutic Monitoring,* Singapore: World Scientific, 2005.

26. Li F, Xie Z, Schmidt H, Sielemann S, Baumbach J. Ion mobility spectrometer for online monitoring of trace compounds. *Spectrochim Acta Part B* 2002; **57**: 1563–1574.

27. Spangler G, Carrico J, Campbell D. Recent advances in ion mobility spectrometry for explosives vapor detection. *J Test Eval* 1985; **13**: 234–240.

28. Baumbach J, Eiceman G. Ion mobility spectrometry: arriving on site and moving beyond a low profile. *Appl Spectrosc* 1999; **53**: 338–354.

29. Sielemann S. *Detektion flüchtiger organischer Verbindungen mittels Ionen-mobilitätsspektrometrie und deren Kopplung mit Multi-Kapillar-Gas-Chromatographie.* Dortmund: University of Dortmund, 1999.

30. Sielemann S, Baumbach J, Pilzecker P, Walendzik G. Detection of *trans*-1,2-dichloroethene, trichloroethene and tetrachloroethene using multi-capillary columns coupled to ion mobility spectrometers with UV-ionisation sources. *Int J Ion Mobility Spectrom* 1999; **2**: 15–21.

31. Sielemann S, Xie Z, Schmidt H, Baumbach J. Determination of MTBE next to benzene, toluene and xylene within 90 s using GC/IMS with multi-capillary column. *Int J Ion Mobility Spectrom* 2001; **4**: 69–73.

32. Xie Z, Ruzsanyi V, Sielemann S, Schmidt H, Baumbach J. Determination of pentane, isoprene and acetone using HSCC-UV-IMS. *Int J Ion Mobility Spectrom* 2001; **4**: 88–91.

33. Soppart O, Baumbach J. Comparison of electric fields within drift tubes for ion mobility spectrometry. *Meas Sci Tech* 2000; **11**: 1473–1479.

LASER SPECTROSCOPIC ON-LINE MONITORING OF EXHALED TRACE GASES

G. VON BASUM, D. HALMER, P. HERING, AND M. MÜRTZ

University of Düsseldorf,
Institute for Laser Medicine,
D-40225 Düsseldorf, Germany

1. Introduction

The analysis of hydrocarbons, such as ethane, in exhaled human breath is generally performed via gas chromatography (GC). Due to the insufficient sensitivity of the GC technique, the breath sample must usually undergo a trap-and-purge process before analysis. This is time-consuming and does not enable the time-resolved analysis of single exhalations.[1] Here, we report on our advances in extremely sensitive and specific on-line analysis of exhaled trace gases by means of infrared laser absorption spectroscopy. This optical method has great advantages for sensitive and specific trace gas analysis, since most relevant trace compounds exhibit a characteristic fingerprint spectrum in the mid-infrared. Our measurements are mainly carried out by infrared cavity leak-out spectroscopy (CALOS), which has proved to be a unique and universal tool for rapid and precise medical breath testing.[2] CALOS is an ultra-sensitive laser absorption spectroscopy method which allows rapid analysis of various volatile organic compounds, VOC's, as well as NO, CO, OCS, etc., at the parts-per-trillion, ppt, level.[3] In particular, we have investigated this technique for the quantitative on-line detection of ethane, which is considered to be the most important volatile marker of free-radical induced lipid peroxidation and cell damage in the human body.[4]

2. Experimental

A schematic of the gas set-up for on-line breath analysis is shown in Fig. 1. The breath sampling was performed by means of a modified mouthpiece,

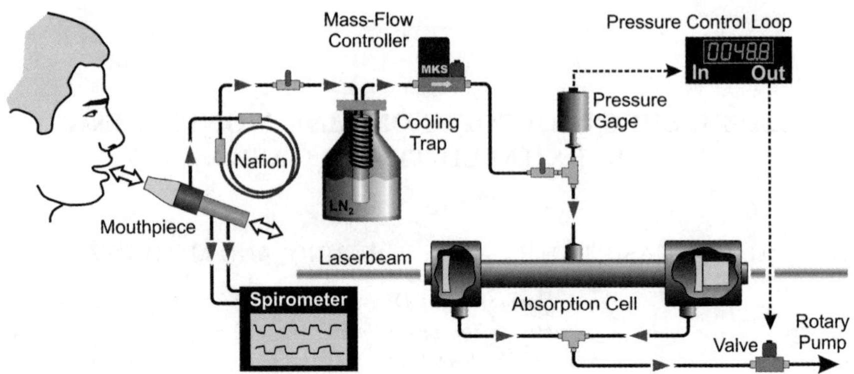

Fig. 1.   Schematic of the gas set-up

which is used to supply the breath sample to the analyzer. Two gas supply lines at the mouthpiece are used to continuously extract portions of the breath into the CALOS analyzer and into a capnograph. The gas flow through the CALOS analyzer is maintained by a rotary pump behind the absorption cell. The breath flow is determined by measuring the pressure difference before and behind a resistance inside the mouthpiece. For monitoring the CO_2 and O_2 concentrations, one portion of the exhaled breath (sample flow rate 200 mL/min) is fed to the capnograph; a second portion of the exhalation flow (1000 mL/min) is directed into the CALOS absorption cell. To avoid contamination with out-gassing materials, all parts that are in contact with the gas flow are made of stainless steel, copper or Teflon. The gas sample is dehumidified by means of a Nafion tube (PermaPure, length: 2 m) and fed through a cooling trap at a temperature of about 160 K to eliminate all interfering molecules (*e.g.* isoprene, pentane). The amount of gas directed into the absorption cell is controlled by means of a mass flow controller. The pressure inside the cell was kept constant at 48.8 mbar independent of the flow rate. This was achieved by means of a control loop consisting of a pressure gage and an electronic valve.

The detection method is based on absorption spectroscopy. For the analysis of traces of ethane and carbon monoxide, the "fingerprint" spectra in the wavelength region near 3.3 μm (for ethane detection) and near 4.8 μm (for CO detection) respectively were used. The trace gas concentrations are determined from the light absorption observed at characteristic wavelengths. The CALOS analyzer consists of a tunable continuous-wave CO sideband laser and an absorption cell containing the gas sample of interest. The absorption cell is a high-finesse ring-down cavity (length: 53 cm), excited by the laser radiation. Figure 2 shows a schematic diagram of the present set-up. The CO laser is line-tunable and operates in the wavelength regions between 2.8 and 4.0 μm, as well as between 4.8 and 8.3 μm. By mixing the laser light with microwave radiation in an electro-optic modulator (EOM), tuneable laser sidebands are generated covering a spectral range of 8 to 18 GHz above and below each laser line with a power of 50 to 150 μW.[5] The sideband radiation excites the fundamental transverse mode of the ring-down cavity. The cavity mirrors have a reflectivity up to 99.996 %, which provides an effective optical absorption path length up to 10 km. Frequency stabilization of the cavity resonance to the laser frequency is accomplished by means of a standard $1f$-lock-in technique. In this way, the laser power is periodically injected into the ring-down cell, twice per modulation period. Each time the transmitted light indicates optimum coincidence of laser frequency and cavity mode, a trigger pulse is provided to turn off the laser sideband radiation via the EOM. The subsequent leak-out of the light is monitored with an InSb photodetector and acquired by means of an analog-to-digital converter. The decay time of the leak-out signal is determined by fitting the data to a single exponential decay. By measuring the decay time of the empty cell, τ_0, and the decay time of the cell filled with the breath sample, τ, the absorption coefficient,

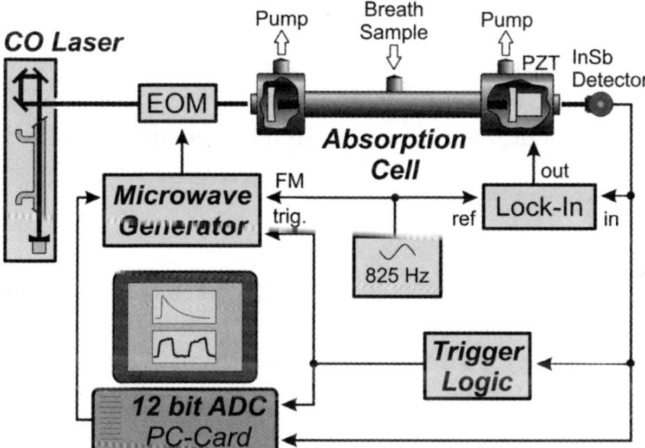

Fig. 2. Schematic of the CALOS analyzer. The CO laser may be replaced by a difference frequency laser or an optical parametric oscillator (OPO). EOM: electro-optic modulator, PZT: piezo-ceramic transducer, ADC: analog-to-digital converter, FM: frequency modulation

and therefore the trace gas concentration, can be directly determined via

$$\alpha(\lambda) = \frac{1}{c}\left(\frac{1}{\tau(\lambda)} - \frac{1}{\tau_0}\right), \tag{1}$$

α is the absorption coefficient, λ the wavelength, and c the speed of light. Calibration is not required if line strength and line broadening data of the absorption line are available.

For the on-line analysis of human breath, a sub-second time resolution is required. Therefore, fast data acquisition and processing are very important if accurate analysis is to be achieved. The recorded exponential decay signals are passed to a state-of-the-art personal computer by means of a 12-bit analog-to-digital converter card with a sample rate of 25 MHz. The modulation of the laser frequency at 825 Hz leads to a signal generation rate of 1.65 kHz. This requires a fast exponential fitting routine that processes a single exponential signal with a sample length of 1536 points within 500 μs. As the internal Levenberg–Marquardt fitting routine from the used programming language (LabView 5.0, National Instruments) needs 100 ms for this task, a new fitting routine based on the method of successive integration (SI) was developed in the group. This fitting routine only needs 150 μs for the same data set. Therefore, it is possible to obtain the decay time from each recorded exponential decay signal. Further details on the new fitting routine have been published in.[6] The measured concentration data is then smoothed by calculating the running average over N data points. N is chosen such that the time resolution is dominated by the gas exchange time and not worsened by the averaging routine. Typical values for N are on the order of 500. The experimental response time (T_{90}) of the analyzer obtained by an instantaneous increase of concentration is less than 800 ms.

3. Results

A representative example of an online recording of exhaled ethane is shown in Fig. 3. The uppermost curve displays the course of the breath ethane concentration detected with the CALOS analyzer. The curves below show the concentration of breath CO_2, O_2, and flow analyzed with the capnograph. For this measurement, a volunteer inhaled synthetic air containing 1 part-per-million, ppm, ethane for a duration of 5 min to enrich the body with ethane (wash-in). During the subsequent wash-out period the subjects inhaled ambient air, which contained 3 to 6 parts-per-billion, ppb, of ethane. The ambient air concentration of ethane (typically 2–5 ppb) was constant during each experiment and was subtracted from the measured exhaled breath fraction.

One goal of this work was to measure the profile of a single exhalation (expirogram). In this case, the recorded concentrations were plotted against the exhaled volume, which was calculated by integrating the expiratory flow (Fig. 4). For further analysis, each expirogram was divided into three parts, the first part in which the concentration is zero (phase I), the second part where the concentration rises rapidly (phase II) and the third part where the

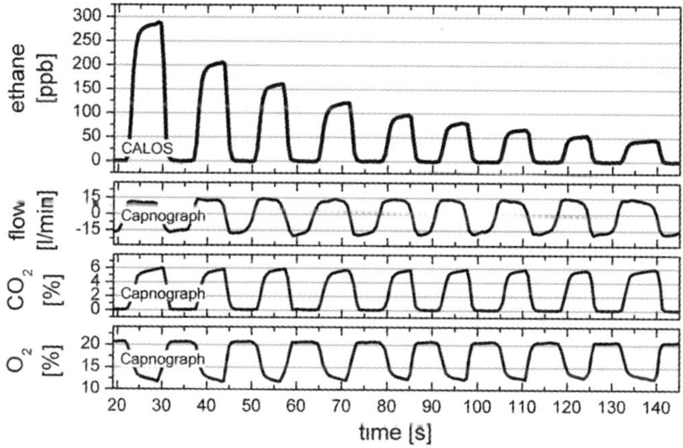

Fig. 3. Representative example of an online recording of ethane, CO_2, and O_2. The subjects performed predefined breathing maneuvers.

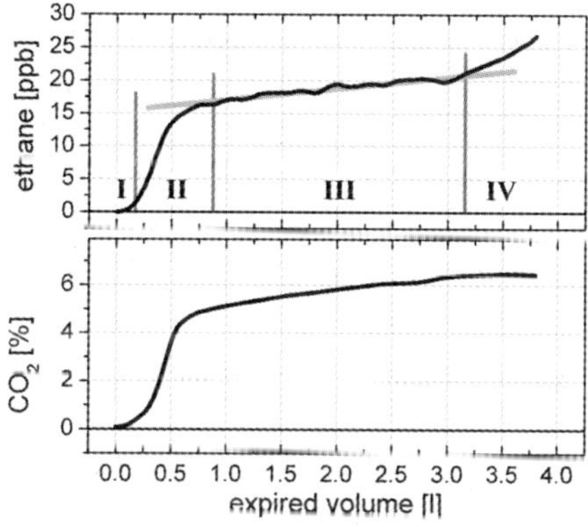

Fig. 4. Recorded single exhalation expirograms for ethane and CO_2. *Above:* expirogram for ethane at a scale of 30 ppb. *Below:* corresponding expirogram for CO_2.

concentration increases linearly (phase III). The observed maximum concentration in the ethane expirograms covered a dynamic range from 800 ppb for the first breathing cycles to 1 ppb for the last recorded expirograms. When the subjects exhaled beyond their functional residual volume, it was noticed that for all subjects an additional increase in ethane concentration (phase IV) occurred within the first 20 breathing cycles. Importantly, this additional increase in concentration was not observed in either the CO_2 or the O_2 curve. The slope of the phase III was determined by means of linear regression and normalized to the mean concentration within the third part. This value is known as the normalized alveolar slope, S_n.

Another aspect focused on was the variation of the breath concentration over a time period of 30 min. So the mean concentration during phase III of each single exhalation was plotted versus time. This resulted in a multi-exponential decay curve representing the wash-out process. These results are described in more detail in Ref. 2.

Recently, the spectrometer has been used to investigate a number of other exhaled trace gases, *e.g.*, carbon monoxide and carbonyl sulfide. Exhaled carbon monoxide (eCO) may be a marker for pulmonary diseases[7] and is commonly detected via non-dispersive infrared spectroscopy. Such analysers are commercially available from various manufacturers. These devices lack sufficient time resolution to allow breath-resolved eCO measurements. However, such measurements with high time-resolution could give additional information about the origin and the exhalation dynamics of carbon monoxide. For this reason, some effort was made to analyze eCO with the laser spectroscopic technique. This molecule exhibits strong absorption lines in the 5 μm spectral region. However, it is essential to choose a spectral window which is not overlapped too much by absorption lines from carbon dioxide and water. A preliminary on-line recording of exhaled carbon monoxide is shown in Fig. 5. The detection limit of CO in a synthetic gas mixture is 90 ppt (1 s averaging time) and 500 ppt in exhaled breath, far below the average exhaled CO concentration of 1 to 10 ppm. It is worth noting that the alveolar plateau exhibits a negative slope. To our knowledge, this has not been previously observed. This variation in the concentration is currently not well-understood and will be the subject of future studies.

Another trace gas of biomedical interest is carbonyl sulfide (OCS),[8,9] which also has some strong absorption features in the 5 μm spectral region. Our current detection limit for OCS is 3 ppt (1 s averaging time) in a synthetic gas mixture. Due to possible interference with water and carbon

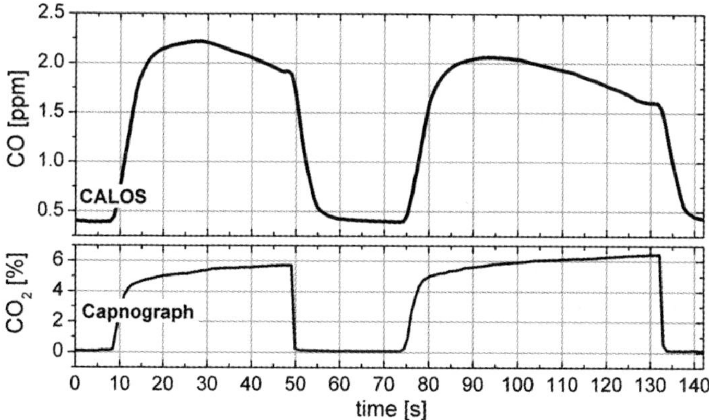

Fig. 5.   Example of an on-line recording of carbon monoxide and CO_2. This is a preliminary result.

dioxide, the detection limit for OCS in breath samples is slightly worse The OCS analysis of exhaled breath is still under investigation in our laboratory.

4. Conclusions

A novel method for the rapid and ultra-sensitive analysis of trace gases in exhaled human breath has been described. The CALOS method enables online quantification of ethane and carbon monoxide at sub-ppb concentrations, with a time resolution better than 800 ms. This unique system is capable of recording ethane expirograms of single exhalations and has proved to be well suited for the precise investigation of the sloping alveolar plateau. As ethane is a volatile marker for lipid peroxidation, this analyzer provides a promising non-invasive tool for on-line monitoring of oxidative stress status. For example, the analyzer could be connected to a mechanical ventilator for continuous monitoring. Since the method is based on infrared spectroscopy, it may be used with slight modifications for many other constituents of exhaled breath that are present in trace concentrations.

Acknowledgement

This work is financially supported by the Deutsche Forschungsgemeinschaft.

References

1. Risby T. Breath markers in normal and diseased humans. In: Marczin N, Yacoub M, eds. *Disease Markers in Exhaled Breath: Basic Mechanisms and Clinical Applications*, Amsterdam: Washington, DC: IOS Press, 2002: 113–122.
2. von Basum G, Dahnke H, Halmer D, Hering P, Mürtz M. Online recording of ethane traces in human breath via infrared laser spectroscopy. *J Appl Physiol* 2003; **95**: 2583–2590.
3. von Basum G, Halmer D, Hering P, Mürtz M, Schiller S, Muller F, Popp A, Kuhnemann F. Parts per trillion sensitivity for ethane in air with an optical parametric oscillator cavity leak-out spectrometer. *Opt Lett* 2004; **29**: 797–799.
4. Andreoni KA, Kazui M, Cameron DE, Nyhan D, Sehnert SS, Rohde CA, Bulkley GB, Risby TH. Ethane: a marker of lipid peroxidation during cardiopulmonary bypass in humans. *Free Radic Biol Med* 1999; **26**: 439–445.
5. Mürtz M, Frech B, Palm P, Lotze R, Urban W. Tunable carbon monoxide overtone laser sideband system for precision spectroscopy from 2.6 to 4.1 μm. *Opt Lett* 1998; **23**: 58–60.
6. Halmer D, von Basum G, Hering P, Mürtz M. Fast exponential fitting procedure for real time instrumental use. *Rev Sci Inst* 2004; **75**: 2187–2191.
7. Kharitonov SA, Barnes PJ. Exhaled markers of pulmonary disease. *Am J Respir Crit Care Med* 2001; **163**: 1693–1722.
8. Sehnert SS, Jiang L, Burdick JF, Risby TH. Breath biomarkers for detection of human liver diseases: preliminary study. *Biomarkers* 2002; **7**: 174–187.
9. Roller C, Kosterev A, Tittel F, Uehara K, Gmachl C, Sivco D. Carbonyl sulfide detection with a thermoelectrically cooled midinfrared quantum cascade laser. *Opt Lett* 2003; **28**: 2052–2054.

EXHALED HUMAN BREATH ANALYSIS WITH QUANTUM CASCADE LASER-BASED GAS SENSORS

G. WYSOCKI, M. MCCURDY, S. SO, C. ROLLER, AND F. K. TITTEL

Department of Electrical and Computer Engineering,
Rice University,
6100 Main Street, Houston TX 77251, USA

1. Introduction

The analysis of the many volatile molecular trace gas species in human breath in the low-ppb (parts-per-billion) concentration range presents a challenge for clinical breath analysis applications, which ideally requires rapid, *in situ* analysis. High molecular selectivity and sensitivity can be achieved using mid-infrared (mid-IR) tunable diode laser absorption spectroscopy (TDLAS) based gas sensors. This technique does not require the sample preparation or pre-concentration techniques associated with gas chromatography,[1-3] which is the most frequently used method for trace detection in various applications (also for human breath analysis[4,5]). TDLAS in combination with quantum cascade lasers (QCLs), which are efficient and reliable mid-IR sources operating within thermoelectric cooling ranges with minimal component requirements,[6] permit the design of selective, sensitive, compact and consumables-free (*e.g.* liquid nitrogen) trace-gas sensors suitable for field applications. In this work a trace gas sensor based on pulsed QCL will be described. The sensor was designed for simultaneous concentration measurement of OCS at the ppb level and CO_2 at the per cent level. A description of the sensor design and performance is reported in detail in Ref. 7. Elevated OCS concentrations in exhaled breath have been reported in lung transplant recipients suffering from acute rejection,[4] as well as in patients with liver disease.[5] In contrast to the currently used invasive diagnostic methods (*e.g.* bronchoscopic lung biopsies to assess lung transplant acute rejection), rapid analysis of expired breath using mid-IR TDLAS is a desirable non-invasive alternative. The thermoelectrically cooled QC laser used in this work operates in a pulsed mode at 4.85 μm and can access a number of strong absorption lines (line intensities about 1×10^{-18} cm^{-1}/molecule cm^{-2}) in the P branch of the OCS fundamental rotational-vibrational spectrum.[8] The availability of a neighboring CO_2 line within the tuning range of the QCL allows ventilation monitoring simultaneously with an OCS measurement and can be used to normalize the resulting OCS concentrations, and to standardize measurement conditions.[9,10] To address space and safety constraints relating to a medical setting, a digital signal processing (DSP) platform for pulsed QCL-based biogenic trace gas sensors is being developed to provide fast data acquisition (faster than 1 MHz), standalone data processing functions, increased reliability, and enhanced sensor portability.

2. Experimental

2.1. *Gas Sensor Configuration*

The optical configuration of the sensor is schematically shown in Fig. 1a. The beam of a thermoelectrically cooled pulsed distributed feedback (DFB) QCL is divided into sample and reference beams in the ratio of 2 to 1 respectively using a ZnSe beam splitter. The sample beam passes through the multipass astigmatic Herriott cell (New Focus, model: 5611) with a 36 m optical path length, and upon exiting is focused onto a fast (50 MHz bandwidth) mercury cadmium telluride (MCT) detector (Kolmar Technologies Inc., model KMPV8-1-J1) by an off-axis parabolic mirror. The reference beam is directed onto the same detector. Due to the difference in the optical path length between the channels, the sample optical pulse arrives about 120 ns later than the reference pulse.[11,12] Fast electronics is used for time resolved capture of peak optical intensity of the sample and reference laser pulses, which are subsequently digitized and processed using a laptop computer equipped with a 500-kilosample/s PCMCIA data acquisition card (National Instruments, model: DAQ 6062E). The reference channel is important for spectroscopic applications employing pulsed QCLs, since pulse-to-pulse fluctuations of the laser optical power degrade the signal-to-noise ratio (SNR) of measured absorption data. The wavelength of the QCL used can be tuned thermally between 2054.5 and 2060.5 cm^{-1} by changing the temperature of the QCL chip from -36 to $+10$ °C. Absorption features of several molecules such as OCS, CO_2, H_2O, and CO are within the tuning range of this laser and can be used for chemical sensing applications. To perform fast QCL wavelength scanning across the target spectroscopic line, a modulation of the sub-threshold laser current at a fixed operating temperature of the QCL heat sink was applied.[13] The laser was supplied with 25 ns injection current pulses at a repetition rate of 125 kHz with the maximum frequency limited by the sampling rate of the data acquisition electronics. The prototype of the sensor was constructed as a table-top platform using commercially available vacuum parts, optical mounts, and optical components (1 inch in diameter). A three dimensional model is depicted in Fig. 1b. This construction can be further optimized and miniaturized to achieve a compact portable instrument for field applications.

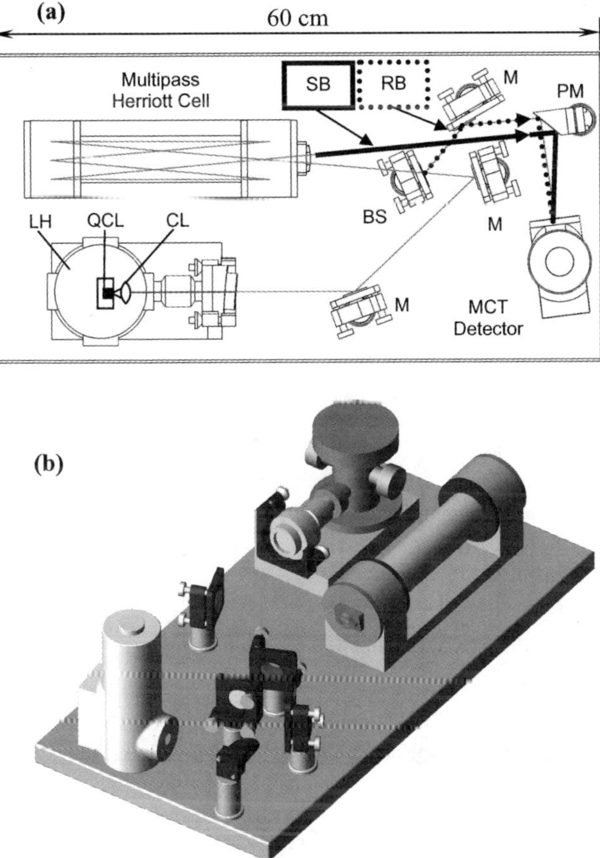

Fig. 1. (a) Schematic optical configuration and (b) three-dimensional drawing of the QCL-based gas sensor. QCL: quantum cascade laser chip; LH: laser housing; CL: collimating lens; SB: sample beam; RB: reference beam; M: mirror; BS: beam splitter; PM: off-axis parabolic mirror

2.2. *Selection of the Spectral Lines Suitable for Breath Analysis*

Human breath is a complex gas mixture, and thus low concentrations measurement of exhaled trace gases requires a careful selection of target molecular transitions, which should be strong and free of spectral interference from other gases (*e.g.* CO_2 and H_2O average level of about 5 % and about 7 % respectively). For measurements of OCS, the $P(11)$ (line strength: 7.49×10^{-19} cm^{-1}/molecule cm^{-2}) in the ν_3 band was selected. This spectroscopic line has minimal spectral interference by CO_2 and H_2O and has several neighboring CO_2 lines within the fast tuning range of the QCL, which can be used for simultaneous ventilation monitoring.[9,10] Fig. 2 shows OCS, CO_2 and H_2O spectral lines in the region of the OCS $P(11)$ line simulated for expected operating conditions using the HITRAN 2000 database.[14] To minimize contribution of wing effects from the very strong $\nu_1 + \nu_2$ CO_2 lines $P(24)$ and $P(26)$, which can affect the OCS measurement at the $P(11)$ line, a reduced gas cell pressure of 60 Torr was chosen.

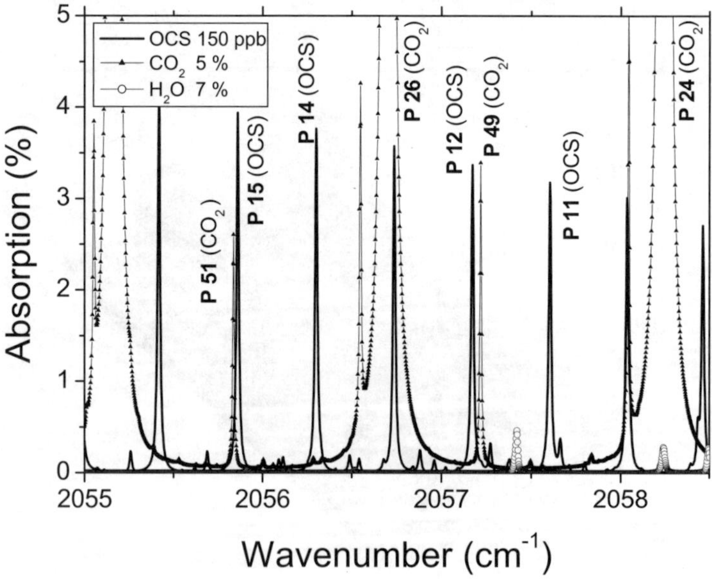

Fig. 2.   Absorption spectra of OCS, CO_2 and H_2O within the QCL spectral range, simulated using the HITRAN 2000 database, for assumed operating conditions (pressure: 60 Torr, optical path length: 36 m, OCS concentration: 150 ppb, CO_2 concentration: 5 %, and H_2O: 7 %)

2.3. *Gas Sensor Calibration*

The QCL was biased with a sub-threshold current sawtooth waveform at a frequency of 250 Hz and a peak-to-peak amplitude of about 35 mA, which provides complete coverage of the measured spectral lines. Calibration of the gas sensor was performed using a permeation tube-based precision gas standard generator (Kin-Tek, model: 491M). Reference 7 includes a detailed description of the concentration retrieval procedure, which result in a minimum detection limit, $C(1\sigma)$, of 0.76 ppb Hz$^{-1/2}$. As depicted in Fig. 3, the gas sensor shows a linear relationship between the measured concentration and the reference mixture concentration produced by the gas standard generator. A quasi real-time concentration plot for several generated concentration levels is shown in the inset to Fig. 3. Each data point in this plot was derived utilizing post-processing of the 100 averages of 400-point scans (acquired within 0.4 s), which results in a spread of the concentration measurements of 1.2 ppb.

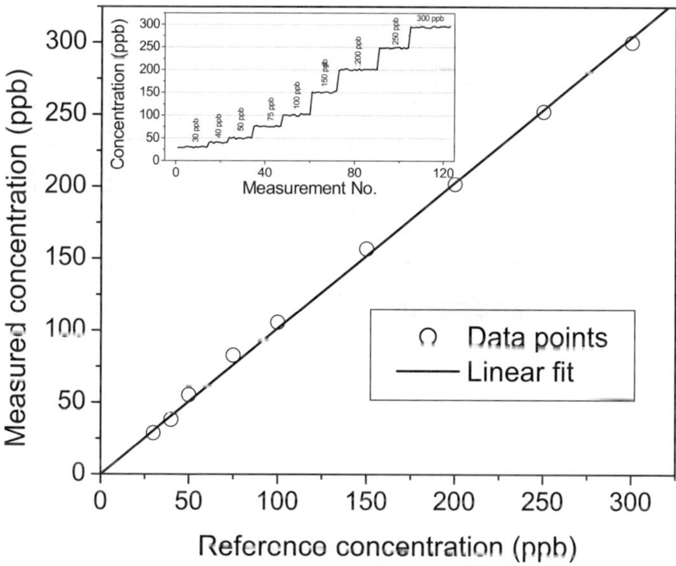

Fig. 3. Calibration curve for OCS concentration measurements obtained with a precision gas standard generator. The inset plot shows OCS concentrations calculated in quasi-real-time (0.4 sec single point acquisition time).

2.4. Breath Sample Collection

For this project a compact, portable breath collection apparatus was developed that can be used to measure alveolar, conducting airway, nasal and headspace air for clinical and research studies. The subject exhales into a mouthpiece through a high efficiency particulate air (HEPA) grade, low pressure drop biological filter, and into a custom T-piece (see Fig. 4). A discard bag connected to the T-piece preferentially fills, because it is the path of least resistance. Once the discard bag is filled, the exhaled breath passes through a flow meter (TSI Model 41211) and into the Tedlar sample collection bag (SKC Model 233-01). A pressure meter (Autotran Series 860) ensures that adequate mouth pressure is maintained during sample collection. The desired mouth pressure is achieved by adjusting the resistance through a stopcock valve. The flow rate is displayed in real time on a computer screen. The subject uses this feedback to maintain a specified flow rate. Several single exhalations were collected into one bag.

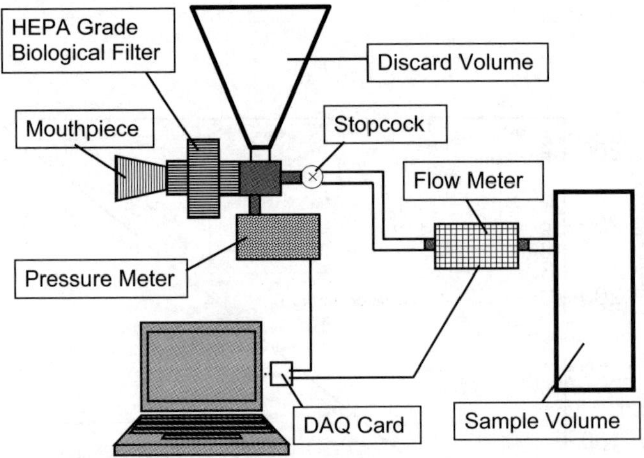

Fig. 4.   Schematic of a breath sampling system

2.5. Example Measurements of Breath Samples

The QCL-based sensor was used to measure exhaled OCS concentration in human breath. This kind of analysis was previously demonstrated using gas chromatography.[4,5,15] In the present work, breath samples were collected from lung transplant recipients using the collection method described above and analyzed within 2 hours after collection. A small portion of the gas sample was injected into the initially evacuated multipass cell, and its spectrum was measured at a total pressure of 60 Torr. Figure 5 shows measurements of samples taken from two different patients. Figures 5(a) and (b) show an OCS and CO_2 spectrum respectively, which were measured in the sample taken from the patient with suspected bronchiolitis. The OCS concentration detected in this sample was estimated to be at the level of about 8.4 ppb. The CO_2 concentration in this sample was determined to be on the level of about 5.1 %. For comparison, Figs. 5(c) and (d) show analogous measurements performed using a breath sample that did not contain any OCS at levels detectable by the instrument. The CO_2 concentration in this sample was found to be at a level of about 5.7 %, as shown in Fig. 5(d). This off-line analysis of human breath samples demonstrates

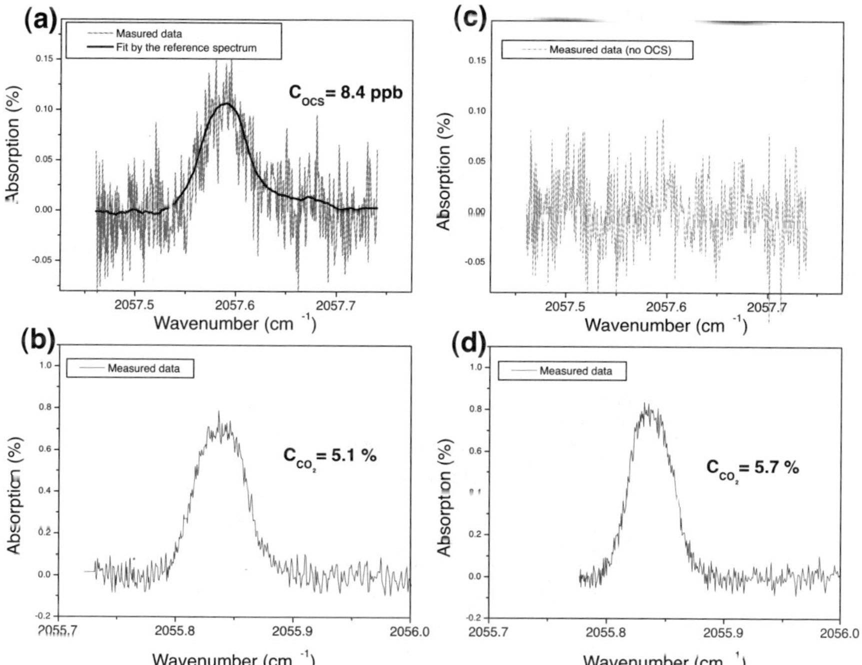

Fig. 5.   Measured spectra of OCS (a), and CO_2 (b), contained in a breath sample of a lung transplant recipient with a detected OCS concentration of 8.4 ppb. (c) and (d) are the same as (a) and (b) respectively, but no OCS was detected in the collected breath sample.

the feasibility of concentration measurement of low ppb OCS levels, as well as the multi-species (OCS and CO_2) detection capability of a QCL-based breath analyzer.

2.6. *Sensor Integration*

Current sensors based on TDLAS frequently require a personal computer (PC) based data acquisition system to process data, and assorted non-integrated support electronics to control the system. Application of digital signal processors (DSP) allows for system integration to develop compact, stand-alone sensors. Currently, custom DSP-based electronics for pulsed QCL-based systems is being developed to provide integrated control and processing functions without sacrificing sensors performance. Such a DSP platform (as shown in Fig. 6) is based on the commercially available DSP (Texas Instruments Inc., Model: TMS320F2812) embedded into an evaluation board (developed by Spectrum Digital Inc., Model: eZdsp F2812) and a custom made plug-in daughter card, which implements all the control functions (replacing modular stand-alone electronic devices), and directly interfaces with the sensor measurement signals. DSPs are (*i*) more suited to mathematics intensive signal processing applications than general purpose PC processors due to optimized arithmetic units (as opposed to graphics, web browsing, multimedia optimization for PCs), (*ii*) provide a simple programming platform due to optimized programming compilers, (*iii*) are very compact, (*iv*) drain much less power than PCs, (*v*) can provide higher data acquisition rates than PCs, and (*vi*) can perform all required functionality

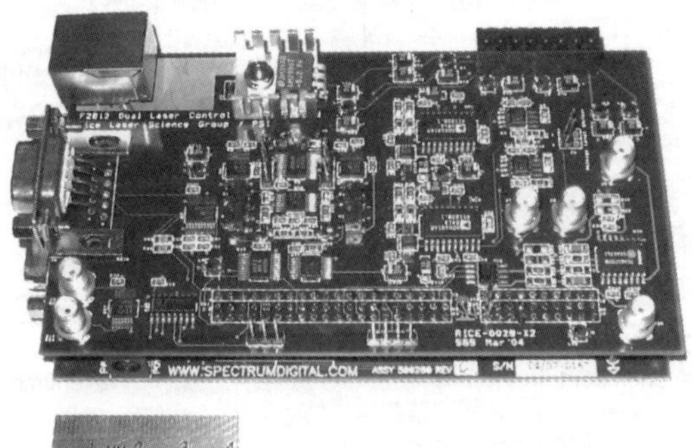

Fig. 6.   Integrated custom stand-alone pulsed tunable diode laser DSP controller with integrated RS232 and Ethernet communication. All processing and control functions are performed by the embedded processor.

autonomously. Furthermore, the custom system also provides integrated standard Ethernet and RS232 ports for remote communication with standard data loggers, PCs, or even other sensors, and can aid in tele-diagnostics or remote/quarantined monitoring.

3. Summary

The requirement of sensitive and compact instrumentation for the measurement of the low concentrations of volatile molecular species in exhaled breath makes QCL-based spectroscopic trace-gas detectors suitable for breath analysis in medical diagnostics. An off-line analysis of human breath samples from lung transplant recipients by means of the developed QCL-based breath analyzer demonstrates its feasibility for OCS concentration measurement with a minimum detection limit , $C(1\sigma)$, of 0.76 ppb Hz$^{-1/2}$, as well as the multi-species (OCS and CO_2) detection capability of the instrument. The development of an advanced pulsed QCL-based system control and data acquisition unit using DSP-based technology has been demonstrated. Such a sensor enhancement will result in faster data acquisition and a shorter processing time (thus decreasing system response time), as well as improved trace gas sensor portability, which is of importance in point-of-care medical applications.

Acknowledgements

The authors wish to thank Dr. Remzi Bag and Carolyn M. Paraguaya (Baylor College of Medicine, Houston, TX) for supplying breath samples. The authors also gratefully acknowledge financial support from the Texas Advanced Technology Program, the Robert Welch Foundation, the National Science Foundation, and the Office of Naval Research via a sub-award from Texas A&M University and the National Aeronautics and Space Administration. Matt McCurdy is the recipient of NASA Graduate Student Researchers Program (GSRP) fellowship award administered by the NASA John Space Center (JSC).

References

1. Steudler P, Kijowski W. Determination of reduced sulfur gases in air by solid absorbent preconcentration and gas chromatography. *Analytical Chemistry* 1984; **65**: 1432–1436.
2. Wardencki W. Problems with the determination of environmental sulphur compounds by gas chromatography. *J Chromatography A* 1998; **793**: 1–19.

3. Inomata Y, Matsunaga K, Murai Y, Osada K, Iwasaka Y. Simultaneous measurement of volatile sulfur compounds using ascorbic acid for oxidant removal and gas chromatography — flame photometric detection. *J Chromatography A* 1999; **864**: 111–119.

4. Studer SM, Orens JB, Rosas I, Krishnan JA, Cope KA, Yang S, Conte JV, Becker PB, Risby TH. Patterns and significance of exhaled-breath biomarkers in lung transplant recipients with acute allograft rejection. *J Heart Lung Transplant* 2001; **20**: 1158–1166.

5. Sehnert SS, Jiang L, Burdick JF, Risby TH. Breath biomarkers for detection of human liver diseases: preliminary study. *Biomarkers* 2002; **7**: 174–187.

6. Kosterev A, Tittel F. Chemical Sensors Based on Quantum Cascade Lasers. *IEEE Journal of Quantum Electronics* 2002; **38**: 582–591.

7. Wysocki G, McCurdy M, So S, Weidmann D, Roller C, Curl R, Tittel F. Pulsed quantum cascade laser based sensor for trace-gas detection of carbonyl sulfide. *Applied Optics* 2004; **43**: 6040–6046.

8. Roller C, Kosterev A, Tittel F, Uehara K, Gmachl C, Sivco D. Carbonyl sulfide detection with a thermoelectrically cooled mid-infrared quantum cascade laser. *Optics Letters* 2003; **28**: 2052–2054.

9. Niu HC, Schoeller DA, Klein PD. Improved gas chromatographic quantitation of breath hydrogen by normalization to respiratory carbon dioxide. *J Lab Clin Med* 1979; **94**: 755–763.

10. Roller C, Namjou K, Jeffers JD, Camp M, Mock A, McCann PJ, Grego J. Nitric oxide breath testing by tunable-diode laser absorption spectroscopy: application in monitoring respiratory inflammation. *Appl Opt* 2002; **41**: 6018–6029.

11. Nelson D, Shorter J, McManus J, Zahniser M. Sub-part-per-billion detection of nitric oxide in air using a thermoelectrically cooled mid-infrared quantum cascade laser spectrometer. *Applied Physics B* 2002; **75**: 343–350.

12. Weidmann D, Kosterev A, Roller C, Curl R, MP F, Tittel F. Pulsed Quantum Cascade Laser based Ethylene Monitoring. *Applied Optics* 2004; **43**: 3329–3334.

13. Namjou K, Cai S, Whittaker E, Faist J, Gmachl C, Capasso F, Sivco D, Cho A. Sensitive absorption spectroscopy with a room-temperature distributed-feedback quantum-cascade laser. *Optics Letters* 1998; **23**: 219–221.

14. Rothman L, Barbe A, Benner D, Brown L, Camy-Peyret C, Carleer M, Chance K, Clerbaux C, Dana V, Devi V, Fayt A, Flaud J, Gamache R, Goldman A, Jacquemart D, Jucks K, Lafferty W, Mandin J, Massie S, Nemtchinov V, Newnham D, Perrin A, Rinsland C, Schroeder J, Smith K, Smith M, Tang K, Toth R, Vander Auwera J, Varanasi P, Yoshino K. The HITRAN molecular spectroscopic database: edition of 2000 including updates through 2001. *J Quant Spectroscopy Radiative Transfer* 2003; **82**: 5–44.

15. Cope KA, Watson MT, Foster WM, Sehnert SS, Risby TH. Effects of ventilation on the collection of exhaled breath in humans. *J Appl Physiol* 2004; **96**: 1371–1379.

TCNQ DERIVATIVES-BASED SENSORS
FOR BREATH GAS ANALYSIS

G. V. KAMARCHUK

B. Verkin Institute for Low Temperature Physics & Engineering,
NAS of Ukraine,
47 Lenin Ave., Kharkov 61103, Ukraine

O. P. POSPYELOV AND YU. L. ALEXANDROV

National Technical University "Kharkov Polytechnical Institute",
21 Frunze Str., Kharkov 61002, Ukraine

A. V. YEREMENKO

B. Verkin Institute for Low Temperature Physics & Engineering,
NAS of Ukraine,
47 Lenin Ave., Kharkov 61103, Ukraine

A. V. KRAVCHENKO

V. Karazin Kharkov National University,
4 Svobody Sq., Kharkov 61077, Ukraine

E. G. KUSHCH AND L. V. KAMARCHUK

Institute for Children and Adolescents Health Care,
AMS of Ukraine,
52-A, 50 let VLKSM Avenue, Kharkov 61153, Ukraine

E. FAULQUES

Institut des Matériaux Jean Rouxel,
2 rue de la Houssinière, F-44322, Nantes, France

1. Introduction

The interest in sensor technology has considerably increased recently.[1] One
of the most prospective trends in this field is the creation of sensor devices for the control of gas media. The improvement of these devices may
be reached either by developing new methods for the production of sensor
elements, or by synthesizing new materials with unique physical-chemical

parameters which are able to provide high metrological characteristics. Synthetic organic conductors are of special significance among such prospective materials. Their importance is due to the wide spectrum of properties and perspectives of practical usage that they have exhibited so far (see, for example, Ref. 2). Synthetic conductors may not only increase the possibilities of the already existing electronic devices but may also widen the arsenal of sensor techniques.[3]

7,7,8,8-tetracyano-quinodimethane's (TCNQ) derivatives are representatives of one of the well-known classes of organic conductive compounds.[4] The peculiarity of their typical crystal structure lies in the stacked packing of TCNQ molecules. The distance between the TCNQ molecules inside stacks is much less than that between stacks. Thus, from a structural aspect, TCNQ complexes are represented by a system of linear conductive chains, which are regularly packed in the crystal. Electrical conductivity of these compounds is due to the motion of electrons along the stacks. The probability of electron hopping between the stacks is much weaker. Such a quasi-one-dimensional type of crystal conductivity causes strong anisotropy in the electron density distribution, which, in turn, might change considerably during adsorption processes. This feature is one of the main reasons why investigations towards the tailoring of sensors based on the TCNQ compounds are of great interest.[5] We found high sensitivity and selectivity of TCNQ-based sensors when they are exposed to the influence of external agents of different nature.[6] This finding stimulated intensive research to unravel many specific properties for this class of substances, namely a high sensitivity to the components of breath exhaled by humans. The results of these investigations are presented in this paper.

The problem of breath gas analysis is currently of special interest, because of its potential value in medical diagnostics.[7] There is no doubt that breath gas analysis will take a leading position amongst the new methods for non-invasive diagnostics, in view of the great number of markers which reflect the state of the human organism. At the present time different techniques are being applied to breath gas analysis. For example, many kinds of spectroscopy and mass spectrometry are widely used to record isotope-markers introduced into the body.[8-10] This has been achieved, for instance, with the successful exploitation of modified mass spectrometry.[11] The majority of spectroscopic techniques are based on chemiluminescence. For instance, the reaction of NO with ozone, which is generated in the analyzer, produces excited molecules of nitrogen dioxide that emit photons.[12] But a most useful approach would be to develop simple and non-expensive technologies, which allows one to obtain diagnostic results immediately when breath gas is exhaled. This should be done without injecting any chemicals into the body or without any additional operations that can influence the breath trace gas concentrations. Such demands may be fulfilled by using specifically designed gas sensors, which may now be possible in view of the rapid progress in modern sensor techniques. This is clearly exemplified, for example, by the sensor targeted at the determination of small NO gas concentrations.[13] Novel gas sensors can yield drastic improvements in measurements of exhaled gases and highly sensitive "electronic nose" devices surpass human and animal olfactory senses.[14,15]

The work described in this paper focuses at the description of new gas sensors based on the TCNQ derivatives and investigations of their response to human exhaled breath.

2. Experimental Technique

The design of our sensitive elements (transformers) is based on the principle of the modification of conductivity and interface properties. The sensor response is performed by electrical conductivity measurement. The output signal of the transformer is based on the variation of the conductive properties of the organic compound as a result of its interaction with the components of the gas mixture to be analyzed. In this case, the maximal relative change of the sample sensor conductivity during its interaction with the gas is registered in samples of minimal thickness. This is associated with modifications of the superficial properties of the sensor material, which yields the output signal. Taking into account this fact the active parts of the sensitive elements were designed by making thin films of the organic conductor deposited onto a dielectric substrate (Fig. 1). The size of each film was 1.0 mm × 0.2 mm with a thickness of 1 to 100 μm. The opposite sides of the thin film were connected to current-feeding copper or silver wires. The sensitive films were prepared by two methods. The first one was based on the ability of the compounds to undergo molten state

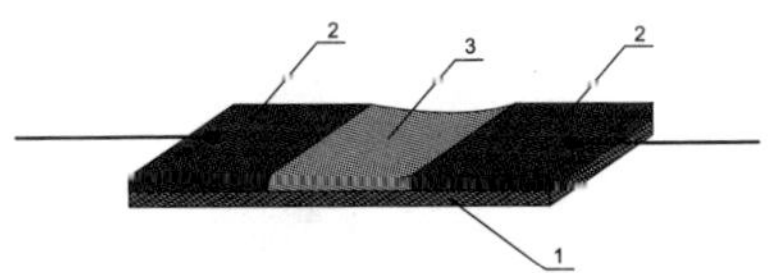

Fig. 1.   General view of a sensitive element. 1: dielectric substrate, 2: current electrodes, 3: gas-sensitive material

transition without degradation.[16] This allowed gas-sensitive film material to be obtained by overlay melting. The second method involved dropping a suspension of the active material onto a substrate, subsequently vaporizing the solvent. A solvent with a low boiling point was used in order to obtain quick evaporation under normal conditions.

The gas-sensitive film of the transformer was manufactured from complex TCNQ salts with N-alkylquinolinium (N-Alk-Qn) and N-alkyliso-quinolinium (N-Alk-iso-Qn) cations. The general formulae of the compounds used are [N-Alk-Qn](TCNQ)$_2$ and [N-Alk-iso-Qn](TCNQ)$_2$. We managed to produce both active and passive sensor samples. As is known,[17] an active sensor generates a current signal, while a passive sensor requires an external power supply to give the output signal — current or voltage. In our case the electrical conductivity was changed under the influence of the gas to be analyzed, and was, therefore, used as the main parameter to test if the sample was working. The influence of gas substances on the TCNQ compound led to an increase of its conductivity and, accordingly, to current growth in the passive sensor circuit which caused the change of the output signal. The samples of the active sensors, produced by us, demonstrated the behavior, which is characteristic of the systems containing an internal source of electrical energy. To obtain reproducible results, an autonomous compact measuring setup was manufactured. It included the sensor, the power supply (for passive modification), recording potentiometer and a special sensor holder for investigating breath gas.

The use of this setup with a standardized approach minimized the variation coefficient when good reproducibility of the metrological characteristics of the sensor samples was obtained. The setup of an active sensor is shown in the Fig. 2. When the gas to be analyzed comes into contact with the gas-sensitive material of sensor S1, a current is generated, which depends on the intensity of the interaction. At this time a bias drop on the resistor R occurs, which is the output signal of the device. To decrease the noise level

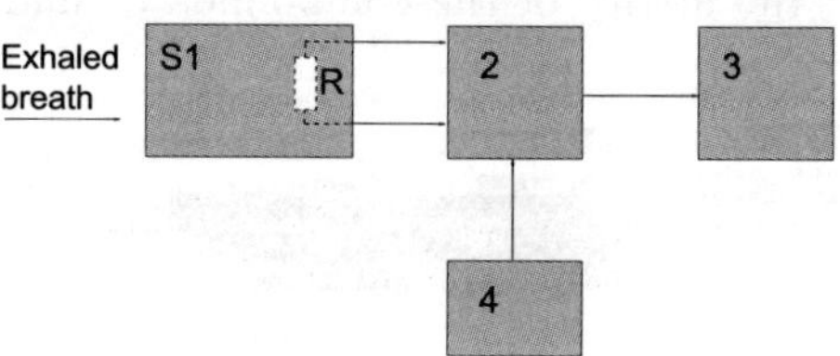

Fig. 2.   Scheme of the setup.   S1: sensor, 2: instrumentation amplifier, 3: recording potentiometer, 4: power supply

and the interferences, the signal from the resistor R enters the differential input of the instrumentation amplifier 2 before registration. It should be emphasized that the level of the output signals produced by the sensors was high enough to be faithfully recorded by potentiometer 3 and did not require any additional amplification. Thus, an amplification coefficient of unity was set in the amplifier in order to decrease the noise level. As the measured signals were rather low, the bodies of the recorder and sensor holder were grounded. In this case, the grounding busbars and the "zero" wire of the amplifier power supply are connected at a single point.

The experimental procedure included several essential formalities. Before the experiment, each volunteer included in the study (breath analysis) filled in a special form, concerning his/her habits (smoking; alcoholic and drug abuse), any known disorders, chronic somatic diseases, chronic infections at the time of the investigation, and any previous diseases. To standardize the measurement procedure, a standard methodology for breath gas sampling was established. It was determined that maximal reproducibility of results was obtained when the sensor response was registered after an exhalation delay of 20 seconds following deep inhalation. This could be easily done by all volunteers. The experiments were carried out at least 2 hours after a meal in order to exclude any influence of volatile components of food and volatile compounds produced during the gastric digestion phase. The record of the sensor response consisted of two periods: the exhalation period, corresponding to the stepped action of the breath gas on the sensor, and the relaxation period when the exhalation was finished. When the influence of the breath gas ceased, the relaxation of the sensor towards the initial state occurred in the ambient atmospheric air. The sensor's response and its relaxation time dependence on the current I, flowing through the sample was measured. The data were used to determine the maximum speed of the output signal change and the relaxation time t of sensor.

3. Results and Discussion

In this work we built laboratory samples of sensors based on TCNQ salts with N-alkylquinolinium (N-Alk-Qn) and alkylisoquinolinium (N-Alk-iso-Qn) cations. Five series of sensors were manufactured, each containing 10 samples. Among them two series were fabricated by means of solvent evaporation from a suspension of the gas-sensitive substance. The first series included active sensors, the second series passive sensors. The other three series of samples were prepared by the melting overlay method (passive modification). Figure 3 revealed for the first time the appearance of an output signal resulting from the interaction of human exhaled breath on TCNQ derivatives-based sensors.

Subsequent experiments showed high selectivity of the TCNQ derivatives-based sensors to the breath gas components. We did not observe a significant response during exposure of sensors to a number of different gases with concentration up to 10^4 ppm. Gases such as nitric and sulfur oxides, hydrogen sulfide, saturated hydrocarbons and vapors of methanol, ethanol, acetone, chloroform and benzene were tested. Temperature and water vapor action only caused a weak sensor response. These did not exceed 5–10 % of the amplitude of the sensor signal exposed in the breath gas. So the interaction of the sensor with breath moisture is insignificant and may be neglected. Thus, the TCNQ derivatives-based sensors, created in this work provide an opportunity to detect the gas components in exhaled air.

The metrological characteristics of samples were estimated by the speed of the response parameters. In the case of stepped changes of the response during the signal increase period (breath exposure), there were two kinds of time parameters that are typical for the process:

- the time delay of the signal increase t_{id} — time interval, which is necessary for the output signal to rise from the initial value to 10 % of its full change;
- the time of the signal increase t_i — time interval of the output signal growth from 10 to 90% of its full change.

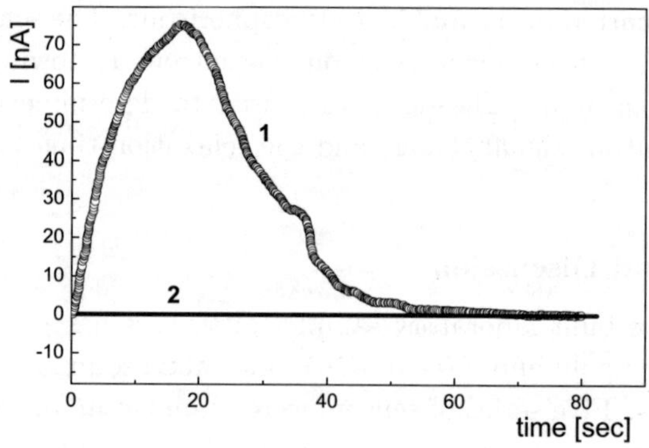

Fig. 3.   Output signal resulting from the interaction of human exhaled breath on TCNQ derivatives-based sensors. Curve 1: influence of the exhaled breath medium. Line 2: carbon dioxide of 50 % concentration in noble gas. I: current flowing through the sensor; t: time

In the case of the stepped changes in the measured value, which cause the decrease of the output signal (relaxation), there were also two kinds of time parameters characterizing the process:

- the time delay of the signal decrease t_{dd} — time interval, necessary for the output signal to decrease from the initial value to 10 % of its full change;
- the signal decrease time t_d — time interval of the output signal to decrease from 10 to 90 % of its full change.

It was shown that the time variation of the sensor output signal under a stepped increase of the gas sample to be analyzed can be accurately represented by a first-order differential equation.[17] The solution of this equation gives the time dependence of the output signal. Thus, the $I(t)$ function can be written as:

$$I = I_0 \left[1 - \exp(-t/\tau)\right];\qquad(1)$$

I_0 is the current intensity flowing through the sensor, which has already reached stationary state after a stepped action in time t, and τ is the time constant for the process. The limits for the variation of the time constants have been calculated according to this equation using the experimental data (see Table 1).

It should be noted that in freshly prepared sensors there was a speed drift of the response parameters. That is why all the samples made soon after production were so-called "trained". Such training included a number of exposure-relaxation cycles, which were repeated until the value of the signal growth speed became constant. Usually this took 10–12 cycles to stabilize the sensor parameters (Fig. 4). After this procedure all the sensors demonstrated reproducible results.

Table 1. Metrological characteristics of the sensors

Way of produ-cing the sensor	Modifi-cation	t_{id} (s)	t_i (s)	t_{dd} (s)	t_d (s)	τ (s)	I_0 (nA)
Overlay melting	Passive	6–20	120–180	2–15	40–95	55–90	900–1500
Evaporation of the solvent	Passive	4–10	60–85	2–8	15–42	28–42	1000–2200
Evaporation of the solvent	Active	2–3	14–18	4–8	40–55	8–10	6–10

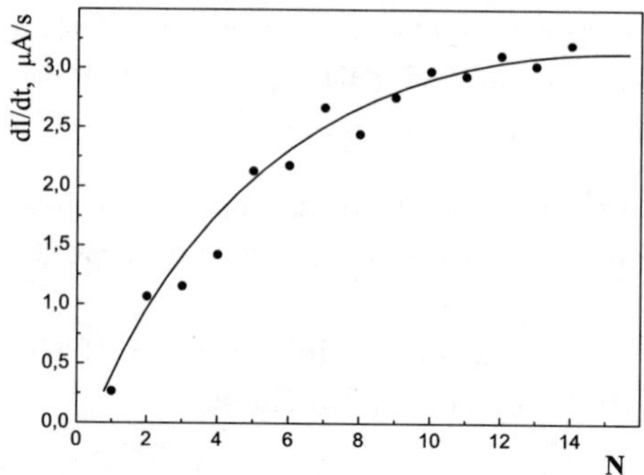

Fig. 4.   The process of "training" of the active sensor sample. dI/dt: velocity of signal growth, N: the number of the cycle

The samples of passive sensors obtained by solvent evaporation surpassed the overlay samples with response parameter speeds more than 2 times higher (see Table 1). This may be due to differences in the structure of material on the interface between the gas-sensitive substance and the gas to be analyzed. The state of the material influences considerably the dynamics of the adsorption process and, consequently, the time necessary to reach a stable sensor regime. Active sensors, in view of their technological peculiarities, had a thinner layer of gas-sensitive material than the passive ones. Their thickness was smaller by more than one order-of-magnitude. The output signal of the active sensors was 200 times smaller than that of the passive sensors. The saturation process in thinner films of active sensors was faster, which was reflected in higher response speed parameters (see Table 1).

The dependence of the sensor output signal on the behaviour of homologic complex cations of the TCNQ salts were studied. It was found out that the level of the output signal is directly proportional to the length of the hydrocarbon radical of the complex cation (Fig. 5). Output signals up to 3 μA in a passive and 100 nA in an active work regime were recorded after exposing the sensors with a gas-sensitive surface area of about 0.2 mm^2 to exhaled breath.

In our investigation of TCNQ compounds it was discovered for the first time that the sensor response essentially depended on the differences in the exhaled breath of different people. The response curves demonstrated high reproducibility in each case (Fig. 6) and differed a lot for various volunteers (see Fig. 7). This result influenced the direction of the subsequent study of sensors based on TCNQ derivatives. It was consideration that the gas to be

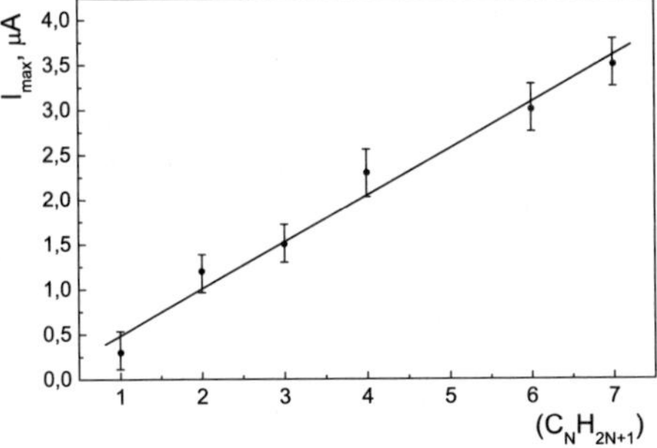

Fig. 5. Dependence of the maximal output signal ($I_{\max}$) of the passive sensors *vs.* the number of carbon atoms (N) in the alkylisoquinolinium cations

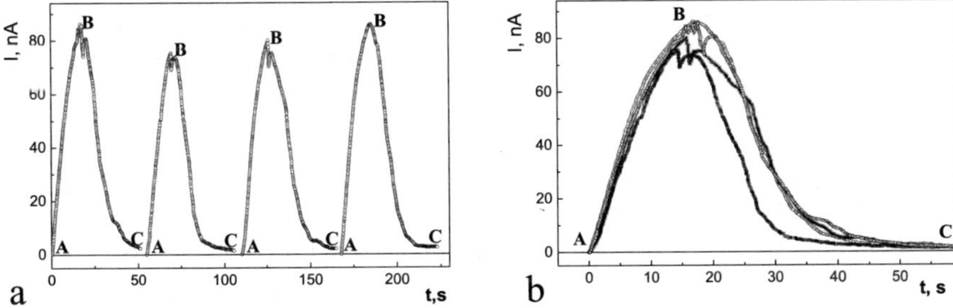

Fig. 6. **a:** Sensor response for four sequential breath exhalations. **b:** The four curves from **a** overlapped. Sections AB correspond to the exhalation periods, sections BC: the relaxation periods.

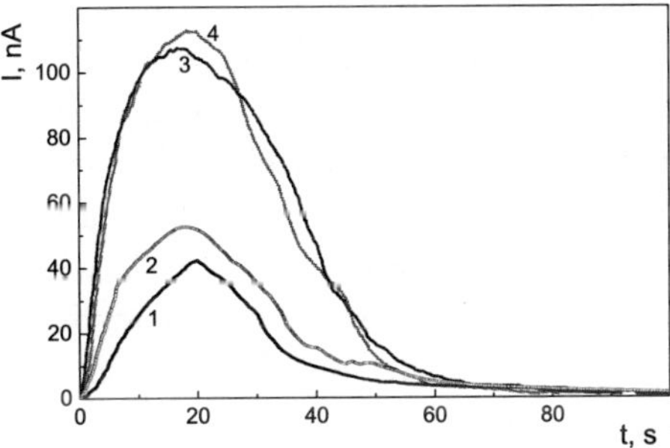

Fig. 7. The response of a sensor to the breath gas of different volunteers. 1: response for the breath gas of volunteer of the 1st group; 2: breath of the volunteers of the 2nd group; 3, 4: breath of the volunteers of the 3rd group; see the text.

analyzed, when exhaled air, might be an indicator of the volunteers' health and could be a biological marker of some diseases.[18] A phenomenological model of the system under investigation was used for the correct selection of the output signal parameter, which properly reflects the concentration of the particular substance. According to this model, the decrease in the conductivity activation energy of a gas-sensitive material and the interface transformations are basic parameters when definite groups of chemical compounds are adsorbed. This phenomenon may be caused both by the increase of conductivity of surface layers of a gas-sensitive material and by the induced influence of adsorbing molecules. The influence of adsorbing molecules may lead to space transformations with a redistribution of electron density of superficial layers of TCNQ compounds, structuring the linear conductive TCNQ chains with high electronic conductivity, and, as a result, to the formation of additional conductivity channels. The effect of the proportional dependence of the sensor electrical conductivity on the hydrocarbon radical length of the complex cation, revealed by us, may be an indirect confirmation of this model (Fig. 5). The increase of the complex radical size is likely to lead to considerably more space transformations of the superficial layer during molecular adsorption.

The adsorption–desorption equilibrium on a sensor surface, which is established on the surface of the sensitive substance during contact with the atmosphere, is disturbed under the action of breath gas. Those molecules in breath gas with adsorption energy exceeding that of the atmospheric components occupy active adsorption centers. Because of this, the composition and the structure of the superficial layer of the gas-sensitive material change. Thus, the exposition curve, recorded in our investigations, characterizes the combined action of two processes: (i) diffusion of gaseous products of breath gas into the sensor surface and (ii) adsorption of some of them onto the surface of the sensitive substance. In our investigations we used an open-type sensor in which direct contact of the sensitive material with the gas to be analyzed is possible. That is why the process of gas diffusion mainly determines the speed of sensor response during the exposure (exhalation) phase. This effect is clearly demonstrated by the form of the curves in Fig. 7. The original, flatter parts of the curves reflect the combined diffusive and adsorption effects on the output signal. It does not exceed 1–3 seconds. Then a sharp rise of the response signal is observed. Consequently, as a first approximation, it can be concluded that the action of the exhaled air has a stepped character and the basic part of the exposure curve reflects the dynamics of the adsorption process. According to the theory of the absolute speed of heterogeneous reactions,[19] the speed of adsorption is directly proportional to the product of concentration of the adsorbing gas molecules and the surface concentration of the vacant active centers. Now consider that the number of active adsorption centers on the surface of sensitive material is constant. Then the maximal value of the first derivative of the exposure curve can be used to estimate the concentration of the adsorbing molecules in the gas mixture. Thus, the adsorbed molecule concentration can be evaluated by taking the maximum speed of the signal increase during the exposure phase:

$$v_e = \left(\frac{dI}{dt}\right)_{\max} \ [\mathrm{nA/s}] \, .$$

Continuous exposure of the sensor to the breath gas leads to a smoother variation of the response signal curve. This is caused by an adsorption speed reduction because of the decrease of the free active center concentration.

In the framework of the adopted experimental procedure, the condition of full saturation, *i.e.*, total occupation of active centers, was not reached. This is connected with the limited exposure time (lasting 20 seconds). Experiments showed that the required saturation period was about 30 seconds (Fig. 8) for comparatively high concentration of the adsorbing molecules in the breath. In the saturation state the specific conductivity of the superficial layer of the sensor active zone increased by more than 2 orders-of-magnitude and reached up to 100 $\Omega^{-1}\,\mathrm{cm}^{-1}$. This corresponds to the maximum conductivity of other TCNQ salts.[20,21] There were also small variations in the maximum conductivity of the sensitive material for a constant composition of the gas mixture. This may indicate the stochastic

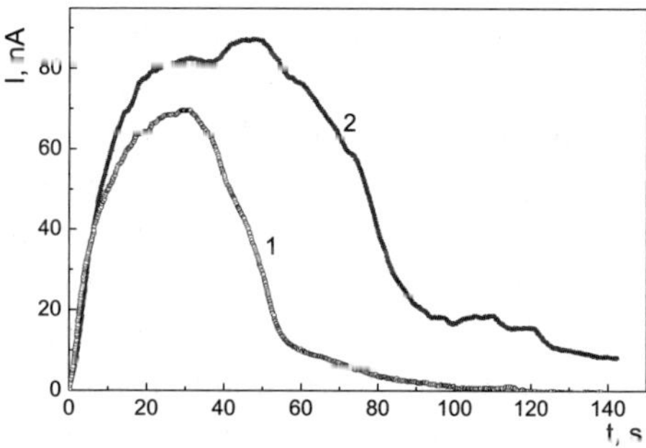

Fig. 8. Demonstration of the absorbing saturation of the gas-sensitive material: sensor response for long breath exhalation for two different volunteers 1 and 2

nature of the process of absorption layer formation. These variations did not exceed 10 percent for the breath of any volunteer.

The relaxation curve (sections BC of the curves in Fig. 6) reflects the opposite process, namely, desorption of the gas mixture molecules when they are in contact with the ambient atmosphere. The form of the curves during the relaxation period is characterized by more variations than the exposure curves. After exposure to the exhaled breath, an abrupt transition of the sensor output signal to the relaxation phase is observed. This may indicate the prevalence of low-energy, physical adsorption of an outer layer of adsorbed molecules. The further course of the relaxation curves is characterized by a decrease of their inclination reaching sometimes zero level, caused by a considerable deceleration of the desorption process. Such a deceleration may be due to the high energy of adsorption links between sensor adsorption centers and adsorbed gas molecules. Formation of structures with high adsorption energy is characteristic of molecules of different types. Thus, the evaluation of the holding time duration (quantity factor) and of the ordinate of each singularity (energetic factor) in the relaxation curves allows the origin and concentration of adsorbing molecules to be identified, *i.e.*, it reveals the nature of the breath gas composition in each volunteer. This holds promise for future investigations and applications of the TCNQ-based sensors for exhaled breath analysis.

The studies of the breath gas of 30 volunteers showed high reproducibility for each person. We found a clear marker in the response signal, which may reflect the individual metabolic profile of each volunteer. Both relaxation and exposure curves contain specific features. Their behavior corresponds to the physical and chemical processes occurring during the first and second periods of the experiment. Depending on the character of the curves obtained and on the maximum speed of the signal increase v_e, which reflects the concentration of the adsorbed breath gas molecules, the group of volunteers was divided into three separate groups. The exhaled air of volunteers of the first group (14 persons) contained low concentration of compounds that could be detected by the sensor ($v_e = 2.5 \ldots 3.0$). The second group (11 persons) had a medium concentration of compounds ($v_e = 4.0 \ldots 6.0$). The third group (5 persons) had a high concentration ($v_e = 8.0 \ldots 12.0$). The curves presented in Fig. 7 are examples of the dependences typical for each group of volunteers. It should be pointed out that all persons from the third group previously suffer from stomach ulcers in anamnesis. This allows one to speculate that their breath gas could contain the products of vital metabolism of the anaerobic bacteria *Helicobacter pylori*,[22] which is

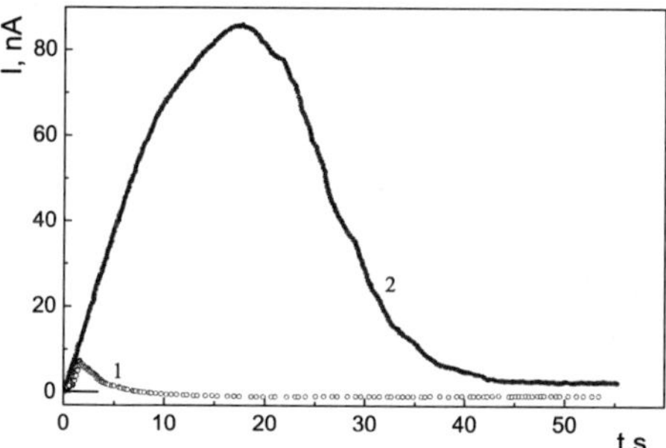

Fig. 9.   TCNQ derivatives-based sensor response to the action of ammonia (curve 1) of concentration of 10^5 ppm and breath gas (curve 2)

now recognized to be a basic etiology factor of stomach ulcers. It is known that ammonia is produced by *Helicobacter pylori* metabolites and can be a biomarker of this infection (see the article by Penault *et al.*[23] on page 393 of this book). Taking this into account, additional investigations were carried out concerning the interaction of the sensors with ammonia. Experiments were performed over a wide range of gas concentrations. One should note that the usual ammonia concentration in the breath gas of ulcerous patients is about 1–10 ppm.[24] However, the sensor did not produce a signal even for ammonia concentration up to 10^4 ppm. Further increase in the ammonia concentration resulted in just a weak response. The amplitude of the sensor output signal was about 4–6 nA for an ammonia concentration of 10^5 ppm. This is about 10 % of the sensor output signal when exposed to breath gas (Fig. 9). This comparison appears to indicate that the sensor response is not connected with the ammonia component in breath gas. The influence of ammonia molecules on the sensor response was also studied at various humidities. This approach should reveal any influences of NH_4^+ ions. Variations of the response amplitude did not exceeded 5 % of the exhaled air sensor output. The influence of the water vapour on the response signal was about 5–10 %. Hence an influence of the ammonium ion was not found. Probably, the obvious response of the TCNQ derivatives-based sensor to breath gas of volunteers suffering from gastric ulcers is caused by the influence of other metabolites or their complex action.

4. Conclusions

To use the sensors presented in this paper for application in medical diagnostics it is necessary to carry out additional experiments in order to obtain much more data to allow meaningful statistical analyses. Experiments are planned to determine which of known breath gas components interact with the sensor active substance. But the results of this work have already indicated that TCNQ complex salts can serve as prospective sensor materials for the analysis of breath gas composition. Application of these sensors in medical practice would be very simple. It could offer a non-invasive method for diagnosis and thus assist in early clinical diagnosis.

Acknowledgement

The authors thank V. Gudimenko for assistance with the treatment of results and A. Zaika for the building the experimental setup. This work was partly supported by the Science and Technology Center in Ukraine and by the Ministry of Education and Science of Ukraine.

References

1. Fraden J. *Handbook of Modern Sensors: Physics, Designs, and Applications.* 3rd ed. New York: Springer, 2004.
2. Faulques E, Perry DL, Yeremenko AV. *Spectroscopy of Emerging Materials.* NATO Science Series II, Mathematics, physics, and chemistry; Vol. 165. Boston: Kluwer Academic Publishers, 2004.
3. Richardson T. *Functional Organic and Polymeric Materials: Molecular Functionality — Macroscopic Reality.* New York: John Wiley & Sons, 2000.
4. Schegolev I. Electric and magnetic properties of linear conducting chains. *Phys Stat Sol Ser a* 1972; **12**: 9–45.
5. Ho K, Liao J. NO_2 gas sensing based on vacuum-deposited TTF-TCNQ thin films. *Sensors and Actuators B: Chemical* 2003; **93**: 370–378.
6. Pospelov A, Ved M, Sakhnenko N, Alexandrov Y, Shtefan V, Kravchenko A, Kamarchuk G. High-conductivity organic metals as electrode materials. *Materials Science* 2002; **20**: 65–72.
7. Marczin N, Yacoub M. *Disease Markers in Exhaled Breath: Basic Mechanisms and Clinical Applications.* NATO Science Series I, Life and behavioural sciences, Vol. 346. Amsterdam, Washington DC: IOS Press, 2002.
8. Kharitonov SA, Barnes PJ. Exhaled markers of pulmonary disease. *Am J Respir Crit Care Med* 2001; **163**: 1693–1722.
9. Braden B, Haisch M, Duan LP, Lembcke B, Caspary WF, Hering P. Clinically feasible stable isotope technique at a reasonable price: analysis of $^{13}CO_2/^{12}CO_2$-abundance in breath samples with a new isotope selective-nondispersive infrared spectrometer. *Z Gastroenterol* 1994; **32**: 675–678.
10. Corradi M, Montuschi P, Donnelly LE, Pesci A, Kharitonov SA, Barnes PJ. Increased nitrosothiols in exhaled breath condensate in inflammatory airway diseases. *Am J Respir Crit Care Med* 2001; **163**: 854–858.

11. Smith D, Španěl P. SIFT applications in mass spectrometry. In: Lindon JC, Tranter GE, and Holmes JL, eds. *Encyclopedia of Spectroscopy and Spectrometry*, San Diego: Academic Press, 2000: 2092–3106.

12. Voznesensky N, Chuchalin A, Antonov N. Nitrogen oxide and lungs (in Russian). *Pulmonology* 1998; **2**: 6–10.

13. Wu D, Cahen D, Graf P, Naaman R, Nitzan A, Shvarts D. Direct determination of low-concentration NO in physiological solutions by a new GaAs-based sensor. *Chem Eur J* 2001; **7**: 1743–1749.

14. Gardner JW, Bartlett PN. *Electronic Noses: Principles and Applications*. Oxford, New York: Oxford University Press, 1999.

15. Pavlou AK, Turner AP. Sniffing out the truth: clinical diagnosis using the electronic nose. *Clin Chem Lab Med* 2000; **38**: 99–112.

16. Bocer K, Starodub V, Swietlik R. Melting of conducting organic composites based on TCNQ and methyl-TCNQ salts studies by IR spectroscopy. *Adv Mater Opt Electron* 1998; **8**: 97–99.

17. Asch G, Desgoutte P. *Les capteurs en instrumentation industrielle*. Paris: Dunod, 1999.

18. Risby T. Breath markers in normal and diseased humans. In: Marczin N, Yacoub M, eds. *Disease Markers in Exhaled Breath. Basic Mechanisms and Clinical Applications*, Amsterdam, Washington DC: IOS Press, 2002: 113–122.

19. Thomas JM, Thomas WJ. *Introduction to the Principles of Heterogeneous Catalysis*. London, New York: Academic Press, 1967.

20. Shibaeva R. Structure of the quasi-one-dimensional organic conductors (in Russian). *Science Tech Ser Crystallochemistry* (VINITI publishers, Moscow) 1981; **15**: 189–264.

21. Starodub V, Gluzman E, Kaftanova Y, Olejniczak I. Melting conducting TCNQ salts as materials for microelectronics (in Russian). *Theor Exper Chem* 1997; **33**: 111–114.

22. Perederiy V, Shvets N, Tkach S, Kliaritskaya I, Gdal V, Perederiy O, Shvets O. The role of breath tests for the diagnostics of the digestive tract diseases (in Russian). *Contemporary Gastroenterology and Hepatology* 2001; **1**: 21–25.

23. Penault C, Španěl P, Smith D. Detection of *H. pylori* infection by breath ammonia following urea ingestion. In: Amann A, Smith D, eds. *Breath Analysis for Clinical Diagnosis and Therapeutic Monitoring*, Singapore: World Scientific, 2005.

24. Smith D , Španěl P. The novel selected-ion flow tube approach to trace gas analysis of air and breath. *Rapid Commun Mass Spectrom* 1996; **10**: 1183–1198.

PART B

NITRIC OXIDE, CARBON MONOXIDE, AND ETHANE

EXHALED NITRIC OXIDE:
HOW AND WHY WE KNOW IT IS IMPORTANT

L. E. GUSTAFSSON

Centre for Allergy Research
and Department of Physiology & Pharmacology,
Karolinska Institutet,
S-17177 Stockholm, Sweden

1. Introduction

The discovery of nitric oxide (NO) in exhaled breath[1] was the result of
a proposal that NO might regulate the pulmonary circulation in a fashion where it counteracts the hypoxic pulmonary vasoconstriction.[2] This
constriction is the normal endogenous mechanism whereby the blood flow
through the lungs is diverted to well-ventilated areas so that a matching
is obtained between ventilation and perfusion.[3] At this time there was a
debate whether NO formation would be increased or not by hypoxia in the
lungs, and therefore the proposal by Persson *et al.* met with considerable
criticism. A joint effort between the Stockholm group and Dr Moncada's
laboratory at the Wellcome Research Laboratories was undertaken to measure nitric oxide in lung perfusates by monitoring its primary metabolite,
nitrite. An NO/nitrite analysis system designed at Wellcome was successfully transferred to Stockholm. However, the efforts were thwarted by severe
interference from the minute, but still significant, seeping of stagnant red
blood cells from the perfused lungs, interfering with the NO/nitrite assay.
On the assumption that NO might be present in the gas phase (breath)
in the lung, attempts were made to measure NO in the exhaled breath of
humans. This also met with considerable difficulties, due to the contamination of room air with NO from environmental pollution; at times exhaled
breath contained lower amounts of NO than the inhalate. Nevertheless,
at times reproducible signals could be obtained (Fig. 1), but animal experiments were required to substantiate these. A decisive experiment was
performed in anesthetised and ventilated rabbits where clean synthetic air

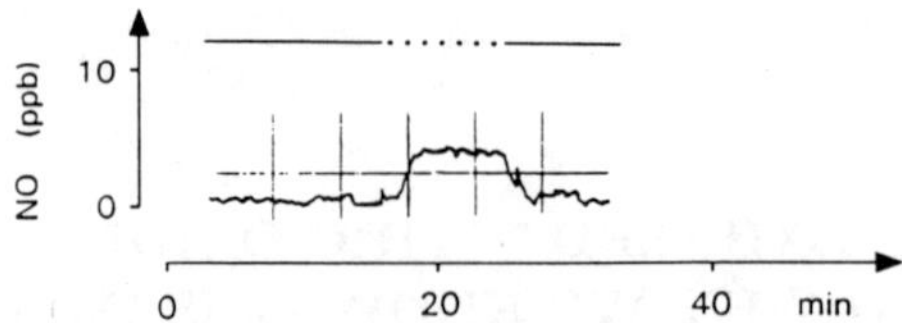

Fig. 1.   Exhaled nitric oxide measurement in mixed exhaled air from a healthy human subject.   Determination in the room (solid marker line) and from mixed exhaled air (dotted marker line). From Ref. 1.

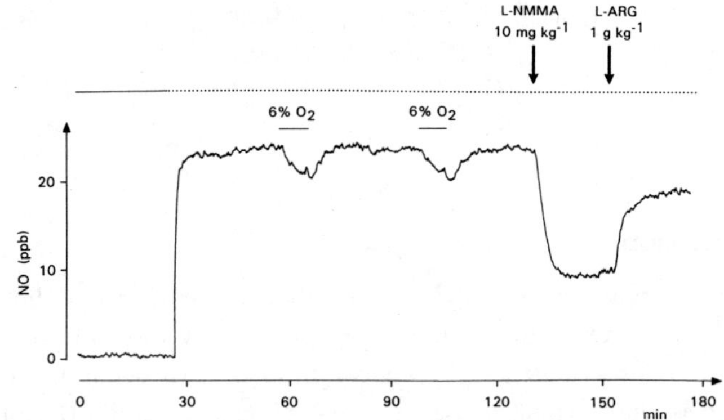

Fig. 2.   Exhaled nitric oxide measurement from inspired synthetic air (solid marker line) and from mixed exhaled air (dotted marker line) in an anesthetised ventilated rabbit. From Ref. 1.

could be used (Fig. 2). In these experiments it was definitely demonstrated that NO was present in the breath originating from L-arginine dependent synthesis (Fig. 2). Furthermore, it was found that NO was decreased by hypoxia, but only significantly at inspired concentrations of oxygen at or below 10 %. This means that NO formation will be maintained as long as the oxygen concentration in the alveolar air is sufficient for normal oxygenation of the blood. Below these oxygen concentrations, NO formation decreases, and lowering of the NO concentration will now work to enhance the hypoxic vasoconstriction. Thus, NO will act as a servo mechanism for hypoxic vasoconstriction, aiding in optimizing ventilation–perfusion matching, which supports the initial suggestion[2] that endogenous NO formation is necessary for normal oxygenation of the blood. To argue that NO improves perfusion in hypoxic lung areas, or that the lack of NO decreases perfusion, or that NO synthase inhibitors are pulmonary vasoconstrictors is thus far too simplistic. Instead, the dynamics of the system must be considered. For example, a pulmonary vasoconstrictor might act to decrease pulmonary perfusion in general, whereas an NO synthase inhibitor will decrease pulmonary perfusion more in areas where NO synthesis is high, levelling out the regional differences in pulmonary perfusion, a notion supported by recent data in humans.[4]

2. Exhaled NO in Asthma; Initial Studies

In the initial publication on exhaled NO[1] it was suggested that NO in breath might originate both from regulatory (constitutive) systems as well as being induced by external influences. Thus, it was conceived by several groups that changes in exhaled NO might be seen in asthma. This has been demonstrated both in an animal model,[5] and in humans.[6-8] Interestingly, the study by Persson *et al.*[8] demonstrated a tentative clinical value of these observations in that increased NO was observed in a patient group measured for breath NO during routine visits to a specialist outpatient clinic. An important observation was also made at that time, namely that exhaled NO was decreased by administration of inhaled corticosteroids.[7]

3. Identity of Exhaled NO

How do we know that we measure NO in breath and not something else? The first publication established the presence of NO by three independent methods: (1) chemiluminescence from its reaction with ozone, (2) formation of nitrite when captured into water, and (3) mass spectrometry after capture by a reagent. The stereoselective nitric oxide synthase (NOS) inhibitor that abolishes the chemiluminescence reactivity was also strong supportive evidence. The discovery of exhaled NO in breath was also confirmed by another research group[9] working independently and initially without knowledge of the results of the first group. Finally, a direct demonstration of NO in breath was made by gas chromatography–mass spectrometry (GC-MS)[10] by separating the NO from other gaseous species with molecular weight of 30 dalton (*e.g.* $^{15}N^{15}N$ nitrogen gas present in ppm-amounts in normal air) using sub-zero temperature gradients for the gas chromatographic separations. It might be that the GC-MS identification of exhaled NO is the first unequivocal demonstration of the presence of the gas NO in biological systems, a matter of much debate in the late '80s and early '90s when the effects of EDRF (endothelium-derived relaxing factor, the bioactivity preceding the discovery of biological NO formation) by several investigators was argued to be a nitrosothiol or an ionized form of NO.[11-19]

4. Impact of the Discovery of Exhaled NO

Since the discovery of the value of exhaled NO measurements in asthmatics, the field has exploded and there is now more than 1000 papers on exhaled nitric oxide in the literature. Thus, it is beyond the scope of this chapter to give a detailed review of the whole field, and the reader is referred to some recent publications[20-22] and to other chapters in this book. A potentially very important development is the realisation of the secretion of and the possibility to measure NO and other gases in naturally or intentionally gas-filled compartments of the body other than the lung.[23,24] A summary of some important steps in the development of exhaled NO measurements are given in Table 1, which is presented for the convenience of the reader and on the condition that the reader accepts that important work, more likely than not, has been omitted due to the lack of space. Additional tabulated summaries on exhaled NO and which the reader might find useful are available.[25-27]

The announcement in 1991 that NO is present in exhaled breath has lead to an intensive development in exhaled breath analysis. The main goal has been to explore the utility of exhaled NO, especially in the field of asthma research. Other markers have also been studied with the aim of improving the diagnosis of pulmonary disease. Only modest attention has been paid to the criteria for identification of exhaled breath markers. Furthermore, when a method has been developed to identify an exhaled breath marker it should be realised that the instruments or methods used are still experimental. Only when methods and instruments fully validated for clinical use are at hand can the necessary clinical trials be performed that will determine if a marker gives useful clinical information in a regular clinical setting. Today, this has only been achieved for exhaled NO as an indicator of inflammation in asthma. Thus, a registered value for NO outside of the normal limits should not be regarded as a diagnostic criterion, but rather as an aid or complementary to monitoring and diagnosis. The same will apply *e.g.* for ammonia in renal disease and acetone in diabetes.

5. What Characterizes an Exhaled Respiratory System Marker?

It has to be realised that rather rigid criteria have to be applied for a marker of airway disease, discriminating it from other endogenous body gases or from exhaled gases of exogenous origin excreted after prior environmental exposure. Furthermore, the marker method has to offer advantages compared with presently used methods for diagnosis or monitoring. Some

Table 1. Selected first and other important early publications on exhaled nitric oxide

Nitric oxide present in exhaled breath of animals and man
  Gustafsson *et al.*, 1991[1]
  Borland *et al.*, 1993[9]

Nitric oxide demonstrated to be present in breath by more than one technique or by gas chromatography-mass spectrometry:
  Gustafsson *et al.*, 1991[1]
  Leone *et al.*, 1994[10]

Exhaled nitric oxide measured in single exhalations and identification of airway origin
  Persson *et al.*, 1993[28]

Exhaled nitric oxide concentrations increased in human asthma
  Alving *et al.*, 1993[6]
  Kharitonov *et al.*, 1994[7]
  Persson *et al.*, 1994[8]

Nasal and sinus origin of NO and the decrease in Kartagener's syndrome
  Lundberg *et al.*, 1994[29]
  Lundberg *et al.*, 1995[23,30]

Exhaled nitric oxide increased by allergen challenge in animals or man
  Persson & Gustafsson, 1993[5]
    (acute effects in guinea-pigs)
  Kharitonov *et al.*, 1995[31]
    (late phase reaction in humans)

Exhaled nitric oxide decreased by inhaled steroids and correlated with eosinophils
  Kharitonov *et al.*, 1994[7]
  Jatakanon *et al.*, 1998[32]

Increased nitric oxide in gas sampled from the lower airways of asthmatics
  Massaro *et al.*, 1996[33]

Flow regulation and exhaled nitric oxide
  Högman *et al.*, 1997[34]
  Silkoff *et al.*, 1997[35]

Guidelines for standardised measurements of exhaled nitric oxide
  Kharitonov *et al.*, 1997[36]
  ATS recommendations, 1999[37]

Nitric oxide present in exhaled gas from isolated lungs, and regulated by respiratory gases
  Gustafsson *et al.*, 1991[1]
  Cremona *et al.*, 1994[38]
  Persson *et al.*, 1994[39]
  Adding *et al.*, 1999[40]

Exhaled nitric oxide excretion increased by exercise
  Persson *et al.*, 1993[28]
  Mills *et al.*, 1996[41]

Stretch or high frequency ventilation stimulating exhaled nitric oxide
  Persson *et al.*, 1995[42]
  Strömberg *et al.*, 1997[43]
  Artlich *et al.*, 1999[44]

Increase in ventilation, but not in cardiac output, increases exhaled nitric oxide
  Mehta *et al.*, 1997[45]

Decrease in exhaled nitric oxide by inhalation of nitric oxide inhibitor in humans
  Kharitonov *et al.*, 1994[7]
  Yates *et al.*, 1995[46]

Decrease in exhaled nitric oxide by more than 50% in humans by systemic nitric oxide inhibition
  Krejcy *et al.*, 1995[47]
  Albert *et al.*, 1997[48]
  Schmetterer *et al.*, 1997[49]
  Jilma *et al.*, 1998[50]
  Rimcika *et al.*, 2004[4]

Tuberculosis increases exhaled nitric oxide
  Wang *et al.*, 1998[51]

Increase in exhaled nitric oxide by endotoxin in humans
  Soop *et al.*, 2003[52]

Table 2.   Criteria for an airway-specific exhaled marker

Optimal marker characteristics
- Relation to (but not identical with) other more difficult markers/methods
- Clinical value (correlation to disease/treatment efficacy)
- Patient friendly = "noninvasive"
- Rapid method
- Immediate results

Necessary marker characteristics
- Defined molecule and its formation
- Identity in breath confirmed by two independent methods
- Airway specific
  - Airway "peak concentration" (dead space > alveolar concentration), especially upon breath hold
  - Airflow-dependent breath concentration
- Not excreted from distant organs ("gut/liver" problem)
- Not excreted from environmental pre-exposure/contamination

---

optimal and necessary breath marker criteria or characteristics may be suggested (Table 2) for an exhaled marker of airway disease.

Correspondingly, the necessary characteristics may be changed for a marker of alveolar or otherwise localised disease. Thus, excretion of the airway marker NO is dependent on exhalation flow rate, whereas an alveolar marker should be flow-independent in its concentration, and should only increase in concentration during breath hold in proportion to its formation rate in alveoli or its delivery by the blood to the lung. An alveolar marker should be independent of airflow in single exhalations made from breathing at rest. A defined formation process should be demonstrable at the claimed site of formation. Even so, other sources of exhaled marker have to be considered (Fig. 3). For example, salivary contribution can be considerable, especially after ingestion of certain foodstuffs. In the case of NO, ingested nitrite can be non-enzymatically reduced to NO or, in saliva, nitrate can through bacterial action and pH cycle to nitrite and then NO.[53,54] Inhalation of NO synthase inhibitor markedly reduces exhaled NO,[7,46] and recent data show that in normal individuals more than 70 % of exhaled NO is blocked by systemic administration of a submaximal dose of NO synthase inhibitor,[4] underlining the usefulness of exhaled NO measurements if precautions are taken concerning nitrite/nitrate ingestion.

By mathematical modeling of NO excretion employing within-breath or between-breath changes of exhalation flow rates, it has been argued that alveolar concentrations of NO can be determined[55] and separated from airway excretion. In the mind of the present author these calculations need to take into consideration the fractal division of the airways and the different surface-to-volume ratios in the central and peripheral airways, and if so done it could well be that it is realized that what is now described as alveolar NO is in fact NO from very peripheral airways, at least in healthy individuals. This does not exclude that such calculations can be of value in the detection of pulmonary disease, but the origin of the change in peripheral NO will then have to be further elucidated. If alveolar NO

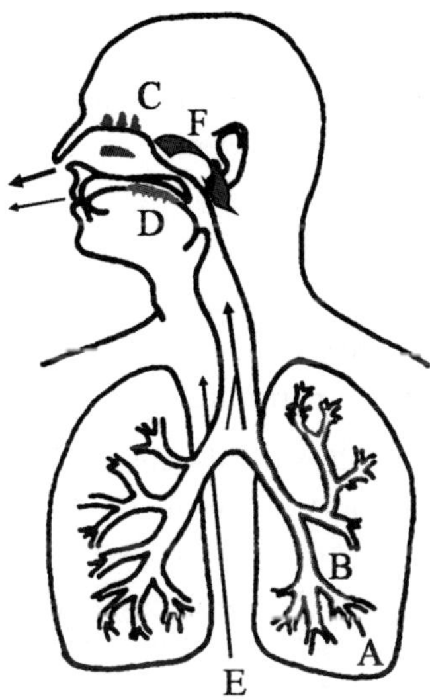

Fig. 3.   Sources of exhaled NO. Nitric oxide in expired air originates from enzymatically-formed NO (NO synthases; NOS) in alveoli (A), small and medium-sized airways (bronchioli and bronchi; B), enzymatically formed NO (mainly iNOS) from the paranasal sinuses and to some extent the nasal cavity (C), enzymatic (NOS) and non-enzymatic-derived NO (nitrite conversion to NO) from the oral cavity (D), and high concentrations of non-enzymatically-formed NO (salivary nitrite converted to NO by gastric acidity) can be intermittently regurgitated from stomach gas (E) via the esophagus, especially during strong forced expiration or exercise. Sinus-derived NO is auto inhaled during inspiration (F) and is rapidly taken up in the alveoli. Alveolar air is usually very low in NO due to the rapid uptake and scavenging of NO by red blood cell hemoglobin in pulmonary capillaries. Nasal and gastric NO contamination is minimized by exhalation against moderate resistance (soft palate closure) and by dumping of initial (dead space) exhalate gas during a single expiration. An adequate sampling of lower airway NO can thus be obtained, but requires that the expiration is not unduly forced, to minimize (E). Non-enzymatic oral NO formation can be minimized by avoiding nitrate/nitrite-rich foodstuffs and/or by mouthwash. Allergic airway inflammation (right-hand lung) will give a reproducible increase in lower airway NO measurable at the mouth if exhalations with standardized controlled exhalation rate[37] are performed. In the ideal case, orally exhaled NO is mainly derived from NOS activity, which is supported by recent data.[4]

appears in exhaled air, this probably requires that the alveoli in question are very poorly perfused or have a severely decreased diffusion capacity, preventing NO uptake into the blood. The importance of studying flow variations in exhaled gas concentrations is evident from recent data, which suggest that exhaled carbon monoxide is not a marker of airway inflammation in asthma,[56] despite several reports suggesting its usefulness for this,[57–59] which would seem logical since CO-forming heme oxygenase is induced in inflamed airways. An explanation for the differences in results may be that patients included in the early studies were inadvertently exposed to environmental CO, or had severe lung pathology preventing CO uptake to alveolar capillaries. If environmental exposure be excluded, and if more highly time-resolved single breath measurements can be made, the situation might again turn in favor of some role of CO measurements in airway inflammation.

6. Some Notes on Technique and Technologies for Exhaled NO Measurements

In 1993 the technique of single breath measurements (Fig. 4) was introduced,[28] and this still prevails as the method of choice. The method of controlling exhalation flow rate is a further improvement.[34,35] Consensus documents with specifications on how a standardized technique is obtained have been published.[36,37] Apart from the currently dominant chemiluminescence technique a recent advancement has been made in electrochemical detection, allowing miniaturized hand-held devices.[60] This will at least

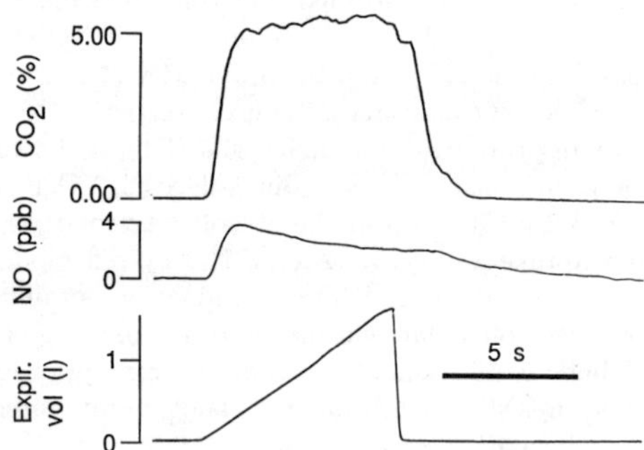

Fig. 4.   Single-breath measurement of exhaled CO_2 (top trace) and NO (middle trace) concomitant with recording of exhaled volume (bottom trace) in a healthy male individual exhaling at approximately 200 mL/s (from Ref. 28).

take the exhaled NO measurements into the "doctor's office" setting and most likely also into home use, and must be regarded as a unique event in diagnostic methods, since it is the first breath method that aims at diagnosing or treating disease in the general population. Another detection technology has been tried, using conversion of NO to NO_2 combined with the hydrogen peroxide-enhanced luminescence reaction.[61] Laser technologies have been used for measurements of particles in exhaled breath[62] and are currently being investigated for detection of exhaled NO, CO, ammonia, ethane, and other volatiles[63–72] and this book contains further references thereto. The final target will be personal hand-held monitors, an objective under realization, but will require extensive documentation.[73] The capital investments for such endeavours should not be underestimated, and require patent protection to be commercially feasible so that they can reach the patient. Thus, the only EU Medical Devices Directive and FDA approved equipments for exhaled NO so far marketed have (November 2004) required investments exceeding 26 million euro, including costs for proof of concept studies and studies required by regulatory authorities. The technological advancement during such development is illustrated in Fig. 5, where it should be noted that the original instrument from 1991 is still one of the most sensitive (sensitivity below 1 ppb) but lacking in time resolution, impossible to adapt for clinical measurements and very demanding in user knowledge. The hand-held device weighs less than 1/100 of the 1991 equipment and is so user-friendly that it most likely can be used by patients in the home setting.

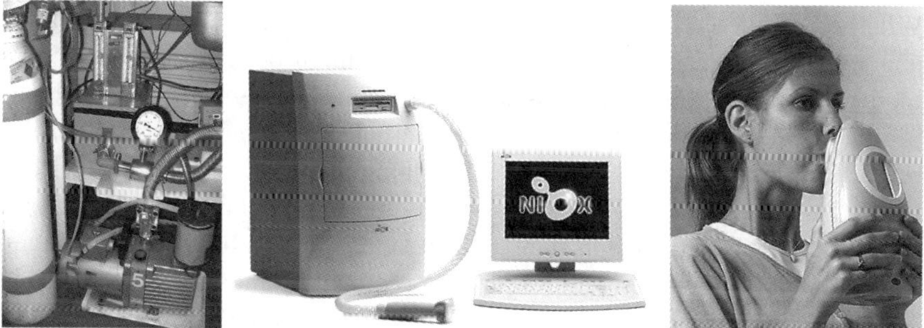

Fig. 5.   Development in exhaled NO measurement technologies; from purely experimental equipment in 1991 (left-hand panel; from Ref. 1), to clinically approved equipment in the EU and USA (middle panel, from Ref. 73), and hand held device (right hand panel; from Ref. 60) approved for clinical use in the EU. (Copyrights: Left-hand panel: the author; middle and right panels: Aerocrine AB)

7. Why Should We Measure Exhaled Nitric Oxide?

The clinical utility of exhaled NO measurements lies both as an adjunct to asthma diagnosis and in monitoring of treatment; see Table 1 and the reviews cited in the Introduction. Despite many publications on this subject we are only beginning to realize its practical impact and we should bear in mind that the true usefulness of exhaled measurements can only be evaluated by appropriate clinical trials, using equipment approved for such trials or for clinical use. The evaluation requires establishment of reproducibility criteria and of clinical cut-off limits for the intended population.[74,75] If NO measurements prove to be a useful aid in asthma control management[76] a whole new therapeutic scenario will evolve, using the exhaled measurements rather than symptom scores as the guiding index, the NO being measured by a personal NO monitor. In favour of such a development are reports that exhaled NO increase precedes bronchoconstriction.[77] Beyond asthma, there are several other conditions where exhaled NO measurements (either nasally or orally) will be of use, for example in Kartagener's syndrome, cystic fibrosis, and perhaps even in sinusitis.[23,25,29,30,78] Coughing is a trivial symptom in the mind of the healthy layman, but to the afflicted individual and the treating physician it can — in its chronic forms — be a severe problem. Exhaled NO measurements may well become a mainstay in evaluating coughing.[79]

8. Is Airway Production of NO a Protective System?

The increase in exhaled NO preceding asthma symptoms might suggest that exhaled NO is beneficial in asthma. Animal data are so far not conclusive. Whether an increase in airway NO production is protective or not might depend on the severity of the disease, where it might be protective in mild to moderate disease, but as the disease worsens an increase in oxygen radical production in more severe disease and lack of L-arginine substrate can be important decisive events leading to damaging peroxynitrite formation from the NO synthesis.[80–85] A detailed discussion is beyond the scope of this chapter and the challenge in such a discussion is illustrated by observations that inhaled NO synthesis inhibitor does not acutely modify asthma,[46] but NO inhibition may attenuate thermally induced asthma.[86]

9. Conclusions

The discovery of exhaled nitric oxide has opened a whole new field of research. The main reason is that it has been shown to constitute an organ-specific on-line biochemical measurement, and has been shown to be useful in a common disease, asthma, where a clinical need for evaluation of airway inflammation was already at hand and where NO measurement promises to fulfill this need, as seen from emerging technologies for personalized monitoring. As other exhaled markers are discovered the clinical need for their use has to be defined, as well as the technology and standardized procedures for their measurement. Fore-sighted patent protection and significant investor capital will be needed, as well as a structured regulatory strategy, in order for the new methods to reach larger patient groups.

Acknowledgements

Supported by the Swedish Science Council and the Swedish Heart-Lung Foundation. Competing interests: The author holds patents on exhaled nitric oxide technologies and is a minority shareholder in Aerocrine AB (publ.).

References

1. Gustafsson LE, Leone AM, Persson MG, Wiklund NP, Moncada S. Endogenous nitric oxide is present in the exhaled air of rabbits, guinea pigs and humans. *Biochem Biophys Res Commun* 1991; **181**: 852–857.
2. Persson MG, Gustafsson LE, Wiklund NP, Moncada S, Hedqvist P. Endogenous nitric oxide as a probable modulator of pulmonary circulation and hypoxic pressor response *in vivo*. *Acta Physiol Scand* 1990; **140**: 449–457.
3. von Euler U, Liljestrand G. Observations on the pulmonary arterial blood pressure in the cat. *Acta Physiol Scand* 1946; **12**: 301–320.
4. Rimeika D, Nyren S, Wiklund NP, Koskela LR, Torring A, Gustafsson LE, Larsson SA, Jacobsson H, Lindahl SG, and Wiklund CU. Regulation of regional lung perfusion by nitric oxide. *Am J Respir Crit Care Med* 2004; **170**: 450–455.
5. Persson MG, Gustafsson LE. Allergen-induced airway obstruction in guinea-pigs is associated with changes in nitric oxide levels in exhaled air. *Acta Physiol Scand* 1993; **149**: 461–466.
6. Alving K, Weitzberg E, Lundberg JM. Increased amount of nitric oxide in exhaled air of asthmatics. *Eur Respir J* 1993; **6**: 1368–1370.
7. Kharitonov SA, Yates D, Robbins RA, Logan-Sinclair R, Shinebourne EA, Barnes PJ. Increased nitric oxide in exhaled air of asthmatic patients. *Lancet* 1994; **343**: 133–135.
8. Persson MG, Zetterstrom O, Agrenius V, Ihre E, Gustafsson LE. Single-breath nitric oxide measurements in asthmatic patients and smokers. *Lancet* 1994; **343**: 146–147.
9. Borland C, Cox Y, Higenbottam T. Measurement of exhaled nitric oxide in man. *Thorax* 1993; **48**: 1160–1162.

10. Leone AM, Gustafsson LE, Francis PL, Persson MG, Wiklund NP, Moncada S. Nitric oxide is present in exhaled breath in humans: direct GC-MS confirmation. *Biochem Biophys Res Commun* 1994; **201**: 883–887.

11. Myers PR, Minor RL, Jr., Guerra R, Jr., Bates JN, Harrison DG. Vasorelaxant properties of the endothelium-derived relaxing factor more closely resemble *S*-nitrosocysteine than nitric oxide. *Nature* 1990; **345**: 161–163.

12. Vanin AF. Endothelium-derived relaxing factor is a nitrosyl iron complex with thiol ligands. *FEBS Lett* 1991; **289**: 1–3.

13. Vedernikov YP, Mordvintcev PI, Malenkova IV, Vanin AF. Similarity between the vasorelaxing activity of dinitrosyl iron cysteine complexes and endothelium-derived relaxing factor. *Eur J Pharmacol* 1992; **211**: 313–317.

14. Stamler JS, Singel DJ, Loscalzo J. Biochemistry of nitric oxide and its redox-activated forms. *Science* 1992; **258**: 1898–1902.

15. Mulsch A, Vanin A, Mordvintcev P, Hauschildt S, Busse R. NO accounts completely for the oxygenated nitrogen species generated by enzymic L-arginine oxygenation. *Biochem J* 1992; **288** (Pt 2): 597–603.

16. Kukreja RC, Wei EP, Kontos HA, Bates JN. Nitric oxide and *S*-nitroso-L-cysteine as endothelium-derived relaxing factors from acetylcholine in cerebral vessels in cats. *Stroke* 1993; **24**: 2010–2014; discussion 2014–2015.

17. Lipton SA, Choi YB, Pan ZH, Lei SZ, Chen HS, Sucher NJ, Loscalzo J, Singel DJ, Stamler JS. A redox-based mechanism for the neuroprotective and neurodestructive effects of nitric oxide and related nitroso-compounds. *Nature* 1993; **364**: 626–632.

18. Gibson A, Brave SR, McFadzean I, Tucker JF, Wayman C. The nitrergic transmitter of the anococcygeus — NO or not? *Arch Int Pharmacodyn Ther* 1995; **329**: 39–51.

19. Arnelle DR, Stamler JS. NO^+, NO, and NO^- donation by *S*-nitrosothiols: implications for regulation of physiological functions by *S*-nitrosylation and acceleration of disulfide formation. *Arch Biochem Biophys* 1995; **318**: 279–285.

20. Ricciardolo FL, Sterk PJ, Gaston B, Folkerts G. Nitric oxide in health and disease of the respiratory system. *Physiol Rev* 2004; **84**: 731–765.

21. Kharitonov SA. Exhaled markers of inflammatory lung diseases: ready for routine monitoring? *Swiss Med Wkly* 2004; **134**: 175–192.

22. Silkoff PE, Robbins RA, Gaston B, Lundberg JO, Townley RG. Endogenous nitric oxide in allergic airway disease. *J Allergy Clin Immunol* 2000; **105**: 438–448.

23. Lundberg JO, Lundberg JM, Settergren G, Alving K, Weitzberg E. Nitric oxide, produced in the upper airways, may act in an 'aerocrine' fashion to enhance pulmonary oxygen uptake in humans. *Acta Physiol Scand* 1995; **155**: 467–468.

24. Lundberg JO. Airborne nitric oxide: inflammatory marker and aerocrine messenger in man. *Acta Physiol Scand Suppl* 1996; **633**: 1–27.

25. Lundberg JO, Weitzberg E, Lundberg JM, Alving K. Nitric oxide in exhaled air. *Eur Respir J* 1996; **9**: 2671–2680.

26. Adding LC, Gustafsson LE. Physiology of exhaled nitric oxide. In: Marczin N, Kharitonov S, Yacoub M, Barnes P, eds. *Disease Markers in Exhaled Breath,* New York: Marcel Dekker Inc, 2002: 29–72.

27. Törnberg D. *Exhaled Nitric oxide — Influence of Mechanical Ventilation and Vasoactive Agents.* diss.kib.ki.se/info/database_content_en.html, Karolinska Institutet 2004: Stockholm.

28. Persson MG, Wiklund NP, Gustafsson LE. Endogenous nitric oxide in single exhalations and the change during exercise. *Am Rev Respir Dis* 1993; **148**: 1210–1214.

29. Lundberg JO, Weitzberg E, Nordvall SL, Kuylenstierna R, Lundberg JM, Alving K. Primarily nasal origin of exhaled nitric oxide and absence in Kartagener's syndrome. *Eur Respir J* 1994; **7**: 1501–1504.

30. Lundberg JO, Farkas-Szallasi T, Weitzberg E, Rinder J, Lidholm J, Anggaard A, Hokfelt T, Lundberg JM, Alving K. High nitric oxide production in human paranasal sinuses. *Nat Med* 1995; **1**: 370–373.

31. Kharitonov SA, O'Connor BJ, Evans DJ, Barnes PJ. Allergen-induced late asthmatic reactions are associated with elevation of exhaled nitric oxide. *Am J Respir Crit Care Med* 1995; **151**: 1894–1899.

32. Jatakanon A, Lim S, Kharitonov SA, Chung KF, Barnes PJ. Correlation between exhaled nitric oxide, sputum eosinophils, and methacholine responsiveness in patients with mild asthma. *Thorax* 1998; **53**: 91–95.

33. Massaro AF, Mehta S, Lilly CM, Kobzik L, Reilly JJ, Drazen JM. Elevated nitric oxide concentrations in isolated lower airway gas of asthmatic subjects. *Am J Respir Crit Care Med* 1996; **153**: 1510–1514.

34. Högman M, Strömberg S, Schedin U, Frostell C, Hedenstierna G, Gustafsson LE. Nitric oxide from the human respiratory tract efficiently quantified by standardized single breath measurements. *Acta Physiol Scand* 1997; **159**: 345–346.

35. Silkoff PE, McClean PA, Slutsky AS, Furlott HG, Hoffstein E, Wakita S, Chapman KR, Szalai JP, Zamel N. Marked flow-dependence of exhaled nitric oxide using a new technique to exclude nasal nitric oxide. *Am J Respir Crit Care Med* 1997; **155**: 260–267.

36. Kharitonov S, Alving K, Barnes PJ. Exhaled and nasal nitric oxide measurements: recommendations. The European Respiratory Society Task Force. *Eur Respir J* 1997; **10**: 1683–1693.

37. Recommendations for standardized procedures for the on-line and off-line measurement of exhaled lower respiratory nitric oxide and nasal nitric oxide in adults and children-1999. This official statement of the American Thoracic Society was adopted by the ATS Board of Directors, July 1999. *Am J Respir Crit Care Med* 1999; **160**: 2104–2117.

38. Cremona G, Wood AM, Hall LW, Bower EA, Higenbottam T. Effect of inhibitors of nitric oxide release and action on vascular tone in isolated lungs of pig, sheep, dog and man. *J Physiol* 1994; **481** (Pt 1): 185–195.

39. Persson MG, Midtvedt T, Leone AM, Gustafsson LE. Ca^{2+}-dependent and Ca^{2+}-independent exhaled nitric oxide, presence in germ-free animals, and inhibition by arginine analogues. *Eur J Pharmacol* 1994; **264**: 13–20.

40. Adding LC, Agvald P, Persson MG, Gustafsson LE. Regulation of pulmonary nitric oxide by carbon dioxide is intrinsic to the lung. *Acta Physiol Scand* 1999; **167**: 167–174.

41. Mills PC, Marlin DJ, Demoncheaux E, Scott C, Casas I, Smith NC, Higenbottam T. Nitric oxide and exercise in the horse. *J Physiol* 1996; **495** (Pt 3): 863–874.

42. Persson MG, Lönnqvist PA, Gustafsson LE. Positive end-expiratory pressure ventilation elicits increases in endogenously formed nitric oxide as detected in air exhaled by rabbits. *Anesthesiology* 1995; **82**: 969–974.

43. Strömberg S, Lönnqvist PA, Persson MG, Gustafsson LE. Lung distension and carbon dioxide affect pulmonary nitric oxide formation in the anaesthetized rabbit. *Acta Physiol Scand* 1997; **159**: 59–67.

44. Artlich A, Adding C, Agvald P, Persson MG, Lönnqvist PA, Gustafsson LE. Exhaled nitric oxide increases during high frequency oscillatory ventilation in rabbits. *Exp Physiol* 1999; **84**: 959–969.

45. Mehta S, Magder S, Levy RD. The effects of changes in ventilation and cardiac output on expired nitric oxide. *Chest* 1997; **111**: 1045–1049.

46. Yates DH, Kharitonov SA, Robbins RA, Thomas PS, Barnes PJ. Effect of a nitric oxide synthase inhibitor and a glucocorticosteroid on exhaled nitric oxide. *Am J Respir Crit Care Med* 1995; **152**: 892–896.

47. Krejcy K, Schmetterer L, Kastner J, Nieszpaur-Los M, Monitzer B, Schutz W, Eichler HG, Kyrle PA. Role of nitric oxide in hemostatic system activation *in vivo* in humans. *Arterioscler Thromb Vasc Biol* 1995; **15**: 2063–2067.

48. Albert J, Schedin U, Lindqvist M, Melcher A, Hjemdahl P, Frostell C. Blockade of endogenous nitric oxide production results in moderate hypertension, reducing sympathetic activity and shortening bleeding time in healthy volunteers. *Acta Anaesthesiol Scand* 1997; **41**: 1104–1113.

49. Schmetterer L, Krejcy K, Kastner J, Wolzt M, Gouya G, Findl O, Lexer F, Breiteneder H, Fercher AF, Eichler HG. The effect of systemic nitric oxide-synthase inhibition on ocular fundus pulsations in man. *Exp Eye Res* 1997; **64**: 305–312.

50. Jilma B, Pernerstorfer T, Dirnberger E, Stohlawetz P, Schmetterer L, Singer EA, Grasseli U, Eichler HG, Kapiotis S. Effects of histamine and nitric oxide synthase inhibition on plasma levels of von Willebrand factor antigen. *J Lab Clin Med* 1998; **131**: 151–156.

51. Wang CH, Liu CY, Lin HC, Yu CT, Chung KF, Kuo HP. Increased exhaled nitric oxide in active pulmonary tuberculosis due to inducible NO synthase upregulation in alveolar macrophages. *Eur Respir J* 1998; **11**: 809–815.

52. Soop A, Sollevi A, Weitzberg E, Lundberg JO, Palm J, Albert J. Exhaled NO and plasma cGMP increase after endotoxin infusion in healthy volunteers. *Eur Respir J* 2003; **21**: 594–599.

53. Zetterquist W, Pedroletti C, Lundberg JO, Alving K. Salivary contribution to exhaled nitric oxide. *Eur Respir J* 1999; **13**: 327–333.

54. Lundberg JO, Weitzberg E, Cole JA, Benjamin N. Nitrate, bacteria and human health. *Nat Rev Microbiol* 2004; **2**: 593–602.

55. George SC, Högman M, Permutt S, Silkoff PE. Modeling pulmonary nitric oxide exchange. *J Appl Physiol* 2004; **96**: 831–839.

56. Zetterquist W, Marteus H, Johannesson M, Nordval SL, Ihre E, Lundberg JO, Alving K. Exhaled carbon monoxide is not elevated in patients with asthma or cystic fibrosis. *Eur Respir J* 2002; **20**: 92–99.

57. Paredi P, Leckie MJ, Horvath I, Allegra L, Kharitonov SA, Barnes PJ. Changes in exhaled carbon monoxide and nitric oxide levels following allergen challenge in patients with asthma. *Eur Respir J* 1999; **13**: 48–52.

58. Yamaya M, Sekizawa K, Ishizuka S, Monma M, Sasaki H. Exhaled carbon monoxide levels during treatment of acute asthma. *Eur Respir J* 1999; **13**: 757–760.

59. Zayasu K, Sekizawa K, Okinaga S, Yamaya M, Ohrui T, Sasaki H. Increased carbon monoxide in exhaled air of asthmatic patients. *Am J Respir Crit Care Med* 1997; **156**: 1140–1143.

60. Hemmingsson T, Linnarsson D, Gambert R. Novel hand-held device for exhaled nitric oxide-analysis in research and clinical applications. *J Clin Monit Comput* 2005: in press.

61. Robinson JK, Bollinger MJ, Birks JW. Luminol/H_2O_2 chemiluminescence detector for the analysis of nitric oxide in exhaled breath. *Anal Chem* 1999; **71**: 5131–5136.

62. Fairchild CI, Stampfer JF. Particle concentration in exhaled breath. *Am Ind Hyg Assoc J* 1987; **48**: 948–949.

63. Lee PS, Majkowski RF, Perry TA. Tunable diode laser spectroscopy for isotope analysis — detection of isotopic carbon monoxide in exhaled breath. *IEEE Trans Biomed Eng* 1991; **38**: 966–973.

64. Skrupskii VA, Stepanov VE, Shulagin Iu A. Monitoring of endogenous carbon monoxide elimination in exhaled air of rats in hyperoxia. *Aviakosm Ekolog Med* 1995; **29**: 49–52.

65. Mürtz P, Menzel L, Bloch W, Hess A, Michel O, Urban W. LMR spectroscopy: a new sensitive method for on-line recording of nitric oxide in breath. *J Appl Physiol* 1999; **86**: 1075–1080.

66. Menzel L, Kosterev AA, Curl RF, Tittel FK, Gmachl C, Capasso F, Sivco DL, Baillargeon JN, Hutchinson AL, Cho AY, Urban W. Spectroscopic detection of biological NO with a quantum cascade laser. *Appl Phys B* 2001; **72**: 859 863.

67. Roller C, Namjou K, Jeffers JD, Camp M, Mock A, McCann PJ, Grego J. Nitric oxide breath testing by tunable-diode laser absorption spectroscopy: application in monitoring respiratory inflammation. *Appl Opt* 2002; **41**: 6018–6029.

68. von Basum G, Dahnke H, Halmer D, Hering P, Mürtz M. Online recording of ethane traces in human breath via infrared laser spectroscopy. *J Appl Physiol* 2003; **95**: 2583–2590.

69. Webber ME, Pushkarsky M, Patel CK. Fiber-amplifier-enhanced photoacoustic spectroscopy with near-infrared tunable diode lasers. *Appl Opt* 2003; **42**: 2119–2126.

70. Bakhirkin YA, Kosterev AA, Roller C, Curl RF, Tittel FK. Mid-infrared quantum cascade laser based off-axis integrated cavity output spectroscopy for biogenic nitric oxide detection. *Appl Opt* 2004; **43**: 2257–2266.

71. Menzel L, Hess A, Bloch W, Michel O, Schuster KD, Gabler R, Urban W. Temporal Nitric Oxide Dynamics in the Paranasal Sinuses during Humming. *J Appl Physiol* 2005.

72. Tanahashi T, Kodama T, Yamaoka Y, Sawai N, Tatsumi Y, Kashima K, Higashi Y, Sasaki Y. Analysis of the ^{13}C-urea breath test for detection of Helicobacter pylori infection based on the kinetics of delta-[13]CO_2 using laser spectroscopy. *J Gastroenterol Hepatol* 1998; **13**: 732–737.

73. Silkoff PE, Carlson M, Bourke T, Katial R, Ögren E, Szefler SJ. The Aerocrine exhaled nitric oxide monitoring system NIOX is cleared by the US Food and Drug Administration for monitoring therapy in asthma. *J Allergy Clin Immunol* 2004; **114**: 1241–1256.

74. Kharitonov SA, Gonio F, Kelly C, Meah S, Barnes PJ. Reproducibility of exhaled nitric oxide measurements in healthy and asthmatic adults and children. *Eur Respir J* 2003; **21**: 433–438.

75. Olin AC, Alving K, Toren K. Exhaled nitric oxide: relation to sensitization and respiratory symptoms. *Clin Exp Allergy* 2004; **34**: 221–226.

76. Delgado-Corcoran C, Kissoon N, Murphy SP, Duckworth LJ. Exhaled nitric oxide reflects asthma severity and asthma control. *Pediatr Crit Care Med* 2004; **5**: 48–52.

77. Steerenberg PA, van Amsterdam JG. Measurement of exhaled nitric oxide. *Methods Mol Biol* 2004; **279**: 45–68.

78. Maniscalco M, Sofia M, Weitzberg E, De Laurentiis G, Stanziola A, Rossillo V, Lundberg JO. Humming-induced release of nasal nitric oxide for assessment of sinus obstruction in allergic rhinitis: pilot study. *Eur J Clin Invest* 2004; **34**: 555–560.

79. Chatkin JM, Ansarin K, Silkoff PE, McClean P, Gutierrez C, Zamel N, Chapman KR. Exhaled nitric oxide as a noninvasive assessment of chronic cough. *Am J Respir Crit Care Med* 1999; **159**: 1810–1813.

80. Ricciardolo FL, Geppetti P, Mistretta A, Nadel JA, Sapienza MA, Bellofiore S, Di Maria GU. Randomised double-blind placebo-controlled study of the effect of inhibition of nitric oxide synthesis in bradykinin-induced asthma. *Lancet* 1996; **348**: 374–377.

81. Ricciardolo FL, Di Maria GU, Mistretta A, Sapienza MA, Geppetti P. Impairment of bronchoprotection by nitric oxide in severe asthma. *Lancet* 1997; **350**: 1297–1298.

82. Ricciardolo FL, Timmers MC, Geppetti P, van Schadewijk A, Brahim JJ, Sont JK, de Gouw HW, Hiemstra PS, van Krieken JH, Sterk PJ. Allergen-induced impairment of bronchoprotective nitric oxide synthesis in asthma. *J Allergy Clin Immunol* 2001; **108**: 198–204.

83. Meurs H, Maarsingh H, Zaagsma J. Arginase and asthma: novel insights into nitric oxide homeostasis and airway hyperresponsiveness. *Trends Pharmacol Sci* 2003; **24**: 450–455.

84. Ricciardolo FL, Timmers MC, Sont JK, Folkerts G, Sterk PJ. Effect of bradykinin on allergen induced increase in exhaled nitric oxide in asthma. *Thorax* 2003; **58**: 840–845.

85. Ricciardolo FL. Multiple roles of nitric oxide in the airways. *Thorax* 2003; **58**: 175–182.

86. Kotaru C, Skowronski M, Coreno A, McFadden ER, Jr. Inhibition of nitric oxide synthesis attenuates thermally induced asthma. *J Appl Physiol* 2001; **91**: 703–708.

NITRIC OXIDE IN EXHALED BREATH: A WINDOW ON LUNG PHYSIOLOGY AND PULMONARY DISEASE

R. A. DWEIK

Department of Pulmonary, Allergy, and Critical Care Medicine,
The Cleveland Clinic Foundation, A90,
9500 Euclid Ave, Cleveland, OH 44195, USA

1. Introduction

In 1987, endothelial derived relaxing factor, EDRF, was identified as nitric oxide (NO).[1,2] Since then, there has been an explosion in our knowledge about the role of NO in mammalian physiology and pathology. NO is present in virtually all mammalian organ systems and is present in the exhaled breath of humans. While NO has long been known as an atmospheric pollutant present in vehicle exhaust emissions and cigarette smoke, its clinical importance as a biological mediator in animals and humans has recently been the focus of intensive research. NO is a gaseous molecule that contains an unpaired electron (a free radical). It is extremely lipophilic and readily diffuses across membranes down its concentration gradient. As a result of its chemical structure, the unpaired electron confers considerable reactivity to the molecule, which accounts for many of its biological effect.[3,4]

NO is endogenously synthesized by nitric oxide synthases (NOSs) which convert L-arginine to L-citrulline and NO in the presence of oxygen and several cofactors. Three NOSs (NOS I, NOS II, and NOS III) have been identified and are widely expressed in various tissues including the lungs. Once produced, NO is freely diffusible and enters target cells activating soluble guanylate cyclase to produce guanosine $3',5'$-cyclic monophosphate (cGMP) which mediates the majority of NO effects. NO also diffuses into the airway and can be detected in exhaled breath of all humans. NO is formed in high concentrations in the upper respiratory tract (nasopharynx and paranasal sinuses). Our studies have also conclusively demonstrated that the lower respiratory tract is a significant source of NO in exhaled breath. Furthermore, we demonstrated that the pulmonary circulation serves as a biologic sink for NO, and is not likely to contribute to NO in exhaled breath.

The functions and effects of NO in the lung/airways reflect its key roles as a vasodilator, bronchodilator, neurotransmitter, and inflammatory mediator. The unique lung anatomy with the close proximity of the airways to the blood vessels allows NO that is produced in high levels in the upper and lower airways by NOS II to affect the pulmonary vascular tone in concert with the low NO levels that are produced by NOS III in the vascular endothelium. We have demonstrated that endogenous NO levels in the lung change rapidly in direct proportion to inspired oxygen which strongly supports a critical role for NO as mediator of ventilation–perfusion coupling in the lung.

NO also plays a major role in the pathophysiology of lung disease. Patients with pulmonary hypertension have low levels of NO while patients with asthma have high levels of exhaled NO in their exhaled breath suggesting a role for NO in the pathogenesis of these diseases.

2. Nitric Oxide Synthesis and Metabolism

NO is synthesized from the semi-essential amino acid L-arginine in a reaction that is catalyzed by nitric oxide synthases (NOS). These enzymes convert the amino acid L-arginine to NO and L-citrulline (Fig. 1) in the presence of oxygen and other cofactors which include nicotinamide adenine dinucleotide phosphate (NADPH), flavin adenine dinucleotide (FAD), flavin mononucleotide (FMN), tetrahydrobiopterin, and calmodulin.[3–6]

Three distinct isoforms of NOS have been identified (Table 1). The genes for these NOS isoforms have been localized to chromosomes 7 (eNOS), 12 (nNOS) and 17 (iNOS). NOS I or nNOS is a constitutive form, which is dependent on Ca^{2+} and calmodulin and found in neuronal tissue, both centrally and peripherally. NOS III or eNOS is a Ca^{2+}/calmodulin requiring constitutive enzyme present in vascular endothelial cells. NOS II or iNOS is a Ca^{2+}-independent form isolated from respiratory epithelial cells or other cells following induction with specific cytokines. Type I and III are termed constitutive nitric oxide synthases (cNOS) and release picomoles of NO within seconds or minutes in response to receptor stimulation by agonists such as acetylcholine, bradykinin, and histamine. Agonists activate cNOS via a rapid increase in intracellular calcium concentration. NOS II is the major NOS protein expressed in normal human airway epithelium, and generates up to 1,000 times more NO than cNOS (nanomolar levels).[3–7]

Table 1. Nitric oxide synthase enzymes

NOS Isoforms	Other Designation	Expression	Sources	Regulation	NO Output	Chromosome
Type I	nNOS	Constitutive	Cytosol of neuronal cells	Calcium/CaM	Low (picomol)	12
Type II	iNOS	Inducible	Macrophages, vascular smooth muscle, vascular endothelium, myocardium, endocardium hepatocytes, immune cells	Induced by cytokines, endotoxin, and oxidants	High (nanomol)	17
Type III	eNOS	Constitutive	Vascular endothelial cells, platelets, myocardium endocardium, mast cells, neutrophils	Calcium/CaM	Low (picomol)	7

NO: nitric oxide; NOS: nitric oxide synthase; nNOS: neural nitric oxide synthase; iNOS, inducible nitric oxide synthase; eNOS: endothelial nitric oxide synthase; CaM: Calmoduline

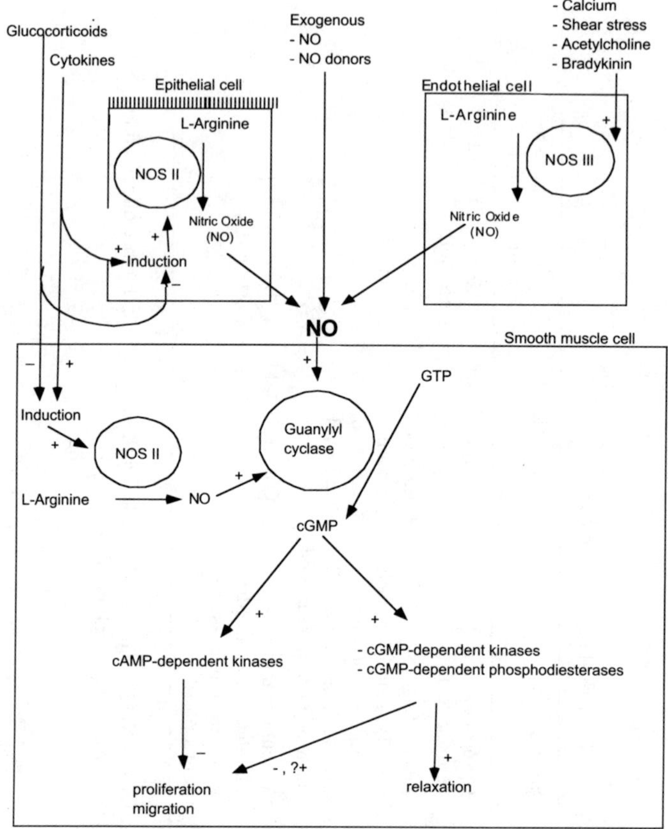

Fig. 1.   Arginine-NOS-NO-cGMP pathway

NOS converts L-arginine to citrulline and NO in the presence of NADPH and molecular oxygen as cosubstrates. Flavoproteins (FAD, FMN) and tetrahydrobiopterin (BH_4) are the other cofactors which the reaction requires. NOS I and NOS III are expressed in neuronal and endothelial cells, and are dependent on increases in intracellular calcium to bind calmodulin (CaM), which result in enzyme activation. NOS II is calcium independent, binds CaM intracellularly, even at low calcium concentrations. All NOS can be inhibited by arginine analogs. NO activates guanylyl cyclase, leading to an increase in intracellular cGMP concentration, which then causes smooth muscle relaxation.

NOS I and NOS III are expressed in neuronal and endothelial cells, and are dependent on increases in intracellular calcium to bind calmodulin (CaM), which result in enzyme activation. NOS II is calcium independent, binds CaM even at low calcium concentrations intracellularly. All NOS can be inhibited by arginine analogs. NO activates guanylyl cyclase, leading to an increase in intracellular cGMP concentration, which then causes smooth muscle relaxation.

Following an appropriate stimulus, such as IFN-γ, interleukin (IL)-1β, tumor necrosis factor-alpha (TNF-α), endotoxin or exotoxin, NOS II is induced in the relevant cell type by gene transcription. This process can be inhibited by glucocorticosteroids (Fig. 1).

Once NO is formed it diffuses into the effector cell and activates guanylate cyclase resulting in increased amounts of cyclic guanosine monophosphate (cGMP) which leads to activation of the cGMP-dependent protein kinase, the mediator of smooth muscle relaxation (Fig. 1). These biochemical events mediate the potent vasodilatory effects of nitric oxide and provide a signaling mechanism by which intravascular stimuli modulate vascular tone and blood flow.[8] NO can also activate soluble guanylate cyclase in platelets, attenuating platelet aggregation and adhesion. In contrast, the reaction of NO with protein bound iron in the mitochondrial respiratory chain and nuclear DNA synthesizing enzymes of microorganisms inhibits their activities and contributes to microbial killing and host defense.[4,5] Table 2 lists selected biologic functions of NO in different biologic systems.

Table 2.   Selected biologic functions of nitric oxide

Target System	Biologic Function	Mechanism
Vascular system	Vascular smooth muscle relaxation	Increased cGMP formation
Brain	Neural messenger	Mediates the action of glutamate acting at N-methyl-D-aspartate (NMDA) receptors
Inflammatory system	Anti-inflammatory effect	Decrease in lymphocyte (Th1) activation, scavenging superoxide
	Pro-inflammatory effect	Increase in leukocyte migration, indirect increase in Th2 lymphocytes and eosinophils, peroxynitritrite-mediated tissue injury
Host defense	Participate host defense	NO and/or its oxides such as NO_2 (nitrogen dioxide), N_2O_3 (dinitrogen trioxide) and $ONOO^-$ (peroxynitrite) can produce bactericidal and cytotoxic effects
Lungs (see Table 3)	Bronchodilation	Functions as a neurotransmitter of the iNANC bronchodilator response
	Airway obstruction	Airway blood vessel dilatation and edema
	Vasodilation	Increased cGMP formation

NO: nitric oxide; cGMP: cyclic guanosine monophosphate; Th: T-helper; iNANC: inhibitory non-adrenergic non-cholinergic

Nitric oxide has a short half-life. It is rapidly inactivated by hemoglobin, and this built-in feature of NO chemistry is probably the most important mechanism for keeping the action of NO localized.[7–10] NO is also inactivated by the free radical superoxide. Thus, scavengers of the superoxide anion, such as superoxide dismutase, may protect nitric oxide, enhancing its potency and prolonging its duration of action. Interaction of NO with superoxide generates peroxynitrite ($ONOO^-$), which is a mediator of potent tissue damage.

The development of substances that inhibit NOS isoforms has been an important strategy in understanding the physiological and pathophysiological roles of nitric oxide. Analogues of L-arginine act as false substrates for the enzyme and therefore block the formation of endogenous nitric oxide.[9] Several arginine analogues have been developed, including N^G-monomethyl-L-arginine (L-NMMA), N^G-nitro-L-arginine (L-NOARG), N^G-nitro-L-arginine methyl ester (L-NAME), and N^G-iminoethyl-L-ornithine (L-NIO), all of which were useful in revealing the role of endogenous nitric oxide in various processes.[8–10]

3. NO in the Lung

NO is produced in the human lung, evidenced by NO detectable in the exhaled air of humans (5–10 parts-per-billion, ppb) and NO metabolites detectable in the bronchoalveolar lavage fluid from human lungs.[6,7,10] NO is recognized to play key roles virtually in all aspects of lung biology and has been implicated in the pathophysiology of lung diseases (Table 3).[4,5,10–13]

Table 3.   Functions of nitric oxide in the lung

Function	Potentially Beneficial Effects	Potentially Harmful Effects
Vasodilation	Vasodilation of pulmonary vessels improves ventilation–perfusion matching	Vasodilation of bronchial vessels increases airway edema and mucus secretion
Mucus secretion	Regulates mucociliary clearance and ciliary mobility	May directly stimulate mucus secretion from submucosal glands
Inflammation	Host defense: toxic effects on bacteria, viruses and parasites	Indirect activation of T-helper lymphocytes
	Antiinflammatory: scavenging oxidants like superoxide	Proinflammatory: through toxic metabolites like peroxynitrite
Neurotransmission	Bronchodilation	

Cellular sources of NO in the lung include epithelial cells, endothelial cells of pulmonary arteries and veins, inhibitory nonadrenergic noncholinergic neurons, smooth muscle cells, mast cells, mesothelial cells, fibroblasts, neutrophils, lymphocytes, and macrophages.[3-9,14] All three NOS isoforms are present in the human lung (Table 4).[6-9] Specifically, NOS I is located in inhibitory nonadrenergic noncholinergic neurons in the lung, while NOS III is found in endothelial cells and the brush border of ciliated epithelial cells.[6-9] NOS II is found in the epithelial cells of the airway. Although NOS II may be induced in several types of cells in response to cytokines, endotoxin, or reactive oxygen species, NOS II is continuously expressed in normal human airway epithelium at basal airway conditions.[14] Once produced, NO is freely diffusible and enters target cells activating soluble guanylate cyclase to produce guanosine 3′,5′-cyclic monophosphate (cGMP) which mediates the majority of NO effects.[8] NO also diffuses into the airway and can be measured in the gas phase.[7]

Potential anatomic sources of NO in exhaled breath include the pulmonary circulation, the lower airways, and the upper airways and paranasal sinuses.[7,8,15] NO is formed in high concentrations in the upper respiratory tract (nasopharynx and paranasal sinuses),[15] but several studies have conclusively demonstrated that NO is also produced in the lower respiratory tract.[7,8] Considering the high diffusibility of NO, the extremely rapid rate of scavenging by hemoglobin (about 3000 times that of oxygen), and the

Table 4.   Sources and effects of nitric oxide in the airways

NOS Isoform	Source	Target	Effects
nNOS, NOS I	NANC nerves	Airway smooth muscle	Bronchodilation
eNOS, NOS III	Vascular endothelium in the bronchial and pulmonary circulation	Vascular smooth muscle	Vasodilation
iNOS, NOS II	Airway epithelium	Epithelium	Epithelial shedding (peroxynitrite, etc)
		Submucosal gland	Mucus secretion
		Arteriole	Vasodilation
		Post-capillary venule	Plasma leakage
		Airway smooth muscle	Bronchodilation
		Vascular smooth muscle	Vasodilation

NOS: nitric oxide synthase; nNOS: neural nitric oxide synthase; iNOS: inducible nitric oxide synthase; eNOS: endothelial nitric oxide synthase; NANC: non-adrenergic noncholinergic rich supply of blood vessels found in the lung, the pulmonary circulation serves as a biologic sink for NO, and is not likely to contribute to NO in exhaled breath.

The functions and effects of NO in the lung/airways reflect its key roles as a vasodilator, bronchodilator, neurotransmitter, and inflammatory mediator (Table 3).

3.1. *Vascular Effects of NO*

NO has a well-established role in the endothelial-dependent control of vascular tone and mediating vascular smooth muscle relaxation in the pulmonary circulation. NO is a potent vasodilator in the bronchial circulation as well and may play an important role in regulating airway blood flow, as in the pulmonary circulation. NO may also modulate systemic vascular tone through its vasodilator property and excess amounts of NO may cause the hypotension associated with sepsis. A diminution of NO within the lungs is implicated in pathological states associated with pulmonary hypertension.[11,12] NO also has antithrombotic functions[16] and inhaled NO is a selective pulmonary vasodilator and can improve ventilation–perfusion matching.

3.2. *Airway Effects of NO*

Similar to its effects on the vascular smooth muscle, NO can also promote bronchodilation by directly relaxing the smooth muscles of the airway. Produced continuously by the overlying airway epithelium, NO can diffuse easily into the bronchial smooth muscle and result in smooth muscle relaxation through activation of cGMP (Fig. 1).

NO can also affect the bronchial tone indirectly as the neurotransmitter of the inhibitory non-adrenergic, non-cholinergic (i-NANC) bronchodilator nerves. NO generated by constitutive NOS in these nerves is thought to have bronchoprotective/bronchodilating effects.[17] There are three types of neural mechanisms in the airways. Cholinergic (ACh: Acetylcholine), alpha-adrenergic (NE: Norepinephrine), and excitatory non-adrenergic non-cholinergic (e-NANC) (NK: Neurokinin) are neural mechanism resulting in bronchoconstriction. Beta-adrenergic (Epinephrine), and inhibitory non-adrenergic non-cholinergic (i-NANC) (VIP: VIP, NO: Nitric oxide) are neural mechanisms resulting in bronchodilation. In proximal human airways there is a prominent i-NANC bronchodilator neural mechanism, which assumes particular functional importance, as it is the only endogenous bronchodilator pathway in human airways. The neurotransmitter of this i-NANC pathway in human airways is NO.

Patients with asthma have higher levels of NOS II expression in their airway epithelium and produce higher levels of NO. Several types of autonomic defects have been proposed in asthma, including enhanced cholinergic, alpha-adrenergic and NANC excitatory mechanism, or reduced beta-adrenergic and i-NANC bronchodilator mechanisms. Furthermore, airway blood vessel dilatation and edema have also been proposed to account for the airway obstruction in asthma.

3.3. *The Role of NO in Matching Ventilation and Perfusion*

Oxygen is the major physiologic regulator of ventilation–perfusion matching in the lung, through vasoconstriction of pulmonary vessels in regions of low ventilation containing low oxygen levels.[7,18–20] Oxygen regulation of pulmonary vascular tone may be mediated in part by NO.[7,18–20] Studies in pulmonary endothelial cells, isolated pulmonary vascular rings, isolated perfused lungs, whole animals, and humans support an important role for NO in modulating the pulmonary vascular response to oxygen.[7] Due to the free diffusion of NO and the close apposition of airways to medium sized pulmonary vessels which modulate pulmonary vessel tone,[7] endogenous NO production in airways proximal to the alveolus may modulate pulmonary vasodilatation. Furthermore, hemoglobin in blood vessels may serve as a natural biologic sink for NO, creating a continuous concentration gradient for NO to move toward perivascular myocytes and thus regulate blood flow. Endogenous NO levels in the lung change rapidly in direct proportion to inspired oxygen which strongly supports a critical role for NO as mediator of ventilation–perfusion coupling in the lung.[7]

4. NO in Lung Disease

NO also plays a major role in the pathophysiology of lung disease. Patients with pulmonary hypertension have low levels of NO in their exhaled breath. Patients with asthma have high levels of exhaled NO in their exhaled breath and high levels of NOS II enzyme expression in the epithelial cells of their airways.

4.1. *NO in Lung Inflammation*

NO can modulate acute and chronic inflammation, producing either pro-inflammatory or anti-inflammatory effects.

NO is a highly reactive molecule/free radical and may have oxidant properties directly or in the form of the more noxious peroxynitrite. These properties give NO its bactericidal and cytotoxic effects and may participate in host defense by mediating antimicrobial activity and cytotoxicity for tumor cells.[4,5,8] These same properties, however, may also promote an inflammatory response for NO that can result in airway inflammation and obstruction, the hallmarks of asthma.[17,21] Many of the harmful effects of NO depend upon the production of peroxynitrite ($ONOO^-$), a potent oxidant and mediator of epithelial damage that results from the reaction of NO with a superoxide anion. The generation of peroxynitrite from nitric oxide and superoxide radicals during inflammatory processes induces epithelial damage, mediator release, and hence airway hyperresponsiveness. All these conditions are very important characteristic features in patients suffering from asthma. Peroxynitrite leads to nitrosylation of tyrosine residues on proteins, and nitrotyrosine may be detected immunocytochemically. The amount of nitrotyrosine immunostaining is correlated with airway hyperresponsiveness, as measured by methacholine challenge.[17] Thus, NO and/or its oxides can nitrosate proteins or thiols altering protein functions. Free radicals/ROS may cause airway inflammation by promoting irreversible lipid perooxidation or by initiating reactions which then become self-sustaining through the generation of propagating radicals. In either case, this can result in deleterious effects on the cell.

The increase in eNO in asthmatics seems to be closely related to airway inflammation, a concept that is supported by several observations. Inflammatory cytokines, especially IFN-γ induce and maintain the gene expression of NOS II in the airway epithelium, the major source of NO in the lung.[7,8,14,22,23] In addition to having increased levels of NOS II expression, airways of asthmatics also have high levels of L-arginine, the NOS substrate and precursor of NO production (Fig. 1).[23] Administration of anti-inflammatory drugs (corticosteroids, leukotriene antagonists) result in decrease in exhaled NO,[24,25] while viral upper respiratory infections and allergen challenge are associated with increased exhaled NO levels.[13,26] NOS II expression in the airway epithelium of asthmatics is also significantly reduced by anti-inflammatory therapy with corticosteroids. Furthermore, through its vasodilating properties, endogenous NO may increase the exudation of plasma by increasing blood flow to the bronchial circulation, thus increasing airway edema.[27] Excessive production of NO in asthma may also contribute to the ventilation–perfusion mismatch that occurs in asthmatic patients particularly during asthma exacerbations.[17]

On the other hand, NO can also have anti-inflammatory properties. Although NO itself is a radical, many of the same chemical and physical properties of NO that allow it to exert oxidant effects can also result in antioxidant actions. The most effective protection against oxidant mediated tissue damage is to scavenge the initiating radical. Due to its high reactivity with several ROS and its ability to traverse membranes and lipoproteins, NO can effectively terminate radical species throughout all aspects of membrane and lipoprotein microenvironments[28] giving NO its antioxidant properties. For example, by reacting with superoxide to form peroxynitrite, NO may serve as scavenger of superoxide resulting in a net antioxidant effect.[28] Thus, NO may exert anti-oxidant (anti-inflammatory) or oxidant (inflammatory) effects depending on the biochemical and physiologic conditions in the tissue milieu. In situations where the oxidant load is high (like asthma),[29] NO may play an antioxidant role by scavenging superoxide and other ROS. In an environment where the oxidant load is low, however, the highly reactive properties of NO give the molecule oxidant properties. In this context, the high NO levels seen in asthma may be necessary to serve a protective antioxidant function.[28–30]

4.2. *Asthma*

Asthma is a disease characterized by airway hyper-responsiveness and inflammation. Although the precise mechanism of airway hyper-responsiveness remains unknown, it is thought to be dependent on and the result of the other main feature of asthma, airway inflammation. Due to its multiple functions, NO may be involved in both aspects of asthma. Since NO is a bronchodilator, increased levels of NO could have beneficial effects on the airway reactivity to bronchoconstrictive stimuli. Furthermore, since NO has both pro- and anti-inflammatory properties, it can modulate the underlying inflammation in asthma. Thus, the explanation for the elevated levels of NO in asthma turned out to be much more difficult than it was initially thought. NO could be involved in the pathogenesis of asthma by modifying bronchial hyper-responsiveness or the underlying airway inflammation or it may be a simple overall marker of inflammation. In either case, measuring exhaled NO has potential clinical importance in monitoring the inflammatory component of asthma.[24,31–38]

Patients with asthma have high levels of exhaled NO in their airways (Fig. 2) and exhaled breath and high levels of NOS II enzyme expression in the epithelial cells of their airways. Both exhaled NO and NOS II expression

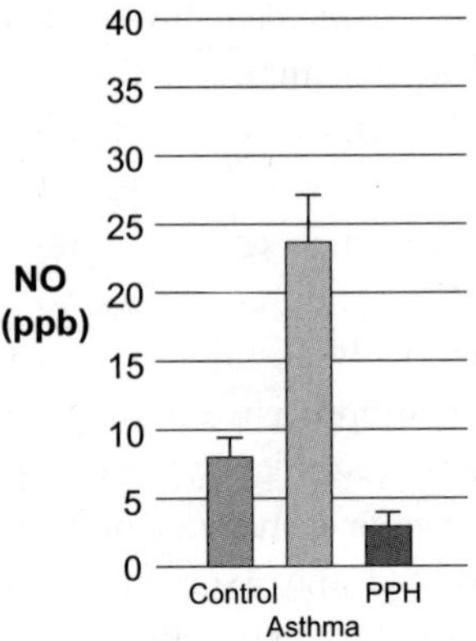

Fig. 2.   NO in lung disease. Lower airway levels of NO measured by bronchoscopy are high in asthma and low in patients with pulmonary hypertension.

return to normal levels after treatment with corticosteroids, making exhaled NO a potentially useful marker of airway inflammation. Although these findings suggest a role for NO in asthma pathogenesis, the exact role of NO in asthma and airway reactivity remains elusive despite intense research in this area. Whether NO is beneficial through its bronchodilator and antioxidant effects or harmful by inducing inflammation remains unclear. It is also possible that it may play both roles depending on the level and the airway milieu in a particular patient or at a particular stage of the disease.

4.3. *Pulmonary Hypertension*

NO plays an integral role in the pathogenesis of pulmonary hypertension. Pulmonary hypertension refers to a group of diseases characterized by high pulmonary artery pressures and pulmonary vascular resistance. It is a progressive disease that affects predominantly young and productive individuals, is more common in females, and has a mean survival between 2 to 3 years from the time of diagnosis. The management of pulmonary hypertension is limited by poor understanding of its pathogenesis. Discoveries in the nitric oxide field, however, are providing major insights in this area. Interestingly, patients with pulmonary hypertension have low levels of NO in their lungs (Fig. 2) and exhaled breath. In fact, the severity of pulmonary hypertension inversely correlates with NO levels estimated by measurement of NO reaction products in the lungs. Although this is a more complex issue than the simple lack of a vasodilator, replacement of NO seems to work well in treating the problem. Exogenous administration of NO gas by inhalation is probably the most effective and specific therapy for pulmonary hypertension. Although cost and unresolved technical difficulties in the delivery system of inhaled NO have prevented its widespread use so far, recent evidence suggests that other therapies for pulmonary hypertension may exert their beneficial effect at least, in part, through endogenous NO.[11,39,40]

4.4. *NO in Other Lung Diseases*

Endogenous NO levels are affected in several other lung diseases and conditions[11,41−45] (Table 5). Low levels of exhaled NO are seen in smokers, which is probably due to the fact that cigarette smoke contains high levels of NO that suppress endogenous production. NO levels are also low in patients with cystic fibrosis but the significance of this is not clear.[41] High NO levels are seen in inflammatory lung diseases like bronchiectasis and chronic beryllium disease.[42,43] NO levels are also high in patients with lymphangioleiomyomatosis (LAM) which may be related to NOS III expression in the smooth muscles of LAM lesions.[8,45]

Table 5. Exhaled NO (eNO) levels in some lung diseases and conditions

High	Low
Asthma	Smoking
Bronchiectasis	Primary pulmonary hypertension
COPD	Cystic fibrosis
Lymphangioleiomyomatosis	NOS inhibitors
Upper respiratory infection	Leukotriene antagonists
Chronic beryllium disease	Corticosteroids
L-arginine ingestion	

5. Measuring NO in Exhaled Breath

Since NO levels in exhaled breath are in the parts-per-billion (ppb) range, a sensitive method utilizing chemiluminescence is needed to detect these low levels. Electrochemical methods[46,47] detect levels in the parts-per-million (ppm) range, while the chemiluminescence method is far more sensitive. The chemiluminescence method depends on the reaction of NO with ozone to form NO_2^* in an excited state which then emits the extra energy as light that can be detected by a photomultiplier tube. The amount of light energy released is proportionate to NO levels in the gas sample.[36,37,48−50]

There are several methods to collect exhaled gas for measurement. These methods are generally classified into off-line or on-line methods. In the off-line method, exhaled gas is collected into an inert reservoir for measurement at a different time or location. In the on-line method, the expired gas is continuously sampled in real-time by the NO analyzer as the individual exhales. Details describing on-line, off-line, and bronchoscopic methods are published in the literature.[7,48,50] Measurements from the different collection techniques are not identical but they correlate well with one another.[36,37,48–50] Table 6 provides a comparison between on-line and off-line measurements.

The American Thoracic Society (ATS) has published standards for performing on-line and off-line measurements of exhaled NO. The guidelines recommend the use of the term FE_{NO} (the fractional exhaled NO concentration) to describe levels of NO in exhaled breath in both the on-line and the off-line methods. FE_{NO} is expressed in parts per billion which is equivalent to nanoliters per liter (nL/L).[50] Several commercial analyzers are available to measure NO levels in exhaled breath based on the ATS guidelines. One such device was approved by the FDA in 2003.[51]

6. Summary and Conclusions

The ability to measure NO levels in exhaled breath has provided us with a unique opportunity to gain insights into lung physiology and to better understand the pathophysiology of lung disease.

In the clinical application arena, the use of exhaled NO is particularly promising in monitoring asthma. It is non-invasive, it can be performed repeatedly, and it can be used in children and patients with severe airflow obstruction where other techniques are difficult or cannot be performed. Exhaled NO may also be more sensitive than currently available tests in detecting airway inflammation, which may allow for the rapid assessment of airway inflammation and for monitoring the response to anti-inflammatory therapy.

Table 6.   Comparison between on-line and off-line NO measurements

	On-line	Off-line
General technique	– Inhale orally to TLC – Perform a vital capacity maneuver into NO analyzer	– Inhale orally to TLC – Perform a vital capacity maneuver into reservoir bag
Specific recommendations	– If ambient NO is high, need to watch for initial peak and allow it to washout (better to use NO-free air for inhalation) – Constant expiratory flow rate (0.05 L/s) – Expiratory resistance (> 5 and < 20 cm H_2O) – Nose clips are not necessary – Exhalation duration of at least 6 s with a plateau of NO *vs.* time of at least 3 s	– If ambient NO in > 20–40 ppb a source of NO-free air should be used for inhalation – Constant expiratory flow rate (0.35 L/s) – Expiratory resistance (> 5 cm H_2O) – Nose clips are not necessary – Reservoir should be nonreactive and impermeable to NO
Advantages	– Suboptimal exhalations can be immediately identified and discarded or repeated – Less affected by high ambient NO levels – Less likely to be contaminated by nasal NO	– Samples can be collected from sites remote from the analyzer – Less dependent on analyzer response times – More efficient use of analyzer (less analyzer time per patient) – Allows for measurement of other gases in the same sample
Disadvantages	– Requires more stringent analyzer specifications – Patient and analyzer need to be at the same place at the same time – Less efficient use of analyzer (more analyzer time per patient)	– Possible errors due to sample storage – Suboptimal exhalations cannot be immediately identified – More likely to be contaminated by nasal and ambient air NO

References

1. Palmer RM, Ferrige AG, Moncada S. Nitric oxide release accounts for the biological activity of endothelium-derived relaxing factor. *Nature* 1987; **327**: 524–526.
2. Ignarro LJ, Buga GM, Wood KS, Byrns RE, Chaudhuri G. Endothelium-derived relaxing factor produced and released from artery and vein is nitric oxide. *Proc Natl Acad Sci USA* 1987; **84**: 9265–9269.
3. Moncada S, Higgs A. The L-arginine-nitric oxide pathway. *N Engl J Med* 1993; **329**: 2002–2012.
4. Nathan C. Nitric oxide as a secretory product of mammalian cells. *Faseb J* 1992; **6**: 3051–3064.
5. Schmidt HH, Walter U. NO at work. *Cell* 1994; **78**: 919–925.
6. Kobzik L, Bredt DS, Lowenstein CJ, Drazen J, Gaston B, Sugarbaker D, Stamler JS. Nitric oxide synthase in human and rat lung: immunocyto-chemical and histochemical localization. *Am J Respir Cell Mol Biol* 1993; **9**: 371–377.
7. Dweik RA, Laskowski D, Abu-Soud HM, Kaneko F, Hutte R, Stuehr DJ, Erzurum SC. Nitric oxide synthesis in the lung. Regulation by oxygen through a kinetic mechanism. *J Clin Invest* 1998; **101**: 660–666.
8. Dweik R, Erzurum S. Effects of nitric oxide and cGMP on smooth muscle proliferation., In: Moss J, ed. *LAM and other diseases characterized by smooth muscle proliferation*, New York: Marcel Dekker, 1999: 333–349.
9. Gaston B, Drazen JM, Loscalzo J, Stamler JS. The biology of nitrogen oxides in the airways. *Am J Respir Crit Care Med* 1994; **149**: 538–551.
10. Ellis JL, Undem BJ. Inhibition by L-NG-nitro-L-arginine of nonadrenergic-noncholinergic-mediated relaxations of human isolated central and peripheral airway. *Am Rev Respir Dis* 1992; **146**: 1543–1547.
11. Ghamra ZW, Dweik RA. Primary pulmonary hypertension: an overview of epidemiology and pathogenesis. *Cleve Clin J Med* 2003; **70** Suppl 1: S2–8.
12. Raychaudhuri B, Dweik R, Connors MJ, Buhrow L, Malur A, Drazba J, Arroliga AC, Erzurum SC, Kavuru MS, Thomassen MJ. Nitric oxide blocks nuclear factor-kappaB activation in alveolar macrophages. *Am J Respir Cell Mol Biol* 1999; **21**: 311–316.
13. Khatri SB, Hammel J, Kavuru MS, Erzurum SC, Dweik RA. Temporal association of nitric oxide levels and airflow in asthma after whole lung allergen challenge. *J Appl Physiol* 2003; **95**: 436–440; discussion 435
14. Guo FH, Uetani K, Haque SJ, Williams BR, Dweik RA, Thunnissen FB, Calhoun W, Erzurum SC. Interferon gamma and interleukin 4 stimulate prolonged expression of inducible nitric oxide synthase in human airway epithelium through synthesis of soluble mediators. *J Clin Invest* 1997; **100**: 829–838.
15. Lundberg JO, Farkas-Szallasi T, Weitzberg E, Rinder J, Lidholm J, Anggaard A, Hokfelt T, Lundberg JM, Alving K. High nitric oxide production in human paranasal sinuses. *Nat Med* 1995; **1**: 370–373.

16. Cheung PY, Salas E, Schulz R, Radomski MW. Nitric oxide and platelet function: implications for neonatology. *Semin Perinatol* 1997; **21**: 409–417.

17. Barnes P. Nitric Oxide. In: Barnes P, Rodger I, Thomson N, eds. *Asthma: Basic Mechanisms and Clinical Management*, London: Academic Press, 1998: 369–388.

18. Voelkel NF. Mechanisms of hypoxic pulmonary vasoconstriction. *Am Rev Respir Dis* 1986; **133**: 1186–1195.

19. McQueston JA, Cornfield DN, McMurtry IF, Abman SH. Effects of oxygen and exogenous L-arginine on EDRF activity in fetal pulmonary circulation. *Am J Physiol* 1993; **264**: H865–871.

20. Cornfield DN, Reeve HL, Tolarova S, Weir EK, Archer S. Oxygen causes fetal pulmonary vasodilation through activation of a calcium-dependent potassium channel. *Proc Natl Acad Sci USA* 1996; **93**: 8089–8094.

21. Sadeghi-Hashjin G, Folkerts G, Henricks P, Verheyen A, van der Linde H, van Ark I, Coene A, Nijkamp F. Peroxynitrite induces airway hyperresponsiveness in Guinea pigs *in vitro* and *in vivo*. *Am J Respir crit care Med* 1996; **153**: 1697–1701.

22. Dweik RA, Guo FH, Uetani K, Erzurum SC. Nitric oxide synthase in the human airway epithelium. *Zhongguo Yao Li Xue Bao* 1997; **18**: 550–552.

23. Guo FH, Comhair SA, Zheng S, Dweik RA, Eissa NT, Thomassen MJ, Calhoun W, Erzurum SC. Molecular mechanisms of increased nitric oxide (NO) in asthma: evidence for transcriptional and post-translational regulation of NO synthesis. *J Immunol* 2000; **164**: 5970–5980.

24. Bisgaard H, Loland L, Oj JA. NO in exhaled air of asthmatic children is reduced by the leukotriene receptor antagonist montelukast. *Am J Respir Crit Care Med* 1999; **160**: 1227–1231.

25. Yates DH, Kharitonov SA, Robbins RA, Thomas PS, Barnes PJ. Effect of a nitric oxide synthase inhibitor and a glucocorticosteroid on exhaled nitric oxide. *Am J Respir Crit Care Med* 1995; **152**: 892–896.

26. Kharitonov SA, O'Connor BJ, Evans DJ, Barnes PJ. Allergen-induced late asthmatic reactions are associated with elevation of exhaled nitric oxide. *Am J Respir Crit Care Med* 1995; **151**: 1894–1899.

27. Bernareggi M, Mitchell JA, Barnes PJ, Belvisi MG. Dual action of nitric oxide on airway plasma leakage. *Am J Respir Crit Care Med* 1997; **155**: 869–874.

28. Rubbo H, Darley-Usmar V, Freeman BA. Nitric oxide regulation of tissue free radical injury. *Chem Res Toxicol* 1996; **9**: 809–820.

29. Comhair SA, Bhathena PR, Dweik RA, Kavuru M, Erzurum SC. Rapid loss of superoxide dismutase activity during antigen-induced asthmatic response. *Lancet* 2000; **355**: 624.

30. Schuiling M, Meurs H, Zuidhof AB, Venema N, Zaagsma J. Dual action of iNOS-derived nitric oxide in allergen-induced airway hyperreactivity in conscious, unrestrained guinea pigs. *Am J Respir Crit Care Med* 1998; **158**: 1442–1449.

31. Jatakanon A, Lim S, Kharitonov SA, Chung KF, Barnes PJ. Correlation between exhaled nitric oxide, sputum eosinophils, and methacholine responsiveness in patients with mild asthma. *Thorax* 1998; **53**: 91–95.

32. Kharitonov SA, Yates D, Robbins RA, Logan-Sinclair R, Shinebourne EA, Barnes PJ. Increased nitric oxide in exhaled air of asthmatic patients. *Lancet* 1994; **343**: 133–135.

33. Persson MG, Zetterstrom O, Agrenius V, Ihre E, Gustafsson LE. Single-breath nitric oxide measurements in asthmatic patients and smokers. *Lancet* 1994; **343**: 146–147.

34. Crater SE, Peters EJ, Martin ML, Murphy AW, Platts-Mills TA. Expired nitric oxide and airway obstruction in asthma patients with an acute exacerbation. *Am J Respir Crit Care Med* 1999; **159**: 806–811.

35. Dupont LJ, Rochette F, Demedts MG, Verleden GM. Exhaled nitric oxide correlates with airway hyperresponsiveness in steroid-naive patients with mild asthma. *Am J Respir Crit Care Med* 1998; **157**: 894–898.

36. Deykin A, Halpern O, Massaro AF, Drazen JM, Israel E. Expired nitric oxide after bronchoprovocation and repeated spirometry in patients with asthma. *Am J Respir Crit Care Med* 1998; **157**: 769–775.

37. Ozkan M, Laskowski D, Erzurum S, Dweik R. Standardization of exhaled nitric oxide measures in healthy controls and individuals with airway disease. *Am J Respir Crit Care Med* 2000; **161**: A920.

38. Silkoff PE, Sylvester JT, Zamel N, Permutt S. Airway nitric oxide diffusion in asthma: Role in pulmonary function and bronchial responsiveness. *Am J Respir Crit Care Med* 2000; **161**: 1218–1228.

39. Arroliga AC, Dweik RA, Kaneko FJ, Erzurum SC. Primary pulmonary hypertension: update on pathogenesis and novel therapies. *Cleve Clin J Med* 2000; **67**: 175–178, 181–185, 189–190.

40. Dweik RA. Pulmonary hypertension and the search for the selective pulmonary vasodilator. *Lancet* 2002; **360**: 886–887.

41. Balfour-Lynn IM, Laverty A, Dinwiddie R. Reduced upper airway nitric oxide in cystic fibrosis. *Arch Dis Child* 1996; **75**: 319–322.

42. Kharitonov SA, Wells AU, O'Connor BJ, Cole PJ, Hansell DM, Logan-Sinclair RB, Barnes PJ. Elevated levels of exhaled nitric oxide in bronchiectasis. *Am J Respir Crit Care Med* 1995; **151**: 1889–1893.

43. Dweik R, Laskowski D, Farver C, Erzurum S. Increased nitric oxide in lymphangioleiomyomatosis. *Am J Respir Crit Care Med* 2000; **161**: A376.

44. Dweik R, Laskowski D, Erzurum S. High levels of nitric oxide (NO) in exhaled breath in patients with chronic beryllium disease. *Am J Respir Crit Care Med* 2000; **161**: A731.

45. Dweik RA. The promise and reality of nitric oxide in the diagnosis and treatment of lung disease. *Cleve Clin J Med* 2001; **68**: 486, 488, 490, 493.

46. Schedin U, Frostell CG, Gustafsson LE. Formation of nitrogen dioxide from nitric oxide and their measurement in clinically relevant circumstances. *Br J Anaesth* 1999; **82**: 182–192.

47. Nelin LD, Christman NT, Morrisey JF, Dawson CA. Electrochemical nitric oxide and nitrogen dioxide analyzer for use with inhaled nitric oxide. *J Appl Physiol* 1996; **81**: 1423–1429.

48. Silkoff PE, Stevens A, Pak J, Bucher-Bartelson B, Martin RJ. A method for the standardized offline collection of exhaled nitric oxide. *Chest* 1999; **116**: 754–759.

49. Silkoff PE, McClean PA, Slutsky AS, Furlott HG, Hoffstein E, Wakita S, Chapman KR, Szalai JP, Zamel N. Marked flow-dependence of exhaled nitric oxide using a new technique to exclude nasal nitric oxide. *Am J Respir Crit Care Med* 1997; **155**: 260–267.

50. Recommendations for standardized procedures for the on-line and off-line measurement of exhaled lower respiratory nitric oxide and nasal nitric oxide in adults and children-1999. This official statement of the American Thoracic Society was adopted by the ATS Board of Directors, July 1999.. *Am J Respir Crit Care Med* 1999; **160**: 2104–2117.

51. Silkoff PE, Carlson M, Bourke T, Katial R, Ogren E, Szefler SJ. The Aerocrine exhaled nitric oxide monitoring system NIOX is cleared by the US Food and Drug Administration for monitoring therapy in asthma. *J Allergy Clin Immunol* 2004; **114**: 1241–1256.

NASAL NITRIC OXIDE MEASUREMENTS AS A DIAGNOSTIC TOOL: READY FOR CLINICAL USE?

J. O. LUNDBERG

Department of Physiology and Pharmacology,
Karolinska Institutet,
S-17177 Stockholm, Sweden

1. Background

In healthy subjects, a large proportion of nitric oxide (NO) found in exhaled air originates from the upper airways with only a minor contribution from the lower respiratory tract and the lungs.[1-3] The role of NO in the upper airways is not entirely known but may involve host defense functions including direct toxic effects on microorganisms[4] and regulation of mucociliary activity.[4,5] Nasal NO is altered in several respiratory disorders, *e.g.* primary ciliary dyskinesia (PCD),[2] cystic fibrosis,[6,7] and allergic rhinitis,[8-10] and this has led to the proposal that a nasal NO test could be clinically useful in diagnosis and monitoring of these diseases. This is a brief summary of what is known about nasal NO. More extensive reviews of nasal NO are available elsewhere.[10,11]

2. Why Measure Nasal NO?

Nasal NO measurements are rapid, completely non-invasive, and can be performed easily even in infants. Because nasal NO is altered in certain airway disorders the measurements could be clinically beneficial to aid in the diagnosis and monitoring of therapy. There is a great difference in background NO output between the upper and the lower airways.[2,3,10] Background lower airway NO output is normally low which makes it easy to find increases (*e.g.* asthma) but more difficult to detect decreases. In the upper airways there is a high background output, and so an increase (*e.g.* in allergic rhinitis) can be obscured, while a decrease is usually easy to reveal. Adding to the complexity is the fact that swelling of the mucosa or secretions during inflammation may lead to less passage of NO from the mucosa of the paranasal sinuses to the nasal cavity where it is measured. In such cases the net change in nasal NO will be variable and difficult to predict.

3. In Which Conditions Might Nasal NO Be Clinically Applicable?

As of today there is one condition for which nasal NO measurements could be considered as a useful diagnosis, namely primary ciliary dyskinesia (PCD). This is a rare disorder characterized by non-functioning cilia, which results in chronic airway infections including sinusitis and bronchiectasis.[12] Several independent studies have now consistently indicated extremely low nasal NO in PCD and in recent trials the sensitivity and specificity of this test in PCD has proven to be excellent.[2,13–15] This makes the nasal NO test attractive for screening of PCD. A simple non-invasive test for PCD could indeed be very useful. Diagnosis of PCD is often delayed despite the presence of typical symptoms early in life.[12] The presently used diagnostic procedure for suspected PCD is quite cumbersome and often involves ultra-structural examination of airway epithelial ciliary structure.[12,16,17] The use of nasal NO in diagnosis and monitoring of other respiratory disorders *e.g.* allergic rhinitis, sinusitis, nasal polyposis and cystic fibrosis is potentially of great interest but more research is needed before we know how clinically useful this test can be for these disorders.

4. How to Measure Nasal NO

The American Thoracic Society and the European Respiratory Society have agreed on a highly standardized procedure for measurements of lower res-piratory tract exhaled NO.[18] Such guidelines are extremely helpful for re-searchers when comparing results and they have been of great value in the process of moving exhaled NO measurements into clinical application. For nasal NO measurements however, one single standardized measurement procedure has not yet been defined. Several techniques for measuring nasal NO have been used. The most commonly presented way to measure nasal NO is to sample nasal air directly from one nostril. Using the intrinsic sampling flow of a chemiluminescent analyzer or an external pump, air is aspirated from (or insufflated into) one nostril.[2,8] Because of its simpli-city the aspiration method is still by far the most used technique for nasal

NO. Another technique to measure nasal NO includes, nasal single-breath exhalation using a face mask.[19]

If the nasal NO test should become a part of future clinical practice it will of course be great importance to standardize the method carefully. However, the recommendation at this time is to allow maximum freedom for nasal NO measurements. The chosen method must however be carefully described including reporting of flow rate and ambient NO levels. It is likely that several methods for nasal NO will be used depending on the situation and the patient population. For example, breath-holding or single-breath measurements are not possible in non-cooperating individuals *e.g.* infants and sedated patients.

5. Nasal NO and Paranasal Sinus Function

One of the more recent findings in this field is the discovery that nasal NO increases dramatically (5- to 15-fold) during humming compared to a silent nasal exhalation.[20] The oscillating sound waves speed up the exchange of gases over the sinus ostium resulting in a rapid washout of NO from the sinuses.[20] This NO peak is transient and the levels decrease gradually during repeated humming maneuver. However, nasal NO levels fully recovers after a short period of silence, allowing for sinus NO to accumulate again. In a model of the nose and sinus it was found that the sinus ostium size was the main determinant of the humming-induced increase in NO. In addition, in patients with CT proven complete sinus ostial obstruction (bilateral nasal polyposis), the nasal NO increase during humming was abolished.[21] This suggests that the increase in nasal NO during humming correlates to ostial function. Ostium obstruction is central in the pathogenesis of sinusitis and one goal in medical as well as surgical therapy of chronic sinusitis is to improve sinus ventilation. Future studies will show if a nasal NO humming test could be used to monitor ostium function in risk patients or in subjects with established sinus disease.

6. Summary and Future Directions

About a decade ago it was found that NO is released in large quantities in the nasal passages of healthy humans. Especially large concentrations of NO have been found in the paranasal sinuses. The physiological role of this NO has still not been clarified but may include important local host-defense mechanisms. Nasal NO can be measured on-line using different non-invasive techniques. Using these methods it has been found that nasal

NO is altered in several airway disorders including allergic rhinitis, PCD, cystic fibrosis and sinusitis. For most indications nasal NO is still to be regarded as an interesting research tool with potential clinical importance. However, in PCD the situation is different because nasal NO is uniformly extremely low. The sensitivity and specificity of a nasal NO test in PCD are so good that this test now should be considered for routine use in specialized centers. To facilitate this process we need to quickly establish guidelines for a simple standardized nasal NO test in PCD.

References

1. Alving K, Weitzberg E, Lundberg JM. Increased amount of nitric oxide in exhaled air of asthmatics. *Eur Respir J* 1993; **6**: 1368–1370.
2. Lundberg JO, Weitzberg E, Nordvall SL, Kuylenstierna R, Lundberg JM, Alving K. Primarily nasal origin of exhaled nitric oxide and absence in Kartagener's syndrome. *Eur Respir J* 1994; **7**: 1501–1504.
3. Schedin U, Frostell C, Persson MG, Jakobsson J, Andersson G, Gustafsson LE. Contribution from upper and lower airways to exhaled endogenous nitric oxide in humans. *Acta Anaesthesiol Scand* 1995; **39**: 327–332.
4. Lundberg JO, Farkas-Szallasi T, Weitzberg E, Rinder J, Lidholm J, Anggaard A, Hokfelt T, Lundberg JM, Alving K. High nitric oxide production in human paranasal sinuses. *Nat Med* 1995; **1**: 370–373.
5. Runer T, Cervin A, Lindberg S, Uddman R. Nitric oxide is a regulator of mucociliary activity in the upper respiratory tract. *Otolaryngol Head Neck Surg* 1998; **119**: 278–287.
6. Lundberg JO, Nordvall SL, Weitzberg E, Kollberg H, Alving K. Exhaled nitric oxide in paediatric asthma and cystic fibrosis. *Arch Dis Child* 1996; **75**: 323–326.
7. Balfour-Lynn IM, Laverty A, Dinwiddie R. Reduced upper airway nitric oxide in cystic fibrosis. *Arch Dis Child* 1996; **75**: 319–322.
8. Kharitonov SA, Rajakulasingam K, O'Connor B, Durham SR, Barnes PJ. Nasal nitric oxide is increased in patients with asthma and allergic rhinitis and may be modulated by nasal glucocorticoids. *J Allergy Clin Immunol* 1997; **99**: 58–64.
9. Arnal JF, Didier A, Rami J, M'Rini C, Charlet JP, Serrano E, Besombes JP. Nasal nitric oxide is increased in allergic rhinitis. *Clin Exp Allergy* 1997; **27**: 358–362.
10. Lundberg JO, Weitzberg E. Nasal nitric oxide in man. *Thorax* 1999; **54**: 947–952.
11. Djupesland PG, Chatkin JM, Qian W, Haight JS. Nitric oxide in the nasal airway: a new dimension in otorhinolaryngology. *Am J Otolaryngol* 2001; **22**: 19–32.
12. Coren ME, Meeks M, Morrison I, Buchdahl RM, Bush A. Primary ciliary dyskinesia: age at diagnosis and symptom history. *Acta Paediatr* 2002; **91**: 667–669.

13. Narang I, Ersu R, Wilson NM, Bush A. Nitric oxide in chronic airway inflammation in children: diagnostic use and pathophysiological significance. *Thorax* 2002; **57**: 586–589.

14. Wodehouse T, Kharitonov SA, Mackay IS, Barnes PJ, Wilson R, Cole PJ. Nasal nitric oxide measurements for the screening of primary ciliary dyskinesia. *Eur Respir J* 2003; **21**: 43–47.

15. Horvath I, Loukides S, Wodehouse T, Csiszer E, Cole PJ, Kharitonov SA, Barnes PJ. Comparison of exhaled and nasal nitric oxide and exhaled carbon monoxide levels in bronchiectatic patients with and without primary ciliary dyskinesia. *Thorax* 2003; **58**: 68–72.

16. Bush A, Cole P, Hariri M, Mackay I, Phillips G, O'Callaghan C, Wilson R, Warner JO. Primary ciliary dyskinesia: diagnosis and standards of care. *Eur Respir J* 1998; **12**: 982–988.

17. Bush A. Primary ciliary dyskinesia. *Acta Otorhinolaryngol Belg* 2000; **54**: 317–324.

18. *Recommendations for standardized procedures for the on-line and off-line measurement of exhaled lower respiratory nitric oxide and nasal nitric oxide in adults and children — 1999.* This official statement of the American Thoracic Society was adopted by the ATS Board of Directors, July 1999. *Am J Respir Crit Care Med* 1999; **160**: 2104–2117.

19. Palm JP, Graf P, Lundberg JO, Alving K. Characterization of exhaled nitric oxide: introducing a new reproducible method for nasal nitric oxide measurements. *Eur Respir J* 2000; **16**: 236–241.

20. Weitzberg E, Lundberg JO. Humming greatly increases nasal nitric oxide. *Am J Respir Crit Care Med* 2002; **166**: 144–145.

21. Lundberg JO, Maniscalco M, Sofia M, Lundblad L, Weitzberg E, Maniscalo M. Humming, nitric oxide, and paranasal sinus obstruction. *Jama* 2003; **289**: 302–303.

EXHALED NITRIC OXIDE
IN HEPATOPULMONARY SYNDROME

G. ROLLA

Allergologia e Immunologia Clinica,
Università di Torino & Ospedale Mauriziano,
Largo Turati 62, I-10128 Turin, Italy

1. Introduction

The term Hepatopulmonary Syndrome (HPS) is used to indicate abnormal oxygenation (at least alveolar arterial oxygen gradient, $Aa\Lambda_{O_2}$, higher than 20 mm Hg) due to intrapulmonary vascular dilatations (IPVD) in a patient with hepatic disease, most commonly liver cirrhosis. Clinical symptoms typically include shortness of breath, which may either worsen on standing (platypnea) and/or be accompanied by a 10 % fall in $P_{a\,O_2}$ (orthodeoxia). It is well known that hypoxemia may be associated with liver disease in the absence of cardiac or pulmonary disease. Right-to-left intrapulmonary shunting, alveolar capillary diffusion limitation, or alveolar ventilation–perfusion $(\dot{V}_A/\dot{Q})$ mismatch have been the physiopathologic mechanisms to which hypoxemia of liver cirrhosis has been variously attributed.[1] The frequency of oxygenation abnormalities has not been established in the cirrhotic population as a whole. While severe hypoxemia ($P_{a\,O_2} < 60$ mm Hg) is found in 5–7 % of patients referred for liver transplantation, a widened alveolar-arterial oxygen gradient has been reported in up to 70 % of patients undergoing pre-transplant assessment of pulmonary function.[2] Intrapulmonary vascular dilatations (IPVD, see below) may lead to impaired oxygen exchange as a result of an increase in O_2 diffusion distance across the dilated pulmonary capillaries (diameter ranging from 15 to 500 μm, compared to the diameter ranging from 8 to 15 μm of normal capillaries) and a decreased transit time of blood through the pulmonary circulation due to hyperdynamic circulation (the so-called diffusion–perfusion defect).[3] Moreover, as a result of vasodilation, there is excess perfusion $(\dot{Q})$ in relation to ventilation $(\dot{V})$ that is most marked in the low $\dot{V}/\dot{Q}$ units of the basal regions of the lung .

1.1. *Intrapulmonary Vascular Dilatations (IPVD)*

intrapulmonary vascular dilatations can be observed using contrast-enhanced echocardiography or fractional brain uptake after lung perfusion of technetium-99m macroaggregated albumin lung scanning.[3] IPVD may be easily identified by contrast enhanced echocardiography. Microbubbles (mean diameter 35 μm), which are simply obtained by shaking normal saline, are the mostly used contrast. When injected in a peripheral vein, microbubbles appear normally in the right heart chambers and, after 4–6 beats, they appear also in the left heart chambers if there are IPVD or anatomical shunts (Figure 1). An earlier appearance of contrast in the left heart chambers is suggestive of intracardiac right-to-left shunt. IPVDs may be identified also by lung scintigraphic perfusion scanning with ^{99m}Tc albumin macroaggregates (diameter 20–80 μm), which normally are trapped in the pulmonary circulation but, in case of right-to-left shunt or IPVD, abnormal uptake of ^{99m}Tc can be observed in other organs such as the brain or the spleen. Fractional brain uptake of radioisotope has been found to be related to hypoxemia.[4] The method cannot discriminate between intracardiac and intrapulmonary shunting.

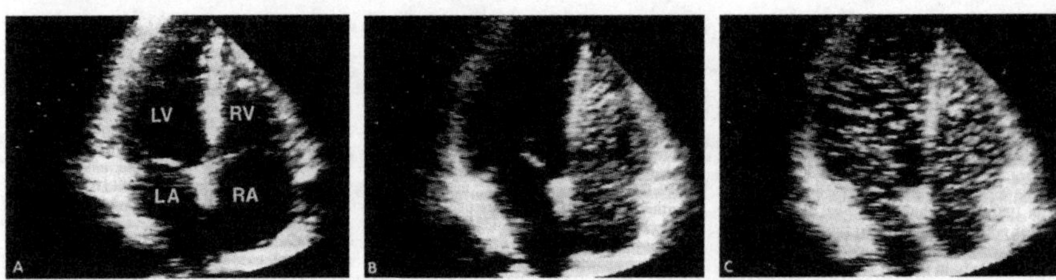

Fig. 1.   Contrast-enhanced echocardiography in HPS. **A**: Cardiac four chambers: left atrium (LA), right atrium (RA), left ventricle (LV), right ventricle (RV). **B**: Microbubbles opacification of right heart chamber after *i.v.* injection of agitated saline. **C**: Delayed (4–6 beats) microbubbles opacification of left heart cavities in the same patient.

1.2. *NO Theory*

Studies concerning the pathogenesis of HPS have focused on the theory that an imbalance between vasodilating and vasoconstrictive mediators, favouring the first one, should play the most important role in causing intrapulmonary vasodilatation. Nitric oxide (NO), one of the most potent and prominent endogenous pulmonary vasodilators, appeared as a very likely candidate, not only for the hyperdynamic circulatory syndrome in cirrhosis, but also for HPS. Vallance and Moncada[5] postulated that an increased production of NO may account for the hyperdynamic circulation of liver cirrhosis. Actually, serum levels of stable NO metabolites (NO_2^-/NO_3^-) have been found to be elevated in cirrhosis, particularly in biliary cirrhosis.[6] The increased levels of circulating NO metabolites have been related to the elevated concentration of endotoxin. The potential causes for systemic endotoxemia in cirrhosis are many, including decreased clearance function of the liver, increased gut permeability and small intestinal bacterial overgrowth, which is associated with bacterial translocation.[7] Exposure to bacteria and their endotoxins, directly or involving cytokines such as TNFα, has been associated with increased synthesis of NO. Nitric oxide is synthesized by different isoforms of nitric oxide synthase, NOS. Two such isoforms have been investigated extensively in the vasculature. NOS II, or iNOS, is induced by LPS, endotoxins, and inflammatory cytokines, and produces large amounts of NO for extended periods of time, and NOS III, or eNOS, which releases NO for short periods in response to physical stimuli such as flow or pressure induced shear stress. Recent investigations have shown that eNOS is the major enzymatic source for NO overproduction in splanchnic circulation of portal hypertensive rats. It is interesting that endotoxin and TNFα, which are well known stimulators of iNOS, can also directly increase the activity of eNOS,[8] which is the major enzymatic source for NO overproduction in splanchnic circulation of portal hypertensive rats. Supporting the important role of endotoxin and bacteria in promoting vasodilation through NO overproduction is the anedoctical report of improved oxygenation in HPS following antibiotic treatment.[9] In a recent double-blind placebo controlled study, selective intestinal decontamination with norfloxacin partially reverse the hyperdynamic circulatory state in 14 patients with alcohol-related cirrhosis.[10]

1.3. *Experimental Model of HPS*

Common bile duct ligation (CBDL) in the rat is the only recognized experimental model of HPS, even if it is distinct from human HPD in that animals reliably develop intrapulmonary vasodilations and gas exchange abnormalities as liver injury progresses, while only 8–15 % of cirrhotic patients are affected.[11] By using this model of HPS, Rabiller *et al.*[12] reported that prophylactic treatment with norfloxacin decreased the incidence of gramnegative bacterial translocation, the number of macrophages sequestered in pulmonary microvessels, the expression and activity of lung iNOS, and the severity of HPS. In a similar rat model of liver cirrhosis, obtained by ligation of common bile duct, Fallon *et al.*[13] found overactivity of eNOS in endothelial cells of lung vasculature, possibly due to stimulation of endothelin-1 B type receptors by increased circulating levels of ET-1. The model implies that HPS develops when both portal hypertension and liver damage coexist, the first by promoting overexpression of ET-B receptors in the lung vasculature, the second by increasing liver and circulating ET-1 levels.[14] While ET-A receptors, which are present in vascular smooth muscle cells, mediate vasoconstriction and proliferation, the ET-B receptor, which is found in endothelium and smooth muscle cells, mediates endothelium dependent vasodilation through the release of NO (Figure 2). Actually, increased plasma ET-1 levels have been reported in patients with liver cirrhosis, both with and without HPS.[15]

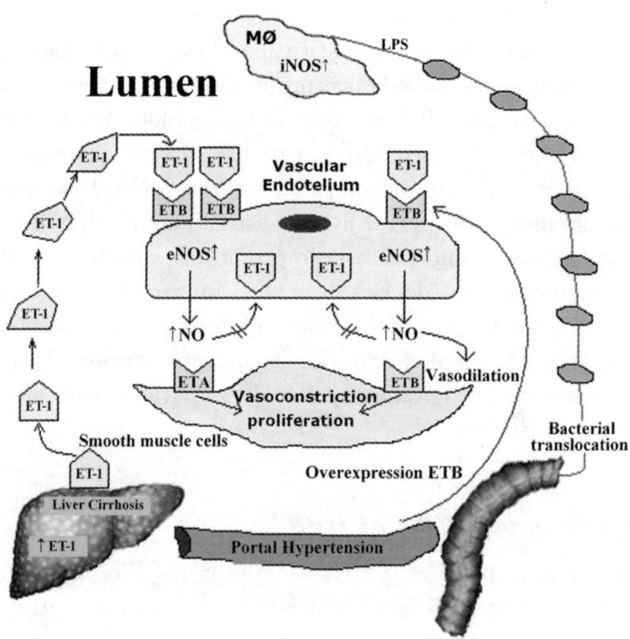

Fig. 2.   Increased production of NO in the alveolar region in hepatopulmonary syndrome (partially modified by Rolla in Ref. 29)

2. Exhaled NO

2.1. *Measurement of NO in Exhaled Air*

The detection of NO in exhaled air was first reported by Gustafsson *et al.* in 1991,[16] and later Alving and coworkers[17] found that NO in exhaled air was elevated in patients with asthma. The most widely used and most sensitive method for measurement of exhaled NO is chemiluminescence after reaction with ozone, which allows measurements down to approximately 1 part per billion. As NO is continuously formed in the airways, the concentration of NO will vary with the flow of exhaled air. Since the publication of the ATS guidelines,[18] most authors have been using the recommended breath flow rate of 50 mL/s. Exhaled NO is usually determined during single breath exhalations. The recommended technique involves inhalation of NO-free air via a mouthpiece to total lung capacity, followed immediately by full exhalation at an even rate through the mouthpiece into the apparatus. During exhalation, an excess pressure is created in the oral cavity, which ensures closure of the velum and prevents contamination of the sample with nasal air. This is important as nasal air contains high concentrations of NO, probably derived from paranasal sinuses.[19]

2.2. *Exhaled NO in HPS*

Increased NO output in exhaled air has been reported in patients with advanced cirrhosis, in whom exhaled NO was positively correlated to cardiac index.[20] In a study of 45 cirrhotic patients, exhaled NO output and serum NO_2^-/NO_3^- have been shown to be significantly higher than in normal controls and in all the patients a significant correlation between exhaled NO and alveolar-arterial oxygen gradient was found.[21] In the same study, the nine patients who met the criteria for the diagnosis of HPS had also the highest values of exhaled NO. By using the technique of multiple flows analysis of NO output, Delclaux *et al* [22] have recently demonstrated that the increased levels of exhaled NO reported in cirrhosis is of alveolar origin and that it was correlated with $AaΔ_{O_2}$. These observations reinforce the hypothesis that NO locally produced in the lung may play an important role in determining oxygenation abnormalities in patients with cirrhosis. A few clinical studies have investigated the relationship between changes in NO produced in the lung and changes in oxygenation abnormalities in liver cirrhosis. In one case of severe HPS, Rolla *et al.*[23] reported that *i.v.* methylene blue (a dye that inhibits the effect of NO on soluble guanylate cyclase and thereby prevents the cascade of events leading to vasodilation) acutely improved oxygenation through a marked decrease in pulmonary shunting. The observation was confirmed by Schenk,[24] who showed that *i.v.* methylene blue improved hypoxemia and hyperdynamic circulation in 7 patients with liver cirrhosis and severe HPS. A significant correlation between the decrease in exhaled NO after liver transplantation and the improvement in oxygenation has been reported in 18 patients with cirrhosis who did not have obvious cardio-respiratory diseases.[25] Five of these patients met the criteria for the diagnosis of HPS before transplantation and the syndrome was cured by transplantation. The correlation between the decrease in exhaled NO after liver transplantation and the improvement in oxygenation reinforces the hypothesis that NO is an important mediator of impaired oxygenation in patients with cirrhosis. Very recently, in a case of HPS associated with HCV related cirrhosis, nebulized N^{G}-nitro-L-arginine methyl ester (L-NAME), an inhibitor of NO synthesis, acutely improved oxygenation, because of a decrease of intrapulmonary vascular dilatations, as evaluated by contrast-enhanced echocardiogram.[26]

3. Concluding Remarks

Many clinical observations support the theory that NO plays a major role in oxygenation abnormalities of patients with liver cirrhosis, complicated by hepatopulmonary syndrome. Alveolar NO concentration might be used to assess the development and the severity of HPS. However, the enthusiasm for inhibiting NO as therapeutical strategy in HPS has been mitigated by the observation of Carter, who showed that the vasodilatory action of NO alone did not completely account for the abnormal vasoreactivity of cirrhotic rat lungs. There is evidence that NO can induce heme oxygenase-1 (HO-1) expression and HO-1-derived CO may contribute significantly to pulmonary vasodilation. A partial reversal of HPS was obtained by inhibiting HO-1 in rats with HPS induced by common bile duct ligation.[27] These observations suggest that the development of HPS is a multifactorial process, involving not only NO, but, at least, HO-1 and carbon monoxide also.[28]

References

1. Wagner PD. Impairment of gas exchange in liver cirrhosis. *Eur Respir J* 1995; **8**: 1993–1995.
2. Battaglia SE, Pretto JJ, Irving LB, Jones RM, Angus PW. Resolution of gas exchange abnormalities and intrapulmonary shunting following liver transplantation. *Hepatology* 1997; **25**: 1228–1232.

3. Krowka MJ, Cortese DA. Hepatopulmonary syndrome. Current concepts in diagnostic and therapeutic considerations. *Chest* 1994; **105**: 1528–1537.

4. Abrams GA, Nanda NC, Dubovsky EV, Krowka MJ, Fallon MB. Use of macroaggregated albumin lung perfusion scan to diagnose hepatopulmonary syndrome: a new approach. *Gastroenterology* 1998; **114**: 305–310.

5. Vallance P, Moncada S. Hyperdynamic circulation in cirrhosis: a role for nitric oxide? *Lancet* 1991; **337**: 776–778.

6. Hokari A, Zeniya M, Esumi H, Kawabe T, Gershwin ME, Toda G. Detection of serum nitrite and nitrate in primary biliary cirrhosis: possible role of nitric oxide in bile duct injury. *J Gastroenterol Hepatol* 2002; **17**: 308–315.

7. Bauer TM, Schwacha H, Steinbruckner B, Brinkmann FE, Ditzen AK, Aponte JJ, Pelz K, Berger D, Kist M, Blum HE. Small intestinal bacterial overgrowth in human cirrhosis is associated with systemic endotoxemia. *Am J Gastroenterol* 2002; **97**: 2364–2370.

8. Wiest R, Das S, Cadelina G, Garcia-Tsao G, Milstien S, Groszmann RJ. Bacterial translocation in cirrhotic rats stimulates eNOS-derived NO production and impairs mesenteric vascular contractility. *J Clin Invest* 1999; **104**: 1223–1233.

9. Anel RM, Sheagren JN. Novel presentation and approach to management of hepatopulmonary syndrome with use of antimicrobial agents. *Clin Infect Dis* 2001; **32**: E131–136.

10. Rasaratnam B, Kaye D, Jennings G, Dudley F, Chin-Dusting J. The effect of selective intestinal decontamination on the hyperdynamic circulatory state in cirrhosis. A randomized trial. *Ann Intern Med* 2003; **139**: 186–193.

11. Fallon MB, Abrams GA, McGrath JW, Hou Z, Luo B. Common bile duct ligation in the rat: a model of intrapulmonary vasodilatation and hepatopulmonary syndrome. *Am J Physiol* 1997; **272**: G779–784.

12. Rabiller A, Nunes H, Lebrec D, Tazi KA, Wartski M, Dulmet E, Libert JM, Mougeot C, Moreau R, Mazmanian M, Humbert M, Herve P. Prevention of gram-negative translocation reduces the severity of hepatopulmonary syndrome. *Am J Respir Crit Care Med* 2002; **166**: 514–517.

13. Fallon MB, Abrams GA, Luo B, Hou Z, Dai J, Ku DD. The role of endothelial nitric oxide synthase in the pathogenesis of a rat model of hepatopulmonary syndrome. *Gastroenterology* 1997; **113**: 606–614.

14. Luo B, Liu L, Tang L, Zhang J, Stockard CR, Grizzle WE, Fallon MB. Increased pulmonary vascular endothelin B receptor expression and responsiveness to endothelin-1 in cirrhotic and portal hypertensive rats: a potential mechanism in experimental hepatopulmonary syndrome. *J Hepatol* 2003; **38**: 556–563.

15. Bruno CM, Neri S, Sciacca C, and Caruso L. Plasma endothelin-1 levels in liver cirrhosis. *Int J Clin Lab Res* 2000; **30**: 169–172.

16. Gustafsson LE, Leone AM, Persson MG, Wiklund NP, Moncada S. Endogenous nitric oxide is present in the exhaled air of rabbits, guinea pigs and humans. *Biochem Biophys Res Commun* 1991; **181**: 852–857.

17. Alving K, Weitzberg E, Lundberg JM. Increased amount of nitric oxide in exhaled air of asthmatics. *Eur Respir J* 1993; **6**: 1368–1370.

18. Recommendations for standardized procedures for the on-line and off-line measurement of exhaled lower respiratory nitric oxide and nasal nitric oxide in adults and children-1999. This official statement of the American Thoracic Society was adopted by the ATS Board of Directors, July 1999. *Am J Respir Crit Care Med* 1999; **160**: 2104–2117.

19. Lundberg JO, Farkas-Szallasi T, Weitzberg E, Rinder J, Lidholm J, Anggaard A, Hokfelt T, Lundberg JM, Alving K. High nitric oxide production in human paranasal sinuses. *Nat Med* 1995; **1**: 370–373.

20. Matsumoto A, Ogura K, Hirata Y, Kakoki M, Watanabe F, Takenaka K, Shiratori Y, Momomura S, Omata M. Increased nitric oxide in the exhaled air of patients with decompensated liver cirrhosis. *Ann Intern Med* 1995; **123**: 110–113.

21. Rolla G, Brussino L, Colagrande P, Dutto L, Polizzi S, Scappaticci E, Bergerone S, Morello M, Marzano A, Martinasso G, Salizzoni M, Bucca C. Exhaled nitric oxide and oxygenation abnormalities in hepatic cirrhosis. *Hepatology* 1997; **26**: 842–847.

22. Delclaux C, Mahut B, Zerah-Lancner F, Delacourt C, Laoud S, Cherqui D, Duvoux C, Mallat A, Harf A. Increased nitric oxide output from alveolar origin during liver cirrhosis versus bronchial source during asthma. *Am J Respir Crit Care Med* 2002; **165**: 332–337.

23. Rolla G, Bucca C, Brussino L. Methylene blue in the hepatopulmonary syndrome. *N Engl J Med* 1994; **331**: 1098.

24. Schenk P, Madl C, Rezaie-Majd S, Lehr S, Muller C. Methylene blue improves the hepatopulmonary syndrome. *Ann Intern Med* 2000; **133**: 701–706.

25. Rolla G, Brussino L, Colagrande P, Scappaticci E, Morello M, Bergerone S, Ottobrelli A, Cerutti E, Polizzi S, Bucca C. Exhaled nitric oxide and impaired oxygenation in cirrhotic patients before and after liver transplantation. *Ann Intern Med* 1998; **129**: 375–378.

26. Brussino L, Bucca C, Morello M, Scappaticci E, Mauro M, Rolla G. Effect on dyspnoea and hypoxaemia of inhaled N(G)-nitro-L-arginine methyl ester in hepatopulmonary syndrome. *Lancet* 2003; **362**: 43–44.

27. Zhang J, Ling Y, Luo B, Tang L, Ryter SW, Stockard CR, Grizzle WE, Fallon MB. Analysis of pulmonary heme oxygenase-1 and nitric oxide synthase alterations in experimental hepatopulmonary syndrome. *Gastroenterology* 2003; **125**: 1441–1451.

28. Rolla G. Is nitric oxide the ultimate mediator in hepatopulmonary syndrome? *J Hepatol* 2003; **38**: 668–670.

29. Rolla G. Hepatopulmonary syndrome: role of nitric oxide and clinical aspects. *Dig Liver Dis* 2004; **36**: 303–308.

EXHALED NITRIC OXIDE
AND PULMONARY COMPLICATIONS
AFTER ALLOGENEIC STEM CELL TRANSPLANTATION

C. BUCCA, L. BRUSSINO, AND E. PANARO

Department of Biomedical Sciences and Human Oncology,
University of Turin, San Giovanni Battista Hospital,
Via Genova 3, I-10126 Turin, Italy

G. AITORO, L. GIACCONE, AND B. BRUNO

Division of Haematology,
University of Turin, San Giovanni Battista Hospital,
Via Genova 3, I-10126 Turin, Italy

1. Introduction

At present, allogeneic hematopoetic stem cell transplantation (AST) is the only potentially curative treatment for multiple myeloma. Its action is most likely due to an *allogeneic graft-versus-myeloma* effect. Unfortunately AST carries a high risk of complications and toxicities related to the intensive preparative regimen which is traditionally used for pre-transplant myeloablation and to the graft versus host disease (GVHD), which may be life threatening.[1]

Pulmonary complications after AST are common[2] and different in nature, ranging from opportunistic infections, such as invasive pulmonary aspergillosis, vascular abnormalities, such as pulmonary veno occlusive disease and diffuse alveolar hemorrhage, and immune-mediated pulmonary processes, such as idiopathic pneumonia syndrome and bronchiolitis obliterans. The last is a nonspecific inflammatory injury of the small airways that was recognized in early 1980s, particularly among patients with acute and chronic GVHD and in those with respiratory infections. Non-myeloablative AST (NST) has the advantage of using low dose total body irradiation, less chemotherapy and more specific immune-modulation. For these reasons it is feasible in elderly patients with almost no upper age limit, in patients heavily pre-treated, and in those with organ dysfunction or other comorbidities precluding standard ablative conditioning. Thus NST is rapidly becoming the treatment of choice in these indications where toxicity of standard ablative therapy is unacceptable. Unfortunately, also for NST, GVHD and disease recurrence remain major obstacles to successful treatment, although existing clinical data demonstrate lowered incidence and severity of GVHD.[3]

It has been observed that pulmonary complications after AST may be predicted by abnormalities in lung function tests.[4] However, these abnormalities do not discriminate between different complications. Exhaled nitric oxide (eNO) is considered a reproducible marker of airway inflammation[5] and its increase has been found to be an early indicator of chronic rejection and of obliterans bronchiolitis in lung transplant[6–9] and of the development of GVHD in allogeneic bone marrow transplantation.[10]

The aim of this study was to evaluate if the measurement of eNO, together with lung function tests, may help in predicting the morbidity and mortality after NST.

2. Methods

We examined 26 consecutive patients with multiple myeloma, followed by the Haematology Clinic of the University of Turin, who had been scheduled for NST. The patients were examined before and 3 and 6 months after NST. All gave their informed consent to participate into the study.

Before transplantation, the patients received induction chemotherapy, autologous transplantation, low dose total body irradiation (200 cGy), fludarabine (30 mg/m^2 daily) and started the treatment with cyclosporine (6 mg/kg *b.d.*), which was continued for 6 months after NST, and with mycophenolate mofetil (15 mg/kg *b.d.*) continued for 1 month.

At each examination the subjects underwent the following measurements:

- eNO, measured offline, using a chemiluminescence analyser (Sievers 280 NOA, Boulder, CO), according to the American Thoracic Society recommendations.[11] Exhaled air was collected using a pressure-regulated flow-restricted apparatus (Sievers, Boulder, CO). In brief, subjects were asked to inhale NO-free air, without a nose clamp, from residual volume to total lung capacity, and, without breath holding, to exhale their whole vital capacity into an impermeable 5-L collection Mylar bag, maintaining a mouth pressure of 10 mm Hg. At this pressure, the flow through the valve apparatus is 350 mL/s. The NO levels were measured within 4 hours from collection.

- Lung function tests. Lung volumes and flow-volume loop were measured using the computerized spirometer Baires (Biomedin, Padua, Italy), using the standardized methods and the reference values proposed by the European Respiratory Society.[12] The tests recorded were: vital capacity (VC), forced expiratory volume in one second (FEV_1), forced expiratory flow between 25 % and 75 % of forced exhaled VC (FEF_{25-75}) and forced mid-expiratory flow (FEF_{50}), residual volume, assessed with the inert gas (helium) dilution method, and total lung capacity (TLC). FEF_{25-75} and FEF_{50} were used as indices of bronchiolar potency.
- Single breath carbon monoxide diffusion capacity, using the diffusion constant (KCO) as index of alveolar-capillary diffusion capacity.
- Arterial blood gases, measured with the ABL 330 analyser (Radiometer, Copenhagen, Denmark).
- Evaluation of infective complications, using: chest X-rays (every 2 weeks), serial dosages of *Aspergillus*, *Cytomegalovirus*, *Legionella* and *Pneumococcus* antigens in blood and/or urine, microbiological cultures of sputum, nasal and pharyngeal tampons, or, when appropriate, of bronchoalveolar lavage.

3. Statistical Analysis

The changes in eNO and lung function tests throughout the follow-up were analysed using the analysis of variance for repeated measures. Linear regression analysis was used to compare the changes in eNO with those of lung function tests. The comparison between patients dead and those survived after 6 months was analysed using the Student's *t* test for unpaired data. For each test a *p* value below 0.05 was considered statistically significant.

4. Results

Out of the 26 patients selected, 8 (31 %) died within one month from transplantation (5 due to disease progression, 2 due to infection and 1 due to severe acute GVHD) while 18 patients completed the 6 months follow-up.

Before NST, 15 of the 18 patients had normal lung volumes and airflow rates, one had lung restrictive pattern and two had mild to moderate airway obstruction. 8 patients had decreased KCO (severe in 2), 9 had mild to moderate arterial hypoxemia. The eNO was increased (over 10 ppb) in 10 patients

12 patients showed chronic GVHD, that in 5 was limited to two organs and in 7 was extensive and involved the lungs. 40 % of the patients

Table 1. Mean values (with SEM) of the measured variables throughout the follow-up for the 18 patients who completed the 6 months follow-up

Variable		Baseline	3 months	6 months
TLC	L	5.51 (1.25)	5.39 (1.25)	5.19 (1.26)
VC	L	3.46 (0.87)	3.32 (0.80)	3.27 (0.88)
FEV_1	L	2.68 (0.71)	2.58 (0.64)	2.53 (0.81)
FEF_{25-75}	L/s	2.83 (1.10)	2.56 (1.0)	2.55 (1.5)
FEF_{50}	L/s	3.66 (1.4)	3.53 (1.2)	3.34 (1.6)
KCO	units	3.40 (0.81)	2.94 (0.62)*	3.57 (1.07)
$P_{a\,O_2}$	mm Hg	80.1 (13)	87.9 (9)	84.5 (10)
$P_{a\,CO_2}$	mm Hg	39.0 (4)	36.3 (4)	36.0 (5)
eNO	ppb	24.5 (18)	18.2 (11)	23.3 (14)

$*p = 0.03$

had infectious complications that consisted of *Cytomegalovirus* reactivation (40%), *Aspergillus* (9%) and *Pneumocystis carinii* (3%). Despite these complications, in the overall patients, the mean values of eNO, lung function tests, and arterial blood gases, showed no significant change throughout the follow-up, apart from a transient decrease in KCO occurred 3 months post-transplantation and totally recovered at the next examination (see Table 1). At the 6 months examination the changes in eNO (as percent of the pretransplant value) were significantly inversely related to the changes in FEF_{50} ($r = 0.521$, $p = 0.026$) and in FEF_{25-75} ($r = 0.554$, $p = 0.017$).

Four patients died after the 6 months visit and before completing the one year follow-up; two had severe extensive GVHD and two had disease progression. All these patients had pulmonary complications and showed ground-glass opacities at lung CT-scan, three of them had *Aspergillus* infection. At the 6 month visit, the comparison between the 14 patients who survived (G1) with those who died (G2) showed that dead patients had significantly higher eNO, lower FEF_{50}, FEF_{25-75} and KCO, see Table 2.

Table 2. Mean values (with SEM) of FEF_{25-75}, FEF_{50}, KCO and exhaled NO at 6 months in subjects who survived and those who had died before the one year visit

Variable		Alive	Dead	p
FEF_{25-75}	L/s	2.79 (0.4)	1.44 (0.4)	0.039
FEF_{50}	L/s	3.62 (0.4)	2.15 (0.5)	0.05
KCO	units	3.80 (0.25)	2.11 (0.36)	0.004
eNO	ppb	19.5 (2.09)	36.3 (8.01)	0.028

5. Discussion

The preliminary results of this study indicate that the measurement of eNO may be useful for the detection of pulmonary complications following NST. In fact, eNO increased in those patients who showed a decrease in the airflow rates and those who reflected peripheral airway patency FEF_{50} and in FEF_{25-75}. Moreover, severe pulmonary complications leading to death were predicted by increases in exhaled NO, as well as by decreases in FEF_{50} and FEF_{25-75} and in KCO. These findings are in agreement with prior observations of Gabbay *et al.* in lung transplantation.[9] They found that eNO is a marker of bronchiolar narrowing (bronchiolitis obliterans) and that, in this circumstance, the major source of eNO is epithelial inducible nitric oxide synthase. Recently, Verleden *et al.*[8] confirmed the accuracy of eNO in the assessment of bronchiolitis obliterans post lung transplant.

Similar findings were reported by Weiss *et al.*[10] in allogeneic bone marrow transplantation, in that the development of GVHD was preceded, by up to 3 days, by a significant rise in nitrite/nitrate in the blood circulation.

The precise role of nitric oxide in pulmonary damage after transplantation is not known. Experimental observations[13] indicate that eNO may be the cause rather than the effect of posttransplant lung damage, in that it might promote obliterative bronchiolitis by destroying airway epithelium, through peroxynitrite formation, and by stimulating fibroblast activity. This reaction might be prevented by binding reactive molecules with superoxide dismutase.

In conclusion, our findings indicate that serial measurements of exhaled NO after NST may be useful to reveal ongoing airway damage and may be predictive of life threatening complications.

References

1. McSweeney PA., Niederwieser D, Shizuru JA, Sandmaier BM, Molina AJ, Maloney DG, Chauncey TR, Gooley TA, Hegenbart U, Nash RA, Radich J, Wagner JL, Minor S, Appelbaum FR, Bensinger WI, Bryant E, Flowers ME, Georges GE, Grumet FC, Kiem HP, Torok-Storb B, Yu C, Blume KG, Storb RF. Hematopoietic cell transplantation in older patients with hematologic malignancies: replacing high-dose cytotoxic therapy with graft-versus-tumor effects. *Blood* 2001; **97** (11): 3390–400.
2. Soubani AO, Miller KB, Hassoun PM. Pulmonary complications of bone marrow transplantation. *Chest* 1996; **109** (4): 1066–77.
3. Crawford SW, Pepe M, Lin D, Benedetti F, Deeg HJ. Abnormalities of pulmonary function tests after marrow transplantation predict nonrelapse mortality. *Am J Respir Crit Care Med* 1995; **152** (2): 690–695.

4. Shimoni A, Nagler A. Non-myeloablative hematopoietic stem cell transplantation (NST) in the treatment of human malignancies: from animal models to clinical practice. *Cancer Treat Res* 2002; **110**: 113–136.

5. Deykin A, Massaro AF, Drazen JM, Israel E. Exhaled nitric oxide as a diagnostic test for asthma: online versus offline techniques and effect of flow rate. *Am J Respir Crit Care Med* 2002; **165** (12): 1597–601.

6. Verleden GM, Dupont LJ, Van Raemdonck D., Vanhaecke J. Effect of switching from cyclosporine to tacrolimus on exhaled nitric oxide and pulmonary function in patients with chronic rejection after lung transplantation. *J Heart Lung Transplant* 2003; **22** (8): 908–913.

7. Verleden GM, Dupont LJ, Delcroix M, Van Raemdonck D, Vanhaecke J, Lerut T, Demedts M. Exhaled nitric oxide after lung transplantation: impact of the native lung. *Eur Respir J* 2003; **21** (3): 429–432.

8. Verleden GM, Dupont LJ, Van Raemdonck DE, Vanhaecke J. Accuracy of exhaled nitric oxide measurements for the diagnosis of bronchiolitis obliterans syndrome after lung transplantation. *Transplantation* 2004; **78** (5): 730–733.

9. Gabbay E, Walters EH, Orsida B, Whitford H, Ward C, Kotsimbos TC, Snell GI, Williams TJ. Post-lung transplant bronchiolitis obliterans syndrome (BOS) is characterized by increased exhaled nitric oxide levels and epithelial inducible nitric oxide synthase. *Am J Respir Crit Care Med* 2000; **162** (6): 2182–2187.

10. Weiss G, Schwaighofer H, Herold M, Nachbaur D, Wachter H, Niederwieser D, Werner ER. Nitric oxide formation as predictive parameter for acute graft-versus-host disease after human allogeneic bone marrow transplantation. *Transplantation* 1995; **60** (11): 1239–1244.

11. American Thoracic Society. Recommendations for standardized procedures for the on-line and off-line measurement of exhaled lower respiratory nitric oxide and nasal nitric oxide in adults and children-1999. This official statement of the American Thoracic Society was adopted by the ATS Board of Directors, July 1999. *Am J Respir Crit Care Med* 1999; **160** (6): 2104–2117.

12. Quanjer PH, Tammeling GJ, Cotes JE, Pedersen OF, Peslin R, Yernault JC. Lung volumes and forced ventilatory flows. Report Working Party Standardization of Lung Function Tests, European Community for Steel and Coal. Official Statement of the European Respiratory Society. *Eur Respir J Suppl* 1993; **16**: 5–40.

13. Salminen US, Maasilta PK, Harjula AL, Romanska HM, Bishop AE, Polak JM. Nitric oxide in the development of obliterative bronchiolitis in a heterotopic pig model. *Transplantation* 2002; **73** (11): 1724–1729.

ISOTOPE SELECTIVE DETECTION OF NITRIC OXIDE IN HUMAN EXHALATION

J. LAUENSTEIN AND K.-H. GERICKE

Institut für Physikalische und Theoretische Chemie,
Technische Universität Braunschweig,
Hans-Sommer-Straße 10, D-38106 Braunschweig, Germany

1. Introduction

Nitric oxide, NO, is a molecule with several different attributes. It interacts toxically with the human body[1] and plays an important role in atmospheric chemistry.[2,3] NO generated by combustion processes[4] catalytically increases the decay of the ozone layer in the stratosphere.[5] Since R. F. Furchgott, L. J. Ignarro and F. Merid were awarded the Nobel Prize for medicine in 1998, the number of scientists studying NO is constantly increasing. Today, the important role of nitric oxide in humans, animals and plants is well established. The main problem when investigating the effects of NO in the human body is to detect it accurately, because its lifetime in the human body is very short due to its reactivity.[6] Ideally, a method is needed to measure NO non-invasively. If these goals can be achieved, NO can be detected in human breath, which is normally at a concentration of about 10 parts per billion (ppb).[7] These low concentrations require an extremely sensitive technique which should also be selective, accurate and rapid. To achieve this, one photon laser induced fluorescence (LIF) is used. In this paper the detection of NO in exhaled human breath using LIF is described.

2. Theory

The ground state of nitric oxide has the configuration $X^2\Pi$, which is split into $^2\Pi_{1/2}$ and $^2\Pi_{3/2}$ states. Figure 1 illustrates a simulated absorption spectrum of NO that contains the γ-band (A $\leftarrow$ X), β-band (B $\leftarrow$ X), δ-band (C $\leftarrow$ X) and ε-band (D $\leftarrow$ X). The spectrum is simulated by LifBase[8] and does not contain all possible transitions. In these experiments, the molecule is excited in the $\gamma(0, 0)$-band around 226 nm. From the γ state the molecule relaxes by emitting a photon. This fluorescence can be measured by a photomultiplier tube. The possible transitions and resulting branches are presented in Fig. 2. The probabilities of the different fluorescence transitions are described by the appropriate Franck–Condon factors.[9,10] For detection, the $(0, 2)$ transition occurring at 247.4 nm was chosen because of the relatively high Franck–Condon factor and the possibility to filter out scattered light around 226 nm.

Nitrogen and oxygen atoms have the following stable isotope distributions: ^{14}N (99.63 %), ^{15}N (0.37 %), ^{16}O (99.76 %), ^{17}O (0.04 %), ^{18}O (0.20 %). The possible combinations of nitrogen and oxygen in NO are: ^{14}N^{16}O (99.390888 %), ^{15}N^{16}O (0.369112 %), ^{14}N^{18}O (0.19926 %), ^{14}N^{17}O (0.039852 %), ^{15}N^{18}O (0.00074 %) and ^{15}N^{17}O (0.000148 %). In that which follows, only on the two most frequently occurring isotopomers ^{14}N^{18}O and ^{15}N^{18}O are considered. The spectra of these isotopomeres are slightly different due to their differing reduced masses; therefore, it is possible to detect both isotopomers with the same optical setup, but according to the natural abundances the ^{14}NO absorption is about 270-fold greater than the ^{15}NO absorption. So a spectral region must be chosen where only ^{15}NO absorbs the laser radiation, taking into account spectral laser linewidth and

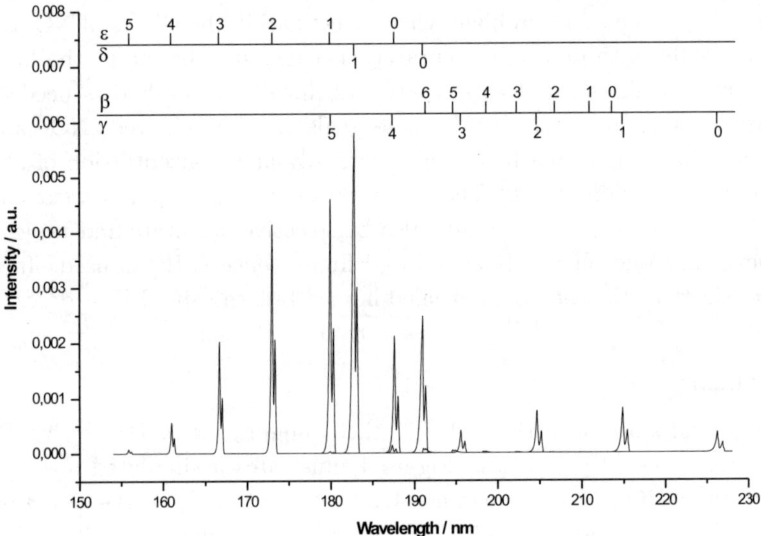

Fig. 1.   Simulated absorption spectrum of nitric oxide in the ultraviolet region. Not all possible transitions are displayed

Doppler broadening of the peaks. For this purpose the absorption spectra of ^{14}NO and ^{15}NO is simulated. One candidate for ^{15}NO detection is the spectral region between 226.369 nm and 226.387 nm that contains four peaks: $P_{11}(6.5;11.5)/R_{22}(10.5)$, $P_{11}(7.5;10.5)$, $Q_{22}(15.5)/R_{12}(15.5)$ and $P_{11}(8.5;9.5)$. The $Q_{22}(15.5)/R_{12}(15.5)$ transition is not resolved by LIF due to the weak transition probability and the closeness to the $P_{11}(7.5;10.5)$

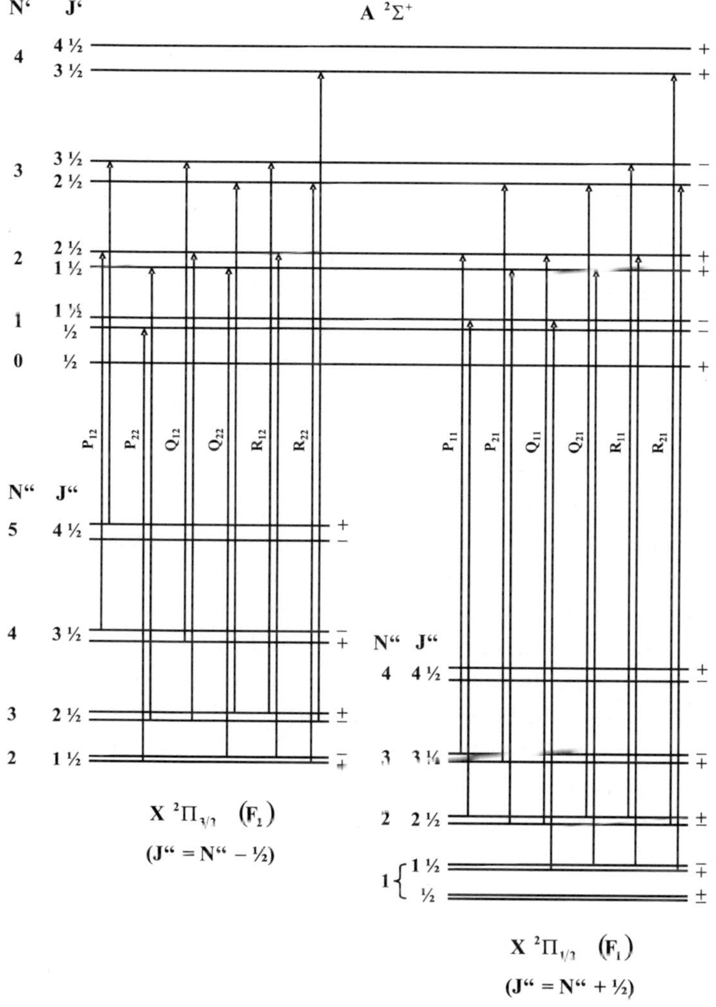

Fig. 2.   Energy level diagram of the $A^2\Sigma^+ \leftarrow X^2\Pi$ transition of nitric oxide

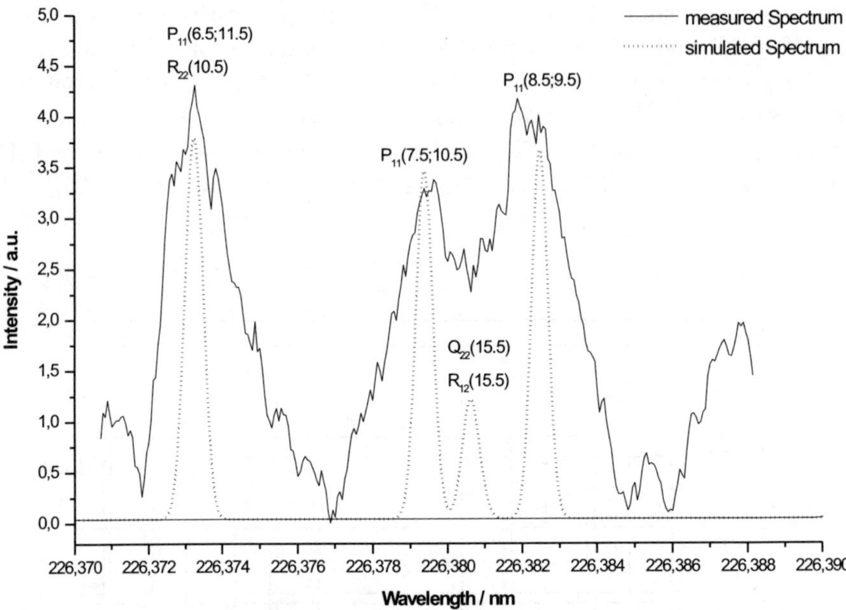

Fig. 3.   Comparison of measured and simulated ^{15}NO spectra. The additional broadening of the experimental line is due to the linewidth of the dye laser radiation.

transition. Fig. 3 illustrates this region with the four ^{15}NO transitions in more detail. It contains a simulated and a measured spectrum. The peak width is due to Doppler broadening and the linewidth of the laser radiation. A spectral width of less than 2 cm^{-1} is required to detect ^{15}NO, because of the surrounding ^{14}NO peaks that conceal the ^{15}NO peaks at broader linewidth. In addition, the pulse length should be short compared to the fluorescence lifetime in order to discriminate between the excitation light and the fluorescence using appropriate gating techniques.[11]

The maximum fluorescence intensity is obtained at a pressure of 10 mbar, because quenching interferes at higher pressures[12,13] and too few fluorescing species are produced at lower pressures. The optimal pressure was determined theoretically and experimentally.

3. Experimental Setup

Figure 4 presents a schematic drawing of the experimental setup used to detect ^{14}NO and ^{15}NO. A XeCl-excimer laser (Lambda Physik LPX600) pumps a dye laser (Lambda Physik LPD2000) that was operated by Coumarine 47.[14] The laser beam was frequency doubled by a BBO crystal to generate UV radiation between 225 nm and 227 nm. The maximum energy of the resulting ultraviolet radiation was 800 μJ at a pulse width of 0.2 cm^{-1} and a repetition rate of 5 Hz. The UV beam was separated from the visible beam by a Pellin Broca prism and then entered the cell through a quartz window at the Brewster angle. After passing through the cell, the laser power is monitored by a joulemeter (Laser Precision Corp., Model RJP-735). The detection optics were arranged perpendicular to the beam axis: two $f/1$ lenses focus the fluorescence to the photomultiplier tube (Hamamatsu R3788), whereas between the two lenses, a bandpass filter blocks the scattered light. The filter (Andover Corporation, 248FS10-50) had a centre wavelength at 248 ± 3 nm with a transmission of 17 %. The signals of the photomultiplier and the joulemeter were integrated by a gated integrator and boxcar averager (Stanford Research Systems SR250, SR280), transferred to a personal computer via an I/O controller card (National Instruments DAQ PCI-1200) and acquired by LabView 5.0. The resulting data were analysed by Origin.

The sample gas mixtures were formed from pure nitrogen (6.0, Linde) and an NO/N$_2$ mixture (2.5 ppm $\pm$ 5 %, Westfalen) using two mass flow controllers (MKS 1179). The total gas flow was established at 100 sccm, while the pressure in the chamber was automatically maintained at 10 mbar via an automatic valve and a pressure gauge (MKS 248AC/221A). The system was evacuated by a rotary vane pump (Edwards RV12) with a cryotrap arranged in line to prevent oil particles reaching the cell which can be fragmented by the laser radiation.

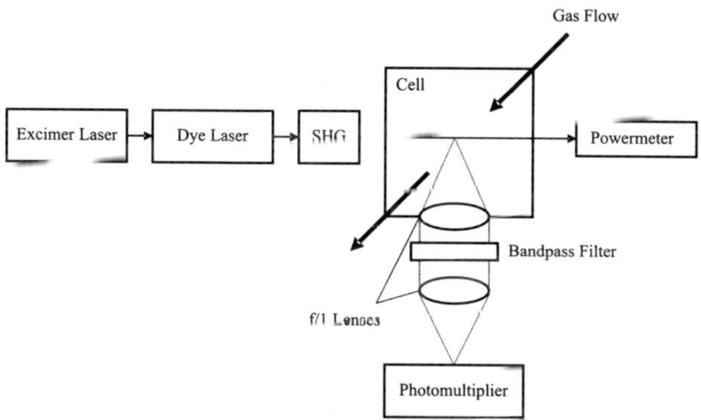

Fig. 4.   Schematic view of the experimental setup

4. Results

Since LIF is not an absolute method, the system has to be calibrated using known NO concentrations. Different ^{14}NO and ^{15}NO concentrations were produced by mixing the 2.5 ppm NO test gas with pure nitrogen via the mass flow controllers. The results are illustrated in Fig. 5. Using these calibration curves, ^{14}NO and ^{15}NO concentrations in a sample could be determined performing only one calibration exercise each day. To measure low NO isotopomer concentrations very accurately, the standard addition method was used.[15] Thus, known NO isotopomer concentrations were added to the sample and the resulting signal intensity was monitored. The resulting straight line is fitted and extrapolated to the abscissa; the intercept (see Fig. 6) provides the absolute value of the concentration of NO isotopomer in the sample. The advantages of the standard addition method are the very high accuracy due to signal averaging and the independence on laser power, photo-multiplier voltage and boxcar sensitivity, as long as these parameters remain constant during the measurement.

To demonstrate the validity of this NO detection system, tracer experiments were performed using ^{15}N-labelled arginine. L-arginine is known to be the precursor for nitric oxide in the human body,[16] so 7.5 mg/kg body weight of ^{15}N-labelled L-arginine were administered orally to a male and a female volunteer. 95 % of the nitrogen atoms were ^{15}N. The time

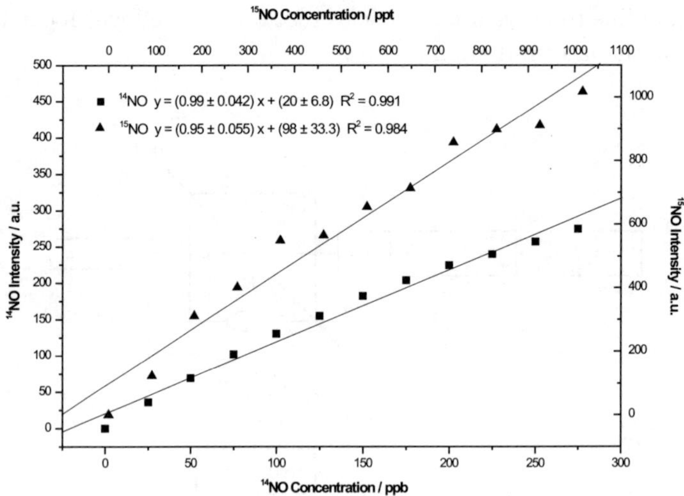

Fig. 5.   Calibration curves for ^{14}NO and ^{15}NO

dependence of the ^{15}NO content of the exhaled air was monitored. The volunteers blew up sample bags made of polyvinyl fluoride (PVF) which were coupled to the mass flow system. The results are shown in Fig. 7. Both volunteers were healthy non-smokers and filled the sample bags in one breath exhalation. The male was 59 years old, the female 23 years old.

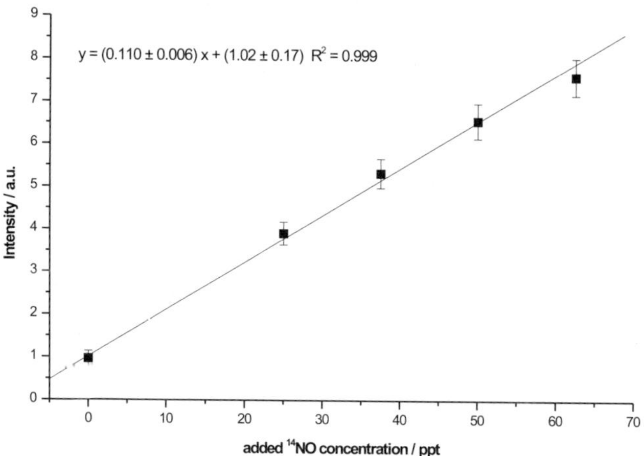

Fig. 6.   Measurement of ^{14}NO via the standard addition method. The ^{14}NO content of the sample is 9.3 ppb $\pm$ 0.2 ppb.

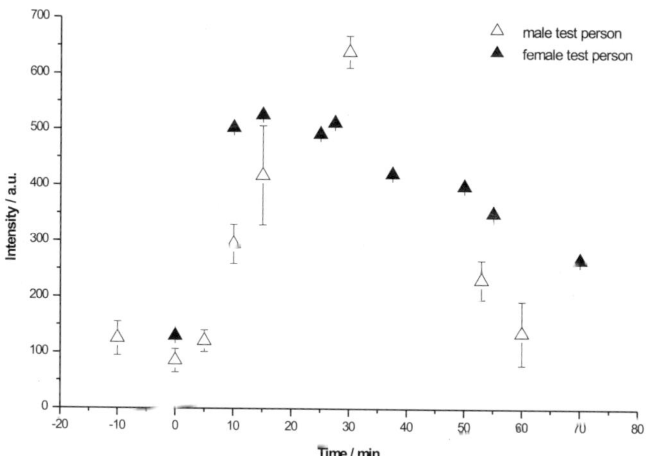

Fig. 7.   Monitoring the ^{15}NO concentration in exhaled breath after ingestion of ^{15}N labelled arginine. Time zero characterises the moment of intake.

Surprisingly, the amount of ^{15}NO increases rapidly following ingestion. The maximum concentration is reached after 10 minutes and falls back to normal levels after about one hour. The experiments with the male volunteer were not performed using the standard addition method; therefore the uncertainties are much higher compared to those for the female volunteer, which are less than 1 %. Currently, the practical detection limit of the apparatus is better than 1 ppt, but this is expected to be reduced to below 0.1 ppt.

5. Conclusions

Our results demonstrate that LIF is a reliable method for measuring nitric oxide traces in gas samples with respect to sensitivity, selectivity, accuracy and time resolution. The sensitivity and selectivity is sufficiently high to detect different isotopomers of nitric oxide down to sub-ppt levels. Hence, experiments using isotopically labelled NO precursor compounds can be carried out to investigate the generation of NO in the body. The high time resolution enables online measurements of nitric oxide in human breath just as in animal breath,[17] plant and soil emissions,[18,19] and combustion exhaust gases.[4]

References

1. Hess D. Adverse effects and toxicity of inhaled nitric oxide. *Respir Care* 1999; **44**: 315–329.
2. Bloss W, Gravestock T, Heard D, Ingham T, Johnson G, Lee J. Application of a compact all solid-state laser system to the in situ detection of atmospheric OH, HO$_2$, NO and IO by laser-induced fluorescence. *J Environ Monit* 2003; **5**: 21–28.
3. Bradshaw J, Rodgers M, Davis D. Single photon laser-induced fluorescence detection of NO and SO$_2$ for atmospheric conditions of composition and pressure. *Appl Opt* 1982; **21**: 2493–2500.
4. Reisel J, Laurendeau N. Quantitative LIF measurements and modeling of nitric oxide in high-pressure C$_2$H$_4$/O$_2$/N$_2$ flames. *Combust Flames* 1995; **101**: 141–152.
5. Birks J, Shoemaker B, Leck T, Hinton D. Studies of reactions of importance in the stratosphere. I. Reaction of nitric oxide with ozone. *J Chem Phys* 1976; **65**: 5181–5185.
6. Thomas D, Liu X, Kantrow S, Lancaster JJ. The biological lifetime of nitric oxide: implications for the perivascular dynamics of NO and O$_2$. *Proc Nat Acad Scienc USA* 2001; **98**: 355–360.

7. Robinson J, Bollinger M, Birks J. Luminol/H_2O_2 chemiluminescence detector for the analysis of nitric oxide in exhaled breath. *Anal Chem* 1999; **22**: 5131–5136.

8. Luque J, Crosley D. *LIFBASE: Database and spectral simulation (version 1.5)*. SRI International Report MP 99-009, 1999.

9. Spindler RJ, Isaacson L, Wentink TJ. Franck–Condon factors and r-centroids for the gamma system of NO. *J Quant Spectrosc Radiat Transfer* 1970; **10**: 621–628.

10. Luque J, Crosley D. Transition probabilities and electronic transition moments of the $A^2\Sigma^+ \leftarrow X^2\Pi$ and $D^2\Sigma^+ \leftarrow X^2\Pi$ systems of nitric oxide. *J Chem Phys* 1999; **111**: 7405–7415.

11. Huber K, Herzberg G. *Molecular spectra and molecular structure IV: Constants of diatomic molecules*. New York: Van Nostrand Reinhold, 1979.

12. McDermid I, Laudenslager J. Radiative lifetimes and electronic quenching rate constants for single-photon-excited rotational levels of NO ($A^2\Sigma^+$, $v' = 0$). *J Quant Spectrosc Radiat Transfer* 1982; **27**: 483–492.

13. Paul P, Gray J, Durant JJ, Thoman JJ. Collisional electronic quenching rates for NO $A^2\Sigma^+$ ($v' = 0$). *Chem Phys Lett* 1996; **259**: 508–514.

14. Brackmann U. *Lambdachrome Laser Dyes*. Goettingen: Lambda Physik, 1997.

15. Ingle JJ, Crouc S. *Spectrochemical analysis*. New Jersey: Prentice-Hall, 1988.

16. Schmidt HH, Klein MM, Niroomand F, Bohme E. Is arginine a physiological precursor of endothelium-derived nitric oxide? *Eur J Pharmacol* 1988; **148**: 293–295.

17. Marlin DJ, Young LE, McMurphy R, Walsh K, Dixon P. Effect of two anaesthetic regimens on airway nitric oxide production in horses. *Br J Anaesth* 2001; **86**: 127–130.

18. Rockel P, Strube F, Rockel A, Wildt J, Kaiser WM. Regulation of nitric oxide (NO) production by plant nitrate reductase *in vivo* and *in vitro*. *J Exp Bot* 2002; **53**: 103–110.

19. Bollmann A, Koschorreck M, Meuser K, Conrad R. Comparison of two different methods to measure nitric oxide turnover in soils. *Biol Fertil Soils* 1999; **29**: 104–110.

DIAGNOSTIC ASPECTS OF EXHALED NITRIC OXIDE IN CARDIOTHORACIC ANAESTHESIA

A. SZABÓ, T. KÖVESI, J. GÁL, AND D. ROYSTON

Department of Anaesthetics,
Royal Brompton and Harefield NHS Trust,
Harefield Hospital, Harefield, Middlesex, UB9 6JH, UK

N. MARCZIN

Department of Anaesthetics,
Royal Brompton and Harefield NHS Trust,
Harefield Hospital, Harefield, Middlesex, UB9 6JH, UK
and
Department of Anaesthetics and Intensive Care,
Faculty of Medicine, Imperial College London,
Chelsea and Westminster Hospital, 369 Fulham Road, London, SW10 9NH, UK

1. Introduction

Basic and clinical research on nitric oxide (NO) has been fascinating and extremely rewarding. Since the original discovery of this remarkable molecule as an endothelium-derived relaxing factor, more than 6500 articles reported the many facets of its regulation and physiological and pathogenic roles in conditions as diverse as acute cardiovascular collapse in septic shock and penile erectile dysfunction. It seems that NO is important in every organ system and it has major relevance to all clinical specialties either as a therapeutic modality or diagnostic tool. In anaesthetics and critical care, our practiced specialty, NO had a roller coaster ride. As we reviewed recently,[1] it was totally condemned initially as a toxic gas killing patients by causing lung injury, as a contaminant of nitrous oxide during anaesthetic accidents.[2] The wheel then turned and we advocated inhalation of NO as a therapeutic magic bullet[3,4] to treat life-threatening acute lung injury. However, we soon realised that this therapy had only a transient and cosmetic effect.[4,5] Recent years have seen a more careful approach to clinical aspects of NO, and its role as a therapeutic agent is more critically analysed by international consensus guidelines based on the outcome of randomized controlled trials.[6]

Parallel to these activities, it has been recognised that production of NO, and concentrations of NO at different anatomical locations, is characteristically altered in different pathologies. Remarkably, NO has been detected in the exhaled breath, and the recognition that its levels are increased in many forms of asthma has lead to its approval as a diagnostic test to monitor airway inflammation and response to anti-inflammatory therapy in asthma.

These developments ignited interest in the anaesthetic community regarding the role of NO as a mediator of different forms of pulmonary and systemic inflammation relevant to high risk surgery and critical illness, and also in elucidating the potential role of exhaled NO as a marker of these events. In light of the importance of surgery-related inflammation to postoperative complications, and the experience of anaesthetists as exhaled breath analyzing professionals, this course of events is not surprising.

An acute systemic or organ specific inflammatory response is one of the most frequent causes of critical illness.[7,8] Major surgery including cardiac, thoracic and abdominal procedures are frequently complicated with this response causing significant morbidity and mortality.[9,10] These surgical procedures, and a multitude of medical conditions can lead to acute lung injury, sepsis and septic shock that are characterized by severe biological and structural injury of endothelial and epithelial cells in the lung, due to activation of inflammatory cells and release of their regulatory and effector products.[11,12] Among these, cytokines and reactive oxygen and reactive nitrogen species appear to play a critical role to initiate, amplify and perpetuate inflammatory processes on a local and systemic basis.[13-16]

Although currently the assessment of disease severity and progression in these patients is based on clinical symptoms and lung function tests, it is widely agreed that monitoring the nature, extent and intensity of inflammation would be highly desirable in offering a timely window of opportunity for early detection and rational basis for novel therapeutic interventions.[16-18] Thus, recent investigations have increasingly focused on suitable methods of assessing inflammation in high-risk surgical and critically ill patients. Among these, several types of samples have been studied, including blood, urine and samples directly obtained from the airways through bronchoalveolar lavage.[17,19-21]

The analysis of exhaled breath has major advantages, since it is non-invasive, represents minimal risk to patient and personnel collecting the samples, and can be sampled repeatedly and frequently during dynamically changing situations. The development of these techniques for use in critically ill and mechanically ventilated patients provides exciting opportunities, although presents unique challenges. The anaesthetic and critical care community has unprecedented expertise with breath analysis in making capnography and anaesthetic gas monitoring everyday standards of patient care. Thus, the term "gas man" in our view not only reflects our basic task of administering anaesthetic gases to the patient, but the equally sophisticated task of obtaining useful medical information by analysis of exhaled breath. Extension of this expertise to exhaled breath markers of inflammation would provide the anaesthetic and intensive care speciality with valuable new window onto metabolic alterations potentially contributing to critical illness.[22] Thus, parallel to increased understanding of the role of breath markers in spontaneously breathing patients, a number of marker molecules have been identified in the breath of mechanically ventilated patients that has been postulated useful in following disease progression, or in monitoring efficacy of therapeutic interventions.[23–29] Such role of exhaled NO is increasingly being recognized.[30,31]

The aims of this chapter are manifold. Firstly, we shall elaborate on current clinical practice of cardiac surgery and arrive at the conclusion that clinically important ischaemia–reperfusion injury is a common scenario of many forms of these surgical procedures. We shall conclude this part by establishing the clinical need for biomarkers of inflammation in cardiothoracic surgery. We shall then take a closer look at mechanisms of ischaemia–reperfusion injury and will propose the role of reactive oxygen and nitrogen species as mediators and biomarkers of acute lung injury. This analysis will provide a good opportunity to highlight major potential mechanisms of altered NO production and bioactivity of NO. We shall conclude that multiple relevant mechanisms may either lead to increased production of NO, or enhance consumption of NO, leaving us with the paradigm that NO maybe used either as a *positive or negative biomarker* of inflammation. In order to explore this dilemma further, we will investigate the dominant effect of oxidative stress on NO bioactivity in cell culture models of ischaemia–reperfusion injury. We will then turn to animal models of ischaemia–reperfusion injury to elucidate the ultimate effects of this condition on lung NO production and concentrations of NO in the lung. Finally, we shall complete this journey by highlighting the human relevance of these observations by reviewing our own experience at Harefield Hospital, UK, regarding exhaled NO in ischaemia–reperfusion injury associated with cardiac surgery and lung transplantation.

2. The Role of Ischaemia–Reperfusion Injury in Complications Following Cardiothoracic Surgery and the Need for Biomarkers of Lung Injury

Modern open-heart surgery utilizing cardiopulmonary bypass (CPB) is predicated on a Faustian bargain and an interesting hierarchical sacrifice as far as vital organs are concerned.[31,32] Extraordinary procedures are now routinely performed in order to restore congenital and acquired anatomical defects of the heart, and advanced surgical techniques are used as revascularization procedures to restore blood flow to areas of the ischaemic myocardium.

However, in order to ultimately improve the heart, this organ and nearly all other vital organs have to sustain severe stresses that cause biochemical and cellular alterations without exception. Although generally subclinical, these changes frequently manifest in organ dysfunction such as myocardial insults, pulmonary dysfunction, renal insufficiency, bleeding complications, immunosuppression and related post-operative infections, stroke, and abdominal events, collectively termed the systemic inflammatory response.[33–40]

From the moment of institution of CPB, the lungs are subjected to severe stresses that result from reduction of pulmonary vascular blood flow. Although the entire output of the right ventricle is directed away from the pulmonary arterial circulation during full CPB, complete lung ischaemia is thought to be avoided by the preserved bronchial circulation. Interestingly, recent studies question this relatively narrow window of safety by showing that bronchial blood flow is dramatically reduced during routine CPB.[41] Thus, CPB is inevitably associated with a defined period of incomplete lung ischaemia, which is followed by reperfusion at the end of CPB.

The combination of this ischaemia–reperfusion induced stress, the systemic inflammatory response caused by the CPB circuit, and the effect of the major surgical stress have important consequences for the lungs. Gas exchange is altered in nearly all patients postoperatively, associated with radiological abnormalities on chest X-ray films. For instance, about sixty percent of the patients exhibit alveolar collapse and eight percent of them develop clinically significant lung dysfunction. A subgroup (about 25 percent) of these latter patients develop life-threatening lung problems, fulfilling the criteria of acute lung injury or ARDS that carries around 50 % mortality.[34,42–44]

The magnitude of this problem worldwide cannot be underestimated. Given the fact that open-heart surgery is routinely performed on the scale of a million patients worldwide every year, 1 to 2 percent mortality due to lung injury in an otherwise successful surgical procedure amounts to more death than caused by the September 11 tragedy in New York in 2001. Moreover, cardiac surgery repeats this tragedy every year! This dramatic analogy fits even better when considering that, on an individual basis, this response and outcome is never really anticipated, the true events leading to the disaster remain largely obscure and our response to these happenings are rather limited. In summary, lung injury after CPB remains a significant clinical problem with high morbidity and mortality. It is presumed that ischaemia–reperfusion injury contributes to the development of post-CPB lung injury and we need a better approach to successfully combat these complications.

Heart and lung transplantation are more heroic aspects of cardiothoracic surgery, which is also frequently complicated by lung injury. There are two major challenges in this regard. Firstly, lung injury occurs quite predictably in the donors, both as a consequence of brain death and medical interventions aimed at saving the patient's life prior to the development of brain death. This lung injury significantly contributes to critical shortage of usable donor organs for lung transplantation, leading to the current situation where nearly fifty percent of patients on the waiting list die before an organ becomes available.[45] Secondly, lung injury in the donor needs to be carefully evaluated in order to prevent transplantation of an already damaged lung, or to avoid rejection of a potentially suitable lung. It appears that current medical practice is less than optimal in both selecting donor lungs and protecting the lungs that are considered ideal for transplantation by the transplant team during the procedure.

The problems of organ acceptance and rejection for transplantation are highlighted by the recent study of Ware and colleagues.[46] They comprehensively evaluated 29 pairs of rejected lungs by physiological, microbiological and histological methods, in order to establish evidence of lung injury. More than eighty percent of these lungs had no or only mild pulmonary oedema and more than sixty percent of these lungs had normal or only mildly abnormal histology. In addition, nearly two thirds exhibited intact alveolar fluid clearance suggesting that these lungs had a considerable physiological reserve to overcome a mild pulmonary oedema. Overall, the authors concluded that at least forty percent of these lungs would have been potentially suitable. Since, currently, more than eighty five percent of the donor lungs are excluded, acceptance of these lungs could have tripled lung transplantation in that region. In contrast, the clinical decision to reject these functionally good lungs appears to contribute to critical organ shortages. The authors have definitely established the urgent need for prospective scientific assessment of the selection of donors for lung transplantation.

Unfortunately, current practice of lung transplantation appears to damage even the ideal donor lungs. Complete and prolonged lung ischaemia for up to several hours is unavoidable during lung transplantation, with dire consequences. Transbronchial biopsies performed after lung transplantation showed characteristic histological features of diffuse alveolar damage in more than thirty percent of patients.[47] This is associated with severe graft dysfunction in about twenty percent of lung transplant recipients, with the clinical manifestation of progressive hypoxemia, decreased pulmonary compliance, high permeability pulmonary oedema, and widespread alveolar densities on chest radiographs.[48–50] This early lung allograft dysfunction, termed "primary graft failure," remains the primary cause of early mortality in lung transplantation.[51] Although severe graft dysfunction can be reversible, it is often associated with the need for prolonged mechanical ventilation, intensive care and hospital stay, and compromised recovery among survivals. In addition to this morbidity, ischaemia–reperfusion injury may also predispose grafts to acute and chronic rejection via upregulation of class II major histocompatibility complex antigens, release of endothelial cell antigens, potentially triggering anti-endothelial antibody production, and via generation of pro-inflammatory mediators, including cytokines and growth factors.[52–54]

Thus, we can conclude that the current practice of lung transplantation presents a number of challenges, both in evaluating donor lungs and managing the accepted organs. It is presumed that better diagnostic tools, perhaps based on molecular analysis of major players involved in the evolution of lung injury, are required for early and more accurate detection of subclinical or impending lung injury. We believe that appropriate biomarkers — among these measures of nitric oxide, perhaps in the exhaled breath — may be helpful in these efforts.

3. Scope of Biomarker Research Applicable to Lung Injury Associated with Cardiothoracic Surgery

At the recent ERS meeting in Glasgow, we proposed a framework involving necessary steps and a basic classification of applicable biomarkers for human lung ischaemia–reperfusion injury and called upon the research community for united efforts to fully develop these concepts. We, and others, believe that despite extensive research in this area, the exact molecular mechanisms of lung injury associated with this condition remain unknown. However, the emerging picture suggests that multiple components and pathways contribute to manifest lung injury. Given this complexity, we believe that further studies are needed to better define the molecular and cellular events that determine ischaemia–reperfusion injury in model systems. However, none of the models represents all aspects of the clinical picture and some of the mechanisms maybe completely irrelevant to human diseases. Thus, it will be crucially important to validate the clinical relevance of the mechanisms observed in the model systems. Such strategies have discovered — and, as new mechanisms are uncovered, will continue to identify — important molecules that are closely linked to the natural history and pathogenesis of the condition. Some of these molecules will fulfil the requirement of "Type 0" biomarkers in that they will correlate longitudinally with organ function and established clinical indices of injury. In order for these biomarkers to be helpful in predicting or following clinical progression of the development of lung injury, the methodology used to monitor these biomarkers should be relatively rapid, preferably applicable at the bedside and not only in the laboratory. In order to be useful in donor selection, which is generally performed in a distant district hospital, portable systems will be required.

It is also anticipated that the molecular, physico-chemical and cellular understanding of the pathogenesis of reperfusion injury will pave the way for novel therapeutic interventions. Currently, apart from preserving the organs in a cold crystalloid solution, little effort is made to interfere with specific biochemical events or physical alterations, either during ischaemia or during the period of reperfusion. This is perhaps due to the fact that some mechanisms that seemed effective in particular models turned out to be ineffective in the clinical scenario. Again, it will be of paramount importance to continue to establish clinical efficacy of these novel therapies. While conducting the therapeutic studies, the influence of new drugs on important intermediate clinical endpoints, such as gas exchange, lung mechanics, pulmonary oedema, metabolic function, will be established. Some of the biomarkers of pathogenesis may also reflect the response to therapy and therefore qualify as a "Type I" biomarker. A selected group of these markers will have a very close relationship with the clinically meaningful intermediate endpoints and/or with the ultimate endpoints of irreversible lung injury leading to irreversible morbidity or mortality, and thereby they can serve as surrogate end points.[55,56] A short review of the current understanding of the pathogenesis of ischaemia–reperfusion injury will enable us to propose a framework for classification of the major potential biomarkers of this condition.

4. Biomarkers of Ischaemia–Reperfusion-Induced Lung Injury Based on Pathogenesis

4.1. *Role of Microvascular Endothelial and Epithelial Cells*

In addition to arteriolar and postcapillary venular alterations, components of the alveolo-capillary unit appear as major targets during acute lung injury with the microvascular endothelium being the most susceptible element. During the injury process, endothelial cells become activated and more permeable with characteristic loss of their normal function as essential regulators of pulmonary vasoreactivity, intravascular coagulation, inflammatory response and gas exchange.[48,57,58] In addition, the composition, function, and metabolism of pulmonary surfactant produced by alveolar type II epithelial cells are increasingly being recognized as important factors in lung injury.[48,59] Although Type I epithelial cells appear to be more resistant to inflammatory response and injury, and their barrier and metabolic function might remain intact even in high permeability pulmonary oedema, long-term outcome might depend upon Type I epithelial cell survival.[60,61]

4.2. *Responses of Endothelial Cells to Hypoxia, Ischaemia and Reperfusion*

It is now established that human endothelial cells are substantially altered either during hypoxia associated with ischaemia or during reestablishment of blood flow and oxygen or in response to inflammatory mediators resulting in an activated phenotype.[62] This includes changes in the profile of vasoregulatory endothelium dependent factors, and the expression of activities that initiate and amplify inflammation and coagulation. Prolonged hypoxia can alter membrane properties, disturb the distribution of ions, increase intracellular volume, and impair the cytoskeletal organization of endothelial cells. Hypoxia may lead to severe depletion of energy stores causing cellular energetic failure.

Immediately after reperfusion, there is a burst of oxidant production within the hypoxic endothelial cells. This, together with complement fragment activation on the surface of these cells, causes transient expression of pre-formed proteins and release of mediators that promote leukocyte-endothelial cell interactions, coagulation and cytoskeletal rearrangement which might underlie transient increase in permeability.[32] Alternatively, this oxidative stress could initiate signal transduction events to activate a delayed transcriptional program of several genes, resulting in the translation and prolonged surface expression of leukocyte adhesion molecules and cytokines that mediate further recruitment of neutrophils to sites of inflammation.[63]

4.3. *Role of Leukocyte Activation*

Recent studies also suggest a crucial role of resident alveolar macrophages in the early phase of ischaemia–reperfusion injury. These cells can be activated by a number of conditions to drive a major pro-inflammatory environment in the alveoli, which includes ischaemia reperfusion injury. Depletion of pulmonary macrophages or treatment with chemical agents that down regulate alveolar macrophage activation, attenuates development of permeability oedema following early reperfusion.[64–67] Proinflammatory cytokines and chemokines could be the major mediators of these activated cells that appear to orchestrate early lung ischaemia–reperfusion injury.

There has been considerable circumstantial evidence both from animal and clinical studies implicating the neutrophil as a potentially important mediator of the changes in lung endothelial and epithelial permeability following ischaemia–reperfusion. The enhanced neutrophil–endothelial interactions might promote microvascular injury by multiple mechanisms. First, activation of neutrophils in the close proximity of endothelial cells might accentuate and prolong oxidative stress, resulting in oxidative stress signalling in endothelial cells, to further enhance pro-inflammatory phenotype and sustain cytoskeletal reorganization.[68–71] Neutrophils can produce significant quantities of a number of pro inflammatory cytokines and potent chemotactic agents that further promote their adherence to the endothelium.[72,73] Finally, they can release elastase and other proteases, which might contribute to direct pulmonary cell injury.[74,75]

Despite many studies suggesting the pivotal role of neutrophils in ischaemia–reperfusion injury, not all investigators have found conclusive evidence for neutrophil involvement. In particular, there are several models where, despite significant decrease in the number of circulating or resident neutrophils, the extent of lung injury remained comparable to that of control situation.[76] Thus, pulmonary ischaemia–reperfusion injury remains a complex process, the initiation of which might occur within the hypoxic endothelial cells, perpetuated by activation of pulmonary macrophage-derived pro-inflammatory cytokines and chemokines. Interaction of these mediators provides a milieu that attracts, sequestrates and activates neutrophils in pulmonary microvessels, amplifying the injury in later phases of reperfusion. While these cellular events cannot readily be monitored at the bedside, a variety of the mediators and related biomarkers can be detected serially from different samples that include plasma, bronchoalveolar lavage fluid, undiluted oedema fluid aspirate and gaseous and fluid phase metabolites in the exhaled breath. Further clinical studies into these biomarkers will significantly enhance our understanding of the pathogenesis of human lung ischaemia–reperfusion injury and the human relevance of different mechanisms identified in animal models. This line of research will be greatly facilitated by international dialogue and consensus on the proposed biomarkers. To facilitate these discussions, we recently proposed a framework for classification of the proposed biomarkers at the Glasgow symposium. Table 1 represents a modified but still preliminary version of this classification.

Table 1.   Proposed biomarkers of ischaemia–reperfusion injury in the setting of cardiothoracic surgery

---

A. Biomarkers reflecting activation of the innate immune system
    a. Markers related to leukocyte activation and their products:
        a1. Neutrophils (adhesion molecule expression, signal transduction, degranulation, elastase, cathepsin G, heparin binding protein, cytokines)
        a2. Monocytes: (adhesion molecules, signal transduction, cytokines)
    b. Coagulation markers
    c. Complement markers
    d. Markers of oxidative stress:
        Reactive oxygen and nitrogen species, isoprostanes

B. Biomarkers of pulmonary macrophage activation:
    Proinflammatory cytokines, chemokines

C. Biomarkers of endothelial cell activation, injury and adaptation:
    Adhesion molecules, vasoactive mediators, apoptosis markers, von Willebrand factor

D. Biomarkers of epithelial cell activation, injury and adaptation:
    Adhesion molecules, KL-6, surfactant and surfactant proteins, apoptosis,

E. Biomarkers of increased permeability and fluid transport:
    BAL albumin, total protein, plasma Clara cell antigen, plasma KL-6, heparin binding protein

F. Biomarkers of resolution and repair:
    Matrix metalloproteinases and their inhibitors, markers of collagen synthesis, markers of fibrosis (procollagen peptide III), TGF-B

---

5. NO as a Mediator and Biomarker of Lung Ischaemia–Reperfusion Injury

NO is produced by many cells within the lung and appears to play a critical role in the pathophysiology of the pulmonary vascular bed and airways.[77–80] Pulmonary vascular endothelial cells and airway epithelial cells continuously generate NO from the amino acid L-arginine via constitutively active NO synthases (NOS). Recent studies suggest that endothelial cells constitutively express a relatively low output NO pathway via Type III NOS, while airway epithelial cells normally express a high output NO pathway via Type II NOS (iNOS), which could be further induced by inflammatory mediators.[81,82] Therefore, under normal conditions, there is a considerable release of NO both in the microvasculature and airways, to elicit a number of bioactivities through either direct signalling or via a guanylate cyclase and cGMP dependent process. In the normal lung these include (1) regulation of pulmonary arteriolar and bronchial tone by relaxing smooth muscle; (2) prevention of platelet aggregation and thrombus formation; (3) modulation of multiple aspects of lung inflammation through attenuation of the adhesive interactions between leukocytes and the endothelial or epithelial cell surface, leukocyte trafficking, and reduction of oxidative stress by effectively scavenging the low intracellular levels of superoxide anion.[57]

NO production and bioactivity is subjected to great alterations during hypoxia, ischaemia and reperfusion. Enzymatic NO production exhibits a characteristic O_2 dependence and, therefore, hypoxia reduces enzyme activity to synthesize NO. This phenomenon has been demonstrated in cells in culture, and in animal and human lungs.[83–86] In addition to basal rates of enzymatic NO production, mechanical forces imposed on the cells by dynamically changing blood-flow and air-flow are also important contributors to both microvascular and airway NO production. These mechanical stimuli are reduced during ischaemia, with a potential effect of decoupling NO synthesis from shear stresses.

Hypoxia, however, might increase NO generation from non-enzymatic sources. This involves non-enzymatic reduction of inorganic nitrite to NO, a reaction that takes place predominantly during acidic/reducing conditions.[87,88] Non-enzymatic NO production has been demonstrated in various organs, including the stomach, on the surface of the skin, in the ischaemic heart, and in infected nitrite-containing urine. The potential relevance of this phenomenon to lung pathology has been demonstrated by showing alteration of acid-base balance and increased NO production from nitrite in the airway lining fluid of asthmatic patients.[89] It has also been suggested that pH changes associated with ischaemia can trigger this chemistry in the heart and aorta.[87,88] Thus, hypoxia and ischaemia might alter NO concentrations and bioactivity by multiple and sometimes opposing mechanisms.

In addition to changes in NO availability during ischaemia, reperfusion can cause further consumption of NO through interactions with superoxide. In this situation, NO undergoes radical–radical reactions with superoxide at near diffusion-limited rates to yield peroxynitrite, a potent oxidizing agent to lipids, aromatic amino acid residues, protein sulfhydryls, and DNA.[90–93] Peroxynitrite has been shown to initiate lipid peroxidation in biological membranes at rates that are a thousand-fold higher than for hydrogen peroxide. However, NO displays a dual action with lipids. In addition to pro-oxidant characteristics through peroxynitrite mediated oxidation reactions, it also has the ability to inhibit lipid radical chain propagation.[94,95] Thus, although NO can serve both as an antioxidant (by inhibiting lipid free radicals) or an oxidant (by contributing to peroxynitrite formation), both of these reactions will lead to consumption of NO and reduced levels of bioactivity to elicit normal signalling and biological functions in the lung.[31]

Following the acute phase of NO-superoxide interactions, the redox milieu is further complicated by transcriptional induction of iNOS and various antioxidant enzymes.[96,97] The resulting reactions will again depend on the relative quantities of NO and superoxide, and the local redox microenvironment. It is conceivable that, in case of continuous ongoing superoxide production, increased NO synthesis may contribute to further peroxynitrite formation. However, increased NO may attenuate the extent of cellular injury through inhibition of apoptosis, or may restore endothelial function if concomitant superoxide generation had subsided.[31]

All these considerations predict that ischaemia–reperfusion injury will be associated with a complicated picture of NOS expression, NO generation and consumption. Actual NO concentrations will be different according to the dynamically changing cytokine environment, the nature of microvascular and airway inflammation, neutrophil activation, concomitant production of reactive oxygen species, and acidity in the immediate environment of endothelial and airway epithelial cells.[98]

These theoretical considerations and experimental observations have important implications in considering reactive oxygen and nitrogen species and their interactions as biomarkers of lung ischaemia–reperfusion injury, and acute lung injury in general. Focusing on NO, it may serve either as a *positive or negative biomarker* of particular stages of lung injury. Considering that it is produced as part of the normal physiological processes, measured levels of NO can either increase due to the above described mechanisms or decrease mainly due to consumption reactions. An increase in NO likely reflects net pro-inflammatory activities in the lung, as the primary mechanism of NO increase is cytokine-mediated induction of the Type II NOS gene. Thus, as a *positive biomarker*, increased NO may ultimately serve as a surrogate end point of inflammation in the lung.

Interestingly, a decrease in NO concentrations, as a *negative biomarker*, may also reflect various aspects of inflammation. As discussed above, steady state levels of NO may decrease due to reduced production and increased consumption. As the primary mechanism of NO consumption is related to superoxide, one can make a reasonable argument that the reduced NO perhaps reflects a degree of superoxide-dominated oxidative stress. Given the increasingly accepted role of oxidative stress in lung injury, this would be an important biomarker function. In addition, because the superoxide-mediated consumption also leads to peroxynitrite formation — a widely confirmed toxic substance to the lung —, decreased NO as a *negative biomarker* may also reflect cytotoxic activities, another important biomarker function. Furthermore, the reduced NO levels may reflect an inability of particular cells to generate this pleitropic mediator. We, and others, have suggested that hydrogen peroxide attenuates NO production in endothelial cells,[99] suggesting another mechanism whereby reduced NO concentrations may reflect oxidative stress. Reduced ability of cells to form and release NO may represent a wide spectrum of epithelial or endothelial cell dysfunction, with irreversible tissue injury representing the most severe form.

The important challenge here is to elucidate how well changes in NO concentrations capture these pathogenic events, and whether or not the opposing effects of various inflammatory events (in inducing *vs.* consuming NO) would make NO concentration an unreliable marker of these processes. For instance, in one scenario, all processes would be occurring with net pro-inflammatory cytokines inducing iNOS that would lead to increased production of NO, which, in turn, would be consumed in superoxide-mediated reactions due to neutrophil activation. These opposing events may result in maintaining NO concentrations in the normal range, producing a false negative result in assessing inflammation, oxidative stress and cytotoxicity. The obvious solution to avoiding such problems would be to assess NO and its metabolites by complimentary means, together with other measures of oxidative stress and cytokine environment.

Finally, there is also a challenge regarding selection of the appropriate biological sample for NO biomarker research. NO is extremely labile with a half-life of only seconds in the fluid phase. Its concentration in fluid samples can only be measured with specific sensors at the surface of the cells or organs, which is currently only applicable to experimental models and perhaps will only be available to surgical conditions in the future. Thus, most assays rely on measuring stable end products such as nitrite and nitrate and footprints of peroxynitrite attack, such as nitrotyrosine. But in lung injury, should these be measured in the plasma, or in samples that are more reflective of pulmonary compartmentalisation? The most frequently used specimen is the bronchoalveolar lavage fluid, which is a very invasive sample collection procedure. A less invasive approach is to collect undiluted lung oedema fluid by direct aspiration or collection of breath condensate, which in some ways represents (to a much- debated extent) airway lining fluid. However, the physico-chemical properties (such as solubility) of NO favours partitioning of NO into the gas phase, and its diffusibility in the gas phase allows detection of gaseous NO far away from its production site.

The mindful discovery of Gustafsson and colleagues, followed by recent technological developments that allow direct measurements of NO in the expired air, have provided an exciting opportunity to evaluate changes in NO production and consumption in the clinical setting.[100,101] It is generally accepted that exhaled NO reflects, at least in qualitative terms, the dynamism of NO production and consumption in the lung.[83]

Accordingly, we, and others, have been pursuing the hypothesis that, similarly to some chronic lung diseases, there is a dominant mechanism that alters NO concentrations in the lung, which lead to either increased or decreased levels of NO, making it a useful biomarkers in the setting of ischaemia–reperfusion-induced lung injury. We were particularly excited about the possibility that these events could be monitored non-invasively, reproducibly, in real time at the bedside by measuring NO in the exhaled breath. In the following, we will review some of our own experience and the relevant investigation of some others in this direction. We will structure this journey according to our postulated framework of biomarker research by focusing on characteristics of NO in cell culture models of oxidative stress first. Then we will move on to animal models and finally will overview the clinical applicability and relevance of these observations, including lung assessment in the donors and recipients following lung transplantation.

6. Endothelial NO Bioactivity in the Setting of Oxidative Stress and Enhanced Endothelial–Leukocyte Interactions: Cell Culture Studies

Our initial studies suggested that several chemical oxidants, including hydrogen peroxide, methylene blue and oxidants generated by xanthine and xanthine oxidase, influenced many aspects of the vascular NO pathways. These included attenuated production and increased consumption of NO, and reduced responsiveness of smooth muscle cells to NO in terms of guanylate cyclase mediated formation of cGMP.[99,102–104] To establish the physiological relevance of these observations, we evaluated endothelium-derived NO bioactivity in the setting of superoxide-mediated oxidative stress induced by activation of neutrophils during coculture with endothelial cells.[104] NO release was estimated in a bioassay using endothelial cell-induced cGMP accumulation in vascular smooth muscle (SM) cells.

Neutrophil activation produced a graded increase in superoxide anion, as measured by cytochrome-c reduction. Associated with this increased superoxide load, endothelial cell-induced and NO-dependent activation of guanylate cyclase was inhibited in a neutrophil concentration-dependent manner. Furthermore, the inhibition of NO action was prevented in the presence of superoxide scavengers, such as superoxide dismutase and Tiron, suggesting that the primary reactive species responsible for loss of NO bioactivity was indeed superoxide anion.[104]

Interestingly, when we compared sensitivity of the NO pathway to other endothelial functions in this model of leukocyte activation and endothelial dysfunction, loss of NO bioactivity was one of the most sensitive biochemical targets of oxidant stress. NO-induced cGMP accumulation was lost earlier and at lower leukocyte concentrations than other cellular responses, such as endothelial ectoenzyme function, changes in permeability and cytotoxicity.[104] These studies indicated that, in the setting of oxidative stress, at least in cell culture models of reperfusion injury, a decrease in NO maybe an extremely sensitive *negative biomarker.*[31]

We also studied the effects of monocytes and monocyte adhesion to endothelial cells on the endothelial NO pathway by estimating release of biologically active NO from cultured endothelial cells and levels of constitutive NO synthase (eNOS).[105] Exposure of smooth muscle cells (SM) cells to porcine aortic endothelial cells (PAECs) and human aortic endothelial cells (HAECs) produced large increases in SM cGMP content. This increase was prevented by N^G-nitro-L-arginine methyl ester, the inhibitor of endothelial NOS. Confluent monolayers of PAECs and HAECs cocultured with monocytes also stimulated SM cGMP formation; however, NO release from these cultures was attenuated in a coculture time (2 to 48 hours)- and monocyte concentration (20 to 200×10^3 per well)-dependent manner. This effect of monocyte adhesion appeared to be selective for NO release, since other biochemical pathways, such as atriopeptin-and isoproterenol-induced cyclic nucleotide accumulation within the endothelial cells, were not altered by monocytes.

The effects of adherent monocytes on NO release were mimicked by monocyte-derived cytokines tumour necrosis factor (TNF)-α and inter-leukin (IL)-1α. Furthermore, the conditioned medium of monocytes contained significant quantities of these cytokines. Conditioned medium, as well as monocytes physically separated from the endothelial cells, attenu-ated NO release, suggesting that soluble factors may mediate the effects of monocytes. An IL-1β neutralizing antibody fully prevented the NO dys-function in response to directly adherent monocytes. Superoxide dismutase, catalase, Tiron, and exogenous L-arginine failed to improve NO release, suggesting that oxidant stress-induced inactivation of NO or limited sub-strate availability were not primarily responsible for the inhibiting effects of monocytes. Western blot analysis revealed reduced quantities of eNOS in monocyte/endothelium cocultures, as well as in HAECs treated with monocyte-conditioned medium or TNF-α. Thus, adhesion of monocytes to endothelial cells and monocyte-derived secretory products down-regulate steady-state levels of ecNOS, an event associated with attenuated release of biologically active NO. Our data are well supported with other studies in this area. Yoshizumi and colleagues also demonstrated cytokine induced down-regulation of eNOS.[106] They discovered that the underlying mecha-nism of such effects of cytokines shortened the half life of eNOS mRNA by destabilization.

Therefore, we, and others, have provided evidence that, similarly to neutrophil-endothelial interactions, monocyte recruitment to endothelial cells and their activation during adhesion also has the capacity to nega-tively influence NO release and steady-state levels. This provides an addi-tional reason for considering decreased NO as a *negative biomarker* of these inflammatory reactions.

Against these observations are the frequent demonstrations of the abil-ity of pro-inflammatory cytokines to induce the high output NO pathways in a variety of cells.[107–109] In the vascular system, our own studies show potent up-regulation of NO release via transcriptional induction of iNOS in rodent vascular smooth muscle cells.[110–113] Although interpretation of these results to human cells is not straightforward, due to the complexity and more stringent regulation of the human iNOS, the appropriate combination of multiple cytokines also has the capacity to induce human iNOS in a variety of conditions in human cells.[114-120]

Consequently, while it appears that the dominant characteristic of the NO system in oxidative stress is reduced steady-state NO, the cytokine environment may modulate this response in two different ways. It may either cause a further decrease in NO response or it may also override these mechanisms by induction of NO-generating enzymes. Figure 1 schematically summarises these regulatory events by depicting the multiple influences of leukocyte-derived oxidants and cytokines on vascular NO pathways. Due to this complexity, it remains crucially important to evaluate the dominant reactions of NO in different phases of clinically relevant *in vivo* models of ischaemia–reperfusion injury, which would be in complete agreement with the necessary steps of general biomarker research, as discussed above. We will focus on two relevant series of experiments: one investigating pul-

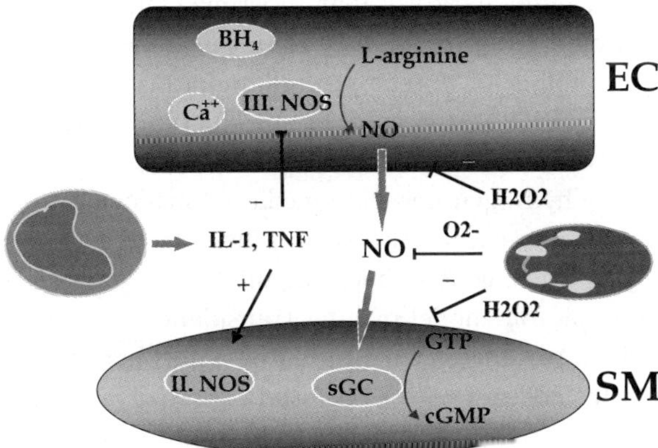

Fig. 1.   Multiple influence of leukocyte-derived mediators on endogenous vascular NO pathways. Under normal conditions, NO is formed by endothelial cells from the amino acid L-arginine by constitutively expressed Type III NO synthase (NOS) utilizing Ca^{2+} and BH$_4$, among others as regulators of enzyme activity. NO acts on smooth muscle cells to produce vasodilation by activating soluble guanylate cyclase (sGC) to increase intracellular cGMP. Activated neutrophils release a mixture of superoxide anion (O_2^-) and hydrogen peroxide (H_2O_2). O_2^- may directly interact with NO and consume NO by peroxynitrite generation. H_2O_2 may act on the endothellum and attenuate NO formation. It may also affect SM and interfere with cGMP formation by NO. Activated monocytes release the cytokines TNF and IL-1. They can downregulate Type III NOS activity in EC. They are also potent inducers of Type II NOS gene in SM.

monary NO pathways following a porcine model of cardiopulmonary bypass and the second investigating NO concentrations following hypothermic ischaemia and reperfusion of rat lungs.

7. Influence of Ischaemia–Reperfusion Injury on NO Pathways: Studies in Animal Models

Morita and colleagues explored the influence of CPB on pulmonary NO production and vasoconstriction in piglets.[121] To study the role of oxidative stress in these alterations, some of the animals were treated with N-mercaptopropionylglycine and catalase, antioxidants that primarily affect hydrogen peroxide metabolism. Cardiopulmonary bypass caused a significant increase in pulmonary vascular resistance, which was associated with a reduction of NO production and depressed right ventricular function. Addition of antioxidants to the CPB allowed a substantial improvement of these deleterious effects of CPB.

This is an important study, which reproduces in a large animal model at least two main components of frequent pulmonary complications of CPB, namely increased pulmonary vascular resistance and consequent strain on the right ventricle. Despite the fact that this condition is characterized by release of a number of potent pro-inflammatory cytokines, and therefore, with the potential of increased NO production via induction of iNOS, the findings of this study indicate that the predominant response in this complex model is hydrogen peroxide-mediated attenuation of NO production. This appears to cause relative insufficiency of NO bioactivity with important physiological consequences manifested in altered vasodilation.

In an orthotopic rat model of lung transplantation, NO release at the surface of the lung was directly measured by a porphyrinic NO microsensor by Pinsky and his colleagues.[122] The study showed that NO levels diminished to one third of the control during 6 hours of hypothermic storage in lactated Ringer solution. Moreover, NO release at the surface of the lung plummeted following reperfusion. This could be partially recovered by administration of superoxide dismutase. This was a landmark study which demonstrated, with sophisticated direct methods, that pulmonary NO production is attenuated by both ischaemia and even more severely during reperfusion. In addition, the authors demonstrated the biological significance of these alterations by showing that attempts to restore the NO pathway, at the level of cGMP, improved functional recovery and graft survival.

We can therefore conclude that, the observations made in cellular studies regarding oxidant-mediated consumption of or reduced production of NO has relevance to *in vivo* situations, at least in animal models of ischaemia–reperfusion injury. But do these have implications to human pathology? Some answers to this question are emerging from studies on bypass surgery, severe acute lung injury and lung transplantation.

8. Studies on Pulmonary NO Metabolism in Human Lung Injury Utilising Analysis of Exhaled Breath

As part of the inflammatory response following CPB for heart surgery, Brett and colleagues at the Royal Brompton Hospital, UK, expected to see increased NO production, due to either increased activity of the constitutive enzyme system or induction of the inflammation-specific systems.[123] While there was a degree of lung dysfunction reflected by reduced oxygenation index, and also some evidence for certain inflammatory reactions, plasma nitrate/nitrite and airway nitric oxide concentrations did not change throughout the course of the study. These observations suggested that the pro-inflammatory events were insufficient to induce the high output NO pathway, but also that the degree of lung injury was not severe enough to attenuate NO release, at least in the compartment contributing to exhaled NO. Two other groups reported different findings.[124,125] In these studies, exhaled NO was reduced after CPB, which was in good agreement with the piglet study on CPB. The reasons for these contradicting results remain unclear and may reflect different patient populations, conduct of the bypass and surgery in different centres, and as a result, different degree of lung injury.

However, a certain degree of caution is required before we accept that no change in exhaled NO fully reflects normal NO metabolism and function in the lung. It is becoming increasingly recognised that airway and microvascular NO pathways contribute to exhaled NO to a different degree.[126,127] Most investigators now accept that, under normal conditions, exhaled NO reflects airway epithelial NO production, and microvascular events only contribute to a significant degree after mechanical or pharmacological stimulation of NO production in this compartment.[128] If this is true, then a decrease in microvascular NO production or consumption of NO in this compartment would not be expected to alter exhaled NO.

In order to further investigate the fate of NO pathways in the microvascular lung compartment, one can deliver exogenous NO to the pulmonary circulation and monitor evolution of this NO in exhaled breath. Shortly after the original observations of Persson *et al.* in animal models, regarding increased exhaled NO levels following vascular metabolism of intravenous NO donors, we have characterized exhaled NO responses produced by intravenous administration of nitroglycerin (GTN) in humans.[129–132] We concluded that a fraction of nitroglycerin is metabolized in the pulmonary microvasculature to NO, which then diffuses into the alveolar space, giving rise to ppb levels of exhaled NO as detected by chemiluminescence. On the basis of these considerations, we have suggested that GTN-induced exhaled NO might be a useful tool to monitor metabolic function of the pulmonary microvasculature, as opposed to endogenous NO in exhaled breath, which would be a marker of production and consumption of NO in the airways.[132]

We have recently applied these methods to evaluate lung NO pathways following CPB and lung transplantation.[31,133,134] Our results agreed with those of Brett and colleagues, showing that endogenous exhaled NO levels remained unchanged 1 and 3 hours after routine CPB.[133] However, we found that there were characteristic changes in GTN-induced response in exhaled NO after CPB. The dose-dependent increases in exhaled NO by GTN were significantly smaller at 1 hour and 3 hours after CPB when compared to levels measured before CPB.[133] These data provide biochemical evidence that, although NO production/consumption in the airway compartment may remain intact following cardiac surgery, consumption reaction may dominate in the microvascular compartment.

There was no characteristic endogenous exhaled NO signal, such as seen with CABG patients, in the majority of the lung transplant recipients during the post CPB period.[134] Since we were able to make measurements both before and after reperfusion of the lung, we could distinguish between an effect of ischaemia and that of reperfusion. In some patients, there was a clear signal before reperfusion, which was attenuated following reperfusion. The majority of patients, however, exhibited no detectable signals even at the end of ischaemia. A comparable NO signal to CABG patients was only seen in two out of the 10 lung transplant recipients during the post reperfusion period. Interestingly, GTN-induced increases in exhaled NO were generally absent or appeared very small in lung transplant recipients after reperfusion. These alterations persisted for several hours after the operation, and recovery of the GTN response appeared particularly slow requiring more than 24 hours.[31]

While some of the observed pattern of NO changes resembled the animal observations, with both ischaemia and reperfusion related alterations

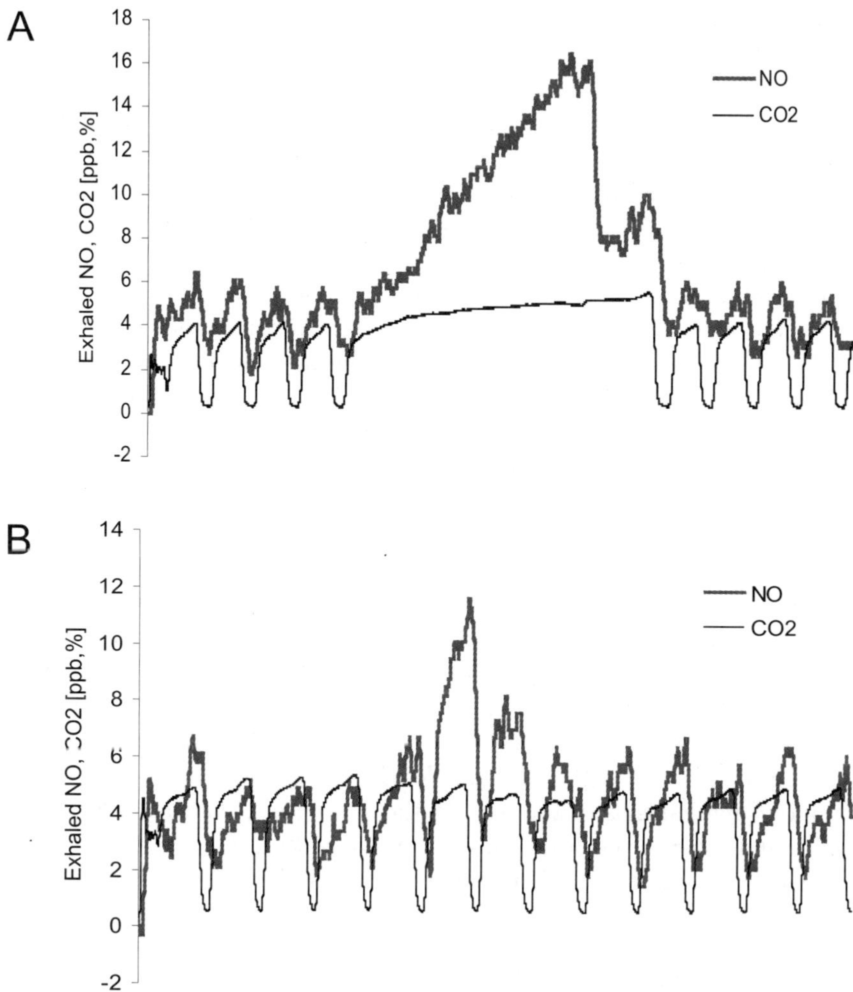

Fig. 2. Representative exhaled NO and CO_2 traces measured under basal conditions (Panel A) before and following a breath-holding maneuvre or following administration of intravenous nitroglycerin (GTN, 2 μg/kg bolus, Panel B) in a mechanically ventilated donor. The measurements were performed in a distant hospital with standardized ventilation utilizing the Logan Research Inc. portable chemiluminescence NO analyzer. Note characteristic exhaled NO tidal traces and increase following the GTN bolus and during breath-holding

in pulmonary NO, a major limitation of our study was that we did not have baseline measurements on exhaled NO in the donor lung prior to retrieval from the donor. This indeed required portable chemiluminescence methodology, which was recently provided by Logan Research Inc. enabling us to perform these measurements. Figure 2 shows representative traces of NO and CO_2 signals during standardised mechanical ventilation, accumulation of these gases in the airways following a breath holding manoeuvre and GTN-induced NO evolution in the exhaled breath in the donors. We believe these measurements will allow calculation of various indices of steady-state NO in the airways and microvasculature. Figure 3 shows changes in peak NO levels in this representative case, clearly demonstrating reduced NO concentration following transplantation. We are now investigating this phenomenon in a larger lung transplant population.

What these studies suggest is that, despite the multiple mechanisms that could potentially affect pulmonary NO pathways in human acute lung injury, consumption reactions appear to dominate the picture. In mild lung injury, such as that following CPB, this may only be evident in the microvascular compartment, and spare the airway compartment. This however, could be affected in more severe injury such as seen in some patients with lung transplantation. Interestingly, while similarly to us, the Brompton group found no alterations in exhaled NO after routine cardiac surgery and CPB, they reported greatly reduced exhaled NO in patients with severe lung injury in ARDS.[135] Thus, exhaled NO may reflect some of the consumption mechanisms in the lung in the setting of ischaemia–reperfusion injury and other forms of lung injury, and may serve as a negative Type 0 biomarker of lung injury. It is remarkable that this characteristic is con-

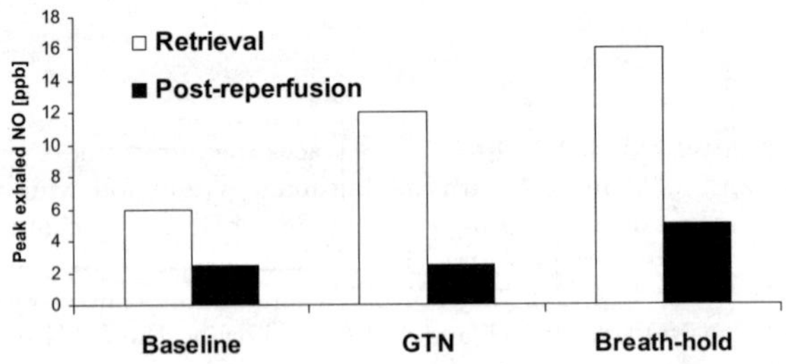

Fig. 3.   Comparison of basal, GTN and breath-holding induced exhaled NO in the donor and following transplantation. Measurements were performed with the same standardized ventilation setting. Note reduced levels of exhaled NO after transplantation and absence of GTN response.

sistently observed in different systems, ranging from simple cellular studies through animal models to human physiology. It is gratifying that the results of our initial cell culture studies seem to be applicable to human conditions.

Further studies are required to elucidate the exact mechanisms of the reduction in steady-state NO levels and whether or not exhaled NO could serve as a Type I biomarker reflecting response to drug therapy. Our working hypothesis is that increased oxidative stress is responsible for NO attenuation and the activity of NO pathways could be restored by appropriate antioxidant therapy. It also remains to be established whether or not exhaled NO could serve as a surrogate end point. Although our initial studies suggest that there may be an association between clinical outcome and different NO pattern following lung transplantation,[134] these results are preliminary and need to be evaluated in larger multi-centre trials. In any case, monitoring of NO in the exhaled breath may become a potentially useful addition in the diagnostic repertoire of the concerning cardiothoracic "gas man."

References

1. Marczin N. Editorial I: Tiny wonders of tiny impurities of nitrous oxide during anaesthesia. *Br J Anaesth* 2004; **93**: 619–623.
2. Clutton-Brock J. Two cases of poisoning by contamination of nitrous oxide with higher oxides of nitrogen during anaesthesia. *Br J Anaesth* 1967; **39**: 388–392.
3. Konstadt S. Nitric oxide: has it progressed from molecule of the year to wonder drug of the decade? *J Cardiothorac Vasc Anesth* 1995; **9**: 625–626.
4. Higenbottam T. Inhaled nitric oxide: a magic bullet? *Q J Med* 1993; **86**: 555–558.
5. Payen DM. Is nitric oxide inhalation a "cosmetic" therapy in acute respiratory distress syndrome? *Am J Respir Crit Care Med* 1998; **157**: 1361–1362.
6. Macrae DJ, Field D, Mercier JC, Moller J, Stiris T, Biban P, Cornick P, Goldman A, Gothberg S, Gustafsson LF, Hammer J, Lonnqviot PA, Sanchez-Luna M, Sedin G, Subhedar N. Inhaled nitric oxide therapy in neonates and children: reaching a European consensus. *Intensive Care Med* 2004; **30**: 372–380.
7. Marshall JC. SIRS and MODS: what is their relevance to the science and practice of intensive care? *Shock* 2000; **14**: 586–589.
8. Payen D, Faivre V, Lukaszewicz AC, Losser MR. Assessment of immunological status in the critically ill. *Minerva Anestesiol* 2000; **66**: 351–357.
9. Royston D, Kovesi T, Marczin N. The unwanted response to cardiac surgery: time for a reappraisal? *J Thorac Cardiovasc Surg* 2003; **125**: 32–35.
10. Asimakopoulos G, Smith PL, Ratnatunga CP, Taylor KM. Lung injury and acute respiratory distress syndrome after cardiopulmonary bypass. *Ann Thorac Surg* 1999; **68**: 1107–1115.

11. Ware LB, Matthay MA. The acute respiratory distress syndrome. *N Engl J Med* 2000; **342**: 1334–1349.
12. Matthay MA. Function of the alveolar epithelial barrier under pathologic conditions. *Chest* 1994; **105**: 67S–74S.
13. Martin TR. Lung cytokines and ARDS: Roger S. Mitchell Lecture. *Chest* 1999; **116**: 2S–8S.
14. Martin TR. Cytokines and the acute respiratory distress syndrome (ARDS): a question of balance. *Nat Med* 1997; **3**: 272–273.
15. Sittipunt C, Steinberg KP, Ruzinski JT, Myles C, Zhu S, Goodman RB, Hudson LD, Matalon S, Martin TR. Nitric oxide and nitrotyrosine in the lungs of patients with acute respiratory distress syndrome. *Am J Respir Crit Care Med* 2001; **163**: 503–510.
16. Marczin N, Royston D. Nitric oxide as mediator, marker and modulator of microvascular damage in ARDS. *Br J Anaesth* 2001; **87**: 179–183.
17. Pittet JF, Mackersie RC, Martin TR, Matthay MA. Biological markers of acute lung injury: prognostic and pathogenetic significance. *Am J Respir Crit Care Med* 1997; **155**: 1187–1205.
18. Dunham CM, Frankenfield D, Belzberg H, Wiles CE, 3rd, Cushing B, Grant Z. Inflammatory markers: superior predictors of adverse outcome in blunt trauma patients? *Crit Care Med* 1994; **22**: 667–672.
19. Pugin J, Ricou B, Steinberg KP, Suter PM, and Martin TR. Proinflammatory activity in bronchoalveolar lavage fluids from patients with ARDS, a prominent role for interleukin-1. *Am J Respir Crit Care Med* 1996; **153**: 1850–1856.
20. Krafte-Jacobs B, Brilli R, Szabo C, Denenberg A, Moore L, Salzman AL. Circulating methemoglobin and nitrite/nitrate concentrations as indicators of nitric oxide overproduction in critically ill children with septic shock. *Crit Care Med* 1997; **25**: 1588–1593.
21. Lieberman JM, Marks WH, Cohn S, Jaicks R, Woode L, Sacchettini J, Fischer B, Moller B, Burns G. Organ failure, infection, and the systemic inflammatory response syndrome are associated with elevated levels of urinary intestinal fatty acid binding protein: study of 100 consecutive patients in a surgical intensive care unit. *J Trauma* 1998; **45**: 900–906.
22. Borner U, Klimek M. Does an analysis of exhaled air indicate the metabolic state of critically ill patients? *Intensive Care Med* 1998; **24**: 403–404.
23. Scholpp J, Schubert JK, Miekisch W, Geiger K. Breath markers and soluble lipid peroxidation markers in critically ill patients. *Clin Chem Lab Med* 2002; **40**: 587–594.
24. Carpenter CT, Price PV, Christman BW. Exhaled breath condensate isoprostanes are elevated in patients with acute lung injury or ARDS. *Chest* 1998; **114**: 1653–1659.
25. Wilson WC, Swetland JF, Benumof JL, Laborde P, Taylor R. General anesthesia and exhaled breath hydrogen peroxide. *Anesthesiology* 1992; **76**: 703–710.
26. Wilson WC, Laborde PR, Benumof JL, Taylor R, Swetland JF. Reperfusion injury and exhaled hydrogen peroxide. *Anesth Analg* 1993; **77**: 963–970.

27. Zegdi R, Perrin D, Burdin M, Boiteau R, Tenaillon A. Increased endogenous carbon monoxide production in severe sepsis. *Intensive Care Med* 2002; **28**: 793–796.

28. Andreoni KA, Kazui M, Cameron DE, Nyhan D, Sehnert SS, Rohde CA, Bulkley GB, Risby TH. Ethane: a marker of lipid peroxidation during cardiopulmonary bypass in humans. *Free Radic Biol Med* 1999; **26**: 439–445.

29. Kazui M, Andreoni KA, Williams GM, Perler BA, Bulkley GB, Beattie C, Donham RT, Sehnert SS, Burdick JF, Risby TH. Visceral lipid peroxidation occurs at reperfusion after supraceliac aortic cross-clamping. *J Vasc Surg* 1994; **19**: 473–477.

30. Brett SJ, Evans TW. Endogenous nitric oxide in exhaled human breath. A new means of monitoring airway disease activity or another no-no? *Chest* 1996; **110**: 873–874.

31. Kovesi T, Royston D, Yacoub M, Marczin N. Exhaled nitric oxide in human lung ischaemia–reperfusion., In: Marczin N, Kharitonov S, Yacoub M, Barnes P, eds. *Disease Markers in Exhaled Breath*, New York, Basel: Marcel Dekker, 2003: 259–279.

32. Boyle EM, Jr., Pohlman TH, Cornejo CJ, Verrier ED. Endothelial cell injury in cardiovascular surgery: ischemia–reperfusion.. *Ann Thorac Surg* 1996; **62**: 1868–1875.

33. Anselmi A, Abbate A, Girola F, Nasso G, Biondi-Zoccai GG, Possati G, Gaudino M. Myocardial ischemia, stunning, inflammation, and apoptosis during cardiac surgery: a review of evidence. *Eur J Cardiothorac Surg* 2004; **25**: 304–311.

34. Ng CS, Wan S, Yim AP, Arifi AA. Pulmonary dysfunction after cardiac surgery. *Chest* 2002; **121**: 1269–1277.

35. Paparella D, Brister SJ, Buchanan MR. Coagulation disorders of cardiopulmonary bypass: a review. *Intensive Care Med* 2004; **30**: 1873–1881.

36. McBride WT, Allen S, Gormley SM, Young IS, McClean E, MacGowan SW, Elliott P, McMurray TJ, Armstrong MA. Methylprednisolone favourably alters plasma and urinary cytokine homeostasis and subclinical renal injury at cardiac surgery. *Cytokine* 2004; **27**: 81–89.

37. Gormley SM, McBride WT, Armstrong MA, Young IS, McClean E, MacGowan SW, Campalani G, McMurray TJ. Plasma and urinary cytokine homeostasis and renal dysfunction during cardiac surgery. *Anesthesiology* 2000; **93**: 1210–1216; discussion 1215A.

38. McBride WT, Armstrong MA, Crockard AD, McMurray TJ, Rea JM. Cytokine balance and immunosuppressive changes at cardiac surgery: contrasting response between patients and isolated CPB circuits. *Br J Anaesth* 1995; **75**: 724–733.

39. Poirier B, Baillot R, Bauset R, Dagenais F, Mathieu P, Simard S, Dionne B, Caouette M, Hould FS, Doyle D, Poirier P. Abdominal complications associated with cardiac surgery. Review of a contemporary surgical experience and of a series done without extracorporeal circulation. *Can J Surg* 2003; **46**: 176–182.

40. Nussmeier NA. A review of risk factors for adverse neurologic outcome after cardiac surgery. *J Extra Corpor Technol* 2002; **34**: 4–10.

41. Schlensak C, Doenst T, Preusser S, Wunderlich M, Kleinschmidt M, Beyersdorf F. Bronchial artery perfusion during cardiopulmonary bypass does not prevent ischemia of the lung in piglets: assessment of bronchial artery blood flow with fluorescent microspheres. *Eur J Cardiothorac Surg* 2001; **19**: 326–331; discussion 331–332.

42. Macnaughton PD, Braude S, Hunter DN, Denison DM, Evans TW. Changes in lung function and pulmonary capillary permeability after cardiopulmonary bypass. *Crit Care Med* 1992; **20**: 1289–1294.

43. Asimakopoulos G, Taylor KM, Smith PL, Ratnatunga CP. Prevalence of acute respiratory distress syndrome after cardiac surgery. *J Thorac Cardiovasc Surg* 1999; **117**: 620–621.

44. Messent M, Sullivan K, Keogh BF, Morgan CJ, Evans TW. Adult respiratory distress syndrome following cardiopulmonary bypass: incidence and prediction. *Anaesthesia* 1992; **47**: 267–268.

45. Fisher AJ, Dark JH, Corris PA. Improving donor lung evaluation: a new approach to increase organ supply for lung transplantation. *Thorax* 1998; **53**: 818–820.

46. Ware LB, Wang Y, Fang X, Warnock M, Sakuma T, Hall TS, Matthay M. Assessment of lungs rejected for transplantation and implications for donor selection. *Lancet* 2002; **360**: 619–620.

47. Gammie JS, Cheul Lee J, Pham SM, Keenan RJ, Weyant RJ, Hattler BG, Griffith BP. Cardiopulmonary bypass is associated with early allograft dysfunction but not death after double-lung transplantation. *J Thorac Cardiovasc Surg* 1998; **115**: 990–997.

48. Novick RJ, Gehman KE, Ali IS, Lee J. Lung preservation: the importance of endothelial and alveolar type II cell integrity. *Ann Thorac Surg* 1996; **62**: 302–314.

49. Khan SU, Salloum J, O'Donovan PB, Mascha EJ, Mehta AC, Matthay MA, Arroliga AC. Acute pulmonary edema after lung transplantation: the pulmonary reimplantation response. *Chest* 1999; **116**: 187–194.

50. Kundu S, Herman SJ, Winton TL. Reperfusion edema after lung transplantation: radiographic manifestations. *Radiology* 1998; **206**: 75–80.

51. Christie JD, Bavaria JE, Palevsky HI, Litzky L, Blumenthal NP, Kaiser LR, Kotloff RM. Primary graft failure following lung transplantation. *Chest* 1998; **114**: 51–60.

52. Serrick C, Giaid A, Reis A, Shennib H. Prolonged ischemia is associated with more pronounced rejection in the lung allograft. *Ann Thorac Surg* 1997; **63**: 202–208.

53. Qayumi AK, Nikbakht-Sangari MN, Godin DV, English JC, Horley KJ, Keown PA, Lim SP, Ansley DM, Koehle MS. The relationship of ischemia–reperfusion injury of transplanted lung and the up-regulation of major histocompatibility complex II on host peripheral lymphocytes. *J Thorac Cardiovasc Surg* 1998; **115**: 978–989.

54. Mal H, Dehoux M, Sleiman C, Boczkowski J, Leseche G, Pariente R, Fournier M. Early release of proinflammatory cytokines after lung transplantation. *Chest* 1998; **113**: 645–651.

55. Lesko LJ, Atkinson AJ, Jr. Use of biomarkers and surrogate endpoints in drug development and regulatory decision making: criteria, validation, strategies. *Annu Rev Pharmacol Toxicol* 2001; **41**: 347–366.

56. Bielekova B, Martin R. Development of biomarkers in multiple sclerosis. *Brain* 2004; **127**: 1463–1478.

57. Carden DL, Granger DN. Pathophysiology of ischaemia–reperfusion injury. *J Pathol* 2000; **190**: 255–266.

58. Granger DN. Ischemia–reperfusion: mechanisms of microvascular dysfunction and the influence of risk factors for cardiovascular disease. *Microcirculation* 1999; **6**: 167–178.

59. Freeman BA, Panus PC, Matalon S, Buckley BJ, Baker RR. Oxidant injury to the alveolar epithelium: biochemical and pharmacologic studies. *Res Rep Health Eff Inst* 1993: 1–30; discussion 31–39.

60. Matthay MA, Fukuda N, Frank J, Kallet R, Daniel B, Sakuma T. Alveolar epithelial barrier. Role in lung fluid balance in clinical lung injury. *Clin Chest Med* 2000; **21**: 477–490.

61. Matthay MA. Alveolar fluid clearance in patients with ARDS: does it make a difference? *Chest* 2002; **122**: 340S–343S.

62. Verrier ED, Boyle EM, Jr. Endothelial cell injury in cardiovascular surgery. *Ann Thorac Surg* 1996; **62**: 915–922.

63. Boyle EM, Jr., Canty TG, Jr., Morgan EN, Yun W, Pohlman TH, Verrier ED. Treating myocardial ischemia–reperfusion injury by targeting endothelial cell transcription. *Ann Thorac Surg* 1999; **68**: 1949–1953.

64. Naidu BV, Woolley SM, Farivar AS, Thomas R, Fraga CH, Goss CH, Mulligan MS. Early tumor necrosis factor-alpha release from the pulmonary macrophage in lung ischemia–reperfusion injury. *J Thorac Cardiovasc Surg* 2004; **127**: 1502–1508.

65. Naidu BV, Farivar AS, Woolley SM, Grainger D, Verrier ED, Mulligan MS. Novel broad-spectrum chemokine inhibitor protects against lung ischemia–reperfusion injury. *J Heart Lung Transplant* 2004; **23**: 128–134.

66. Naidu BV, Krishnadasan B, Farivar AS, Woolley SM, Thomas R, Van Rooijen N, Verrier ED, Mulligan MS. Early activation of the alveolar macrophage is critical to the development of lung ischemia–reperfusion injury. *J Thorac Cardiovasc Surg* 2003; **126**: 200–207.

67. Fiser SM, Tribble CG, Long SM, Kaza AK, Kern JA, and Kron IL. Pulmonary macrophages are involved in reperfusion injury after lung transplantation. *Ann Thorac Surg* 2001; **71**: 1134–1138; discussion 1138–1139

68. Pillai R, Bando K, Schueler S, Zebly M, Reitz BA, Baumgartner WA. Leukocyte depletion results in excellent heart–lung function after 12 hours of storage. *Ann Thorac Surg* 1990, **50**: 211–214.

69. Bando K, Pillai R, Cameron DE, Brawn JD, Winkelstein JA, Hutchins GM, Reitz BA, Baumgartner WA. Leukocyte depletion ameliorates free radical-mediated lung injury after cardiopulmonary bypass. *J Thorac Cardiovasc Surg* 1990; **99**: 873–877.

70. Eppinger MJ, Deeb GM, Bolling SF, Ward PA. Mediators of ischemia–reperfusion injury of rat lung. *Am J Pathol* 1997; **150**: 1773–1784.

71. Eppinger MJ, Jones ML, Deeb GM, Bolling SF, Ward PA. Pattern of injury and the role of neutrophils in reperfusion injury of rat lung. *J Surg Res* 1995; **58**: 713–718.

72. Xing Z, Jordana M, Kirpalani H, Driscoll KE, Schall TJ, Gauldie J. Cytokine expression by neutrophils and macrophages *in vivo*: endotoxin induces tumor necrosis factor-alpha, macrophage inflammatory protein-2, interleukin-1 beta, and interleukin-6 but not RANTES or transforming growth factor-beta 1 mRNA expression in acute lung inflammation. *Am J Respir Cell Mol Biol* 1994; **10**: 148–153.

73. Kunkel SL, Lukacs N, Strieter RM. Expression and biology of neutrophil and endothelial cell-derived chemokines. *Semin Cell Biol* 1995; **6**: 327–336.

74. Binns OA, DeLima NF, Buchanan SA, Mauney MC, Cope JT, Thies SD, Shockey KS, Tribble CG, Kron IL. Neutrophil endopeptidase inhibitor improves pulmonary function during reperfusion after eighteen-hour preservation. *J Thorac Cardiovasc Surg* 1996; **112**: 607–613.

75. Baird BR, Cheronis JC, Sandhaus RA, Berger EM, White CW, Repine JE. O_2 metabolites and neutrophil elastase synergistically cause edematous injury in isolated rat lungs. *J Appl Physiol* 1986; **61**: 2224–2229.

76. Steimle CN, Guynn TP, Morganroth ML, Bolling SF, Carr K, Deeb GM. Neutrophils are not necessary for ischemia–reperfusion lung injury. *Ann Thorac Surg* 1992; **53**: 64–72; discussion 72–73

77. Barnes PJ, Belvisi MG. Nitric oxide and lung disease. *Thorax* 1993; **48**: 1034–1043.

78. Barnes PJ. Nitric oxide and airway disease. *Ann Med* 1995; **27**: 389–393.

79. Pinsky DJ. The vascular biology of heart and lung preservation for transplantation. *Thromb Haemost* 1995; **74**: 58–65.

80. Moncada S, Palmer RM, Higgs EA. Nitric oxide: physiology, pathophysiology, and pharmacology. *Pharmacol Rev* 1991; **43**: 109–142.

81. Guo FH, De Raeve HR, Rice TW, Stuehr DJ, Thunnissen FB, Erzurum SC. Continuous nitric oxide synthesis by inducible nitric oxide synthase in normal human airway epithelium *in vivo*. *Proc Natl Acad Sci USA* 1995; **92**: 7809–7813.

82. Asano K, Chee CB, Gaston B, Lilly CM, Gerard C, Drazen JM, Stamler JS. Constitutive and inducible nitric oxide synthase gene expression, regulation, and activity in human lung epithelial cells. *Proc Natl Acad Sci USA* 1994; **91**: 10089–10093.

83. Dweik RA, Laskowski D, Abu-Soud HM, Kaneko F, Hutte R, Stuehr DJ, Erzurum SC. Nitric oxide synthesis in the lung. Regulation by oxygen through a kinetic mechanism. *J Clin Invest* 1998; **101**: 660–666.

84. Phelan MW, Faller DV. Hypoxia decreases constitutive nitric oxide synthase transcript and protein in cultured endothelial cells. *J Cell Physiol* 1996; **167**: 469–476.

85. Nelin LD, Thomas CJ, Dawson CA. Effect of hypoxia on nitric oxide production in neonatal pig lung. *Am J Physiol* 1996; **271**: H8–14.

86. Ziesche R, Petkov V, Mosgoller W, Block LH. Regulation of human endothelial nitric oxide synthase by hypoxia and inflammation in human pulmonary arteries — implications for the therapy of pulmonary hypertension in COPD patients. *Acta Anaesthesiol Scand Suppl* 1996; **109**: 97–98.

87. Zweier JL, Samouilov A, Kuppusamy P. Non-enzymatic nitric oxide synthesis in biological systems. *Biochim Biophys Acta* 1999; **1411**: 250–262.

88. Modin A, Bjorne H, Herulf M, Alving K, Weitzberg E, Lundberg JO. Nitrite-derived nitric oxide: a possible mediator of 'acidic-metabolic' vasodilation. *Acta Physiol Scand* 2001; **171**: 9–16.

89. Hunt JF, Fang K, Malik R, Snyder A, Malhotra N, Platts-Mills TA, Gaston B. Endogenous airway acidification. Implications for asthma pathophysiology. *Am J Respir Crit Care Med* 2000; **161**: 694–699.

90. Beckman JS, Beckman TW, Chen J, Marshall PA, Freeman BA. Apparent hydroxyl radical production by peroxynitrite: implications for endothelial injury from nitric oxide and superoxide. *Proc Natl Acad Sci USA* 1990; **87**: 1620–1624.

91. Royall JA, Kooy NW, Beckman JS. Nitric oxide-related oxidants in acute lung injury. *New Horiz* 1995; **3**: 113–122.

92. Freeman BA, Gutierrez H, Rubbo H. Nitric oxide. a central regulatory species in pulmonary oxidant reactions. *Am J Physiol* 1995; **268**: L697–698.

93. Freeman BA, White CR, Gutierrez H, Paler-Martinez A, Tarpey MM, Rubbo H. Oxygen radical-nitric oxide reactions in vascular diseases. *Adv Pharmacol* 1995; **34**: 45–69.

94. O'Donnell VB, Freeman BA. Interactions between nitric oxide and lipid oxidation pathways: implications for vascular disease. *Circ Res* 2001; **88**: 12–21.

95. Bloodsworth A, O'Donnell VB, Freeman BA. Nitric oxide regulation of free radical- and enzyme-mediated lipid and lipoprotein oxidation. *Arterioscler Thromb Vasc Biol* 2000; **20**: 1707–1715.

96. Liu M, Tremblay L, Cassivi SD, Bai XH, Mourgeon E, Pierre AF, Slutsky AS, Post M, Keshavjee S. Alterations of nitric oxide synthase expression and activity during rat lung transplantation. *Am J Physiol Lung Cell Mol Physiol* 2000; **278**: L1071–1081.

97. Itano H, Zhang W, Ritter JH, McCarthy TJ, Mohanakumar T, Patterson GA. Adenovirus-mediated gene transfer of human interleukin 10 ameliorates reperfusion injury of rat lung isografts. *J Thorac Cardiovasc Surg* 2000; **120**: 947–956.

98. Marczin N, Kovesi T, Royston D, Yacoub M. Exhaled nitric oxide in acute lung injury: Measurements and Physiological implications., In: Matalon S, Sznajder J, eds. *Etiology and Treatment of Acute Lung Injury: From Bench to Bedside*, Amsterdam, Berlin, Oxford, Tokyo, Washington: IOPS Press, 2001.

99. Marczin N, Ryan US, Catravas JD. Effects of oxidant stress on endothelium-derived relaxing factor-induced and nitrovasodilator-induced cGMP accumulation in vascular cells in culture. *Circ Res* 1992; **70**: 326–340.

100. Gustafsson LE, Leone AM, Persson MG, Wiklund NP, Moncada S. Endogenous nitric oxide is present in the exhaled air of rabbits, guinea pigs and humans. *Biochem Biophys Res Commun* 1991; **181**: 852–857.

101. Recommendations for standardized procedures for the on-line and off-line measurement of exhaled lower respiratory nitric oxide and nasal nitric oxide in adults and children-1999. This official statement of the American Thoracic Society was adopted by the ATS Board of Directors, July 1999.. *Am J Respir Crit Care Med* 1999; **160**: 2104–2117.

102. Marczin N, Ryan US, Catravas JD. Methylene blue inhibits nitrovasodilator- and endothelium-derived relaxing factor-induced cyclic GMP accumulation in cultured pulmonary arterial smooth muscle cells via generation of superoxide anion. *J Pharmacol Exp Ther* 1992; **263**: 170–179.

103. Marczin N, Ryan US, Catravas JD. Sulfhydryl-depleting agents, but not deferoxamine, modulate EDRF action in cultured pulmonary arterial cells. *Am J Physiol* 1993; **265**: L220–227.

104. Marczin N, Chen X, Catravas J. Basal release of EDRF under conditions of oxidant stress., In: Catravas J, Callow A, Ryan U, eds. Vascular Endothelium: Physiological Basis of Clinical Problems II., New York: Plenum Press, 1993: 3–16.

105. Marczin N, Antonov A, Papapetropoulos A, Munn DH, Virmani R, Kolodgie FD, Gerrity R, Catravas JD. Monocyte-induced downregulation of nitric oxide synthase in cultured aortic endothelial cells. *Arterioscler Thromb Vasc Biol* 1996; **16**: 1095–1103.

106. Yoshizumi M, Perrella MA, Burnett JC, Jr., Lee ME. Tumor necrosis factor downregulates an endothelial nitric oxide synthase mRNA by shortening its half-life. *Circ Res* 1993; **73**: 205–209.

107. Cohen J, Evans TJ, Spink J. Cytokine regulation of inducible nitric oxide synthase in vascular smooth muscle cells. *Prog Clin Biol Res* 1998; **397**: 169–177.

108. Szabo C. Alterations in nitric oxide production in various forms of circulatory shock. *New Horiz* 1995; **3**: 2–32.

109. Mitchell RN, Lichtman AH. The link between IFN-gamma and allograft arteriopathy: is the answer NO? *J Clin Invest* 2004; **114**: 762–764.

110. Marczin N, Papapetropoulos A, Catravas JD. Tyrosine kinase inhibitors suppress endotoxin- and IL-1 beta-induced NO synthesis in aortic smooth muscle cells. *Am J Physiol* 1993; **265**: H1014–1018.

111. Marczin N, Papapetropoulos A, Jilling T, Catravas JD. Prevention of nitric oxide synthase induction in vascular smooth muscle cells by microtubule depolymerizing agents. *Br J Pharmacol* 1993; **109**: 603–605.

112. Marczin N, Jilling T, Papapetropoulos A, Go C, Catravas JD. Cytoskeleton-dependent activation of the inducible nitric oxide synthase in cultured aortic smooth muscle cells. *Br J Pharmacol* 1996; **118**: 1085–1094.

113. Marczin N, Go CY, Papapetropoulos A, Catravas JD. Induction of nitric oxide synthase by protein synthesis inhibition in aortic smooth muscle cells. *Br J Pharmacol* 1998; **123**: 1000–1008.

114. Taylor BS, Geller DA. Molecular regulation of the human inducible nitric oxide synthase (iNOS) gene. *Shock* 2000; **13**: 413–424.

115. Kleinert H, Schwarz PM, Forstermann U. Regulation of the expression of inducible nitric oxide synthase. *Biol Chem* 2003; **384**: 1343–1364.

116. Lee SC, Brosnan CF. Cytokine Regulation of iNOS Expression in Human Glial Cells. *Methods* 1996; **10**: 31–37.

117. Denis M. Human monocytes/macrophages: NO or no NO? *J Leukoc Biol* 1994; **55**: 682–684.

118. Chester AH, Borland JA, Buttery LD, Mitchell JA, Cunningham DA, Hafizi S, Hoare GS, Springall DR, Polak JM, Yacoub MH. Induction of nitric oxide synthase in human vascular smooth muscle: interactions between proinflammatory cytokines. *Cardiovasc Res* 1998; **38**: 814–821.

119. Romanska HM, Polak JM, Coleman RA, James RS, Harmer DW, Allen JC, Bishop AE. iNOS gene upregulation is associated with the early proliferative response of human lung fibroblasts to cytokine stimulation. *J Pathol* 2002; **197**: 372–379.

120. Kooguchi K, Kobayashi A, Kitamura Y, Ueno H, Urata Y, Onodera H, Hashimoto S. Elevated expression of inducible nitric oxide synthase and inflammatory cytokines in the alveolar macrophages after esophagectomy. *Crit Care Med* 2002; **30**: 71–76.

121. Morita K, Ihnken K, Buckberg GD, Sherman MP, Ignarro LJ. Pulmonary vasoconstriction due to impaired nitric oxide production after cardiopulmonary bypass. *Ann Thorac Surg* 1996; **61**: 1775–1780.

122. Pinsky DJ, Naka Y, Chowdhury NC, Liao H, Oz MC, Michler RE, Kubaszewski E, Malinski T, Stern DM. The nitric oxide/cyclic GMP pathway in organ transplantation: critical role in successful lung preservation. *Proc Natl Acad Sci USA* 1994; **91**: 12086–12090.

123. Brett SJ, Quinlan GJ, Mitchell J, Pepper JR, Evans TW. Production of nitric oxide during surgery involving cardiopulmonary bypass. *Crit Care Med* 1998; **26**: 272–278.

124. Ishibe Y, Liu R, Hirosawa J, Kawamura K, Yamasaki K, Saito N. Exhaled nitric oxide level decreases after cardiopulmonary bypass in adult patients. *Crit Care Med* 2000; **28**: 3823–3827.

125. Cuthbertson BH, Stott SA, Webster NR. Exhaled nitric oxide as a marker of lung injury in coronary artery bypass surgery. *Br J Anaesth* 2002; **89**: 247–250.

126. Pietropaoli AP, Perkins PT, Perillo IB, Hyde RW. Exhaled nitric oxide does not provide a marker of vascular endothelial function in healthy humans. *Am J Respir Crit Care Med* 2000; **161**: 2113–2114.

127. Marczin N. Exhaled nitric oxide and cardiac surgery with extracorporeal circulation. *J Thorac Cardiovasc Surg* 2003; **126**: 1673–1674; author reply 1674–1675.

128. Sartori C, Lepori M, Busch T, Duplain H, Hildebrandt W, Bartsch P, Nicod P, Falke KJ, Scherrer U. Exhaled nitric oxide does not provide a marker of vascular endothelial function in healthy humans. *Am J Respir Crit Care Med* 1999; **160**: 879–882.

129. Persson MG, Agvald P, Gustafsson LE. Detection of nitric oxide in exhaled air during administration of nitroglycerin *in vivo*. *Br J Pharmacol* 1994; **111**: 825–828.

130. Cederqvist B, Persson MG, Gustafsson LE. Direct demonstration of NO formation *in vivo* from organic nitrites and nitrates, and correlation to effects on blood pressure and to *in vitro* effects.. *Biochem Pharmacol* 1994; **47**: 1047–1053.

131. Husain M, Adrie C, Ichinose F, Kavosi M, Zapol WM. Exhaled nitric oxide as a marker for organic nitrate tolerance. *Circulation* 1994; **89**: 2498–2502.

132. Marczin N, Riedel B, Royston D, Yacoub M. Intravenous nitrate vasodilators and exhaled nitric oxide. *Lancet* 1997; **349**: 1742.

133. Kovesi T, Royston D, Yacoub M, Marczin N. Basal and nitroglycerin-induced exhaled nitric oxide before and after cardiac surgery with cardiopulmonary bypass. *Br J Anaesth* 2003; **90**: 608–616.

134. Marczin N, Riedel B, Gal J, Polak J, Yacoub M. Exhaled nitric oxide during lung transplantation. *Lancet* 1997; **350**: 1681–1682.

135. Brett SJ, Evans TW. Measurement of endogenous nitric oxide in the lungs of patients with the acute respiratory distress syndrome. *Am J Respir Crit Care Med* 1998; **157**: 993–997.

CAN INHALATION CARBON MONOXIDE BE UTILIZED AS A THERAPEUTIC MODALITY IN HUMAN DISEASES?

T. DOLINAY, A. M. K. CHOI, AND S. W. RYTER

Department of Medicine,
Division of Pulmonary, Allergy and Critical Care Medicine,
The University of Pittsburgh School of Medicine,
MUH628NW 3459, 5th ave, Pittsburgh, PA 15213, USA

1. Introduction

Carbon monoxide (CO) and nitric oxide (NO) arise endogenously in humans as products of ordinary metabolism. The variable occurrence of these gases in ambient inspired air, in combination with their systemic metabolic production, which can increase during inflammatory disease states, contribute to their appearance at trace levels in the exhaled breath of humans.[1]

Despite its well-known properties as a lethal chemical asphyxiant and environmental contaminant, CO, like its predecessor NO, shows promise as a potential inhalation therapeutic modality in a number of disease states.[2] *In vivo*, both these diatomic gases originate from the enzymatic oxidation of organic precursor molecules. NO arises during the metabolic conversion of L-arginine to L-citrulline by nitric oxide synthases (NOS; EC 1:14:13:39), while CO originates from the oxidative degradation of heme by the heme oxygenases (HO; EC 1:14:99:3).[3-5] Furthermore, both enzyme systems consist of constitutive and inducible isozymes. The two gases differ, however, in inherent stability and reactivity. CO, which is much more stable than NO, typically reacts only with iron centers of heme-containing proteins.[6] NO, a free radical, displays a broader spectrum of chemical reactivity, and has a much shorter lifetime in biological systems.[7]

Both NO and CO can occur in the environment as atmospheric pollutants, and are thus considered inhalation hazards. CO occurs ubiquitously as a product of the incomplete combustion of hydrocarbons.[8] Common sources of CO include burning coal, wood, tobacco, and fossil fuels. Environmental CO, when accidentally inhaled in poorly ventilated areas, is a common cause of mortality.[8] CO, especially dangerous due to lack of color, odor, or taste, can produce deleterious physiological effects and, with prolonged exposure, can be lethal.[8] The first written accounts regarding the interaction between CO and humans probably date back to Antiquity. Aristotle, the great Greek philosopher, thinker and scientist writes about "Coal fumes that lead to heavy head and death," most likely in reference to CO gas. However, the mechanism of CO toxicity was not revealed until 1857, when the French scientist Claude Bernard described the ability of CO to bind strongly to hemoglobin. CO causes hypoxia in tissues as a consequence of its high affinity binding (more than 240 that of O_2 to hemoglobin), which restricts oxygen delivery. CO may also stabilize oxyhemoglobin, thereby inhibiting the release of oxygen.[9] The clinical toxicology of CO has been reviewed extensively elsewhere.[8,10,11] At present, strict environmental standards are applied to protect humans from poisoning. Current environmental standards are cited in Table 1.

The endogenous occurrence of CO has been known for approximately a half-century. CO normally exists in human blood tightly bound to the oxygen carrier hemoglobin. The majority of blood CO arises from endogenous erythrocyte degradation in the absence of significant environmental contamination.[12–14] An estimated 86 % of endogenous CO arises from endogenous heme metabolism, the majority of which occurs from hemoglobin turnover, with a minor component arising from the turnover of cytochromes

Table 1.   Current regulatory limits for CO

Agency	Exposure Limits
NIOSH	35 ppm (8 h TWA); 200 ppm ceiling
OSHA	50 ppm (8 h TWA)
ACGIH	25 ppm TLV (8 h TWA)
CPSC	15 ppm (1 h); 25 ppm (8 h), ceiling
EPA	9 ppm (8 h), 35 ppm (1 h); outdoor air
WHO	9 ppm (8 h)

ppm – parts-per-million partial pressure in air

Abbreviations: TWA: time weighted average; TLV: Threshold limit value; NIOSH: U.S. Department of Health and Human Services, Public Health Service, Centers for Disease Control, National Institute for Occupational Safety and Health (NIOSH); OSHA: Occupational Safety and Health Administration (OSHA); ACGIH: American Conference of Governmental Industrial Hygienists; CPSC: Consumer Product Safety Commission; EPA: Environmental Protection Agency, U.S. National Ambient Air Quality Standards for Outdoor Air; WHO: World Health Organisation.
(Sources: www.osha.gov; www.epa.gov; www.cpsc.gov; www.coheadquarters.com)

and other hemoproteins in cells and tissues.[15] Tenhunen and colleagues[4,5] identified heme oxygenase (HO) as the principle enzyme system involved in heme breakdown in 1968 (Fig. 1). The HO enzymes convert heme to biliverdin, iron, and CO, and thus represent the major source of endogenous CO production in man.[16] Since the discovery of the HO system, CO has been widely regarded as an undesirable waste product of heme metabolism, and assigned little physiological significance.[4,17] The remaining fraction of CO not associated with heme metabolism arises from poorly characterized sources, which may include the peroxidation of lipids, the photooxidation of organic molecules, and the metabolic conversion of xenobiotics.[15]

In 1998, the Nobel Prize in Physiology was awarded to Drs. Murad, Furchgott, and Ignarro for work leading to the discovery that the endogenous production of a similar small gas, NO, could exert multiple physiological functions. Their discoveries included the identification of endothelial derived relaxing factor, a substance involved in relaxation of vascular smooth muscle, as NO gas.[18,19] These observations led to the realization that endogenously derived gases could participate in the regulation of physiological processes. NO produces its vasodilatory effect by binding to and activating soluble guanylyl cyclase (sGC), leading to the enhanced production of guanosine $3', 5'$-monophosphate (cGMP).[20,21]

Snyder and colleagues, working with models of olfactory neurotransmission were among the first to propose that CO could exert similar physiological functions as NO, also by acting on sGC. Verma *et al.*[22] speculated on CO signaling pathways by observing a co-localization of HO-2 and sGC in distinct brain regions.[22] The authors demonstrated an important role for cGMP in olfactory signaling in the central nervous system, and suggested the involvement of CO in this process by using inhibitors of HO activity.

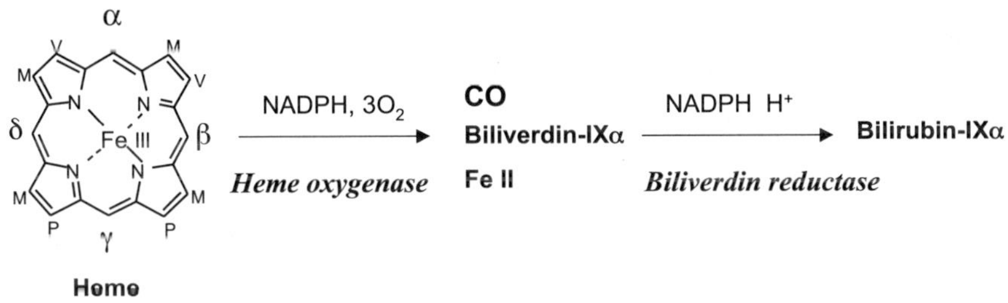

Fig. 1.   Major enzymatic steps in heme metabolism

Despite the well characterized toxicity of CO, recent research has indicated that low concentrations of this gas may exert considerable vasoregulatory, anti-inflammatory, anti-apoptotic, and anti-proliferative activity in cell culture and in animal models, by influencing intracellular signal transduction pathways (reviewed in Ref. 16). Morita *et al.*[23] demonstrated that CO can activate the sGC and cGMP system in vascular smooth muscle cells (SMC), which inhibits the proliferation of these cells.[23–25] Otterbein *et al.* demonstrated an anti-inflammatory effect of CO in macrophages that depended on the cGMP-independent modulation of p38 mitogen activated protein kinase (p38 MAPK) pathways.[2] In other models of CO regulation, however, such as the inhibition of SMC proliferation, links between sGC and p38 MAPK have now been described.[26] The protective effects of exogenously applied CO have been demonstrated in organ transplant, inflammatory and oxidative lung pathologies, ischemia/reperfusion (I/R) injury, vascular injury, and most recently in ventilator-induced lung injury (VILI).[2,26–30] This chapter will therefore summarize recent studies that support the cytoprotective application of CO in experimental models of human disease. The readers are also directed to other recent reviews regarding the cytoprotective effects of CO and HO-1.[16,31–34]

1.1. *Heme Oxygenase Isozymes and Activity*

HO catalyzes the first and rate-limiting step in heme degradation. Tenhunen *et al.*[4,5] first characterized HO as a microsomal monooxygenase system distinct from cytochrome P450.[4,5] The HO enzymatic activity requires molecular oxygen and reducing equivalents from NADPH: cytochrome P450 reductase, to catalyze the oxidation of heme-b to biliverdin-IXα, which is further converted to bilirubin-IXα by an NAD(P)H-dependent reductase.[35] The heme iron is liberated as Fe(II) as a consequence of heme cleavage, while the α-methene bridge carbon escapes as CO.[4] HO plays a principal role in degrading hemoglobin from senescent erythrocytes, in reticuloendothelial tissues such as the spleen, kidney, and liver.[4,36] HO exists in three genetically distinct isoforms (HO-1, HO-2, and HO-3). The transcriptional activation of the *ho-1* gene, and corresponding increases in protein and enzymatic activity, are stimulated in most cells and tissues by exposure to a wide spectrum of chemical and physical stresses, as well as physiological regulators, such as cytokines and growth factors. HO-2, the constitutively expressed isozyme, occurs at high levels in neuronal, vascular, testicular, hepatic, and other tissues.[17,37–39] HO-2 does not respond to transcriptional activation by environmental stress, but may respond to hormonal regulation in the brain. Another constitutive isozyme, HO-3, which has little enzymatic activity, exhibits high sequence similarity with HO-2 and remains incompletely characterized.[40] HO enzymes have been found in lower organisms as well. Variants of HO-1 have been described in bacteria, fungi, plants, and algae.[41-47]

1.2. *Molecular Basis for Regulation of HO-1 in Cells and Tissues*

The agents that induce *ho-1* gene expression include changes in ambient oxygen tension (hypoxia, hyperoxia), ultraviolet-A radiation, NO and its derivatives, heavy metals, sulfhydryl reactive substances, cytokines and growth factors, bacterial lipopolysaccharide (LPS), and the HO enzymatic substrate heme (reviewed in Refs. 48 and 49). Recent studies implicate mitogen activated protein kinases (MAPK) as intermediates in the signaling pathways that link cellular stimulation by many of these environmental agents to the transcriptional regulation of the *ho-1* gene.[49] The three major MAPK families known in mammalian cells include c-Jun-N-terminal kinase (JNK), extracellular regulated kinases (ERK1/ERK2) and p38 MAPK.[50] While each of these kinase families has been implicated in *ho-1* regulation in various models, the specific kinases involved vary in a tissue specific and inducer specific fashion. Recent studies strongly implicate a major role for p38 MAPK in *ho-1* regulation, and have established a link between p38 MAPK activation and transcriptional regulation of *ho-1* through the nrf-2 transcription factor[51] (see below). The *ho-1* gene contains several *cis*-acting elements in its 5′ regulatory region that govern its basal and inducible transcriptional regulation. In particular, two transcriptional enhancer sequences located at −4kb (E1) and −10kb (E2) of the transcriptional start site mediate the induction of *ho-1* in response to cellular stimulation with heavy metals, phorbol esters, LPS, heme, H_2O_2, and others.[51-55] Both enhancer elements contain repeated essential *cis*-acting stress responsive elements (StRE); which contain an intrinsic consensus antioxidant responsive element (ARE), overlapping a Maf recognition element, and an activator protein-1 (AP-1) binding site.[51,55,56]

The NF-E2 related factor (Nrf2), a member of the Cap'n'collar/basic-leucine zipper family, recognizes and binds to the StRE in the *ho-1* promoter, as well as to consensus ARE sequences found in the promoter regions of several other detoxifying enzymes.[56-58] Nrf2 forms stable heterodimers with members of the maf (MafK, MafF, MafG) family.[57] The DNA-binding activity of Nrf2 is markedly induced by electrophilic agents, including polyphenols and plant-derived substances, through a post-translational mechanism. Under basal conditions, a cytoplasmic factor, Keap-1, inhibits the activity of Nrf2 by binding to the negative regulatory domain of Nrf2. Induction by electrophiles releases the inhibitor, allowing the nuclear translocation of Nrf2.[59] Nrf2 plays a critical role in the induction of *ho-1* by a number of agents, including heme, $CdCl_2$, arsenite, and phenolic compounds.[51,55,56,60] A transcriptional repressor of *ho-1* (Bach-1) has also recently been characterized.[60] Bach-1 potentially dimerizes with maf proteins, and antagonizes the effects of Nrf-2/maf dimers at the StRE sites of E1 and E2. The DNA binding activity of Bach-1 is negatively regulated by heme *in vitro*,[62] and this may account for the substrate dependent activation of *ho-1*. In addition to the distal enhancers, the promoter region of *ho-1* also contains a distinct hypoxia response element occurring at -9kb from the transcriptional start site, which comprises two functional binding sites for the hypoxia inducible factor-1, and mediates the *ho-1* response to hypoxia.[63]

1.3. *Cytoprotection by HO-1: An Overview*

HO-1, the major 32-kDa mammalian stress protein, can be induced at the transcriptional level by multiple forms a cellular stress.[64] Keyse *et al.*[64] were among the first to suggest that HO-1 acts as a general cellular defense mechanism against oxidative stress, which has been demonstrated in cell culture[16,65−68] and in animal models of inflammatory or oxidative tissue injury.[2,69−73] Numerous studies have linked HO-1 mediated cytoprotection to the biological activities of its enzymatic reaction products.[34] Both biliverdin and bilirubin display considerable antioxidant properties *in vitro*.[74] The HO-derived heme-iron regulates the synthesis of ferritin, an iron storage molecule, which acts as a cytoprotectant by sequestering and detoxifying the released iron.[65,75] An intracellular iron pump associated with HO-1 has also been associated with detoxification of the released iron.[76,77] To further emphasize the importance of this enzyme, HO-1 gene deficient mice ($ho\text{-}1^{-/-}$) are born abnormal, die before the age of 1 year and suffer from various chronic inflammatory diseases.[78,79] Endothelial cells derived from $ho\text{-}1^{-/-}$ mice display increased sensitivity to oxidative stress in culture. Similar disorders were shown in a unique HO-1 deficient patient described in 1999.[80]

1.3.1. *Antiapoptotic effects of HO-1/CO*

The antiapoptotic potential of CO was first demonstrated in cell culture studies using fibroblasts or endothelial cells. Both the exogenous administration of CO or the over-expression of HO-1, inhibited tumor necrosis factor-α (TNFα)-induced apoptosis in murine fibroblasts.[81] In the endothelial cell model, the inhibitory effect of CO on TNFα-induced apoptosis could be abolished with the selective chemical inhibitor, SB203580, or a p38 MAPK dominant negative mutant, implying a critical role for the p38 MAPK pathway.[82] Furthermore, HO-1 or CO co-operated with NF-κB-dependent anti-apoptotic genes (c-IAP2 and A1) to protect against TNFα-mediated endothelial cell apoptosis.[83] More recently, the anti-apoptotic effects of CO have been demonstrated in disease models including lung I/R injury, and lung transplantation (see sections 2.2 and 4).

2. Protective Effects of CO in Acute Lung Injury Models

Acute lung injury, ALI, is a common disease in medical intensive care units. Although the origins of ALI can be diverse (*e.g.* infection, trauma, ischemia, hyperoxia, mechanical ventilation), they are all associated with cell damage, cell death and inflammation.[84,85] Acute lung injury often leads to acute respiratory distress syndrome (ARDS), which has a 40–50 % mortality rate.[86] Here we describe three clinically relevant models where CO shows potential as a therapeutic agent.

2.1. *HO-1 and CO Protect Against Hyperoxic Lung Injury*

Mechanical ventilation with hyperoxia is commonly used in critical care medicine as supportive care for acute, severe respiratory failure. However, hyperoxia (more than 95 % O_2) generates reactive oxygen species (ROS) that cause cell and organ injury. The damage occurs predominantly in the respiratory endothelium and epithelium. These targeted and damaged barriers can also represent sources of ROS that further exacerbate the injury.[87] Hyperoxia, which evokes symptoms in mice similar to human ARDS,[84] causes cell growth arrest, cell death and inflammation in various *in vitro* and *in vivo* models.[88–90]

The adenoviral mediated gene transfer of *ho 1* into rat lungs protected against the development of lung apoptosis and inflammation during hyperoxia.[69] Intratracheal administration of an adenoviral construct containing *ho-1* cDNA (Ad5-HO-1) resulted in a time-dependent increase in the expression of HO-1 mRNA and protein in the rat lungs, with diffuse immunohistochemical staining in the bronchiolar epithelium. Rats receiving Ad5-HO-1 before exposure to hyperoxia (more than 99 % O_2) exhibited marked reduction in lung injury relative to vector controls, as assessed by volume of pleural effusion and histological analyses (significant reduction of edema, hemorrhage, and inflammation), and a marked increase in survivability against hyperoxic stress when compared control-infected rats. Furthermore, rats treated with Ad5-HO-1 exhibited attenuation of hyperoxia-induced neutrophil inflammation and apoptosis.[69] Exogenous CO, through anti-inflammatory action, also protects the lung in a model of hyperoxia-induced lung injury.[27,91] Rats exposed to a low concentration of CO exhibit a marked tolerance to lethal concentrations of hyperoxia *in vivo*. This increased survival was associated with highly significant attenuation of hyperoxia-induced lung injury as assessed by the volume of pleural effusion, protein accumulation in the airways, and histological analysis. The lungs of rats receiving CO treatment (250 parts per million, ppm) in combination with hyperoxia, were completely devoid of lung airway and parenchymal inflammation, fibrin deposition, and pulmonary edema relative to rats exposed to hyperoxia alone. Furthermore, exogenous CO completely protected against hyperoxia-induced lung injury in rats in which endogenous HO enzyme activity was inhibited with tin protoporphyrin, a selective inhibitor of HO. Rats exposed to CO also exhibited a marked attenuation of hyperoxia-induced neutrophil infiltration into the airways and total lung apoptotic index.[27]

When mice were exposed to a hyperoxic environment (more than 98 % O_2), they displayed signs of lung injury by 64–72 h, and 100 % mortality within 90–100 h of exposure. The presence of CO (250 ppm) initiated prior to the hyperoxia, prolonged the survival of mice in the hyperoxic environment, increasing the LD_{50} to 128 h exposure. Similar to the results observed in the rat model, CO inhibited the appearance of histological markers of lung injury associated with hyperoxia, as well as markers of oxidative damage (*i.e.*, lung lipid peroxidation).[91] CO also inhibited the influx of neutrophils into the airways associated with hyperoxia treatment, as measured in bronchoalveolar lavage fluid (BALF). Hyperoxia induced the expression of pro-inflammatory cytokines including $TNF\alpha$, IL-1β, and IL-6, by 84 h of exposure and activated MAPK in lung tissue including ERK1/2, JNK, p38 MAPK and its upstream kinases MKK3/6. The protection afforded by CO treatment against the lethal effects of hyperoxia correlated with the inhibited release of the pro-inflammatory cytokines, TNFα, IL-1β and IL-6, in the BALF.

MKK3$^{-/-}$ mice displayed the accelerated appearance of tissue damage markers and increased susceptibility to the lethal effects of hyperoxia, relative to wild-type mice. Cytokine mRNA (TNFα, IL-1β and IL-6) expression in response to hyperoxia appeared earlier in the MKK3$^{-/-}$ mice relative the wild-type mice exposed to continuous hyperoxia. CO did not inhibit the expression of the pro-inflammatory cytokines in the MKK3$^{-/-}$ mice and, furthermore, did not confer protection or extend survival against hyperoxia in MKK3$^{-/-}$ mice or in wild-type mice injected with SB203580. In contrast, JNK$^{-/-}$ mice responded like wild-type mice with respect to the anti-inflammatory effects of CO.[91]

The protective effects of CO in this model were also observed *in vitro*. CO treatment of A549 lung epithelial cells increased the activation of MKK3, and specifically the β-isoform of p38 MAPK while suppressing that of the α-isoform. CO exposure increased the survival of A549 cells grown in continuous hyperoxia, relative to cells exposed to hyperoxia alone. Treatment with the SB203580 or transient transfection with dominant negative mutants of p38β or MKK3 abolished the cytoprotective effect of CO against hyperoxia. In summary, these experiments demonstrate that CO protects against the lethal and inflammatory effects of hyperoxia *in vivo* and *in vitro*, by downregulating the expression of pro-inflammatory cytokines, through a mechanism dependent on activation of the p38β/MKK3 pathway.[91]

2.2. *CO Protects Against Ischaemia–Reperfusion Injury*

Ischemia–reperfusion during lung surgery, lung transplantation, after hemorrhagic or cardiogenic shock leads to tissue I/R injury. The massive cell death associated with I/R limits therapeutic options. Animal models have suggested that apoptosis is a major cause of cell death following I/R trauma in lung, heart, kidney and brain.[92–95] Anti-inflammatory effects of CO have been demonstrated in models of I/R injury of the heart, lung, kidney, and small bowel.[96,97] CO protected against liver I/R injury via activation of the p38 MAPK.[96] Homozygous *ho-1* null mice (*ho-1*$^{-/-}$) displayed increased mortality in a model of lung I/R injury. CO inhalation (1,000 ppm) partially compensated for the HO-1 deficiency in *ho-1*$^{-/-}$ mice, and improved survival following I/R.[95] In this model, Fujita *et al.* proposed that the protection provided by CO involved the enhancement of fibrinolysis, by the cGMP-dependent inhibition of plasminogen activator inhibitor-1 (PAI-1), a potent smooth muscle cell proliferation activator produced by macrophages.[95] Mice treated with an sGC inhibitor, ODQ, were not protected from I/R-induced lethality by CO.

Independent investigations, also using the mouse lung I/R model, also demonstrated that CO exposure protected against I/R induced lung injury. A left hilar clamp was placed on mechanically-ventilated rats for 30 minutes. After removing the clamp, a two-hour reperfusion was allowed. CO was introduced through the ventilator for a 1 h pretreatment period and throughout the experiment. TUNEL staining showed decreased number of apoptotic cells in the lungs of CO treated animals. Chemical inhibition of p38 MAPK activity, or deletion of MKK3 as in $MKK3^{-/-}$ mice, abolished the anti-apoptotic effects of CO during I/R by preventing the modulation of caspase-3 activity.[98,99] Exogenously applied CO at concentrations starting at 15 ppm inhibited I/R-induced apoptosis in pulmonary artery endothelial cell (PAEC) cultures, associated with the CO-dependent activation of the p38β MAPK isoform and its upstream MAPK kinase (MKK3), with concomitant suppression of ERK and JNK activation. Inhibition of p38 MAPK with SB203580 abolished the cytoprotective potential of CO in this model. The anti-apoptotic effect of CO also involved inhibition of Fas/FasL expression, and other apoptosis-related factors including caspases (−3,−8,−9) mitochondrial cytochrome-c release, Bcl-2 proteins, and poly (ADP-ribose) polymerase (PARP) cleavage.[98,99] These studies confirmed a link between p38 MAPK and the down-regulation of caspase-3 activity by CO, as previously described for Fas-mediated apoptosis.[100] In addition to I/R, apoptotic pathways play a central part in many models of disease. A better understanding of cytoprotection provided by CO *in vivo* could lead future therapeutic solutions in other illness.

2.3. *Cytoprotective Effect of CO Observed in a Model of Ventilator-Induced Lung Injury*

An average of 39 % of medical intensive care unit patients require mechanical ventilation.[101] Many develop ventilator-induced lung injury (VILI).[102] Eventually, VILI contributes to ARDS. A series of clinical trials showed that ARDS/VILI-related mortality could be reduced with lower tidal volume ventilation, positive end-expiratory pressure (PEEP), and more recently with a recruitment maneuver combined with protective ventilator strategies.[86,103,104] Despite efforts to reduce its mortality, ARDS remains a major problem in intensive care units. Preclinical animal models have shown that the pro- and anti-inflammatory cytokines released during VILI play a significant role in the pathology of the disease by causing biotrauma.[105–107] Our laboratory has observed an anti-inflammatory effect of inhaled CO in a rat model of VILI.[30] Rats were ventilated with a relatively injurious ventilator setting, (26 mL/kg tidal volume without PEEP), complemented with an intraperitoneal bacterial LPS injection to induce inflammation and injury. One hour mechanical ventilation with LPS pretreatment significantly increased both the mRNA and the protein expression of HO-1, suggesting that HO-1 may play a role in the defense against VILI. CO was mixed in the ventilator air in different doses (10–250 ppm) and directly applied to the animals. CO (250 ppm) significantly reduced the inflammatory cell count in the BALF at 2–4 h. Furthermore, CO (100–250 ppm) attenuated the levels of the pro-inflammatory cytokine TNFα in the BALF, while significantly increasing the levels of the anti-inflammatory cytokine IL-10. CO treatment did not alter the arterial blood pressure or blood gas results during ventilation, suggesting that a low dose of CO does not cause significant cardiovascular changes in the animals. To investigate the downstream targets of CO in VILI, we performed electrophoretic mobility shift assays on ventilated lung tissue extracts. The activation of AP-1 and NF-κB transcription factors were not modified by CO in this model. However, the tissue showed increased activation of p38 MAPK following ventilation with CO, similar to findings in other models of ALI. Inhibition of p38 MAPK *in vivo* with SB203580 attenuated IL-10 production in VILI. Based on these findings it is exciting to speculate that CO could represent a potential therapeutic modality in ALI and VILI, though further investigations are needed.[30]

3. Carbon Monoxide (CO):
An Anti-Inflammatory Mediator in Sepsis Models

Sepsis has attracted intensive investigation because it is the leading cause of mortality in intensive care units. Until now, therapeutic approaches have failed to dramatically reduce the incidence of this inflammatory disease. According to statistics, approximately 500,000 new cases occur in the U.S. each year, with a mortality rate of approximately 35 %.[108] By definition, sepsis is a systematic inflammatory response to an infectious insult. Clinically, sepsis is characterized by tachycardia, tachypnoe, leukocytosis, hyper- or hypothermia and positive culture for organisms. On the cellular level, the inflammatory response is mainly mediated by macrophages.

Pro-inflammatory cytokines, such as TNFα, and interleukins (IL-1β, IL-6, IL-8) released from macrophages, exert direct effects on the organs or activate secondary mediators such as prostaglandin E2, thromboxane A2, platelet-activating factor-1, bradykinin, angiotensin, vasoactive intestinal peptide, and complement derived products. These mediators exert overlapping effects on endothelial cell function, vascular function, coagulation, hemodynamics, and the cardiovascular mechanism. At present, it is thought that anti-inflammatory mechanisms can compensate for pro-inflammatory mechanisms in an ideal case. This compensation can take place in an organ, before sepsis occurs, or during healing from sepsis. Anti-inflammatory mediators such as IL-10 and IL-11 limit the inflammatory process. If the balance between pro-and anti-inflammatory responses is compromised due to an overwhelmed immune system, or severe infection, the sepsis further propagates to shock and multiple organ dysfunction syndrome. Only supportive therapy is available to these patients, who have a poor prognosis. Gram-negative bacteria cause approximately 50 % of all sepsis cases, which are more likely to be complicated than Gram-positive infections.[109]

One of the most investigated sepsis models utilizes Gram-negative bacterial lipopolysaccharide (LPS), a constituent of the bacterial cell wall.[110] When administered to cells, rodents or humans, LPS mimics the same inflammatory response as the whole bacterium. LPS activates macrophages, lymphocytes, polymorphonuclear leukocytes, and epithelial cells in different models. Macrophages are the key inflammatory cells in LPS-induced sepsis. LPS binds to their CD14 cell surface protein and toll-like receptor 2/4. The complex activates tyrosine kinases and the major MAPKs (p38, JNK, ERK1/2). In macrophages the LPS mediated stimulation of pro-inflammatory cytokine production involves the activation of the MAPK signaling pathways.[110–113]

3.1. *Anti-Inflammatory Effect of CO in a Macrophage Sepsis Model*

Recent studies have elucidated a novel anti-inflammatory effect of HO-1 mediated by CO generated in the HO reaction.[2] The effectiveness of LPS (1 μg/ml) to stimulate the production of the pro-inflammatory cytokine TNFα was inhibited in transfected RAW 264.7 macrophage cells over-expressing HO-1, compared to that in control transfectants. Exogenously administered CO (250 ppm) inhibited the production of TNFα in RAW 264.7 cells in response to LPS treatment, indicating that CO can substitute for HO activity in mediating these effects. The treatment of RAW 264.7 cells with exogenous CO prior to LPS treatment inhibited the expression of additional pro-inflammatory cytokines (*i.e.*, IL-1β), and the macrophage inflammatory protein-β (MIP-1β), whereas it increased the production of the anti-inflammatory cytokine IL-10. LPS treatment activated the p38 MAPK, ERK1/ERK2 and JNK pathways in RAW 264.7 macrophages. In the presence of LPS, CO increased p38 MAPK activation, but did not modulate ERK1/2 and JNK. Of the MAP kinase kinases (MKK): (MKK3, MKK4, and MKK6) that activate p38 MAPK,[114,115] CO enhanced the LPS-mediated stimulation of MKK3 and MKK6 in RAW 264.7 cells. CO treatment did not significantly modulate cGMP production in RAW 264.7 macrophages. Pretreatment of the RAW 264.7 macrophages with a non-hydrolysable cGMP analog or L-NAME did not compromise the ability of CO to inhibit LPS-inducible TNFα production. These anti-inflammatory effects of CO were substantiated *in vivo*, in experiments where mice received injections of LPS (1 mg/kg) with or without CO pretreatment (250 ppm). CO inhibited LPS-inducible serum TNFα levels and increased LPS-inducible IL-10 production. The responsiveness of TNFα to LPS treatment was inhibited in MKK3$^{-/-}$ mice compared to wild-type mice. CO failed to further inhibit TNFα levels or increase IL-10 levels in LPS treated MKK3$^{-/-}$ mice. In IL-10$^{-/-}$ mice, CO inhibited TNFα levels within the first hour of LPS treatment to a similar extent than in wild-type mice, excluding a role for IL-10 in the early anti-inflammatory effects of CO.[2] These results demonstrate that CO exerts anti-inflammatory effects by inhibiting the synthesis of the pro-inflammatory cytokines under inducing conditions, by a mechanism that involves stimulation of the MKK3/p38 MAPK pathway, but excludes sGC/cGMP, iNOS, or NO-dependent signaling. In contrast, the mechanism for the inhibition of IL-6 production by CO involved the JNK MAPK pathway.[116] JNK regulates several transcription factors including AP-1. The ability of CO to inhibit LPS-induced IL-6 production was abolished when the AP-1 DNA binding site was mutated in the IL-6 promoter. Mutation of the nuclear factor κB (NF-κB) and CCAAT/enhancer-binding protein (C/EBP) binding sites, however, had no effect on the inhibitory effect of CO on IL-6 gene transcription.

Differential effects of CO were also observed in rat pulmonary artery endothelial cells treated with TNF-α, which rapidly increased MAPK activities. CO treatment reduced ERK1/2 activation, increased p38 MAPK activation, and did not affect JNK.[117] The direct physical target of CO in initiating these pathways remains obscure.

3.2. *CO Reduces Granulocyte-Macrophage Colony Stimulating Factor Production in Sepsis*

Granulocyte-macrophage-colony stimulating factor (GM-CSF), a glycoprotein, promotes the proliferation and the differentiation of hematopoetic progenitor cells into neutrophils and macrophages. Besides this function, GM-CSF also plays a critical role in antigen- and complement mediated phagocytosis and anti-tumor immunity. Elevated GM-CSF levels appear in chronic inflammatory pulmonary diseases like asthma, COPD, or sarcoidosis and have been linked to pulmonary alveolar proteinosis. Many cell types produce GM-CSF (*i.e.*, fibroblasts, endothelial cells, airway smooth muscle cells, and T lymphocytes). GM-CSF enhances the secretion of pro-inflammatory cyokines including TNFα, IL-1, interferon (IFN)-γ, as well as inflammatory mediators (*i.e.*, superoxide anion, E-series prostaglandins, leukotrienes, arachidonic acid, plasminogen activator and other colony stimulating factors.[118] Macrophages treated with GM-CSF display a higher TNFα production and cytotoxicity in response to *in vitro* stimulation with IFN-γ than non-treated cells.[119]

RAW 264.7 macrophages treated with LPS produced an increased amount of GM-CSF, which could be attenuated by CO pretreatment. NF-κB, a transcription factor that regulates pro-inflammatory cytokine release, can mediate the expression of the GM-CSF gene in certain cell types.[120] CO inhibited the LPS-induced activation of NF-κB, by preventing the phosphorylation and degradation of the inhibitory subunit I-kBα. Roles for ERK1/2 and cGMP were not established for this model.

3.3. *Conclusion*

CO can interact with LPS/sepsis mediated pathways at several potential targets (Fig. 2). Collectively, CO exerts a potent anti-inflammatory effect in sepsis models.

4. Protective Roles of CO in Organ Transplantation

Increasing survival rates in organ transplantation represents one of the successes of modern medicine. However graft rejection limits its efficacy, especially following lung transplantation. The frequency and severity of acute rejection episodes is a predominant risk for chronic graft rejection. Expression of the stress protein HO-1 in rodent allografts (kidney, heart, and liver) and xenografts (heart) correlates with long-term graft survival in several models of transplantation.[28,121–124] In a rodent model of renal transplantation, HO-1 expression increased in the allograft in response to immune injury.[73,124] The reduced expression of HO-1 in chronic rejection as compared with acute rejection may represent an inadequate response to injury or a consequence of prior injury that sensitizes further tissue response to immune attack.[124] HO-1 gene therapy protected against rejection in rat liver transplants.[125] The induction of HO-1 protected pancreatic islet cells

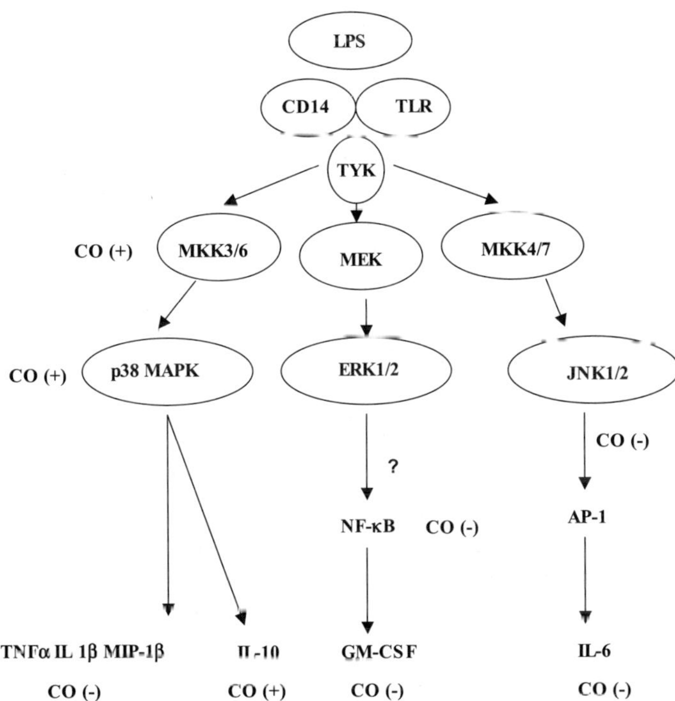

Fig. 2.   Possible targets for carbon monoxide in LPS-induced sepsis in macrophages. Legend: LPS: Gram negative bacteria lipopolysaccharide; CD14: macrophage cell surface adhesion protein; TLR: Toll like receptor (2 or 4); Tyk: tyrosine kinase; MKK or MEK: mitogen activated protein kinase kinase; p38 MAPK: p38 mitogen activated protein kinase; ERK1/2: extracellular regulated kinase-1/2; JNK1/2: c-jun NH$_2$-terminal kinase-1/2; TNFα: tumor necrosis factor-α; IL-1β: interleukin 1β; IL-6: interleukin-6; IL-10: interleukin-10; NF-κB: nuclear factor κB; AP1: activator protein-1; CO: carbon monoxide; (+) stimulatory effect; (−) inhibitory effect.

from Fas-mediated apoptosis in a dose-dependent fashion, supporting an anti-apoptotic role of HO-1 in transplantation models.[126,127] In a rat liver allograft model, HO-1 may confer protection in the early phase after transplantation by inducing Th2-dependent cytokines such as IL-4 and IL-10, while suppressing IFN-γ and IL-2 production.[128] HO-1 gene therapy in rats undergoing liver transplantation resulted in protection against I/R injury and improved survival after transplantation, possibly by suppression of Th1-cytokine production and decreased apoptosis after reperfusion.[94]

Protective effects of HO-1 have also been documented in xeno-transplantation models, where HO-1 gene expression correlates with xenograft survival.[28,129] In a mouse to rat cardiac transplant model, the effects of HO-1 expression could be mimicked by CO administration, suggesting that HO-derived CO suppressed the graft rejection.[28] Sato *et al.* proposed that CO suppressed graft rejection by inhibition of platelet aggregation, a process that facilitates vascular thrombosis and myocardial infarction.[28] The ability of CO to suppress inflammation is likely involved in xenograft transplant models in which 400 ppm CO for 2 days prevented rejection for up to 50 days.[28] The effects of CO on platelet aggregation, vasodilation, and pro-inflammatory cytokines all potentially contribute to the favorable outcome in xenograft transplantation.[26]

4.1. *CO Protected Against Acute Rejection in Lung Transplantation*

Lung transplantation has become an accepted treatment modality for end-stage lung disease. After lung transplantation, there remains a persistent risk of acute and chronic graft failure, as well as of complications of the toxic immunosuppressive regimen used.[130] Compared to other solid organ transplants, the success of lung transplantation has been severely limited by the high incidence of acute and chronic graft rejection. The frequency and severity of episodes of acute rejection are the predominant risk factors for chronic airway rejection, manifested as obliterative bronchiolitis (OB).[131,132] Data from rodent allograft studies as well as from clinical lung transplantation show that the lung, in comparison to other solid organs, is highly immunogenic. Despite advances in immunosuppression, the incidence of acute rejection in lung graft patients can be as high as 60 % in the first postoperative month.[133,134] OB, which may develop during the first months after transplantation, is the main cause of morbidity and death following the first half-year after transplantation despite therapy. Once

OB has developed, re-transplantation remains the only therapeutic option available[135]

Until recently, only very limited research data were available on the possible role for HO-1 in allograft rejection after lung transplantation. Increased HO-1 expression has been detected in alveolar macrophages from lung tissue in lung transplant recipients with either acute or chronic graft failure when compared to stable recipients.[136] The level of HO-1 mRNA and protein expression correlated with the acute rejection grade scores in lung fibroblasts taken from biopsies from a lung transplant patient.[137] The effects of CO were also examined in a rat model of lung transplantation. Orthotopic left lung transplantation was performed in Lewis rat recipients from Brown-Norway rat donors. HO-1 mRNA and protein expression were markedly elevated in transplanted rat lungs at 4 days post-transplantation compared to sham-operated lungs. Animals were exposed to continuous inhalation CO (500 ppm) or air. Transplanted lungs developed severe intralveolar hemorrhage and intravascular coagulation. In the presence of continuous CO exposure, however, the gross anatomy and histology of transplanted lungs showed dramatic preservation relative to air-treated controls, with marked reduction in hemorrhage, fibrosis, and thrombosis on the sixth day after transplantation. Furthermore, transplanted lungs displayed increased apoptotic cell death compared with the transplanted lungs of CO-treated recipients, as assessed by TUNEL and caspase-3 immunostaining. IL-6 expression corresponds to the magnitude of injury during transplantation.[136,138] CO exposure inhibited the induction of IL-6 mRNA expression in lung and serum caused by the transplantation. Gene array analysis revealed that CO also down-regulated other pro-inflammatory genes, including MIP-1α and macrophage migration inhibitory factor (MIF), and growth factors such as PDGF, which were up-regulated as a result of transplantation.[127] In organ transplantation, the I/R injury that occurs leads to rapid endothelial cell apoptosis. The loss of endothelial cells in the vessels serving the organ results in a rapid cascade of events including thrombosis that can ultimately result in the rejection of the organ. These data suggest CO limits lung graft injury by maintaining cell viability and suppressing inflammation.

4.2. *Antiproliferative Effect of CO in Vascular Transplant and Balloon Injury Models*

The vascular injury, intimal hyperplasia, and subsequent arteriosclerosis leading to vessel obliteration during chronic graft rejection remain critical problems in transplantology. Infiltrating leukocytes and smooth muscle cells play key roles in the pathology of the disease. Leukocytes initiate an immune-mediated injury that activates endothelial cells and disturbs their barrier function. Macrophages and T lymphocytes infiltrate the graft. In the meantime smooth muscle cells (SMC) penetrate to the intima of vessels. The hyperproliferation of SMC produces extracellular matrix depositions and leads to luminal stenosis. A potential therapeutic effect of CO in limiting SMC proliferation was shown in two models. First, Brown–Norway rat aortic segments were transplanted into Lewis rats.[26] The most significant changes were seen after 50–60 days characterized by intimal hyperplasia, the loss of SMC in the medial region of the vessels and leukocyte infiltration in the adventitia. A group of rats was pretreated with 250 ppm CO for 2 days and maintained in the CO containing environment until they were sacrificed. These animals displayed significantly less intimal proliferation and a lower magnitude of leukocyte infiltration in the graft. The accumulation of macrophages, helper and cytotoxic T cells was also reduced in the transplanted aortic ring.[26]

In a model of intimal hyperplasia, where smooth muscle cells proliferate uncontrollably following balloon angioplasty of the carotid artery, exposure to CO also completely prevented stenosis of the vessel.[26] Pre-treatment of a rat with CO (250 ppm) for just 1 hour significantly reduced the neointimal proliferation seen at 14 days post-balloon angioplasty relative to control animals that did not receive CO treatment. The mechanisms involved in this effect were attributed to the inhibition of smooth muscle proliferation by CO.[24,26,129] SMC proliferation is regulated by the cyclin dependent kinase inhibitor $p21^{Waf1/Cip1}$. CO treatment induced $p21^{Waf1/Cip1}$ expression in SMC. The antiproliferative effect of CO was compromised in smooth muscle cells from the $p21^{Waf1/Cip1}$ knockout mice ($p21^{-/-}$). Although $p21^{Waf1/Cip1}$ is regulated by p53, the antiproliferative effect of CO occurred in SMC from p53 gene deficient mice ($p53^{-/-}$). CO treatment activated p38 MAPK in SMC. The antiproliferative effect and the induction of $p21^{Waf1/Cip1}$ by CO treatment depended on the activation of p38 MAPK, since these effects were reversed by the p38 MAPK inhibitor SB203580. Treatment of SMC with ODQ, a guanylyl cyclase inhibitor abolished the effects of CO on SMC proliferation and activation of p38 MAPK. The dependence of cGMP in these effects is further supported by the observation that the "cell-permeable" cGMP analog (8-Br-cGMP) activated p38 MAPK, and increased $p21^{Waf1/Cip1}$ expression in SMC. Furthermore 8-Br-cGMP inhibited proliferation in wild type but not $p21^{-/-}$ SMC.[26] Adenoviral mediated expression of HO-1 (AdHO-1) in pigs inhibited vascular cell proliferation and lesion formation in a model of arterial injury. Conversely, $HO-1^{-/-}$ mice subjected to arterial injury displayed increased vascular cell proliferation, and developed hyperplastic lesions in comparison to $HO-1^{+/+}$ controls.[139] The application of HO-1 by adenoviral mediated gene transfer also protected against intimal hyperplasia following vascular balloon injury.[140] In conclusion, the potential use of CO in transplantation remains very promising. In the balloon injury model 1-hour pretreatment was enough to exert a beneficial effect. CO pretreatment of organs prior to transplantation may result in lower rejection rates.

4.3. *Antiproliferative Effect of CO in T-Lymphocytes*

The anti-proliferative effects of CO, as described above, were recently also explored in a model of T-cell proliferation. Cumulating data suggests that caspases, in addition to their role in apoptosis, are also involved in T-lymphocyte activation and proliferation.[141] Both leukemia cell line (Jurkat cells) and primary cultured T-lymphocytes increased caspase activity during proliferation. Song *et al.*[142] demonstrated that CO could reduce caspase activity independent of MAPK in T-lymphocytes.[142] To test the effect of CO on these cells, anti-CD3 antibody-stimulated primary cell cultures were treated with 250 ppm CO, which caused a marked decrease in proliferation as assayed with the $[^3H]$ thymidine incorporation assay. CO did not increase cell death, as measured by annexin V/PI flow cytometry. Primary culture T-lymphocytes display decreased caspase 3 activity in the presence of CO. However, CO did not produce this effect in T-lymphocytes isolated from $MKK3^{-/-}$ mice or $JNK1^{-/-}$ mice. Meanwhile, CD3 antibody stimulated and CO exposed T-lymphocytes demonstrate increased $p21^{Waf1/Cip1}$ cell cycle inhibitor expression. Lymphocytes isolated from $p21^{-/-}$ mice showed a partial decrease in caspase activity. This result suggests that CO can exert anti-proliferative effects via the $p21^{Waf1/Cip1}$ pathway in lymphocytes as well as in SMC. Furthermore, CO can reduce caspase-8 activity in Jurkat T cells, providing further evidence that CO can activate several independent pathways to carry out anti-proliferative effects in different cell types. At present, we do not fully understand the cell-specific variation in signal transduction pathways underlying the principle effects of CO.

5. Asthma

Asthma, a complex chronic inflammatory disease, affects at least 10 million people in the U.S. alone.[143] Due to the high morbidity of the disease, the pathology of asthma has attracted intense investigation. HO-1 induction has been demonstrated in preclinical asthma models. Furthermore, increased exhaled CO levels were measured in asthma patients.[144] These observations have encouraged the application of CO in various asthma models.

5.1. *Chronic Inflammation*

Blood eosinophilia has long been known to represent a major characteristic of inflammation in asthma.[29] The BALF of asthmatics contains elevated levels of many inflammatory cells (eosinophils, basophils, lymphocytes, macrophages, and neutrophils) as well as pro-inflammatory mediators. Th2-like cytokines (IL-4, IL-5, IL-13, and eotaxin) initiate and maintain inflammation and bronchial hyperreactivity. Mice develop an airway hyperresponsiveness, similar to that seen in human asthma, when challenged with aerosolized ovalbumin after initial sensitization. Animals were treated with ovalbumin, with one group receiving CO before and after treatment. The BALF was collected 24 and 48 hours later. Progressive increases in total cell number were detected after 24 and 48 hours of challenge. Differential cell counts showed that ovalbumin challenge activates all inflammatory cells. Macrophages, eosinophils, neutrophils, lymphocytes were detected in the BALF. CO treated mice displayed a significantly lower increase in total cell number. CO was also able to reduce the number of all inflammatory cell types, especially eosinophils and macrophages in the BALF at 24 hours post challenge. Exogenous CO administration significantly reduced IL-5 production at 24 hours, which returned to near control values at 48 hours, but did not affect other cytokines. In this model, eicosanoid mediator levels (IFN-γ, leukotriene B4, and prostaglandin E2) were also reduced by CO. It is not clear whether inflammatory cell numbers and mediator levels seen in BALF can accurately reflect the magnitude of inflammation and/or the outcome of the disease. However, the changes in cell count and mediator levels indicate that CO can regulate inflammation in asthma.[29]

CO can also affect another cytokine, GM-CSF, which is increased in asthma. In a series of experiments human airway smooth muscle cells (HASMC) were treated with cytomix (TNFα, IL-1β, IFN-γ, and LPS). Stimulated HASMC cells can release GM-CSF. IL-1β was able to stimulate GM-CSF release alone, while TNFα and INF-γ stimulated GM-CSF only as components of cytomix. CO inhibited the induction of GM-CSF protein stimulated by cytomix; LPS, and IL-1β alone. Western blotting analysis showed that in IL-1β stimulated HASMC, the ERK1/2 MAPK pathway was activated. The activation was blocked with CO. The inhibitory effect of CO on GM-CSF was reversed with the specific cGMP inhibitor ODQ. These results show that CO can carry out its anti-inflammatory effect by activating ERK1/2 MAPK in a cGMP-dependent fashion[145]

5.2. *Airway Remodeling*

Airway remodeling contributes to hyper-reactivity, another characteristic of asthma. Respiratory tract smooth muscle cells (SMC) respond to inflammatory cell-derived mediators with increased proliferation and further release of inflammatory mediators. Thus, SMC play a central role in asthma pathology. CO treatment suppressed HASMC cell growth. Cell cycle analysis by PI staining showed that CO affected the G0/G1 phase of cell cycle. SMC proliferation is conducted by cell cycle dependent kinases and cyclin complexes, which are regulated by the cell cycle inhibitor $p21^{Waf1/Cip1}$. CO treatment increased the expression of $p21^{Waf1/Cip1}$ and decreased cyclin D1. While CO activated ERK1/2 MAPK in this model, ODQ failed to attenuate the CO effect. These results directly contrast to the observation that the anti-inflammatory effect of CO in HASMC depended on cGMP-dependent regulation of ERK1/2.[146] The signaling pathways affected by CO can vary in a cell-type specific manner, and even in the same cell type in response to different cellular processes (*e.g.*, inflammation and proliferation).[146b,147] A number of pro-inflammatory cytokines utilize the MAPK pathways to propagate inflammation and lung-injury. CO inhalation therapy could add a new dimension to asthma therapy, by contributing to the therapeutic arsenal to reduce inflammation and attenuate airway smooth muscle proliferation in asthma.

6. Challenges Ahead for Therapeutic Use of CO in Human Disease

The recent research described in this monograph strongly supports that CO, when applied exogenously at low concentration, may also protect cells and tissues in a number of disease models, including acute lung injury, ischemia/reperfusion injury, ventilator induced lung injury, sepsis, organ transplantation, and asthma. The protective effects of CO in these models depend on the anti-inflammatory, anti-apoptotic and anti-proliferative activity of this gas. There is growing preclinical evidence (in rodents) that inhaled CO can confer beneficial effects in diverse diseases. In certain models, only a short exposure period and very low concentration of CO inhalation sufficed to yield positive effects. This concentration range may fall within the presently enforced standards.

Potent anti-inflammatory effects of CO have been demonstrated in sepsis models and could be applied to inflammatory lung diseases. The *ex-vivo* application of CO to organ tissue may confer significant benefit in limiting the rejection of organ transplants. The positive therapeutic effects of CO in ALI models show promise in the light of the high mortality of ARDS. However, in most cases, there is little opportunity for pretreatment in acute diseases. The potential success of CO therapy in ALI could be improved if CO could be used promptly in combination with other medication or administered locally to the lung. The potential therapeutic effects of CO need to be tested in other ALI models. Since very low dose (15 ppm) CO was effective in the I/R model, CO therapy may be employed as a short-term pretreatment before major surgery or continuously administrated to critical care patients. The complex anti-inflammatory, anti-apoptotic and anti-proliferative effects of exogenous CO treatment as described in this review could also be promising in disease models such as VILI, COPD, and pulmonary fibrosis. If experiments with higher mammals such as pigs or primates present similar responses as in rodents, CO remains a good candidate for human trials.

Considerable obstacles remain before CO may reach clinical application, including political and regulatory approval, as well as social acceptance of a substance widely regarded as a poison. The duration and dose of exposure is still a subject of evaluation. It remains unclear how to define a safe dose of CO for human therapy. The toxicological consequences of low dose CO application remain incompletely understood. Alternative delivery approaches must also be considered, such as the injection of experimental CO releasing molecules.[147] Despite its reputation as a noxious gas, CO may be well on its way to providing a low cost and effective therapy for a number of disease conditions. Collectively, the body of research described herein heralds the future exploitation of CO in the clinic for the treatment of advanced-stage lung disease, and the improved success of organ transplantation.

Acknowledgements

This work was supported by an award from the American Heart Association (AHA #0335035N), to SWR, and NIH grants R01-HL60234, R01-AI42365, R01-HL55330 awarded to A. M. K. Choi.

Appendix: Abbreviations

ALI	acute lung injury
AP1	activator protein-1
ARDS	acute respiratory distress syndrome
ARE	antioxidant responsive element
BALF	bronchoalveolar lavage fluid
cGMP	guanosine $3', 5'$-monophosphate
CO	carbon monoxide
ERK1/2	extracellular regulated kinase 1/2
GM-CSF	granulocyte-macrophage-colony stimulating factor
HASMC	human airway smooth muscle cell
HO	heme oxygenase
IL	interleukin
INF-γ	interferon-γ
JNK	c-jun NH_2-terminal kinase
LPS	Gram negative bacterial lipopolysaccharide
MAPK	mitogen activated protein kinase
MIF	macrophage migration inhibitory factor
MIP-$1\alpha/\beta$	macrophage inflammatory protein-1α
MKK	mitogen activated kinase kinase
NF-κB	nuclear factor κB
Nrf2	NF-E2 related factor
NO	nitric oxide
$p21^{Waf1/Cip1}$	p21 cell cycle inhibitor
p38 MAPK	p38 mitogen activated protein kinase
PDGF	platelet derived growth factor
ppm	parts per million
sGC	soluble guanylate cyclase
SMC	smooth muscle cells
StRE	stress responsive element
TNFα	tumor necrosis factor-α
TUNEL	terminal deoxynucleotidyl-transferase dUTP nick end-labeling assay
VILI	ventilator induced lung injury

References

1. Horvath I, MacNee W, Kelly FJ, Dekhuijzen PN, Phillips M, Doring G, Choi AM, Yamaya M, Bach FH, Willis D, Donnelly LE, Chung KF, Barnes PJ. "Haemoxygenase-1 induction and exhaled markers of oxidative stress in lung diseases," summary of the ERS Research Seminar in Budapest, Hungary, September, 1999. *Eur Respir J* 2001; **18**: 420–430.
2. Otterbein LE, Bach FH, Alam J, Soares M, Tao Lu H, Wysk M, Davis RJ, Flavell RA, Choi AM. Carbon monoxide has anti-inflammatory effects involving the mitogen-activated protein kinase pathway. *Nat Med* 2000; **6**: 422–428.
3. White KA, Marletta MA. Nitric oxide synthase is a cytochrome P-450 type hemoprotein. *Biochemistry* 1992; **31**: 6627–6631.
4. Tenhunen R, Marver HS, Schmid R. Microsomal heme oxygenase. Characterization of the enzyme. *J Biol Chem* 1969; **244**: 6388–6394.
5. Tenhunen R, Marver HS, Schmid R. The enzymatic conversion of heme to bilirubin by microsomal heme oxygenase. *Proc Natl Acad Sci USA* 1968; **61**: 748–755.
6. Hartsfield CL. Cross talk between carbon monoxide and nitric oxide. *Antioxid Redox Signal* 2002; **4**: 301–307.
7. Wink DA, Mitchell JB. Chemical biology of nitric oxide: Insights into regulatory, cytotoxic, and cytoprotective mechanisms of nitric oxide. *Free Radic Biol Med* 1998; **25**: 434–456.
8. Von Burg R. Carbon monoxide. *J Appl Toxicol* 1999; **19**: 379–386.
9. Smith R. Toxic responses of the blood., In: Klaassen K, Amdur M, Doull J, eds. *Casarett and Doull's Toxicology, the basic science of poisons*, New York: MacMillan Publishing Company, 1986: 223–244.
10. Weaver LK. Carbon monoxide poisoning. *Crit Care Clin* 1999; **15**: 297–317, viii.
11. Gorman D, Drewry A, Huang YL, Sames C. The clinical toxicology of carbon monoxide. *Toxicology* 2003; **187**: 25–38.
12. Sjostrand T. Endogenous production of carbon monoxide in man under normal and pathophysiological conditions. *Acta Physiol Scand* 1949; **26**: 338–344.
13. Sjostrand T. The formation of carbon monoxide by the decomposition of haemoglobin in vivo. *Acta Physiol Scand* 1952; **26**: 338–344.
14. Coburn RF, Blakemore WS, Forster RE. Endogenous carbon monoxide production in man. *J Clin Invest* 1963; **42**: 1172–1178.
15. Vremen H, Wong R, Stevenson D. Carbon monoxide in breath, blood and other tissues., In: Penney D, ed. *Carbon monoxide toxicity*, Boca Raton: CRC Press, 2000: 19–60.
16. Ryter SW, Otterbein LE, Morse D, Choi AM. Heme oxygenase/carbon monoxide signaling pathways: regulation and functional significance. *Mol Cell Biochem* 2002; **234-235**: 249–263.
17. Maines MD. The heme oxygenase system: a regulator of second messenger gases. *Annu Rev Pharmacol Toxicol* 1997; **37**: 517–554.

18. Ignarro LJ, Buga GM, Wood KS, Byrns RE, Chaudhuri G. Endothelium-derived relaxing factor produced and released from artery and vein is nitric oxide. *Proc Natl Acad Sci USA* 1987; **84**: 9265–9269.

19. Ignarro LJ, Byrns RE, Buga GM, Wood KS. Endothelium-derived relaxing factor from pulmonary artery and vein possesses pharmacologic and chemical properties identical to those of nitric oxide radical. *Circ Res* 1987; **61**: 866–879.

20. Ignarro LJ, Degnan JN, Baricos WH, Kadowitz PJ, Wolin MS. Activation of purified guanylate cyclase by nitric oxide requires heme. Comparison of heme-deficient, heme-reconstituted and heme-containing forms of soluble enzyme from bovine lung. *Biochim Biophys Acta* 1982; **718**: 49–59.

21. Furchgott RF, Jothianandan D. Endothelium-dependent and -independent vasodilation involving cyclic GMP: relaxation induced by nitric oxide, carbon monoxide and light. *Blood Vessels* 1991; **28**: 52–61.

22. Verma A, Hirsch DJ, Glatt CE, Ronnett GV, Snyder SH. Carbon monoxide: a putative neural messenger. *Science* 1993; **259**: 381–384.

23. Morita T, Perrella MA, Lee ME, Kourembanas S. Smooth muscle cell-derived carbon monoxide is a regulator of vascular cGMP. *Proc Natl Acad Sci USA* 1995; **92**: 1475–1479.

24. Morita T, Mitsialis SA, Koike H, Liu Y, Kourembanas S. Carbon monoxide controls the proliferation of hypoxic vascular smooth muscle cells. *J Biol Chem* 1997; **272**: 32804–32809.

25. Morita T, Kourembanas S. Endothelial cell expression of vasoconstrictors and growth factors is regulated by smooth muscle cell-derived carbon monoxide. *J Clin Invest* 1995; **96**: 2676–2682.

26. Otterbein LE, Zuckerbraun BS, Haga M, Liu F, Song R, Ushcva A, Stachulak C, Bodyak N, Smith RN, Csizmadia E, Tyagi S, Akamatsu Y, Flavell RJ, Billiar TR, Tzeng E, Bach FH, Choi AM, Soares MP. Carbon monoxide suppresses arteriosclerotic lesions associated with chronic graft rejection and with balloon injury. *Nat Med* 2003; **9**: 183–190.

27. Otterbein LE, Mantell LL, Choi AM. Carbon monoxide provides protection against hyperoxic lung injury. *Am J Physiol* 1999; **276**: L688–694.

28. Sato K, Balla J, Otterbein L, Smith RN, Brouard S, Lin Y, Csizmadia E, Sevigny J, Robson SC, Vercellotti G, Choi AM, Bach FH, Soares MP. Carbon monoxide generated by heme oxygenase-1 suppresses the rejection of mouse-to-rat cardiac transplants. *J Immunol* 2001; **166**: 4185–4194.

29. Chapman JT, Otterbein LE, Elias JA, Choi AM. Carbon monoxide attenuates aeroallergen-induced inflammation in mice. *Am J Physiol Lung Cell Mol Physiol* 2001; **281**: L209–216.

30. Dolinay T, Szilasi M, Liu M, Choi AM. Inhaled carbon monoxide confers antiinflammatory effects against ventilator-induced lung injury. *Am J Respir Crit Care Med* 2004; **170**: 613–620.

31. Ryter SW, Morse D, Choi AM. Carbon monoxide: to boldly go where NO has gone before. *Sci STKE* 2004; **2004**: RE6

32. Ryter SW, Otterbein LE. Carbon monoxide in biology and medicine. *Bioessays* 2004; **26**: 270–280.

33. Slebos DJ, Ryter SW, Choi AM. Heme oxygenase-1 and carbon monoxide in pulmonary medicine. *Respir Res* 2003; **4**: 7.

34. Ryter SW, Tyrrell RM. The heme synthesis and degradation pathways: role in oxidant sensitivity. Heme oxygenase has both pro- and antioxidant properties. *Free Radic Biol Med* 2000; **28**: 289–309.

35. Tenhunen R, Ross ME, Marver HS, Schmid R. Reduced nicotinamide-adenine dinucleotide phosphate dependent biliverdin reductase: partial purification and characterization. *Biochemistry* 1970; **9**: 298–303.

36. Tenhunen R, Marver HS, Schmid R. The enzymatic catabolism of hemoglobin: stimulation of microsomal heme oxygenase by hemin. *J Lab Clin Med* 1970; **75**: 410–421.

37. Maines MD, Trakshel GM, Kutty RK. Characterization of two constitutive forms of rat liver microsomal heme oxygenase. Only one molecular species of the enzyme is inducible. *J Biol Chem* 1986; **261**: 411–419.

38. Trakshel GM, Kutty RK, Maines MD. Purification and characterization of the major constitutive form of testicular heme oxygenase. The noninducible isoform. *J Biol Chem* 1986; **261**: 11131–11137.

39. Maines MD. *Heme oxygenase: clinical applications and functions.* Boca Raton, Fla.: CRC Press, 1992.

40. McCoubrey WK Jr., Huang TJ, Maines MD. Isolation and characterization of a cDNA from the rat brain that encodes hemoprotein heme oxygenase-3. *Eur J Biochem* 1997; **247**: 725–732.

41. Muramoto T, Kohchi T, Yokota A, Hwang I, Goodman HM. The Arabidopsis photomorphogenic mutant hy1 is deficient in phytochrome chromophore biosynthesis as a result of a mutation in a plastid heme oxygenase. *Plant Cell* 1999; **11**: 335–348.

42. Lee BC. Quelling the red menace: haem capture by bacteria. *Mol Microbiol* 1995; **18**: 383–390.

43. Wilks A. Heme oxygenase: evolution, structure, and mechanism. *Antioxid Redox Signal* 2002; **4**: 603–614.

44. Wilks A, Schmitt MP. Expression and characterization of a heme oxygenase (Hmu O) from Corynebacterium diphtheriae. Iron acquisition requires oxidative cleavage of the heme macrocycle. *J Biol Chem* 1998; **273**: 837–841.

45. Beale SI, Cornejo J. Enzymatic heme oxygenase activity in soluble extracts of the unicellular red alga, Cyanidium caldarium. *Arch Biochem Biophys* 1984; **235**: 371–384.

46. Zhu W, Wilks A, Stojiljkovic I. Degradation of heme in gram-negative bacteria: the product of the hemO gene of Neisseriae is a heme oxygenase. *J Bacteriol* 2000; **182**: 6783–6790.

47. Ratliff M, Zhu W, Deshmukh R, Wilks A, Stojiljkovic I. Homologues of neisserial heme oxygenase in gram-negative bacteria: degradation of heme by the product of the pigA gene of Pseudomonas aeruginosa. *J Bacteriol* 2001; **183**: 6394–6403.

48. Ryter SW, Choi AM. Heme oxygenase-1: molecular mechanisms of gene expression in oxygen-related stress. *Antioxid Redox Signal* 2002; **4**: 625–632.

49. Ryter SW, Choi AM. Heme oxygenase-1: redox regulation of a stress protein in lung and cell culture models. *Antioxid Redox Signal* 2005; **7**: 80–91.

50. Kyriakis JM, Avruch J. Sounding the alarm: protein kinase cascades activated by stress and inflammation. *J Biol Chem* 1996; **271**: 24313–24316.

51. Alam J, Wicks C, Stewart D, Gong P, Touchard C, Otterbein S, Choi AM, Burow ME, Tou J. Mechanism of heme oxygenase-1 gene activation by cadmium in MCF-7 mammary epithelial cells. Role of p38 kinase and Nrf2 transcription factor. *J Biol Chem* 2000; **275**: 27694–27702.

52. Alam J. Multiple elements within the 5′ distal enhancer of the mouse heme oxygenase-1 gene mediate induction by heavy metals. *J Biol Chem* 1994; **269**: 25049–25056.

53. Alam J, Camhi S, Choi AM. Identification of a second region upstream of the mouse heme oxygenase-1 gene that functions as a basal level and inducer-dependent transcription enhancer. *J Biol Chem* 1995; **270**: 11977–11984.

54. Camhi SL, Alam J, Wiegand GW, Chin BY, Choi AM. Transcriptional activation of the HO-1 gene by lipopolysaccharide is mediated by 5′ distal enhancers: role of reactive oxygen intermediates and AP-1. *Am J Respir Cell Mol Biol* 1998; **18**: 226–234.

55. Inamdar NM, Ahn YI, Alam J. The heme-responsive element of the mouse heme oxygenase-1 gene is an extended AP-1 binding site that resembles the recognition sequences for MAF and NF-E2 transcription factors. *Biochem Biophys Res Commun* 1996; **221**: 570–576.

56. Alam J, Stewart D, Touchard C, Boinapally S, Choi AM, Cook JL. Nrf2, a Cap'n'Collar transcription factor, regulates induction of the heme oxygenase-1 gene. *J Biol Chem* 1999; **274**: 26071–26078.

57. Itoh K, Chiba T, Takahashi S, Ishii T, Igarashi K, Katoh Y, Oyake T, Hayashi N, Satoh K, Hatayama I, Yamamoto M, Nabeshima Y. An Nrf2/small Maf heterodimer mediates the induction of phase II detoxifying enzyme genes through antioxidant response elements. *Biochem Biophys Res Commun* 1997; **236**: 313–322.

58. Venugopal R, Jaiswal AK. Nrf2 and Nrf1 in association with Jun proteins regulate antioxidant response element-mediated expression and coordinated induction of genes encoding detoxifying enzymes. *Oncogene* 1998; **17**: 3145–3156.

59. Itoh K, Wakabayashi N, Katoh Y, Ishii T, Igarashi K, Engel JD, Yamamoto M. Keap1 represses nuclear activation of antioxidant responsive elements by Nrf2 through binding to the amino-terminal Neh2 domain. *Genes Dev* 1999; **13**: 76–86.

60. Li N, Venkatesan MI, Miguel A, Kaplan R, Gujuluva C, Alam J, Nel A. Induction of heme oxygenase-1 expression in macrophages by diesel exhaust particle chemicals and quinones via the antioxidant-responsive element. *J Immunol* 2000; **165**: 3393–3401.

61. Sun J, Hoshino H, Takaku K, Nakajima O, Muto A, Suzuki H, Tashiro S, Takahashi S, Shibahara S, Alam J, Taketo MM, Yamamoto M, Igarashi K. Hemoprotein Bach1 regulates enhancer availability of heme oxygenase-1 gene. *Embo J* 2002; **21**: 5216–5224.

62. Ogawa K, Sun J, Taketani S, Nakajima O, Nishitani C, Sassa S, Hayashi N, Yamamoto M, Shibahara S, Fujita H, Igarashi K. Heme mediates derepression of Maf recognition element through direct binding to transcription repressor Bach1. *Embo J* 2001; **20**: 2835–2843.

63. Lee PJ, Jiang BH, Chin BY, Iyer NV, Alam J, Semenza GL, Choi AM. Hypoxia-inducible factor-1 mediates transcriptional activation of the heme oxygenase-1 gene in response to hypoxia. *J Biol Chem* 1997; **272**: 5375–5381.

64. Keyse SM, Tyrrell RM. Heme oxygenase is the major 32-kDa stress protein induced in human skin fibroblasts by UVA radiation, hydrogen peroxide, and sodium arsenite. *Proc Natl Acad Sci USA* 1989; **86**: 99–103.

65. Vile GF, Basu-Modak S, Waltner C, Tyrrell RM. Heme oxygenase 1 mediates an adaptive response to oxidative stress in human skin fibroblasts. *Proc Natl Acad Sci USA* 1994; **91**: 2607–2610.

66. Abraham NG, Lavrovsky Y, Schwartzman ML, Stoltz RA, Levere RD, Gerritsen ME, Shibahara S, Kappas A. Transfection of the human heme oxygenase gene into rabbit coronary microvessel endothelial cells: protective effect against heme and hemoglobin toxicity. *Proc Natl Acad Sci USA* 1995; **92**: 6798–6802.

67. Lee PJ, Alam J, Wiegand GW, Choi AM. Overexpression of heme oxygenase-1 in human pulmonary epithelial cells results in cell growth arrest and increased resistance to hyperoxia. *Proc Natl Acad Sci USA* 1996; **93**: 10393–10398.

68. Chen K, Gunter K, Maines MD. Neurons overexpressing heme oxygenase-1 resist oxidative stress-mediated cell death. *J Neurochem* 2000; **75**: 304–313.

69. Otterbein LE, Kolls JK, Mantell LL, Cook JL, Alam J, Choi AM. Exogenous administration of heme oxygenase-1 by gene transfer provides protection against hyperoxia-induced lung injury. *J Clin Invest* 1999; **103**: 1047–1054.

70. Minamino T, Christou H, Hsieh CM, Liu Y, Dhawan V, Abraham NG, Perrella MA, Mitsialis SA, Kourembanas S. Targeted expression of heme oxygenase-1 prevents the pulmonary inflammatory and vascular responses to hypoxia. *Proc Natl Acad Sci USA* 2001; **98**: 8798–8803.

71. Juan SH, Lee TS, Tseng KW, Liou JY, Shyue SK, Wu KK, Chau LY. Adenovirus-mediated heme oxygenase-1 gene transfer inhibits the development of atherosclerosis in apolipoprotein E-deficient mice. *Circulation* 2001; **104**: 1519–1525.

72. Panahian N, Yoshiura M, Maines MD. Overexpression of heme oxygenase-1 is neuroprotective in a model of permanent middle cerebral artery occlusion in transgenic mice. *J Neurochem* 1999; **72**: 1187–1203.

73. Wagner M, Cadetg P, Ruf R, Mazzucchelli L, Ferrari P, Redaelli CA. Heme oxygenase-1 attenuates ischemia/reperfusion-induced apoptosis and improves survival in rat renal allografts. *Kidney Int* 2003; **63**: 1564–1573.

74. Stocker R, Yamamoto Y, McDonagh AF, Glazer AN, Ames BN. Bilirubin is an antioxidant of possible physiological importance. *Science* 1987; **235**: 1043–1046.

75. Vile GF, Tyrrell RM. Oxidative stress resulting from ultraviolet A irradiation of human skin fibroblasts leads to a heme oxygenase-dependent increase in ferritin. *J Biol Chem* 1993; **268**: 14678–14681.

76. Ferris CD, Jaffrey SR, Sawa A, Takahashi M, Brady SD, Barrow RK, Tysoe SA, Wolosker H, Baranano DE, Dore S, Poss KD, Snyder SH. Haem oxygenase-1 prevents cell death by regulating cellular iron. *Nat Cell Biol* 1999; **1**: 152–157.

77. Baranano DE, Wolosker H, Bae BI, Barrow RK, Snyder SH, Ferris CD. A mammalian iron ATPase induced by iron. *J Biol Chem* 2000; **275**: 15166–15173.

78. Poss KD, Tonegawa S. Heme oxygenase 1 is required for mammalian iron reutilization. *Proc Natl Acad Sci USA* 1997; **94**: 10919–10924.

79. Poss KD, Tonegawa S. Reduced stress defense in heme oxygenase-1-deficient cells. *Proc Natl Acad Sci USA* 1997; **94**: 10925–10930.

80. Yachie A, Niida Y, Wada T, Igarashi N, Kaneda H, Toma T, Ohta K, Kasahara Y, Koizumi S. Oxidative stress causes enhanced endothelial cell injury in human heme oxygenase-1 deficiency. *J Clin Invest* 1999; **103**: 129–135.

81. Petracho I, Otterbein LE, Alam J, Wiegand GW, Choi AM. Heme oxygenase-1 inhibits TNF-alpha-induced apoptosis in cultured fibroblasts. *Am J Physiol Lung Cell Mol Physiol* 2000; **278**: L312–319.

82. Brouard S, Otterbein LE, Anrather J, Tobiasch E, Bach FH, Choi AM, Soares MP. Carbon monoxide generated by heme oxygenase 1 suppresses endothelial cell apoptosis. *J Exp Med* 2000; **192**: 1015–1026.

83. Brouard S, Berberat PO, Tobiasch E, Seldon MP, Bach FH, Soares MP. Heme oxygenase-1-derived carbon monoxide requires the activation of transcription factor NF-kappa B to protect endothelial cells from tumor necrosis factor-alpha-mediated apoptosis. *J Biol Chem* 2002; **277**: 17950–17961.

84. Clark JM, Lambertsen CJ. Pulmonary oxygen toxicity: a review. *Pharmacol Rev* 1971; **23**: 37–133.

85. Steinberg KP, Milberg JA, Martin TR, Maunder RJ, Cockrill BA, Hudson LD. Evolution of bronchoalveolar cell populations in the adult respiratory distress syndrome. *Am J Respir Crit Care Med* 1994; **150**: 113–122.

86. Brower R, Matthay A, Morris A, Schoenfeld D, Thompson T, Wheeler A. Ventilation with lower tidal volumes as compared with traditional tidal volumes for acute lung injury and the acute respiratory distress syndrome. The Acute Respiratory Distress Syndrome Network. *N Engl J Med* 2000; **342**: 1301–1308.

87. Lee PJ, Choi AM. Pathways of cell signaling in hyperoxia. *Free Radic Biol Med* 2003; **35**: 341–350.

88. Clement A, Edeas M, Chadelat K, Brody JS. Inhibition of lung epithelial cell proliferation by hyperoxia. Posttranscriptional regulation of proliferation-related genes. *J Clin Invest* 1992; **90**: 1812–1818.

89. Zhang X, Shan P, Sasidhar M, Chupp GL, Flavell RA, Choi AM, Lee PJ. Reactive oxygen species and extracellular signal-regulated kinase 1/2 mitogen-activated protein kinase mediate hyperoxia-induced cell death in lung epithelium. *Am J Respir Cell Mol Biol* 2003; **28**: 305–315.

90. Barazzone C, White CW. Mechanisms of cell injury and death in hyperoxia: role of cytokines and Bcl-2 family proteins. *Am J Respir Cell Mol Biol* 2000; **22**: 517–519.

91. Otterbein LE, Otterbein SL, Ifedigbo E, Liu F, Morse DE, Fearns C, Ulevitch RJ, Knickelbein R, Flavell RA, Choi AM. MKK3 mitogen-activated protein kinase pathway mediates carbon monoxide-induced protection against oxidant-induced lung injury. *Am J Pathol* 2003; **163**: 2555–2563.

92. Hegazy KA, Dunn MW, Sharma SC. Functional human heme oxygenase has a neuroprotective effect on adult rat ganglion cells after pressure-induced ischemia. *Neuroreport* 2000; **11**: 1185–1189.

93. Shimizu H, Takahashi T, Suzuki T, Yamasaki A, Fujiwara T, Odaka Y, Hirakawa M, Fujita H, Akagi R. Protective effect of heme oxygenase induction in ischemic acute renal failure. *Crit Care Med* 2000; **28**: 809–817.

94. Amersi F, Buelow R, Kato H, Ke B, Coito AJ, Shen XD, Zhao D, Zaky J, Melinek J, Lassman CR, Kolls JK, Alam J, Ritter T, Volk HD, Farmer DG, Ghobrial RM, Busuttil RW, Kupiec-Weglinski JW. Upregulation of heme oxygenase-1 protects genetically fat Zucker rat livers from ischemia/reperfusion injury. *J Clin Invest* 1999; **104**: 1631–1639.

95. Fujita T, Toda K, Karimova A, Yan SF, Naka Y, Yet SF, Pinsky DJ. Paradoxical rescue from ischemic lung injury by inhaled carbon monoxide driven by derepression of fibrinolysis. *Nat Med* 2001; **7**: 598–604.

96. Amersi F, Shen XD, Anselmo D, Melinek J, Iyer S, Southard DJ, Katori M, Volk HD, Busuttil RW, Buelow R, Kupiec-Weglinski JW. Ex vivo exposure to carbon monoxide prevents hepatic ischemia/reperfusion injury through p38 MAP kinase pathway. *Hepatology* 2002; **35**: 815–823.

97. Nakao A, Kimizuka K, Stolz DB, Seda Neto J, Kaizu T, Choi AM, Uchiyama T, Zuckerbraun BS, Bauer AJ, Nalesnik MA, Otterbein LE, Geller DA, Murase N. Protective effect of carbon monoxide inhalation for cold-preserved small intestinal grafts. *Surgery* 2003; **134**: 285–292.

98. Zhang X, Shan P, Alam J, Davis RJ, Flavell RA, Lee PJ. Carbon monoxide modulates Fas/Fas ligand, caspases, and Bcl-2 family proteins via the p38alpha mitogen-activated protein kinase pathway during ischemia-reperfusion lung injury. *J Biol Chem* 2003; **278**: 22061–22070.

99. Zhang X, Shan P, Otterbein LE, Alam J, Flavell RA, Davis RJ, Choi AM, Lee PJ. Carbon monoxide inhibition of apoptosis during ischemia-reperfusion lung injury is dependent on the p38 mitogen-activated protein kinase pathway and involves caspase 3. *J Biol Chem* 2003; **278**: 1248–1258.

100. Juo P, Kuo CJ, Reynolds SE, Konz RF, Raingeaud J, Davis RJ, Biemann HP, Blenis J. Fas activation of the p38 mitogen-activated protein kinase signalling pathway requires ICE/CED-3 family proteases. *Mol Cell Biol* 1997; **17**: 24–35.

101. Esteban A, Anzueto A, Alia I, Gordo F, Apezteguia C, Palizas F, Cide D, Goldwaser R, Soto L, Bugedo G, Rodrigo C, Pimentel J, Raimondi G, Tobin MJ. How is mechanical ventilation employed in the intensive care unit? An international utilization review. *Am J Respir Crit Care Med* 2000; **161**: 1450–1458.

102. Aldrich T, Prezant D. Indications for mechanical ventilation., In: Tobin MJ, ed. *Principles and practice of mechanical ventilation*, New York: McGraw-Hill, Inc., 1994: 155–189.

103. Amato MB, Barbas CS, Medeiros DM, Magaldi RB, Schettino GP, Lorenzi-Filho G, Kairalla RA, Deheinzelin D, Munoz C, Oliveira R, Takagaki TY, Carvalho CR. Effect of a protective-ventilation strategy on mortality in the acute respiratory distress syndrome. *N Engl J Med* 1998; **338**: 347–354.

104. Grasso S, Mascia L, Del Turco M, Malacarne P, Giunta F, Brochard L, Slutsky AS, Marco Ranieri V. Effects of recruiting maneuvers in patients with acute respiratory distress syndrome ventilated with protective ventilatory strategy. *Anesthesiology* 2002; **96**: 795–802.

105. Tremblay L, Valenza F, Ribeiro SP, Li J, Slutsky AS. Injurious ventilatory strategies increase cytokines and c-fos m-RNA expression in an isolated rat lung model. *J Clin Invest* 1997; **99**: 944–952.

106. Chiumello D, Pristine G, Slutsky AS. Mechanical ventilation affects local and systemic cytokines in an animal model of acute respiratory distress syndrome. *Am J Respir Crit Care Med* 1999; **160**: 109–116.

107. von Bethmann AN, Brasch F, Nusing R, Vogt K, Volk HD, Muller KM, Wendel A, Uhlig S. Hyperventilation induces release of cytokines from perfused mouse lung. *Am J Respir Crit Care Med* 1998; **157**: 263–272.

108. Parker MM, Parrillo JE. Septic shock. Hemodynamics and pathogenesis. *Jama* 1983; **250**: 3324–3327.

109. Dahlberg P, Dunn D. Endotoxins and sepsis., In: Fein A, Abraham E, Balk R, Bernard G, Bone R, Dantzker D, Fink M, eds. *Sepsis and Multi-organ Failure: Mechanisms for Treatment Strategies*, Baltimore, Md., USA: Williams & Wilkins, 1997.

110. Chow JC, Young DW, Golenbock DT, Christ WJ, Gusovsky F. Toll-like receptor-4 mediates lipopolysaccharide-induced signal transduction. *J Biol Chem* 1999; **274**: 10689–10692.

111. Hambleton J, Weinstein SL, Lem L, DeFranco AL. Activation of c-Jun N-terminal kinase in bacterial lipopolysaccharide-stimulated macrophages. *Proc Natl Acad Sci USA* 1996; **93**: 2774–2778.

112. Han J, Lee JD, Bibbs L, Ulevitch RJ. A MAP kinase targeted by endotoxin and hyperosmolarity in mammalian cells. *Science* 1994; **265**: 808–811.

113. Raingeaud J, Gupta S, Rogers JS, Dickens M, Han J, Ulevitch RJ, Davis RJ. Pro-inflammatory cytokines and environmental stress cause p38 mitogen-activated protein kinase activation by dual phosphorylation on tyrosine and threonine. *J Biol Chem* 1995; **270**: 7420–7426.

114. Derijard B, Raingeaud J, Barrett T, Wu IH, Han J, Ulevitch RJ, Davis RJ. Independent human MAP-kinase signal transduction pathways defined by MEK and MKK isoforms. *Science* 1995; **267**: 682–685.

115. Raingeaud J, Whitmarsh AJ, Barrett T, Derijard B, Davis RJ. MKK3- and MKK6-regulated gene expression is mediated by the p38 mitogen-activated protein kinase signal transduction pathway. *Mol Cell Biol* 1996; **16**: 1247–1255.

116. Morse D, Pischke SE, Zhou Z, Davis RJ, Flavell RA, Loop T, Otterbein SL, Otterbein LE, Choi AM. Suppression of inflammatory cytokine production by carbon monoxide involves the JNK pathway and AP-1. *J Biol Chem* 2003; **278**: 36993–36998.

117. Sethi JM, Otterbein LE, Choi AM. Differential modulation by exogenous carbon monoxide of TNF-alpha stimulated mitogen-activated protein kinases in rat pulmonary artery endothelial cells. *Antioxid Redox Signal* 2002; **4**: 241–248.

118. Reed JA, Whitsett JA. Granulocyte-macrophage colony-stimulating factor and pulmonary surfactant homeostasis. *Proc Assoc Am Physicians* 1998; **110**: 321–332.

119. Bone R. Systemic inflammatory response syndrome: a unifying concept of systemic inflammation., In: Fein A, Abraham E, Balk R, Bernard G, Bone R, Dantzker D, Fink M, eds. *Sepsis and Multiorgan Failure: Mechanisms for Treatment Strategies,* Baltimore, Md., USA: Williams & Wilkins, 1997.

120. Schottelius AJ, Mayo MW, Sartor RB, Baldwin AS, Jr. Interleukin-10 signaling blocks inhibitor of kappaB kinase activity and nuclear factor kappaB DNA binding. *J Biol Chem* 1999; **274**: 31868–31874.

121. Coito AJ, Shaw GD, Li J, Ke B, Ma J, Busuttil RW, Kupiec-Weglinski JW. Selectin-mediated interactions regulate cytokine networks and macrophage heme oxygenase-1 induction in cardiac allograft recipients. *Lab Invest* 2002; **82**: 61–70.

122. DeBruyne LA, Magee JC, Buelow R, Bromberg JS. Gene transfer of immunomodulatory peptides correlates with heme oxygenase-1 induction and enhanced allograft survival. *Transplantation* 2000; **69**: 120–128.

123. Tullius SG, Nieminen-Kelha M, Bachmann U, Reutzel-Selke A, Jonas S, Pratschke J, Bechstein WO, Reinke P, Buelow R, Neuhaus P, Volk H. Induction of heme-oxygenase-1 prevents ischemia/reperfusion injury and improves long-term graft outcome in rat renal allografts. *Transplant Proc* 2001; **33**: 1286–1287.

124. Avihingsanon Y, Ma N, Csizmadia E, Wang C, Pavlakis M, Giraldo M, Strom TB, Soares MP, Ferran C. Expression of protective genes in human renal allografts: a regulatory response to injury associated with graft rejection. *Transplantation* 2002; **73**: 1079–1085.

125. Ke B, Buelow R, Shen XD, Melinek J, Amersi F, Gao F, Ritter T, Volk HD, Busuttil RW, Kupiec-Weglinski JW. Heme oxygenase 1 gene transfer prevents CD95/Fas ligand-mediated apoptosis and improves liver allograft survival via carbon monoxide signaling pathway. *Hum Gene Ther* 2002; **13**: 1189–1199.

126. Pileggi A, Molano RD, Berney T, Cattan P, Vizzardelli C, Oliver R, Fraker C, Ricordi C, Pastori RL, Bach FH, Inverardi L. Heme oxygenase-1 induction in islet cells results in protection from apoptosis and improved in vivo function after transplantation. *Diabetes* 2001; **50**: 1983–1991.

127. Tobiasch E, Gunther L, Bach FH. Heme oxygenase-1 protects pancreatic beta cells from apoptosis caused by various stimuli. *J Investig Med* 2001; **49**: 566–571.

128. Ke B, Shen XD, Melinek J, Gao F, Ritter T, Volk HD, Busuttil RW, Kupiec-Weglinski JW. Heme oxygenase-1 gene therapy: a novel immunomodulatory approach in liver allograft recipients? *Transplant Proc* 2001; **33**: 581–582.

129. Soares MP, Lin Y, Anrather J, Csizmadia E, Takigami K, Sato K, Grey ST, Colvin RB, Choi AM, Poss KD, Bach FH. Expression of heme oxygenase-1 can determine cardiac xenograft survival. *Nat Med* 1998; **4**: 1073–1077.

130. Hosenpud JD, Bennett LE, Keck BM, Boucek MM, Novick RJ. The Registry of the International Society for Heart and Lung Transplantation: seventeenth official report 2000. *J Heart Lung Transplant* 2000; **19**: 909–931.

131. Bando K, Paradis IL, Similo S, Konishi H, Komatsu K, Zullo TG, Yousem SA, Close JM, Zeevi A, Duquesnoy RJ *et al.* Obliterative bronchiolitis after lung and heart-lung transplantation. An analysis of risk factors and management. *J Thorac Cardiovasc Surg* 1995; **110**: 4–13; discussion 13–14.

132. Girgis RE, Tu I, Berry GJ, Reichenspurner H, Valentine VG, Conte JV, Ting A, Johnstone I, Miller J, Robbins RC, Reitz BA, Theodore J. Risk factors for the development of obliterative bronchiolitis after lung transplantation. *J Heart Lung Transplant* 1996; **15**: 1200–1208.

133. Sibley RK, Berry GJ, Tazelaar HD, Kraemer MR, Theodore J, Marshall SE, Billingham ME, Starnes VA. The role of transbronchial biopsies in the management of lung transplant recipients. *J Heart Lung Transplant* 1993; **12**: 308–324.

134. Trulock EP. Management of lung transplant rejection. *Chest* 1993; **103**: 1566–1576.

135. Estenne M, Hertz MI. Bronchiolitis obliterans after human lung transplantation. *Am J Respir Crit Care Med* 2002; **166**: 440–444.

136. Lu F, Zander DS, Visner GA. Increased expression of heme oxygenase-1 in human lung transplantation. *J Heart Lung Transplant* 2002; **21**: 1120–1126.

137. Song R, Kubo M, Morse D, Zhou Z, Zhang X, Dauber JH, Fabisiak J, Alber SM, Watkins SC, Zuckerbraun BS, Otterbein LE, Ning W, Oury TD, Lee PJ, McCurry KR, Choi AM. Carbon monoxide induces cytoprotection in rat orthotopic lung transplantation via anti-inflammatory and anti-apoptotic effects. *Am J Pathol* 2003; **163**: 231–242.

138. Scholma J, Slebos DJ, Boezen HM, van den Berg JW, van der Bij W, de Boer WJ, Koeter GH, Timens W, Kauffman HF, Postma DS. Eosinophilic granulocytes and interleukin-6 level in bronchoalveolar lavage fluid are associated with the development of obliterative bronchiolitis after lung transplantation. *Am J Respir Crit Care Med* 2000; **162**: 2221–2225.

139. Duckers HJ, Boehm M, True AL, Yet SF, San H, Park JL, Clinton Webb R, Lee ME, Nabel GJ, Nabel EG. Heme oxygenase-1 protects against vascular constriction and proliferation. *Nat Med* 2001; **7**: 693–698.

140. Tulis DA, Durante W, Liu X, Evans AJ, Peyton KJ, Schafer AI. Adenovirus-mediated heme oxygenase-1 gene delivery inhibits injury-induced vascular neointima formation. *Circulation* 2001; **104**: 2710–2715.

141. Los M, Stroh C, Janicke RU, Engels IH, Schulze-Osthoff K. Caspases: more than just killers? *Trends Immunol* 2001; **22**: 31–34.

142. Song R, Mahidhara RS, Zhou Z, Hoffman RA, Seol DW, Flavell RA, Billiar TR, Otterbein LE, Choi AM. Carbon monoxide inhibits T lymphocyte proliferation via caspase-dependent pathway. *J Immunol* 2004; **172**: 1220–1226.

143. Lenfant C, Hurd SS. National Asthma Education Program. *Chest* 1990; **98**: 226–227.

144. Horvath I, Donnelly LE, Kiss A, Paredi P, Kharitonov SA, Barnes PJ. Raised levels of exhaled carbon monoxide are associated with an increased expression of heme oxygenase-1 in airway macrophages in asthma: a new marker of oxidative stress. *Thorax* 1998; **53**: 668–672.

145. Song R, Ning W, Liu F, Ameredes BT, Calhoun WJ, Otterbein LE, Choi AM. Regulation of IL-1beta-induced GM-CSF production in human airway smooth muscle cells by carbon monoxide. *Am J Physiol Lung Cell Mol Physiol* 2003; **284**: L50–56.

146. Song R, Mahidhara RS, Liu F, Ning W, Otterbein LE, Choi AM. Carbon monoxide inhibits human airway smooth muscle cell proliferation via mitogen-activated protein kinase pathway. *Am J Respir Cell Mol Biol* 2002; **27**: 603–610.

147. Motterlini R, Clark JE, Foresti R, Sarathchandra P, Mann BE, Green CJ. Carbon monoxide-releasing molecules: characterization of biochemical and vascular activities. *Circ Res* 2002; **90**: E17–24.

BREATH ETHANE IN DISEASE:
METHODS FOR ANALYSIS
BASED ON ROOM AIR CORRECTION*

K. A. COPE

*Department of Environmental Health Sciences,
Bloomberg School of Public Health, Johns Hopkins University,
615 N. Wolfe Street, Baltimore, MD 21205, USA*

1. Introduction

Exhaled hydrocarbons, such as ethylene, ethane and pentane, have been
widely used as non-invasive biomarkers of oxidative stress status. These
molecules are produced following free radical-mediated attack on n-3 or
n-6 polyunsaturated fatty acids found in cellular membranes, and can be
non-invasively collected from exhaled breath samples. In 1974, Riely *et al.*[1]
showed that increased concentrations of ethane and ethylene were produced
in the breath of mice fed a dose of carbon tetrachloride, and that the mechanism for the evolution of these compounds was dependent on lipid peroxidation. Since then, ethane has been demonstrated to be a sensitive *in
vivo* biomarker of lipid peroxidation in humans. It is thought that exhaled
ethane may provide a non-invasive real-time index of total-body oxidative
stress status, since it exhibits low solubility in blood and tissues, is slowly
metabolized, and is rapidly exhaled following oxidative injury.[1-5] For example, an increase in ethane can be detected following putatively pro-oxidative
and free-radical promoting events such as ischemia–reperfusion injury and
during total-body irradiation.[6,7]

Quantification of ethane in conscious subjects is complicated by variations in breathing patterns and room air concentrations. In animal models,
it has been shown that there is rapid diffusion of ethane between the venous

*The copyright of the contribution is a property of the U. S. government. Permission to
publish the contribution as part of this collective work has been granted by Beltsville
Human Nutrition Research Center, U. S. Department of Agriculture. Although this work
was reviewed by EPA and approved for publication, it may not necessarily reflect official
Agency policy.

blood and the alveolar air.[8] Therefore, the exhalation of ethane is perfusion limited and the concentration of exhaled ethane is highest in the end-tidal volume of a breath.[9] A recently described on-line method that uses laser spectroscopy to analyze ethane in real-time allows the quantification of ethane concentration in the end-tidal plateau.[10] However, in the absence of this capability, it is necessary to collect and concentrate breath samples either from multiple breaths over a defined period of time or from a single exhalation of breath.[9,11] Breath ethane concentrations have been shown to correlate with end-tidal carbon dioxide and inter-individual variability can be reduced by normalizing to carbon dioxide. Hyperventilation causes a reduction in end-tidal carbon dioxide and would also be expected to affect the concentration of other endogenous breath molecules. Thus, for breath sampling to be reliable the breathing pattern during breath collection must be carefully controlled and carbon dioxide measurements must be made.[12]

Often, room air concentrations of ethane are higher than endogenously produced concentrations. Breath samples can be corrected for background provided that the subject breathes normally and the exogenous concentration is stable. Under these conditions, the exhaled concentration will reflect the exogenous concentration plus the endogenous concentration. Alternative methods for quantifying endogenous ethane production include sampling breath after a washout of the room air, or re-breathing a known concentration for a defined period of time to establish a steady state.[5] At least 4 minutes of breathing hydrocarbon-free air is required to washout the lung of exogenous ethane.[13] However, hydrocarbon-scrubbed free air can contain as much as 1 part-per-million (ppm) total hydrocarbons, and concentrations of ethane vary between tanks of air.[14] When ethane is present in breathing air tanks, it is still necessary to correct the breath sample for this concentration. Humans exposed to high ethane concentrations (19–29 ppm) can achieve steady state in less than 2 minutes.[15] Von Basum *et al.*[10] found that it took under 30 minutes to washout ethane from the tissues following exposure to 1 ppm ethane for five minutes. Nevertheless, if a steady state is not achieved, high background concentrations of ethane can obscure the endogenous contributions. A negative concentration gradient indicates that the subject did not reach steady state, or that the endogenous production of ethane is not detectable.[16]

Increased exhaled ethane concentrations have been reported in patients with end-stage renal disease,[17] liver disease,[18,19] inflammatory bowel disease,[20] ulcerative colitis,[21] Crohn's disease,[22,23] chronic obstructive pulmonary disease,[24] asthma,[25] and human immunodeficiency virus (HIV) infection.[26] An increased oxidative stress status may follow up-regulation of inflammatory pathways.[27] Systemic scleroderma is characterized by chronic inflammation and vascular disease that can promote oxidative stress and fibrosis to multiple organs.[28] Severe vasoconstriction, due to intimal thickening in small and medium size arteries is a common complication to scleroderma and is associated with incidents of ischemia that are suspected to increase the production of reactive oxygen species.[29] F_2 isoprostanes, another biomarker of lipid peroxidation, have been shown to be increased in scleroderma patients compared to control groups.[30] Unfortunately, current therapies have limited impact on the morbidity and mortality of scleroderma, but it is thought that controlling ischemic events might assist in disease management.[31] A major challenge is to identify sensitive biomarkers of tissue damage that indicate when these events occur.[32] This would require a large number of repeated analyses to be conducted, which is a task that is well suited for breath analysis, because collecting repeated breath samples is far more tolerable than collecting repeated blood samples.

Alzheimer's disease is another disease where inflammation has been implicated in disease progression. Oxidative changes to proteins and lipids in the microvasculature of the brain can promote vasoconstriction similar to blockages found in atherosclerotic plaques and have been correlated with β-amyloid deposition.[33] It has been shown that the neuronal nitric oxide synthase enzyme is overexpressed in the brains of Alzheimer's disease patients.[34] Superoxide radicals can react with nitric oxide radicals to generate peroxynitrite, which is a highly reactive lipid peroxidizing agent. Examination of lipid peroxidation end-points may offer insight into pathological mechanisms involved in Alzheimer's disease.[35] F_2-isoprostanes have been used to analyze oxidative stress status of Alzheimer's disease patients, but have shown mixed results. When measured in the cerebral spinal fluid, F_2-isoprostanes are higher in patients with Alzheimer's disease; however, when assayed in blood and urine there is no such correlation.[36] As of yet, there is no reliable biomarker that is useful as a non-invasive index of oxidative stress status in Alzheimer's disease patients.

Lung cancer pathology involves oxidative stress and enhanced lipid peroxidation. Tumorigenesis, vascularization of tumors (angiogenesis) and inflammation of tissues surrounding the malignancy are potential sources for oxidative stress in lung cancer patients. The center of solid tumors is thought to be relatively anoxic compared to healthy tissues. Nevertheless, it has been demonstrated that non-small cell lung carcinoma cells taken from tumor biopsies have enhanced levels of the lipid peroxidation markers, conjugated dienes and lipid hydroperoxides, when compared to matched biopsies taken from healthy parenchymal tissues.[37] Continued smoking has also been shown to increase lipid peroxidation in lung cancer patients.[38] Thus, biomarkers of oxidative stress may be potentially useful in identifying malignancies among patients in pulmonary clinics.

2. Methods

2.1. *Human Studies Procotols*

Protocols for breath collection were approved by the Johns Hopkins University Bloomberg School of Public Health, Committee on Human Research (principal investigator, Terence H. Risby, Ph. D.). In all cases breath collection was considered to be a minimal risk protocol. Breath was collected only after subjects gave verbal informed consent. In these case-control studies, breath was collected at the Johns Hopkins Hospital from control subjects and patients diagnosed with systemic scleroderma, lung cancer, or Alzheimer's disease.

2.2. *The Collection of Breath Samples*

Breath was collected using two different methods from subjects who were seated at rest in a comfortable position. In the first method, which was used in the scleroderma and lung cancer studies, breath was collected during continuous tidal breathing for a one-minute time period. Subjects breathed through a low resistance bacterial filter that was attached to a two-way non-rebreathing valve, which ensured no inspiratory air was sampled. Exhaled breath was sampled through a port adjacent to the expiratory valve. A constant flow pump was used to sample exhaled breath. The breath sample was collected onto duplicate thermal desorption tubes. The pump flow rate was 80 mL/min and breath was sampled for one minute. The properties of the breath collection system and thermal desorption tubes have been previously described in detail.[12,39] End-tidal carbon dioxide, average carbon dioxide, tidal volume, respiratory rate, and inspiratory mouth pressure were monitored during breath collection.

In the second method, which was used to sample Alzheimer's disease patients, a single exhalation of breath was collected into a 3 liter bag (SKC Inc., Eighty-four, PA). The subject exhaled through a low-resistance bacterial filter that was attached to the bag. A portable carbon dioxide monitor was placed in-line between the bag and the filter. The bag valve was turned open when the subject began to exhale and was closed when a full exhalation was complete. The end-tidal carbon dioxide concentration was determined during exhalation, and the mixed expired carbon dioxide partial pressure was measured in the laboratory. A gas tight syringe was used to sample 80 mL of breath from the bag onto thermal adsorbents. The remaining volume of the bag was measured and recorded.

2.3. *Room Air Measurements*

Room air samples were collected onto duplicate thermal desorption tubes prior to or after collection of the breath sample. A constant flow sampling pump was used to sample 80 milliliters of room air onto the adsorbent beds. The tubes were returned to the laboratory and analyzed within a few hours of collection.

2.4. *Chromatographic Analysis*

Breath molecules were analyzed by automated two-stage thermal desorption gas chromatography. The sample tubes were desorbed at 300 °C for 15 min under a stream of ultrapure helium. In the second stage of desorption, a cold trap that was maintained at −30 °C was heated and the desorbed molecules were injected onto the chromatography column. Separations were performed on a 60-meter fused silica open tubular column (0.32 mm i. d.) with a thick film (5 μm) of cross-bonded dimethyl silicone. The temperature protocol used for chromatography was as follows: isothermal at 35 °C for 5 minutes, temperature programmed 35 to 200 °C at 5 °C/min, and isothermal at 200 °C for 10 minutes. Molecules were detected using a flame ionization detector that was maintained at 300 °C. Quantification of ethane was based on response factors derived from calibration curves using an authentic standard.

2.5. *Data Analysis*

The corrected concentrations were determined as follows:

$$C_{\text{corr}} = \frac{\text{ET}_{\text{CO}_2}(C_{\text{me}} - C_{\text{ra}})}{\text{ME}_{\text{CO}_2}}$$

The dead space corrected endogenous concentration C_{corr} is the difference between the measured ethane concentration C_{me} in breath and room air ethane concentration C_{ra} when multiplied by the ratio of end-tidal CO_2 to mixed expired CO_2. Exhaled molecule concentrations can be converted from pmol/L to pmol/mL CO_2 by normalizing to carbon dioxide output as follows if it is assumed that at STP atmospheric pressure is 760 Torr and temperature is 25 °C.

$$C_{\text{norm}} = \frac{0.76\,C_{\text{corr}}}{\text{ME}_{\text{CO}_2}}$$

Uncorrected concentrations were quantified in pmol/L, adjusted to end-tidal concentrations, and normalized to carbon dioxide output.[12]

3. Results

Table 1 shows that ethane concentrations were increased in the diseased groups compared to controls. Similar levels of exhaled ethane were found in scleroderma patients [Ssc(+)] and Alzheimer's disease patients [AD(+)]. The concentration among the lung cancer patients [LC(+)] was less than it was in Ssc(+) or AD(+), but was significantly increased in comparison to patients without lung cancer in the pulmonary clinic [LC(−)].

The data are presented as "uncorrected" and "corrected" concentrations. In the uncorrected data, the room air contribution has not been subtracted from the endogenous concentration; however, significant differences between patient and control groups were determined. This suggests

Table 1.   Comparison of exhaled ethane concentration in patients with different diseases and controls

Disease type	Number of subjects N	Breath ethane pmol/mL CO_2 uncorrected*	corrected[†]	Ambient ethane pmol/L	Frequency %
Ssc(+)	41	18.1 (5.7)[a]	4.1 (−1.7 ... 7.3)[d]	560 (258)	73[g]
Ssc(−)	20	11.5 (4.5)	−0.9 (−2.4 ... 2.4)	536 (430)	40
AD(+)	25	19.8 (25.6)[b]	4.2 (0.4 ...11.9)[e]	337 (72)	83[h]
AD(−)	22	9.5 (4.4)	−0.65 (−0.32... 3.0)		57
LC(+)	41	12.6 (5.6)[c]	0.72 (−2.87... 2.24)[f]	409 (107)	63[i]
LC(−)	47	10.1 (4.6)	−0.38 (−4.76... 1.8)		38

* Uncorrected concentrations are expressed as means (SD).
† Corrected concentrations are expressed as median (25–75 centiles). Frequency equals the ratio of the number of producers / total number of subjects in the study sample group. Ambient ethane is expressed as the mean (SD) ethane concentration in the room air. Tests for statistical significance are performed using a non-parametric, Mann–Whitney test for corrected concentrations, and uncorrected concentrations that are skewed. A 2-sample Student's t-test is used where the data is normally distributed. A two-sided Fisher's exact test is used to test the significant differences between proportions. A p-value smaller than 0.05 is considered significant. All comparisons are made between the diseased sample group (+) and the control group for that study (−).
p-values for the compared samples are as follows: a: $p < 0.001$, b: $p < 0.009$, c: $p < 0.035$, d: $p < 0.0001$, e: $p < 0.007$, f: $p < 0.024$, g: $p = 0.023$, h: $p = 0.0432$, i: $p = 0.032$.

that enough time was allowed to reach steady state with the room air concentration. The room air concentrations were relatively similar between the Ssc(+) and Ssc(−) groups, but the ambient ethane concentrations were lower in the Alzheimer's disease and the lung cancer studies.

There were several cases where correction generated negative concentration gradients. However, it can be seen that there are significant differences in the proportional frequency of people who had a positive concentration gradient, and those with a negative concentration gradient between the patient and control groups. In each case the diseased groups have a proportionally greater number of people that were found to have breath ethane concentrations above the room air concentration. Similarly, the median values of the corrected concentrations were significantly higher in patients versus controls. In each study, the control groups have median values that are negative compared to the positive values in the diseased groups.

4. Discussion

Breath ethane concentrations have been shown to be affected by smoking, diet, and nutrient status.[40] Ethane concentrations can remain elevated for up to an hour after smoking a cigarette and follow an exponential washout.[41] The increase may be due in part to the systemic absorption of ethane contained in the gas phase of cigarette smoke, but may also result from lipid peroxidation induced by radicals that are present in cigarette smoke.[42,43] In the present investigations, the most significant source of variability in ethane concentrations resulted from exposure to exogenous ethane from excessive room air levels. However, correcting the mixed expired concentration for dead space dilution, subtracting room air concentration, and normalizing concentrations to carbon dioxide output, addresses the key methodological problems in comparing ethane concentrations in different clinical settings.

The "gold standard" for the quantification of ethane is to perform a washout with hydrocarbon-free breathing air prior to breath collection, but this method is not always practical. In previous washout experiments, conducted in our laboratory, it was found that at least four minutes was required to achieve steady state with the ethane concentration in the tank. In one study, breath samples were repeatedly collected from a healthy subject that breathed room air followed by 4 minutes of breathing from a "hydrocarbon-free" breathing air source. It was found that after correcting for the concentration in the breathing air tank (241 pmol/L), this subject's exhaled breath ethane dropped from the concentration in the room air, which was 417 pmol/L, to an endogenous output of 92 pmol/L (2.0 pmol/mL CO_2). A previous study of normal healthy subjects ($n = 16$) showed that the mean ethane concentration was 103 pmol/L (1.99 pmol/mL CO_2) when corrected for room air.[12] This example suggests that similar estimates of exhaled ethane concentrations can be obtained from room air correction as are found from washout experiments.

In the studies presented herein, two different methods for breath collection were successfully applied. The continuous breathing method and single breath method could both be used to determine differences between diseased groups and control groups. There does appear to be evidence to suggest that lipid peroxidation is increased in scleroderma and Alzheimer's disease cases. Concentrations of ethane were less elevated in lung cancer cases, but were significantly different than controls. The lung cancer group included a large number of current smokers, but the Alzheimer's disease and scleroderma groups did not. It might be expected that ethane concentrations would be higher in lung cancer patients due to smoking; however, it is suspected that long waiting periods of several hours in the hospital provided adequate washout times to make the contribution of recent cigarette exposure negligible.

In order to compare concentrations across groups (disease versus disease, or patients versus controls), and to compare concentrations that were collected using these two different methods, it was necessary to normalize the ethane concentrations to carbon dioxide. Doing so allows for a physiologically based comparison that adjusts for potentially spurious results from an inadequate breath sample. In summary, the collection of breath ethane can be dramatically affected by room air concentrations, but physiologically-based inter-individual comparisons can be made if breathing is controlled and a near steady state is reached during breath collection.

Acknowledgements

The research presented herein is derived from the author's doctoral dissertation entitled "Breath Biomarkers of Exposure and Disease". He wishes to acknowledge the collaborations with scientists and clinicians at the Johns Hopkins Medical Institutions that made these investigations possible, especially Terence H. Risby, Ph. D., of the Department of Environmental Health Sciences, in whose laboratory this research was conducted. The scleroderma studies were carried out in cooperation with Steve Solga, M. D., and Anna Mae Diehl, M. D. of the Division of Gastroenterology and Frederick Wigley, M. D. and Laura Hummers, M. D. of the Division of Rheumatology in the

Department of Medicine. Andrew Warren, M.D. of the Department of Psychiatry and Behavioral Sciences coordinated and collected the breath samples for the Alzheimer's disease study. The lung cancer investigations were conducted with Rex C.-W. Yung, M.D. of the Division of Pulmonary and Critical Care Medicine in the Department of Medicine. This research was supported in part by a National Institute of Environmental Health Sciences Grant T32 ES-07141.

References

1. Riely CA, Cohen G, Lieberman M. Ethane evolution: a new index of lipid peroxidation.. *Science* 1974; **183**: 208–210.
2. Kazui M, Andreoni KA, Norris EJ, Klein AS, Burdick JF, Beattie C, Sehnert SS, Bell WR, Bulkley GB, Risby TH. Breath ethane: a specific indicator of free-radical-mediated lipid peroxidation following reperfusion of the ischemic liver. *Free Radic Biol Med* 1992; **13**: 509–515.
3. Matos vanLohensels E, Anderson JC, Hildebrandt J, Hlastala MP. Modeling diffusion limitation of gas exchange in lungs containing perfluorocarbon. *J Appl Physiol* 1999; **86**: 273–284.
4. Remmer H, Hintze T, Frank H, Muh-Zange M. Cytochrome P-450 oxidation of alkanes originating as scission products during lipid peroxidation. *Xenobiotica* 1984; **14**: 207–219.
5. Wade CR, van Rij AM. In vivo lipid peroxidation in man as measured by the respiratory excretion of ethane, pentane, and other low-molecular-weight hydrocarbons. *Anal Biochem* 1985; **150**: 1–7.
6. Arterbery VE, Pryor WA, Jiang L, Sehnert SS, Foster WM, Abrams RA, Williams JR, Wharam MD Jr., Risby TH. Breath ethane generation during clinical total body irradiation as a marker of oxygen-free-radical-mediated lipid peroxidation: a case study. *Free Radic Biol Med* 1994; **17**: 569–576.
7. Risby TH, Maley W, Scott RP, Bulkley GB, Kazui M, Sehnert SS, Schwarz KB, Potter J, Mezey E, Klein AS, *et al.* Evidence for free radical-mediated lipid peroxidation at reperfusion of human orthotopic liver transplants. *Surgery* 1994; **115**: 94–101.
8. Schimmel C, Bernard SL, Anderson JC, Polioor NL, Lakshminarayan S, Hlastala MP. Soluble gas exchange in the pulmonary airways of sheep. *J Appl Physiol* 2004; **97**: 1702–1708.
9. Risby TH, Sehnert SS. Clinical application of breath biomarkers of oxidative stress status. *Free Radic Biol Med* 1999; **27**: 1182–1192.
10. von Basum G, Dahnke H, Halmer D, Hering P, Murtz M. Online recording of ethane traces in human breath via infrared laser spectroscopy. *J Appl Physiol* 2003; **95**: 2583–2590.
11. Zarling EJ, Clapper M. Technique for gas-chromatographic measurement of volatile alkanes from single-breath samples. *Clin Chem* 1987; **33**. 140 141.
12. Cope KA, Watson MT, Foster WM, Sehnert SS, Risby TH. Effects of ventilation on the collection of exhaled breath in humans. *J Appl Physiol* 2004; **96**: 1371–1379.

13. Knutson MD, Handelman GJ, Viteri FE. Methods for measuring ethane and pentane in expired air from rats and humans. *Free Radic Biol Med* 2000; **28**: 514–519.

14. Do BK, Garewal HS, Clements NC, Jr., Peng YM, Habib MP. Exhaled ethane and antioxidant vitamin supplements in active smokers. *Chest* 1996; **110**: 159–164.

15. Dale O, Bergum H, Lund T, Nilsen T, Aadahl P, Stenseth R. A validated method for rapid analysis of ethane in breath and its application in kinetic studies in human volunteers. *Free Radic Res* 2003; **37**: 815–821.

16. Cope KA. Breath Biomarkers of Exposure and Disease., Thesis, Department of Environmental Health Sciences, Johns Hopkins University, Baltimore, 2002

17. Handelman GJ, Rosales LM, Barbato D, Luscher J, Adhikarla R, Nicolosi RJ, Finkelstein FO, Ronco C, Kaysen GA, Hoenich NA, Levin NW. Breath ethane in dialysis patients and control subjects. *Free Radic Biol* Med 2003; **35**: 17–23.

18. Sehnert SS, Jiang L, Burdick JF, Risby TH. Breath biomarkers for detection of human liver diseases: preliminary study. *Biomarkers* 2002; **7**: 174–187.

19. Letteron P, Duchatelle V, Berson A, Fromenty B, Fisch C, Degott C, Benhamou JP, Pessayre D. Increased ethane exhalation, an in vivo index of lipid peroxidation, in alcohol-abusers. *Gut* 1993; **34**: 409–414.

20. Pelli MA, Trovarelli G, Capodicasa E, De Medio GE, Bassotti G. Breath alkanes determination in ulcerative colitis and Crohn's disease. *Dis Colon Rectum* 1999; **42**: 71–76.

21. Sedghi S, Keshavarzian A, Klamut M, Eiznhamer D, Zarling EJ. Elevated breath ethane levels in active ulcerative colitis: evidence for excessive lipid peroxidation. *Am J Gastroenterol* 1994; **89**: 2217–2221.

22. Wendland BE, Aghdassi E, Tam C, Carrrier J, Steinhart AH, Wolman SL, Baron D, Allard JP. Lipid peroxidation and plasma antioxidant micronutrients in Crohn disease. *Am J Clin Nutr* 2001; **74**: 259–264.

23. Aghdassi E, Wendland BE, Steinhart AH, Wolman SL, Jeejeebhoy K, Allard JP. Antioxidant vitamin supplementation in Crohn's disease decreases oxidative stress. a randomized controlled trial. *Am J Gastroenterol* 2003; **98**: 348–353.

24. Paredi P, Kharitonov SA, Leak D, Ward S, Cramer D, Barnes PJ. Exhaled ethane, a marker of lipid peroxidation, is elevated in chronic obstructive pulmonary disease. *Am J Respir Crit Care Med* 2000; **162**: 369–373.

25. Paredi P, Kharitonov SA, Barnes PJ. Elevation of exhaled ethane concentration in asthma. *Am J Respir Crit Care Med* 2000; **162**: 1450–1454.

26. Allard JP, Aghdassi E, Chau J, Salit I, Walmsley S. Oxidative stress and plasma antioxidant micronutrients in humans with HIV infection. *Am J Clin Nutr* 1998; **67**: 143–147.

27. Davi G, Falco A, Patrono C. Determinants of F2-isoprostane biosynthesis and inhibition in man. *Chem Phys Lipids* 2004; **128**: 149–163.

28. Sambo P, Jannino L, Candela M, Salvi A, Donini M, Dusi S, Luchetti MM, Gabrielli A. Monocytes of patients with systemic sclerosis (scleroderma) spontaneously release in vitro increased amounts of superoxide anion. *J Invest Dermatol* 1999; **112**: 78–84.

29. Hummers LK, Wigley FM. Management of Raynaud's phenomenon and digital ischemic lesions in scleroderma. *Rheum Dis Clin North Am* 2003; **29**: 293–313.

30. Morrow JD. The isoprostanes: their quantification as an index of oxidant stress status in vivo. *Drug Metab Rev* 2000; **32**: 377–385.

31. Wigley FM, Flavahan NA. Raynaud's phenomenon. *Rheum Dis Clin North Am* 1996; **22**: 765–781.

32. Simonini G, Cerinic MM, Generini S, Zoppi M, Anichini M, Cesaretti C, Pignone A, Falcini F, Lotti T, Cagnoni M. Oxidative stress in Systemic Sclerosis. *Mol Cell Biochem* 1999; **196**: 85–91.

33. Markesbery WR. Oxidative stress hypothesis in Alzheimer's disease. *Free Radic Biol Med* 1997; **23**: 134–147.

34. Fernandez-Vizarra P, Fernandez AP, Castro-Blanco S, Encinas JM, Serrano J, Bentura ML, Munoz P, Martinez-Murillo R, Rodrigo J. Expression of nitric oxide system in clinically evaluated cases of Alzheimer's disease. *Neurobiology of Disease* 2004; **15**: 287–305.

35. Pratico D, V MYL, Trojanowski JQ, Rokach J, Fitzgerald GA. Increased F2-isoprostanes in Alzheimer's disease: evidence for enhanced lipid peroxidation in vivo. *Faseb J* 1998; **12**: 1777–1783.

36. Montine TJ, Neely MD, Quinn JF, Beal MF, Markesbery WR, Roberts I, L. Jackson, Morrow JD. Lipid peroxidation in aging brain and Alzheimer's disease. *Free Radical Biology and Medicine* 2002; **33**: 620–626.

37. Zieba M, Nowak D, Suwalski M, Piasecka G, Grzelewska-Rzymowska I, Tyminska K, Kroczynska-Bednarek J, Kwiatkowska S. Enhanced lipid peroxidation in cancer tissue homogenates in non-small cell lung cancer. *Monaldi Arch Chest Dis* 2001; **56**: 110–114.

38. Anand U, Agarwal R, Anand CV. Pulmonary lipid peroxidation in cigarette smokers and lung cancer patients. *Chest* 1992; **101**: 290.

39. Risby TH. Volatile organic compounds as markers in normal and diseased states. In: Marczin N, Yacoub M, eds. *Disease markers in exhaled breath: basic mechanisms and clinical applications*, Washington, DC: IOS Press, 2002: 418.

40. Miller ER 3rd, Appel LJ, Risby TH. Effect of dietary patterns on measures of lipid peroxidation: results from a randomized clinical trial. *Circulation* 1998; **98**: 2390–2395.

41. Dahnke H, Kleine D, Hering P, Murtz M. Real-time monitoring of ethane in human breath using mid-infrared cavity leak out spectroscopy. *Appl Phys B* 2001; **72**: 971–975.

42. Miller ER, 3rd, Appel LJ, Jiang L, Risby TH. Association between cigarette smoking and lipid peroxidation in a controlled feeding study. *Circulation* 1997; **96**: 1097–1101.

43. Flicker TM, Green SA. Comparison of gas-phase free-radical populations in tobacco smoke and model systems by HPLC. *Environ Health Perspect* 2001; **109**: 765–771.

PART C

BROADLY-BASED STUDIES

CURRENT STATUS OF CLINICAL BREATH ANALYSIS

T. H. RISBY

Department of Environmental Health Sciences,
Bloomberg School of Public Health, Johns Hopkins University,
615 N. Wolfe Street, Baltimore, MD 21205, USA

1. Introduction

The concept that blood, urine, and other body fluids and tissues can be collected and analyzed to yield information for diagnosis of disease states or to monitor disease progression and/or therapy is the foundation of modern medicine. However, the use of breath as a collectable sample has not received comparable clinical use. This chapter will review the current status of clinical breath analysis, suggest reasons for this status and attempt to identify future directions for the field.

The ability to exchange oxygen for carbon dioxide is essential for many life forms. In animals, this gas exchange occurs at the alveolar-blood capillary membrane in the respiratory tract. Oxygen and carbon dioxide are passively transported from blood to breath or *vice versa* and the diffusion of these gases is governed by their concentration gradients across the alveolar-capillary junction. Any additional molecule present in the blood or in the inspiratory air will also pass into the breath or blood respectively. The only requirement for this transport is that molecules must exhibit significant vapor pressures. The molecular profile of breath will be the product of the composition of the inspiratory air and the volatile molecules that are present in the blood. Cells or tissues in the mouth, nose, sinuses, airway and the gastrointestinal tract will also contribute molecules to exhaled breath. These sources can produce molecules in exhaled breath that are not present in circulating blood (such as nitric oxide). The bulk matrix of breath is a mixture of nitrogen, oxygen, carbon dioxide, water vapor and the inert gases. The remainder of breath (less than 100 ppm) is a mixture of as many as 500 different compounds. These molecules have both endogenous and

Table 1.   Typical concentrations of endogenous breath molecules

Concentration (v/v)	Molecule
Percentage (%)	oxygen, water, carbon dioxide
Parts-per-million (ppm)	acetone, carbon monoxide,methane, hydrogen
Parts-per-billion (ppb)	formaldehyde, acetaldehyde, isoprene, n-pentane, ethane, ethanol, ethylene, other hydrocarbons, nitric oxide, carbon disulfide, methanol, carbonyl sulfide, methanethiol, ammonia, methylamine, dimethyl sulfide

exogenous origins. Normal and abnormal physiological processes are the source for endogenous molecules. The sources of exogenous molecules are inspiratory air, ingested foods and beverages, and any exogenous molecule that has entered the body by other routes (such as dermal absorption). The rates of excretion of molecules in breath are directly related to rates of ventilation. For molecules that are produced systemically their rates of excretion will also be directly related to cardiac output. The physical and chemical properties of the molecules will also affect their rates of excretion. If a molecule is lipid soluble it could be stored in tissues not well perfused by blood, such as adipose tissue, and thereby be released more slowly than a similar molecule with hydrophilic properties that is not stored. For example, we have detected unmetabolized inhalation anesthetics in the breath of patients who have undergone surgery more than six weeks previously. The presence of long-lived exogenous molecules in breath can easily interfere with clinical analysis. Moreover, as a general rule, the concentrations of molecules in breath will be higher when their origins are exogenous. Table 1 summarizes some of the molecules found in human breath and also lists their typical concentrations.

Each of these molecules is endogenously produced or has direct clinical relevance (oxygen).

2. Brief History

The concept that breath contains molecules that originated from normal or abnormal physiology has its origins in the writings of Hippocrates, the father of medicine. Moreover, the detection of the presence of water vapor in breath has been used as a non-invasive monitor of mortality for thousands of years. Additionally, distinctive breath odors have been used for centuries as indicators of "evil humors" that are now diagnosed as uncontrolled diabetes, liver disease, renal disease, bacterial infection, or dental disease.

Lavoisier reported the first quantitative analysis of carbon dioxide in 1784 and demonstrated conclusively that this breath compound was a product of normal respiration. In the interim there were a number of reports of breath analysis for molecules such as ethanol. The earliest publications of modern day breath analysis appeared in the late 1960s and early 1970s, which was the time of nascence for modern analytical chemistry. Researchers such as Pauling,[1] Larsson,[2] Chen,[3] Cohen,[4] and Phillips[5] reported some of these pioneering studies. Many of these studies were only possible as a result of enhanced separation of gaseous molecules by gas chromatography, increased selectivities of mass or optical spectrometers and improved limits of detection from high parts-per-million to parts-per-billion.

A number of investigators have reported on the analysis of breath in the intervening period and the subsequent discussion is based upon a Library of Medicine computer search (`www.ncbi.nlm.nih.gov`) performed on September 10, 2004. More than 5000 citations to breath and clinical tests were found in this search and the distribution of the studies, based upon the identity of the compound, are shown in Table 2.

Table 2. Number of published clinical uses of breath

Compound	Number of publications
Oxygen	2155
Carbon dioxide	2027
Hydrogen	1722
Ethanol	1053
Hydrocarbons	968
Carbon monoxide	849
Water	679
Nitric oxide	638
Pentane	141
Ethane	128
Acetone	126
Ammonia	95
Acetaldehyde	83
Isoprene	66
Methanol	51
Methylamine	47
Ethylene	38
Methanethiol	29
Carbon disulfide	23
Carbonyl sulfide	5

Table 3. Distribution of published studies

Physiological basis	Number of publications
Pulmonary diseases	2983
Asthma	1178
COPD	417
Emphysema	222
Cystic fibrosis	221
ARDS	104
Infectious diseases	1674
Cardiovascular diseases	1551
Cancer	1334
Liver diseases	730
Renal diseases	230
Organ transplantation	221
Gastrointestinal diseases	81
Dental diseases	47
Normal physiology	4453
Alcohol assessment	1858
Exercise	1322
Exposure assessment	1142
Smoking	1004
Anesthesia	556
Nutrition	445

Only breath molecules whose origins are endogenous (except oxygen) have been included in this tabulation. As expected, this distribution of molecules in terms of number of studies is directly related to their concentrations (compare the concentrations of molecules shown in Table 1 to the ranking contained in Table 2). These same publications have been regrouped in terms of their clinical or physiological uses and Table 3 presents this compilation.

Pulmonary diseases, particularly asthma, and the understanding of normal physiology were the most popular published uses of breath analysis. Two endogenously produced molecules dominate this distribution of published studies: nitric oxide deriving from airway tissues and cells, and carbon dioxide originating from normal and abnormal metabolism. A summary of the biochemical or physiological bases for the remaining endogenous molecules is presented in Table 4.

Inspection of this information shows that metabolism of foods or exogenous substances is the major source of breath molecules and therefore the use of odors of breath for clinical diagnosis can be confounded by the characteristic odors that result from the metabolism of foods containing garlic, onions, fish, spices, mints or ethanol. Also, if the origin of a molecule is metabolism then the composition of breath will have a temporal relationship.

Table 4.   Physiological origins of some endogenous breath molecules

Compound	Physiological basis
Acetaldehyde	Ethanol metabolism
Acetone	Decarboxylation of acetoacetate
Ammonia	Protein metabolism
Carbon disulfide	Gut bacteria
Carbon monoxide	Production catalyzed by *heme oxygenase*
Carbonyl sulfide	Gut bacteria
Ethane	Lipid peroxidation
Ethanol	Gut bacteria
Ethylene	Lipid peroxidation
Hydrocarbons	Lipid peroxidation/metabolism
Hydrogen	Gut bacteria
Isoprene	Cholesterol biosynthesis
Methane	Gut bacteria
Methanethiol	Methionine metabolism
Methanol	Metabolism of fruit
Methylamine	Protein metabolism
Nitric oxide	Production catalyzed by *nitric oxide synthase*
Pentane	Lipid peroxidation

3. Current Status

Although modern breath analysis has a history of 35 years, its clinical use has been more limited. This is surprising since the breath test is one of the few clinical laboratory tests that are completely non-invasive. The only requirement to collect a breath sample is that the subject must be breathing (spontaneously or mechanically supported). In our laboratories, we have successfully analyzed breath samples collected from a neonate[6] (600 g, gestation age 28 weeks), and perioperatively during pediatric liver transplantation.[7] We have also demonstrated that it is possible to collect breath from patients suffering from Alzheimer's disease[8] and from conscious 2 year old children.[9] The latter willingly provided breath samples and treated breath collection as a game. Additionally, we have shown that it is possible to collect breath samples easily and reproducibly in the field, in a clinic, in a patient's room in the hospital, or from patients in an intensive care unit. Breath can also be collected multiple times without significant risk to the patient. Moreover, collecting breath samples poses minimum risk to the person that collects the breath sample. So therefore, why are there only six approved breath tests currently in clinical use and a seventh breath test that is widely used by law enforcement officials world-wide (Table 5)?

Furthermore, the FDA has only approved two of these tests within the last 12 months (breath nitric oxide test for asthma therapy, and the breath test for detection of heart transplant rejection).

Perhaps the easiest way to rationalize the current status of clinical breath tests is to examine the tests that currently are in use. Breath tests fall into two basic categories: tests that quantify molecules in breath after administration of a drug or substrate; and tests that quantify molecules in breath without any prior administration of a drug or substrate. The first group of tests is based upon the detection of a metabolite of the drug or substrate. Carbon dioxide is the most popular metabolite; however, since it is

Table 5.   Clinical breath tests that are most developed

Breath Carbon Dioxide Test for capnography
Breath Carbon Monoxide Test for neonatal jaundice
Breath Ethanol Test for blood ethanol (law enforcement)
Breath Hydrogen Test to detect *disaccharidase* deficiency, gastro-
  intestinal transit time, bacterial overgrowth, intestinal statis
Breath Nitric Oxide Test for asthma therapy
Breath Test for detection of heart transplant rejection
Urea Breath Test for detection of *H. pylori* infection

---

one of major products of cellular metabolism, the drug or substrate must be labeled with carbon (^{13}C or ^{14}C). Spectroscopic or radiochemical methods can be used to separate and analyze labeled carbon dioxide in the presence of unlabeled carbon dioxide. The relatively large natural abundance of ^{13}C limits the sensitivity of this method. Breath tests based upon this approach require that the metabolism of the substrate and the excretion of carbon dioxide be well characterized. Moreover, the breath test must be performed under defined conditions based upon the time of administration of the substrate and the time the breath test is administered. Additionally, the ventilation pattern of the patient must be carefully controlled. Table 6 summarizes clinical breath tests that have been proposed based upon the quantification of labeled carbon dioxide.

Most of these breath tests are diagnostic for liver function or for gastrointestinal tract function. The breath hydrogen test (Table 5) is similar to these tests (Table 6), since it involves the metabolism of a substrate (a carbohydrate, usually lactose) by colonic bacteria.[10] In people who are *lactase* deficient, lactose is not absorbed in the small intestine and is therefore, metabolized in the colon. Since the production of hydrogen in a fasting state normal subject is low (resulting in a breath concentration of less than 42 ppm) it is not necessary to isotopically label the diagnostic disaccharide. However, it is important to conduct the breath hydrogen test under carefully controlled conditions, since the time for the maximum evolution of hydrogen will depend upon gut motility and this time is critical to the

Table 6.   Clinical breath tests based upon labeled substrates

Substrate	Clinical test
Acetate	Orocecal transit time
Aminopyrine	Liver function
Caffeine	Liver function
Erythromycin	Liver function
Galactose	Liver function
Glucose	Insulin resistance
Glycosyl ureides	Orocecal transit time
Ketoisocaproate	Liver mitochondrial function
Linoleic acid	Fatty acid metabolism
Methacetin	Liver function
Methionine	Liver mitochondrial function
Phenylalanine	*Phenylalanine hydrolase* activity
Triolein	Fat malabsorption
Uracil	*Dihydropyrimidine dehydrogenase* activity
Urea	*H. pylori* infection

test. The chapter by Ledochowski *et al.*[11] on page 375 of this book focuses on the use of breath hydrogen in medicine. The breath ethanol test is also similar to the other breath tests contained in Table 6, since it involves the measurement of a molecule whose origin is often exogenous. However, this breath test does not involve metabolism of the substrate and the legal basis for its use is that the concentration of breath ethanol can be used as a screening test for the concentration of ethanol in blood. Breath ethanol is an ideal screening test, since it is non-invasive and can easily be performed in the field by law enforcement officers. Since the result of a breath ethanol test may have important legal consequence, the conduct of this test must be rigorously controlled. Metabolism by enteric bacteria can also produce breath ethanol, although the amount generated by this source is orders of magnitude less than an exogenous source. Ethanol in human breath appears to be elevated in obesity or with reduced gut motility.[12]

The second group of breath tests is based upon the detection of molecules that are produced endogenously as a result of normal or abnormal physiologies. Table 4 has listed a number of molecules with known biochemical pathways that have been detected in human breath and yet only four of these endogenously produced molecules are monitored in the tests listed in Table 5. The common feature for most of the tests listed in Table 5 is that breath is collected under carefully controlled conditions that include careful monitoring of the ventilation of the subject. Capnography, real-time measurement of the carbon dioxide concentration profile, is the most widely used clinical breath test. It is used to monitor every patient undergoing surgery or in an intensive care unit. Capnography provides important information on cellular metabolism, carbon dioxide transport and pulmonary ventilation (exchange of carbon dioxide for oxygen, and assessment of airway integrity). Each of these processes is critical to monitoring the well-being of a patient. Another common feature to the tests listed in Table 5 is that most are based upon real time time measurement of the analyte species.

The nitric oxide breath test highlights the need to standardize the method for breath sampling, because without controlling the mouth pressure and the exhalation flow rate through a critical orifice it is impossible to determine airway-derived nitric oxide. Measurement of nitric oxide originating from cells present in the airway is relevant for asthma studies. The sinuses contribute high concentrations of nitric oxide to exhaled breath and the breath sampling protocol separates this source from airway-derived nitric oxide.[13,14] In summary, all the breath tests that are currently the most developed involve the careful control of breathing and breath collection and generally involve the use of real-time monitors. Currently, carbon dioxide is the only breath molecule that can be detected, in real time, with a portable breath monitor.

4. Important Research Gaps to Address

The successful use of the nitric oxide breath test to monitor therapy for the treatment of asthma was only possible as a result of the American Thoracic Society (ATS)[14] and the European Respiratory Society (ERS)[13] generating guidelines for the method to perform nitric oxide breath analysis and the availability of a real time monitor that was able to record the profile of nitric oxide in a single breath.[13,14] The exhalation profile for breath nitric oxide showed that if the velopharyngeal aperture was not blocked then a transitory pulse of nitric oxide originating from the nasopharynx was observed.[13,14] This source of nitric oxide produced major variations in the reported levels of breath nitric oxide when breath over a complete breath cycle was collected and analyzed for nitric oxide. The sinus-derived nitric oxide contribution was eliminated when the ATS/ERS standard maneuver[13,14] was adopted for on-line breath analysis for nitric oxide. An updated consensus statement from these two societies is currently in review and is based upon a joint task force that met in Toronto, Canada in December 2002.

Researchers in the field of breath analysis need to generate comparable guidelines for the collection and analysis for all the other molecules found in breath. Ideally, standard protocols should be generated for the collection and analysis of single breath samples, for the collection and analysis of end-tidal breath samples, and for the analysis of breath samples collected during constant tidal breathing. Also guidelines should be generated for methods of breath collection that involve breath holding. The development of these guidelines will allow breath samples collected and analyzed in different laboratories to be compared and contrasted. At this time it is reasonable to propose that the method for the collection of a single breath could be the same as the ATS/ERS standard method for on-line breath nitric oxide analysis. If the method does not involve the use of a real time monitor for the analyte molecule then an end-tidal concentration of the carbon dioxide should also be monitored. In general when breath is collected under any sampling protocol, mouth pressure, and carbon dioxide should be monitored continuously. The profile of carbon dioxide will define the quality of the breath sample and the variation of mouth pressure with breathing cycle will demonstrate that the patient is maintaining a tight seal at the mouth and is exhaling through the mouthpiece. In addition, volume flow should be monitored continuously during tidal breathing.

Additionally these guidelines should include a definition for the way the results of breath analysis are expressed. Breath analyses data for single breath samples could be expressed in terms of concentration units that are dimensionless (*i.e.* parts-per-million, etc.) or in terms of moles per unit volume (pmol/L). Alternately, single breath analyses could be normalized to a physiological based parameter such as carbon dioxide (*i.e.* pmol/mL of CO_2). Normalization to carbon dioxide allows breath analysis data for subjects with widely different body masses to be compared. This latter method of data expression should definitely be used for reporting analysis of breath collected after breath holding.[15] Collection of breath during tidal breathing presents additional problems, since when human subjects are asked to breathe normally they tend to hypoventilate Hyperventilation will change the distributions of molecules across the alveolar-capillary junction with time. Hyperventilation during breath collection can be prevented by requiring the subject to breathe at a constant defined rate (10 breath/min) and at a constant tidal volume based upon height and body weight.[16] Breath collected during tidal breathing will provide the average composition of all the breaths sampled. The resulting breath analyses can be normalized to minute ventilation per body mass (pmol/kg min), normalized to minute ventilation per body surface area (pmol/m^2 min) or normalized to carbon dioxide production (pmol/mL of CO_2). The latter method of normalization is preferred when cross-sectional breath data are compared for subjects with widely different body weights.

The composition of the inspiratory air is another area of breath analysis that requires study. Many molecules that are important for clinical diagnosis can also be present in the ambient environment. Currently, there is no consensus for a standard method to allow the background levels to be subtracted. At least part of the reason for this deficiency is the fact that there are no data that define how long it takes for a subject to reach steady state with his or her ambient environment. It has been suggested the lung can be washed out in approximately 4 minutes if a subject breathes pure air.[17] However, the washout of the entire body may take days or weeks depending upon the identity of the molecule. Similarly, the body may take a significant time to reach steady state with the composition of inspiratory air. At this time there are few toxicokinetic models that can predict the disposition of molecules present in inspiratory air. Until robust models are generated, a sample of inspiratory air should be collected and if the concentrations of analyte molecules in the inspiratory air are greater than 25 % of the concentrations in breath, then the analytical data should be treated with caution. This limitation is proposed since the study subject may not be in steady state with his or her environment and the resulting analysis will have a significant error.

Finally, when standard techniques for breath collection and procedures for background correction have been adopted, then it should be possible to generate normal concentration ranges for diagnostic breath biomarkers as a function of gender, age and ethnicity. These ranges will allow limits to be set that identify abnormal concentrations of breath biomarkers. Similarly, it will be possible to set limits for concentrations of breath biomarkers not normally present in breath so that breath biomarkers can be used to diagnose abnormal physiology, tissue injury or disease. Once this basic information on the molecules that have been already identified in breath has been obtained, then pioneering studies can be performed to identify new breath biomarkers of normal and abnormal physiologies. These novel breath biomarkers will require concurrent studies aimed at determining the biochemical basis for their production. The future of clinical breath analysis can only be based upon analysis of molecules whose biochemical pathways for their generation are well known.

5. New Directions for Clinical Breath Analysis

There are three directions for future studies in clinical breath analysis: profiling molecules in breath, development of hand held real-time breath monitors for specific molecules, and use of breath condensate as a collectable sample for novel clinical studies. Breath profiling or breath fingerprinting can be considered to be a subfield of human metabolomics, which is a popular new area of research. Analytical instrumentation involved in breath profiling is generally based upon mass spectrometry with or without prior separation by gas chromatography. Soft ionization techniques must be used with direct mass spectrometry in order to perform breath profiling, since these methods of ionization will produce predominantly parent or protonated molecular ions for each breath molecule.[18] Atmospheric pressure ionization mass spectrometry (API-MS)[19] or SIFT-MS, selected ion flow tube mass spectrometry are currently the most popular ionization methods for direct breath analysis. The application of SIFT-MS to breath analysis is discussed elsewhere in this book, *e.g.* in the article by Smith and Španěl[20] on page 3. Breath is the biological media that is the most suitable for direct mass spectrometric profiling or fingerprinting, since the background matrix is a gas (low concentration) and is relatively simple as compared to blood or urine (Table 1). Conclusive identification of molecules in breath based upon the mass-to-charge ratios of protonated molecular ions is difficult, but the ability to perform real-time breath profiling is extremely exciting. More energetic methods of ionization will produce extensive fragmentation of the molecules and make analysis of the breath complex difficult, if not impossible. Separation and analysis of collected breath samples by gas chromatography-mass spectrometry, GC-MS[21] allows more conventional ionization sources to be used such as electron impact. This ionization method produces fragmentation of the analyte molecules and the resulting mass spectrum is often compound specific. Identification of novel breath biomarkers can be made on the basis of chromatographic retention data and mass spectral data. However, generation of breath profiles or breath fingerprints by GC-MS cannot be performed in real-time. Fast gas chromatography is another technique that could be used to generate breath profiles or breath fingerprints. This technique can produce breath profiles or breath fingerprints of single breaths in times that approach real-time (10 seconds). The disadvantage of this latter approach is that only discrete samples of breath can be analyzed and chromatographic retention data cannot be used for conclusive identification of breath molecules.

The development of real-time hand-held breath monitors is an area of research receiving active interest, although currently there are only a few breath monitors available. Moreover, the real-time breath monitors available are transportable but not portable. Monitors based upon electrochemical or mid-infrared technologies are likely to be the most portable devices although mini mass spectrometers or mini gas chromatographs could soon become portable. It is expected that many of these portable monitors will use multipass absorption cells and quantum cascade lasers.[22] Hand-held real-time breath monitors will be designed to analyze specific breath molecules and ideally all these monitors should have an identical platform. The basic platform would contain all the monitors and instrumentation associated with monitoring breath sampling. Real-time breath monitors should be able to respond to the concentration of the analyte species during a normal breath cycle (*i.e.* response time of less than one second). There are a number of clinical applications where real-time breath analysis would have an immediate application such as: monitoring the progress of hemodialysis therapy for patients with end-stage renal disease,[23] identifying pulmonary infections (bacteria, fungus or virus) in patients suffering from cystic fibrosis,[24] identifying pulmonary infections (bacteria, fungus or virus) or acute tissue rejection in patients who are immunocompromised due to receiving lung transplants[25] and for identifying gastrointestinal dysfunction. Currently, breath biomarkers that could be used for some of these applications have been identified, but no real-time portable monitors are available. There are many other clinical applications where breath biomarkers need to be identified or real-time monitors need to be developed.

5.1. *Breath Condensate*

The collection of breath condensate is a new addition to the field of clinical breath analysis.[24] This method of sampling adds new dimensions to the field, since it collects the non-volatile molecules that may be present in exhaled breath. These liquid droplets are produced during normal breathing when turbulent airflow across the airway surface, or the airway cilia, causes the airway-lining fluids to be nebulized. Airway-lining fluids can also be nebulized when closed respiratory bronchioles and alveoli pop open during normal ventilation. The amount of airway fluids that are produced is dependent upon the dynamics of breathing and the composition of the liquid droplets will be similar to the composition of airway-lining fluid. Typically sufficient samples of breath condensate are obtained by chilling the breath that is exhaled during 5–15 minutes. Currently, there are many designs for equipment to chill exhaled breath and the volume of condensate is dependent upon the heat transfer efficiency. Additionally, the ventilation pattern during the sampling period will also affect the volume of condensate that is collected.[26] The volume of breath condensate is dependent upon the efficiency of collection of water vapor from cellular respiration. A summary of the non-volatiles that have been found in breath condensate is shown in Table 7.

Table 7.   Species found in breath condensate

Cytokines and other proteins
Eicosanoids
Isoprostanes
Leukotrienes
Nitrites and nitrates
Prostanoids
Reactive oxygen species

The pulmonary system is the source for the non-volatiles that have been collected from exhaled breath and therefore breath condensate has been used exclusively to study pulmonary diseases.[24] Breath condensate is an exciting new direction for clinical breath analysis and its full potential will be achieved when consensus is adopted for the sampling protocols and equipment is standardized to collect this condensate.

6. Conclusions

Although clinical breath analysis is currently in its infancy it offers unique capabilities to the field of clinical chemistry. Breath can be collected multiple times non-invasively from humans or animals without posing any risk to the subject or the person collecting the sample. Breath can be collected easily in the field and the samples returned to the laboratory for analysis. Breath samples do not require refrigeration and there are many ways to maintain breath sample integrity between collection and analysis. Real-time monitors that detect specific breath biomarkers are currently being developed and these devices are well suited for field and epidemiological studies. Real-time monitors are particularly suited for studies in developing countries where collecting blood and urine samples are difficult without refrigeration. If inexpensive portable real-time monitors can be developed then chronically sick patients could themselves monitor their progress in their home thereby minimizing their exposure to infections during routine visits to clinics.

Breath analysis can be used to detect disease, monitor disease progression, or monitor therapy. Breath analysis can be used for phase 1 and phase 2 clinical trials to monitor new drug therapy or to detect potential adverse effects. Since breath analysis is non-invasive and can be performed easily, it allows larger numbers of study subjects to be studied. Using larger numbers of study subjects, unusual adverse effects are more likely to be identified.

Coupling administration of isotopically-labeled diagnostic substrates with breath analysis will allow phenotyping of subjects to be performed, and allow polymorphisms, genetic abnormalities and susceptible populations to be identified. The use of substrates labeled with stable isotopes is ideally suited to neonatal studies, since it does not involve exposing the infants to radioactive agents. Moreover, it is easier to obtain single or multiple breath samples from these infants than it is to obtain blood or urine samples. Clinical breath analysis is in its infancy and its full potential has yet to be achieved.

Acknowledgements

I wish to thank my colleagues in various medical specialties in the School of Medicine at The Johns Hopkins University who have contributed both intellectually to my research and who have helped to recruit patients for study. I would also like to thank all my former students who have contributed to every aspect of this research. Finally, I would like to acknowledge the National Institutes of Health and the U. S. Air Force Office of Scientific Research who have supported my research into clinical breath analysis.

References

1. Pauling L, Robinson AB, Teranishi R, Cary P. Quantitative analysis of urine vapor and breath by gas-liquid partition chromatography. *Proc Natl Acad Sci USA* 1971; **68**: 2374–2376.

2. Jansson BO, Larsson BT. Analysis of organic compounds in human breath by gas chromatography-mass spectrometry. *J Lab Clin Med* 1969; **74**: 961–966.

3. Chen S, Zieve L, Mahadevan V. Mercaptans and dimethyl sulfide in the breath of patients with cirrhosis of the liver. Effect of feeding methionine. *J Lab Clin Med* 1970; **75**: 628–635.

4. Riely CA, Cohen G, Lieberman M. Ethane evolution: a new index of lipid peroxidation. *Science* 1974; **183**: 208–210.

5. Dannecker JR, Jr., Shaskan EG, Phillips M. A new highly sensitive assay for breath acetaldehyde: detection of endogenous levels in humans. *Anal Biochem* 1981; **114**: 1–7.

6. Schwarz KB, Cox JM, Sharma S, Clement L, Humphrey J, Gleason C, Abbey H, Sehnert SS, Risby TH. Possible antioxidant effect of vitamin A supplementation in premature infants. *J Pediatr Gastroenterol Nutr* 1997; **25**: 408–414.

7. Risby TH, Maley W, Scott RP, Bulkley GB, Kazui M, Sehnert SS, Schwarz KB, Potter J, Mezey E, Klein AS, *et al.* Evidence for free radical-mediated lipid peroxidation at reperfusion of human orthotopic liver transplants. *Surgery* 1994; **115**: 94–101.

8. Cope KA. *Breath Biomarkers of Exposure and Disease.* PhD Dissertation. Baltimore: Johns Hopkins University, Department of Environmental Health Sciences, 2002.

9. Refat M, Moore TJ, Kazui M, Risby TH, Perman JA, Schwarz KB. Utility of breath ethane as a noninvasive biomarker of vitamin E status in children. *Pediatr Res* 1991; **30**: 396–403.

10. Perman JA. Clinical application of breath hydrogen measurements. *Can J Physiol Pharmacol* 1991; **69**: 111–115.

11. Ledochowski M, Amann A, Fuchs D. Breath gas analysis in patients with carbohydrate-malabsorption syndrome. In: Amann A, Smith D, eds. *Breath Analysis for Clinical Diagnosis and Therapeutic Monitoring,* Singapore: World Scientific, 2005.

12. Nair S, Cope K, Risby TH, Diehl AM. Obesity and female gender increase breath ethanol concentration: potential implications for the pathogenesis of nonalcoholic steatohepatitis. *Am J Gastroenterol* 2001; **96**: 1200–1204.

13. Kharitonov S, Alving K, Barnes PJ. Exhaled and nasal nitric oxide measurements: recommendations. The European Respiratory Society Task Force. *Eur Respir J* 1997; **10**: 1683–1693.

14. Recommendations for standardized procedures for the on-line and off-line measurement of exhaled lower respiratory nitric oxide and nasal nitric oxide in adults and children — 1999. This official statement of the American Thoracic Society was adopted by the ATS Board of Directors, July 1999. *Am J Respir Crit Care Med* 1999; **160**: 2104–2117.

15. Furne JK, Springfield JR, Ho SB, Levitt MD. Simplification of the end-alveolar carbon monoxide technique to assess erythrocyte survival. *J Lab Clin Med* 2003; **142**: 52–57.

16. Cope KA, Watson MT, Foster WM, Sehnert SS, Risby TH. Effects of ventilation on the collection of exhaled breath in humans. *J Appl Physiol* 2004; **96**: 1371–1379.

17. Risby TH, Sehnert SS. Clinical application of breath biomarkers of oxidative stress status. *Free Radic Biol Med* 1999; **27**: 1182–1192.

18. Gross J. *Mass spectrometry: a textbook.* Berlin; New York: Springer, 2004.

19. Benoit FM, Davidson WR, Lovett AM, Nacson S, Ngo A. Breath analysis by API/MS — human exposure to volatile organic solvents. *Int Arch Occup Environ Health* 1985; **55**: 113–120.

20. Smith D, Španěl P. Selected ion flow tube mass spectrometry, SIFT-MS, for on-line trace gas analysis of breath. In: Amann A, Smith D, eds. *Breath Analysis for Clinical Diagnosis and Therapeutic Monitoring,* Singapore. World Scientific, 2005.

21. Phillips M, Herrera J, Krishnan S, Zain M, Greenberg J, Cataneo RN. Variation in volatile organic compounds in the breath of normal humans. *J Chromatogr B Biomed Sci Appl* 1999; **729**: 75–88.

22. Wysocki G, McCurdy M, So S, Weidmann D, Roller C, Curl RF, Tittel FK. Pulsed quantum-cascade laser-based sensor for trace-gas detection of carbonyl sulfide. *Appl Opt* 2004; **43**: 6040–6046.

23. Narasimhan LR, Goodman W, Patel CK. Correlation of breath ammonia with blood urea nitrogen and creatinine during hemodialysis. *Proc Natl Acad Sci USA* 2001; **98**: 4617–4621.

24. Kharitonov SA, Barnes PJ. Biomarkers of some pulmonary diseases in exhaled breath. *Biomarkers* 2002; **7**: 1–32.

25. Studer SM, Orens JB, Rosas I, Krishnan JA, Cope KA, Yang S, Conte JV, Becker PB, Risby TH. Patterns and significance of exhaled-breath biomarkers in lung transplant recipients with acute allograft rejection. *J Heart Lung Transplant* 2001; **20**: 1158–1166.

26. McCafferty JB, Bradshaw TA, Tate S, Greening AP, Innes JA. Effects of breathing pattern and inspired air conditions on breath condensate volume, pH, nitrite, and protein concentrations. *Thorax* 2004; **59**: 694–698.

VOC BREATH MARKERS IN CRITICALLY ILL PATIENTS: POTENTIAL AND LIMITATIONS

J. K. SCHUBERT, W. MIEKISCH, AND G. F. E. NÖLDGE-SCHOMBURG

Department of Anaesthesia and Critical Care,
University of Rostock,
Schillingallee 35, D-18057 Rostock, Germany

1. Introduction: Monitoring in the ICU

Vital sign monitoring and various other diagnostic methods play important roles in critical care. Many of the procedures employed for monitoring or diagnostic purposes are invasive and not without risk to the patient (Fig. 1). Bleeding, infection, pneumothorax or damage to intracardial structures are common complications of arterial or venous canulas and central or pulmonary artery catheters. However, despite their invasiveness, these monitoring and diagnostic procedures do not often provide sufficient information

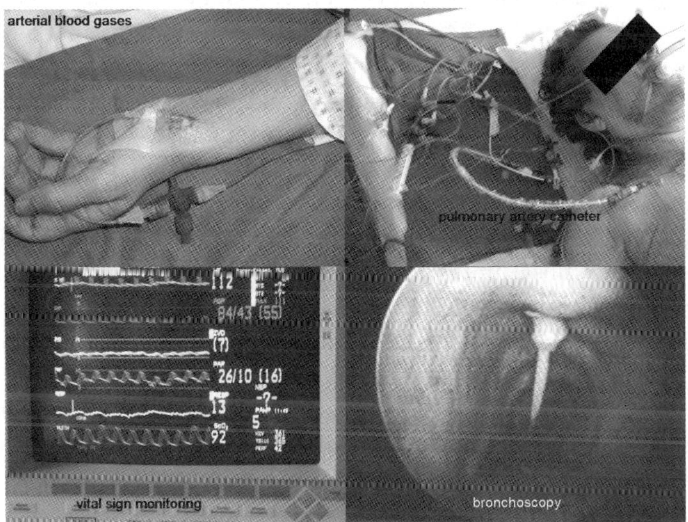

Fig. 1. Monitoring of the critically ill: invasive blood pressure measurement, pulmonary artery catheter, standard vital sign monitor, bronchoscopy

to guide and tailor treatment for critically ill patients. Hence, there is an increasing need for new diagnostic methods in critical care. Tests have to be highly reliable, since any decision based on them can have vital consequences for the patient and tests have to take into account medications, diagnostic and therapeutic actions that are proceeding at the moment of measurement.

In addition, new techniques have to be without risk to the patient, even if repeated frequently, and must provide more information than is obtained from conventional blood and urine analyses. Breath analysis can meet all these requirements. Regarding more than one breath marker compound, we can define marker sets that may have predictive value even in complex diseases such as acute lung failure, pneumonia, lung cancer, sepsis/SIRS, or ischemia/reperfusion injury.

The bulk matrix of breath is a mixture of nitrogen, oxygen, carbon dioxide, water and inert gases. The remaining small fraction of human breath consists of trace components occurring in concentrations in the mmol/L to pmol/L (parts-per-million, ppmv, to parts-per-trillion, pptv) range. Far more than 1000 of these compounds have been tentatively described.[1] These volatile substances may be generated in the body (endogenous) or may be absorbed as contaminants from the environment (exogenous). Endogenous substances include inorganic gases such as NO and CO, as well as various volatile organic compounds (VOCs). NO and a fraction of the exhaled CO are generated in the airways and are looked upon as markers of airway inflammation.[2-5] Volatile compounds can be produced anywhere in the body or in tissues lining the airway and may reflect physiological or pathological biochemical processes. Those compounds that are not generated in the lung are transported via the blood stream and exhaled through the lungs. Alkanes such as ethane and pentane have been linked to lipid peroxidation,[6-14] ketones such as acetone have been linked to dextrose metabolism,[15,16] unsaturated compounds such as isoprene[17] are known to be associated with cholesterol metabolism, sulphur and nitrogen containing compounds such as mercaptans and amines/ammonia are correlated respectively with liver disease[18,19] and renal failure.[20,21]

Critically ill patients can be expected to exhale excessive concentrations of volatile markers, since clinical conditions change rapidly and pathological conditions are profound in these patients. Hence, relationships between the composition of breath and clinical conditions should be easier to detect than in other patients. A non-invasive diagnostic method that facilitates recognition and monitoring of the rapid and often dramatically changing clinical conditions could considerably improve the clinical outcome of critically ill patients.

This chapter is intended to describe the diagnostic potential of endogenous organic volatile substances in the breath of critically ill patients. Results of recent scientific work describing the links between volatile breath markers and patients' clinical status will be discussed. Since many of these patients need ventilators, aspects of breath analysis during mechanical ventilation will be addressed.[22] Then the technical problems related to sampling and analytical procedures and methodology will be assessed.

2. Diagnostic Potential of Volatile Organic Compounds in the Breath of the Critically Ill

2.1. *Inflammation and Oxidative Injury*

Reactive oxygen species (ROS) are supposedly produced in mitochondria through leakage of 2–5 % of the oxygen normally used in respiration.[23,24] In addition, ROS such as the superoxide anion O_2^- or the hydroxyl radical OH represent most effective defence mechanisms against microbial attack.[25] ROS are generated in large concentrations by activated granulocytes and can destroy any cellular structure, including DNA and RNA. For this reason, there are a number of protective mechanisms to prevent the organism from being damaged by those reactive molecules. Important antioxidant (enzyme) systems are glutathione (GSH), superoxide dismutase, catalase and vitamins C and E. Under normal conditions, ROS activity is well controlled and balanced by antioxidant protection by the body. In some diseased states, however, the balance between ROS activity and protection may be impaired when antioxidant systems are overwhelmed or exhausted[26]. This status of oxidative stress is amongst the most frequent pathological conditions in critical illness.[27] This typically happens during systemic inflammatory reaction syndrome (SIRS) or sepsis, when inflammatory reactions are triggered throughout the body by infectious (sepsis) or non-infectious (SIRS) stimuli. Ischemia–reperfusion also leads to the generation of ROS that may locally or systematically exhaust antioxidant defence mechanisms.[28,29] Multi organ dysfunction (MODS) and multi organ failure (MOF), which are among the major reasons for morbidity and mortality in critical care, are caused in this way.[30]

Animal and human studies have demonstrated a close correlation between clinical conditions with high inflammatory or peroxidative activity and the exhalation of hydrocarbons[31] generated through ROS attack on membrane lipid structures. Lipid peroxidation is a chain reaction, which ultimately generates saturated hydrocarbons such as ethane and pentane from ω-3 and ω-6 fatty acids,[32,33] the basic components of cell membranes. Aldehydes, such as malondialdehyde (MDA), are produced along the same pathway.

In vitro studies have shown that ethane and pentane are generated when cell cultures are exposed to ROS. Elevated concentrations of exhaled *n*-alkanes were found following reperfusion of ischemic livers[11] following abdominal ischemia,[34] in ischemic heart disease,[35] in myocardial infarction,[9] following cardio-pulmonary bypass[36] and in acute rejection after heart transplantation.[37] Exhaled pentane concentrations were different in patients with SIRS and sepsis.[38] Using the diagnostic methods actually available, it is difficult to differentiate between infectious and non-infectious inflammation. The differentiation between these pathological inflammatory conditions via breath analysis (Fig. 2) could have important consequences, since SIRS is best treated with anti-inflammatory agents whereas sepsis requires the use of antibiotics.

Furthermore, levels of exhaled pentane and ethane correlate well with other lipid peroxidation markers such as MDA, thiobarbituric acid reactive substances (TBARS) and GSH.[13] Hydrocarbons, as stable end products of lipid peroxidation, show only low solubility in blood and are therefore excreted into breath within minutes of their formation in tissues. Hence, exhaled concentrations of ethane and *n*-pentane can be used to monitor

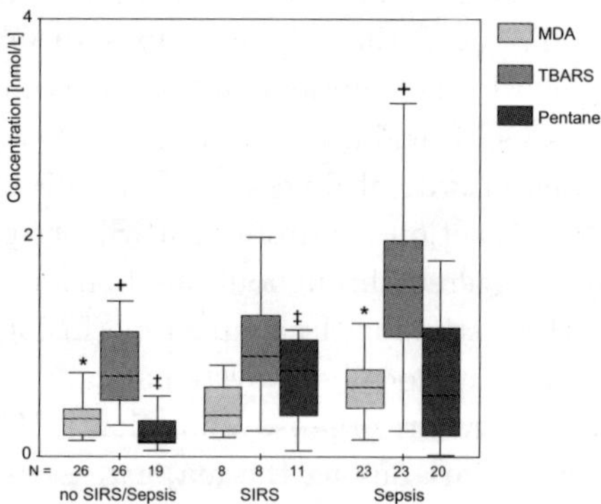

Fig. 2.   Concentrations of lipid peroxidation markers in critically ill patients. Patterns of serum and breath markers could enable differentiation between sepsis and SIRS.[38] The symbols *, †, and ‡ denote significant differences between medians. *n*-pentane was determined in exhaled breath, MDA and TBARS were analyzed in serum.

the degree of oxidative damage in the body.[14,39] Methylated hydrocarbons have also been suggested as lipid peroxidation markers.[40,41] However, the biochemical pathways for their generation and the physiological significance of these compounds have not yet been elucidated in sufficient depth.[42]

Inflammation and oxidative stress are amongst the most important factors in disease and organ damage in critically ill patients. The mechanisms of these diseased states are poorly understood and treatment often remains merely symptomatic. Breath tests involving lipid peroxidation markers, such as ethane and pentane, could provide a better understanding and tailoring of therapy for oxidative stress and inflammation.

2.2. *Acute Lung Injury, ARDS, Pneumonia*

Lung infections such as pneumonia, acute lung injury (ALI) and acute respiratory distress syndrome (ARDS, Fig. 3) are amongst the most frequent reasons for admission to the intensive care unit (ICU). Chronic lung diseases such as asthma, COPD, or pulmonary hypertension can seriously affect outcome.

Many lung diseases, including chronic obstructive pulmonary disease, asthma, bronchiectasis, cystic fibrosis, interstitial lung disease and ARDS, are linked to chronic or acute inflammation. Since ROS-mediated reactions are basic mechanisms of inflammatory processes, lipid peroxidation markers should be elevated under these conditions. In fact, pentane and ethane levels are increased in patients with asthma,[43,44] COPD[45] obstructive sleep apnoea,[46] pneumonia[47] and ARDS.[47,48]

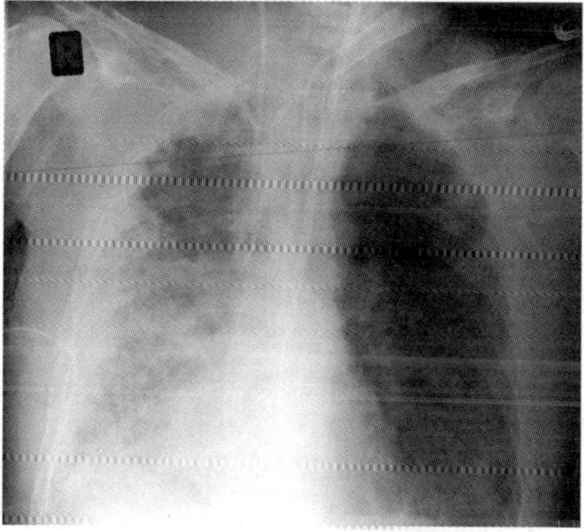

Fig. 3. A typical chest radiography of a patient suffering from ARDS with bilateral interstitial and alveolar infiltrations

Another substance linked to airway inflammation is NO.[49] Exhaled NO concentrations have been extensively studied in asthma and other inflammatory lung diseases and will not be discussed here (they are discussed in detail in Ref. 50, on page 171 of this book, and in Ref. 51, on page 121 of this book). Isoprene (2-methyl-1,3-butadiene) is another marker linked to lung injury, but it is not a lipid peroxidation marker. Isoprene is always present in human breath, and is thought to be formed along the mevalonic pathway of cholesterol synthesis.[17] There is experimental evidence that isoprene exhalation may be related to oxidative damage to the fluid lining of the lung[52] and the body.[53] Exhaled isoprene concentrations are seen to be significantly lower in ARDS patients when compared to any other patient group[38,47] (Fig. 4). Impairment of membrane repair through a decreased cholesterol biosynthesis has been proposed as a possible reason for decreased isoprene concentrations in ARDS.[47]

Breath volatiles are linked to acute lung diseases such as pneumonia and ARDS and to chronic affections such as asthma and COPD. Therefore, breath analysis has considerable potential for diagnostics and surveillance of the critically ill. Since many bacteria produce volatile substances when they are growing,[54,55] even the recognition of infectious agents from exhaled air analysis seems plausible.

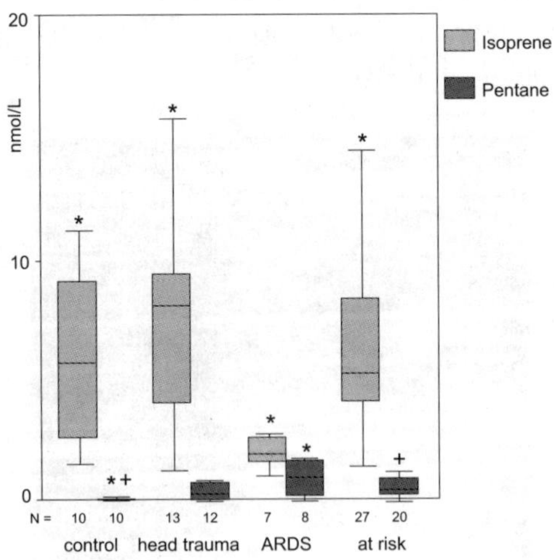

Fig. 4.   Isoprene and pentane concentrations in the breath of healthy volunteers and patients with head injuries, ARDS and patients at risk of developing ARDS. The symbols * and † denote significant differences between medians

2.3. *Metabolism*

Metabolic disorders and starvation are common problems in critical care medicine. Anaerobic dextrose metabolism and protein catabolism cause acidosis, muscle and neurological disorders in the critically ill. Easy to measure and reliable markers for these pathological states are lacking.

Acetone (dimethylketone) is one of the most abundant compounds in human breath. Acetone is produced by hepatocytes via decarboxylation of excess Acetyl-CoA, which derives from lipolysis or lipid peroxidation. Ketone bodies, like acetone, are oxidized via the Krebs cycle in peripheral tissue. Ketone bodies in blood (including acetoacetate and β-hydroxybutyrate) are increased in ketonemic subjects, in times of fasting or starving[56] or during dieting. Breath acetone concentrations are increased in patients with (uncontrolled) diabetes mellitus.[15] 2-propanol is postulated to be a product of an enzyme mediated reduction of acetone. Like acetaldehyde, concentrations of 2-propanol in humans are always lower than acetone concentrations.[56,57]

Ethanol concentrations in breath of human subjects are normally very much lower than the levels found in human breath after alcohol ingestion. The potential source of endogenous ethanol is the intestinal bacterial flora.[58] Acetaldehyde is produced by oxidation of endogenous ethanol. As a consequence, acetaldehyde concentrations in breath are always lower then corresponding ethanol concentrations.[59] Breath volatiles can provide valuable information on metabolic states in the critically ill. Since measurements are non-invasive and can be repeated frequently, a continuous metabolic surveillance seems possible.

2.4. *Organ Function*

2.4.1. *Hepatic and renal failure*

Sulphur containing compounds like methyl mercaptan, ethyl mercaptan, dimethylsulfide or dimethyldisulfide are responsible for the characteristic odour in the breath of cirrhotic patients.[18] They are generated in humans by incomplete metabolism of methionine in the transamination pathway.[19] Their concentrations in human blood and breath are very low under healthy conditions. Impairment of liver function increases the level of sulphur containing compounds.[60]

The characteristic odour of uremic breath due to elevated levels of dimethylamine and trimethylamine has been known for a long time.[20] Significant levels of ammonia will appear in the blood if the removal of ammonia through conversion to urea is limited due to an impairment of liver function. Ammonia has also been identified in the breath of healthy persons and in higher concentrations in uremic patients.[21]

2.4.2. *Transplantation*

After organ transplantation, patients have to be treated in the ICU because of chronic or acute rejection of the transplanted organ and to avoid complications due to infection following immune suppression. Allograft rejection following organ transplantation has been linked to alkane exhalation. Pentane concentration were found to be elevated in acute rejection of transplanted hearts.[61] One has to remember, however, that pentane as a lipid peroxidation marker is linked to inflammation rather than being a specific marker for allograft rejection. Carbonyl sulfide (OCS) seems to be generated as a by-product of methionine metabolism and may act as an acute marker of organ rejection after lung transplantation.[62] This volatile marker is not found in the exhaled breath of healthy individuals. A crucial problem is the distinction between organ dysfunction due to infection or any other complication and organ dysfunction due to organ rejection. Up to now, invasive procedures such as biopsy (heart, liver, kidney) or bronchoscopy (lung) were necessary for that purpose. Non-invasive breath test could, therefore, be of considerable benefit to these patients.

2.5. *Lung Physiology*

Pulmonary gas exchange is mainly determined through ventilation of alveoli and perfusion of pulmonary blood vessels. In the healthy state, the ratio of ventilation and perfusion in the lung $(\dot{V}/\dot{Q})$ is closely controlled and equals about 0.8. If alveoli are ventilated but not perfused dead space ventilation occurs (Fig. 5). This typically happens in asthma, COPD or pulmonary embolism. If alveoli are perfused but not ventilated, intrapulmonary shunt occurs (Fig. 5). This typically happens in atelectasis, pneumonia and acute respiratory distress syndrome (ARDS). In critically ill patients, impairment of pulmonary gas exchange is due almost exclusively to ventilation/perfusion mismatch of the lung.[63]

Respiratory problems are a common cause of morbidity and lengthened stay in the ICU. In today's clinical practice, therapy for pulmonary problems is guided through global parameters such as oxygen saturation, P_{aO_2} and P_{CO_2}, as ventilation perfusion ratios cannot easily be analyzed. Especially in mechanically ventilated patients, this kind of therapy control is not often satisfactory and not efficacious, because the actual reasons for the impairment of pulmonary gas exchange cannot be recognized. Hence, a causative control of respiration and mechanical ventilation could considerably improve treatment in critical care, shorten ICU stay and diminish patient morbidity and mortality.[64−70]

In the mid-seventies Wagner *et al.*[71] developed a method called multiple inert gas elimination technique (MIGET) to quantitatively measure the ventilation/perfusion ratio of the lung.[71−73] Six volatile substances (sulphur hexafluoride, ethane, cyclopropane, diethylether, acetone, halothane) were infused intravenously until a steady state between the concentrations in blood and exhaled breath was reached. Compound concentrations were then determined in arterial and mixed venous blood and in exhaled breath. Sulphur hexafluoride has to be determined by gas chromatography coupled with electron capture detection; the other compounds can be analyzed via gas chromatography and flame ionisation detection. Assuming a 50 compartment lung model, distributions of ventilation and perfusion were calcu-

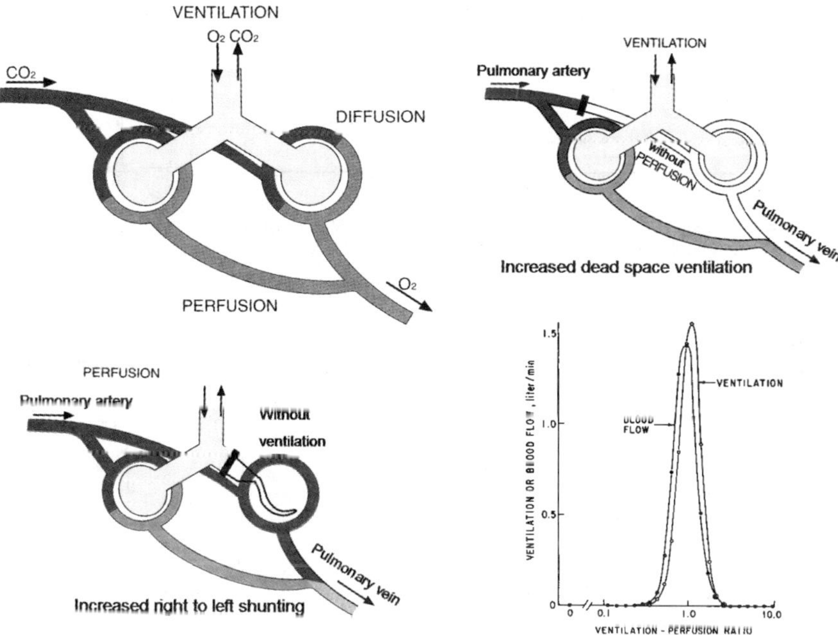

Fig. 5.   Ventilation/perfusion ratio, ventilation/perfusion mismatch (dead space ventilation, intra pulmonary right to left shunting), MIGET diagram of normal ventilation/perfusion[63,69]

lated from these data (Figs. 5 and 6). Obviously, this experimental method is sophisticated and not suitable for routine clinical purposes. If a simplified, reliable and rapid alternative method to determine ventilation–perfusion ratios could be realised, respiratory surveillance and ventilatory support in critical care could be moved from the empirical towards evidence-based and more effective treatment.

Breath analysis can actually meet these requirements. Analytical methods developed for the quantitative analysis of exhaled gases can be employed to determine endogenous volatile substances in blood and breath that have physical properties similar to the MIGET substances used by Wagner *et al.*[71] Instead of infusing substances that might harm the patient, compounds already present in patients' blood and breath in steady state concentrations could be used to do the MIGET calculations. Due to the high sensitivity of modern analytical methods, these analyses could be

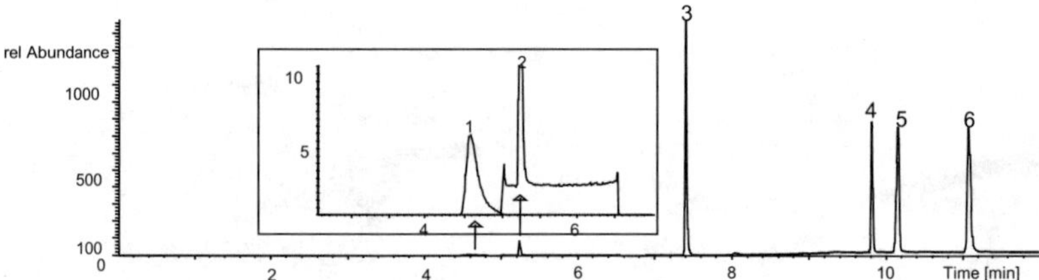

Gas chromatography of a venous sample. Detection by MS (Ion Trap).
1= sulphur hexafluoride 2= ethane, 3= cyclopropane, 4= acetone, 5= ether, 6= halothane.

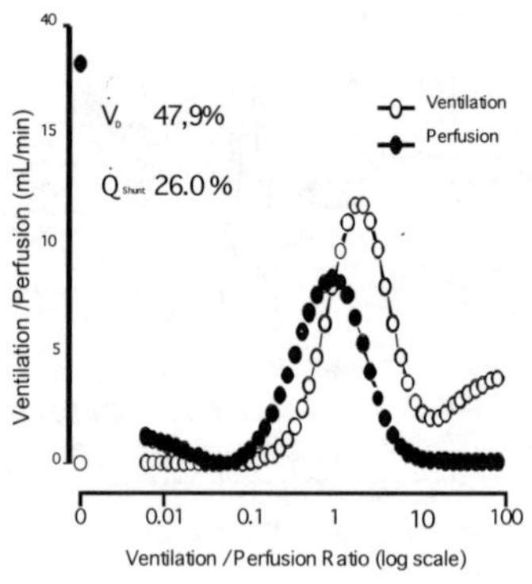

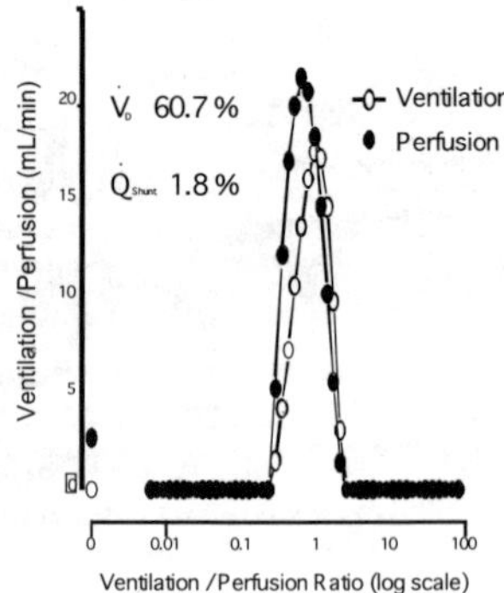

Fig. 6.   Modified MIGET analysis by means of GC-MS (ion trap). Ventilation–perfusion calculation for an isolated rabbit lung model[74]

performed reliably, without risk to the patient and fast enough to enable effective control of therapy.

In a first step, the analytical procedures of conventional MIGET were modified in the way that all six compounds could be determined in a single step using GC-MS. On-going research is aimed at building a set of endogenous volatile markers that can be used for intrinsic MIGET calculations.

3. Limitations and Methodological Aspects

Despite a number of very promising results revealing interesting diagnostic properties of different markers, analysis of volatile compounds in the breath of the critically ill has not yet been introduced into clinical practice. The main obstacles are technical problems such as sampling, preconcentration and analysis as well as basic methodological issues such as normalization, expression of data and the problem of background contamination. Apart from NO, generally accepted standards of sampling, preconcentration and analysis do not exist.

3.1. *Technical Problems*

3.1.1. *Sampling*

Sampling of exhaled air is a crucial issue in breath analysis. Dilution and contamination of samples with dead space gas and loss of analytes through physical or chemical reactions during the sampling procedure may considerably affect the reliability and reproducibility of results. Collection of expired air can be done in a way that pure alveolar breath is sampled or in a way that total breath, including dead space air, is sampled (Figs. 7 and 8).

Mixed expiratory sampling has been used most often, since this method is easy to perform. However, concentrations of endogenous volatile substances in alveolar breath are 2–3 times higher than those found in mixed ex-

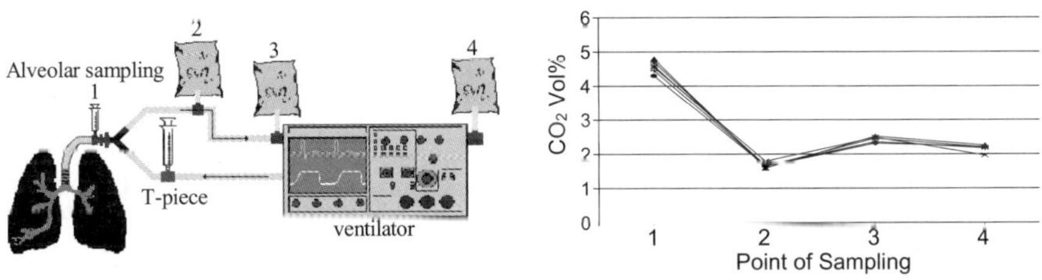

Fig. 7. Dependency of exhaled CO_2 concentrations on the sampling points in the respiratory circuit

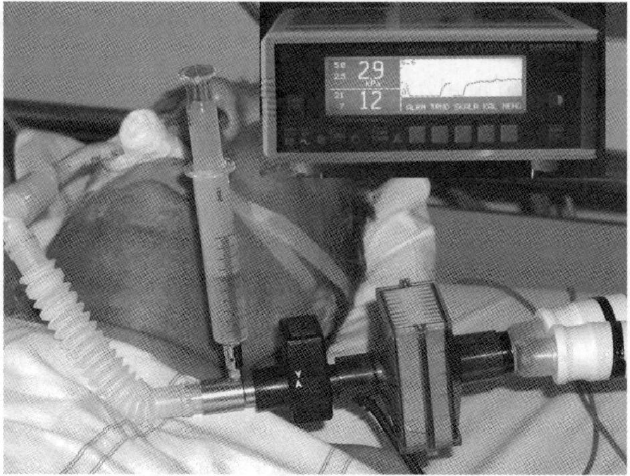

Fig. 8.   Alveolar breath sampling at the bedside. Alveolar gas samples are withdrawn from the circuit under visual control of expired CO_2. Gas collection only takes place during the alveolar portion of the expiration.

piratory samples, because there is no dilution by dead-space gas. Moreover alveolar breath samples have the lowest concentration of contaminants.[75,76] Sampling of a single breath exhalation or for a longer period of time may be performed. For single breath sampling, one has to be sure that the single breath is representative of all subsequent breaths. In spontaneously breathing subjects, breath-to-breath concentrations may vary considerably. Exhaled breath can be collected at the bedside into some sort of receptacle, whence the gaseous samples are pre-concentrated and analyzed in the laboratory.[77] Sampling may also be carried out at the bedside by means of adsorption onto special adsorption materials[78,79] or by direct cryofocussation.[80]

3.1.2. *Preconcentration and desorption*

Pre-concentration is necessary for GC(-MS) methods, since trace gas concentrations in exhaled breath are as low as nmol/L–pmol/L (ppbv–pptv). Pre-concentration can be achieved by adsorption onto sorbent traps, coated fibers (solid phase micro extraction, SPME)[81,82] or by direct cryofocussation.[80]

Adsorbent materials have to be selected carefully to avoid breakthrough, *i.e.* non-quantitative adsorption of analytes, and to avoid memory effects, *i.e.* incomplete desorption with residual substances remaining adsorbed on the trap, thus influencing subsequent adsorptions. Organic polymers (*e.g.* Tenax TA),[83] activated charcoal,[79] different types of graphite (*e.g.* Carbopack X) and carbon molecular sieves (*e.g.* Carboxen 1021) have been used.[84] Organic polymers are least affected by high water content of the samples, but these have low breakthrough volumes, especially for small hydrocarbons. By contrast, carbon molecular sieves and graphites have high breakthrough volumes for these compounds (*e.g.* ethane). The price you pay for these advantages are possible memory effects when these substances are used as the only adsorption materials. This problem can be avoided by using multibed sorbent traps.[84,85]

In the next step the volatile substances have to be released from the adsorption materials. Desorption can be achieved by heating (thermal desorption) or by using microwave energy. Commercially available devices enable automatic thermal desorption. By means of cryofocussation volatile substances can be pre-concentrated directly into the GC inlay. This has been used as an independent sampling method as well as to enhance thermal desorption. SPME[81] represents an alternative method for pre-concentrating breath volatiles. Desorption of volatile compounds from these coated fibers is done by direct heating in the GC inlay. This adsorption technique is not affected by a high water content of the sample and SPME may be automated for adsorption as well as for desorption (Fig. 9).

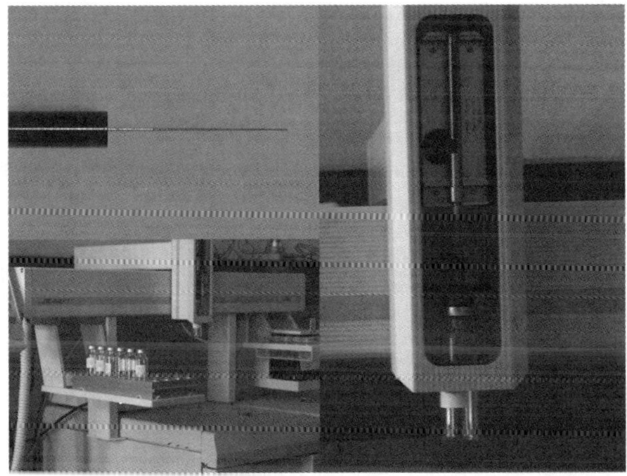

Fig. 9. SPME fiber and SPME autosampler (CTC Multi Purpose Sampler, PAL, Zwingen, Switzerland) with sample tray and automatic adsorption and desorption

3.1.3. *Separation and detection*

Gas–liquid chromatography has most often been employed to separate volatile compounds, but also gas–solid chromatography has been used.[86] A critical issue is the high water content of breath samples, which may affect separation and detection of single compounds. This is especially true for mechanically ventilated patients if active humidifiers are used in the respiratory circuit. Best results have been obtained using thick film columns (*e.g.* 505.5) or porous layer open tubular (PLOT) columns. Hydrocarbons present in exhaled breath in the nmol/L–pmol/L concentration range, such as ethane, *n*-pentane and isoprene, are usually quantified using gas chromatography (GC, Fig. 10) with flame ionization detectors (FID)[14,31,79] or mass spectrometers.[87,88] Mass spectrometric detection must be used for the identification of unknown compounds. Only if a compound had been identified unequivocally by mass spectroscopy and only if separation from all possible contaminants is perfect, can simpler and more economical detection systems like FID be used.

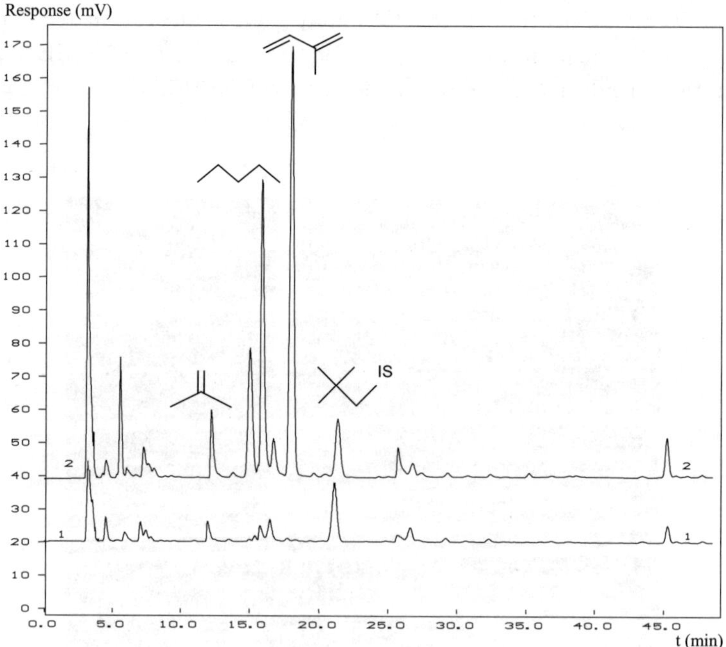

Fig. 10.   Chromatogram (GC-FID) of inspired (1) and expired (2) breath samples of a mechanically ventilated patient. IS = Internal Standard

3.1.4. *Trends and new developments in breath analysis*

As long as sophisticated procedures such as manual sampling, pre-concentration of large breath volumes onto chemical traps, and sophisticated methods like gas chromatography and mass spectrometry are necessary, breath analysis will be limited to special applications carried out in well-equipped laboratories. Recent developments and technical progress, however, show a trend towards improved and simplified analytical techniques, which could be employed for routine clinical use. Regarding the on-going technical progress in the field, one may expect that most of the technical problems will be solved in the near future.

Sampling can be standardized by automatic devices that can separate alveolar air from dead-space and inspiratory gas.[75] Pre-concentration of some volatile substances has already been simplified considerably by the introduction of SPME (Fig. 9),[81] thus facilitating automatic pre-concentration as well as automatic desorption. A very promising new technique is the membrane extraction with sorbent interface (MESI) recently developed by Pawliszyn *et al.*[89] It is based on a selective membrane acting as the interface between the respiratory circuit and the analytical system (GC), and thus it integrates sampling and pre-concentration in one step. Considerable progress has also been made using separation technologies that exploit fast or two dimensional GC.[90,91]

On-going development of real time analysis will further expand the potential of breath analysis for the critically ill. Ethane can already be detected in the pmol/L range via laser spectroscopy.[92] Other compounds have been detected and identified on-line and in real time by means of selected ion flow tube mass spectrometry (SIFT-MS) (see Ref. 93, on page 3 of this book, and Ref. 94) or proton-transfer-reaction mass spectrometry (PTR-MS) (see Ref. 95, on page 305 of this book). On-line analysis of exhaled air coupled to computer-based expert systems could solve crucial problems in critical care such as ischemia detection and the control of mechanical ventilation. Non-specific sensor array technology (electronic noses)[96,97] and ion mobility spectrometry (see Ref. 98, on page 53 of this book) may become useful for diagnostic purposes when specific patterns of disease markers have been defined and disturbing factors can be excluded.

3.2. Methodological Problems

3.2.1. *Normalization and expression of data*

Crucial problems hampering the use of exhaled VOCs in clinical practice are the lack of standardization of analytical methods and the great variation of results obtained from different studies.[1,39,47,78,79] Due to substantially different technical approaches, data cannot be compared to each other if there is no normalization to some generally accepted standard compound and to standard conditions. This issue is still a matter for debate, and the impact of physiological variables such as cardiac output, breathing pattern[99] and ventilation–perfusion ratio of the lung[63] on the results of breath analysis have not been explored in sufficient detail. Under normal conditions (healthy volunteers) these effects may be negligible. In patients with severe hemodynamic or pulmonary dysfunction, however, data should be corrected or normalized *e.g.* by means of end-tidal and/or arterial P_{CO_2} measurement.

3.2.2. *Inspired compounds*

Other parameters that can affect results are the concentrations of inspired compounds. Addition of inhaled concentrations to exhaled concentrations may blur the concentrations present in the blood. Expired samples are diluted or contaminated by inspired and/or dead-space gas, depending on the ratio of alveolar and dead-space ventilation, which itself depends on the breathing pattern.[99] Alveolar concentration gradients are altered through inhaled compounds, and compound elimination is affected accordingly, *i.e.* less compound is eliminated from the blood into the alveoli than venous concentrations would induce in the absence of inhaled compounds. The extent of this influence is controlled by the ventilation–perfusion ratio in the lung.[63,71] In addition, background concentrations of volatile compounds in inspired air have to be taken into account in order to distinguish between endogenous substances and exogenous contaminants (Fig. 11).

Different approaches have been adopted to overcome this problem. Substance concentrations in ambient or inhaled air are measured and exhaled concentrations are corrected by subtracting inspiratory from exhaled concentrations.[100] Others have tried to eliminate ambient concentrations by having patients or volunteers breathe pure air before measurement.[14] This approach is the most effective, but cumbersome and time consuming, and is not practical for routine clinical purposes.

Calculating differences between expired and inspired compound concentrations is easy to perform, but this method does not take into account the complexity of pulmonary adsorption and exhalation of volatile substances. Excretion and intake of volatile compounds depend on the ventilation–perfusion ratio in the lung and on the alveolar concentration gradients of the compounds. Due to the complexity of pulmonary adsorption and exhalation of volatile substances[63,71] these effects are not linear. These complex inter-dependencies cannot be accounted for by simply subtracting the concentrations of inspired from expired compounds. Similar problems occur when breath analysis is performed to assess an individual's exposure to xenobiotic materials.[101] In a study where exposure and body burden of VOCs were to be calculated from results of breath analysis, the present authors found predicted values within 25 % of those observed although solubility, compound distributions in a multi-compartment model and exha-

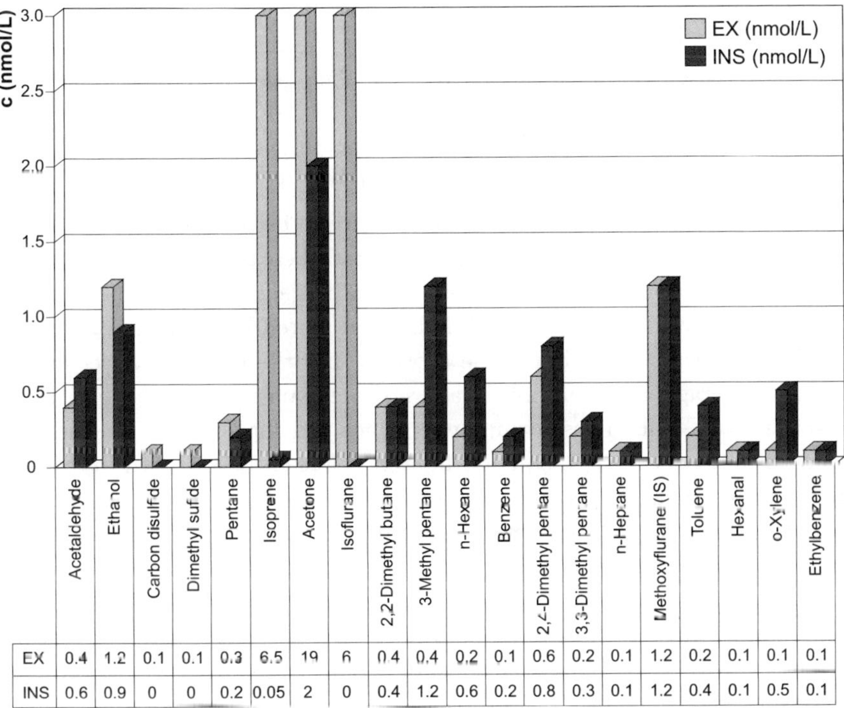

	Acetaldehyde	Ethanol	Carbon disulfide	Dimethyl sulfide	Pentane	Isoprene	Acetone	Isoflurane	2,2-Dimethyl butane	3-Methyl pentane	n-Hexane	Benzene	2,4-Dimethyl pentane	3,3-Dimethyl pentane	n-Heptane	Methoxyflurane (IS)	Toluene	Hexanal	o-Xylene	Ethylbenzene
EX	0.4	1.2	0.1	0.1	0.3	6.5	19	6	0.4	0.4	0.2	0.1	0.6	0.2	0.1	1.2	0.2	0.1	0.1	0.1
INS	0.6	0.9	0	0	0.2	0.05	2	0	0.4	1.2	0.6	0.2	0.8	0.3	0.1	1.2	0.4	0.1	0.5	0.1

Fig. 11. Inspired and expired concentrations of breath volatiles in mechanically ventilated patients

lation kinetics were taken into account. In addition, blood/breath ratios were higher than expected from the blood/air partition coefficients.[102]

This finding is in contrast to the findings of other researchers who use subtraction methods to account for inhaled compound concentrations. The recognition patterns that Phillips *et al.* uses to detect lung cancer,[103] for instance, are based on calculations of "alveolar gradients" regardless of the relative inhaled concentrations. The patients they investigated substantially differed from critically ill patients in that they were spontaneously breathing. Hence, the likelihood of severe deviations from normal breathing patterns and the presence of ventilation–perfusion mismatch are much lower. The non-linear effects of inhaled compound concentrations are most probably linked to the occurrence of dead-space ventilation and shunt perfusion, which is a common and frequent problem in mechanically ventilated patients.[68,70] This may explain why Phillips *et al.*[103] were able to obtain clinically relevant results by using a subtraction method. In addition, no information on the ratio of compound concentrations in blood and breath in their patients is available, since they did not determine marker concentrations in blood. This carries the risk that the results might be different if for any reason the breathing patterns of the patients were modified.[99]

3.2.3. *Physiological meaning, biochemical pathways, exhalation kinetics*

If volatile compounds found in the breath are to be used as markers of disease or health their physiological meaning and their pathways of generation should be known. Volatile compounds can be generated anywhere in the body, may have been previously inhaled and stored in the body or may be produced in the tissues lining the airways. For these reasons, the mechanisms of storage and metabolism as well as exhalation kinetics have to be taken into account. Those compounds which are not generated in the lung are transported via the blood stream and can then be excreted in exhaled air, in urine or faeces or can be metabolized in the body. Renal and intestinal excretions, as well as metabolism, are slow in comparison to loss via exhalation. Hence, if these compounds are to be used as markers of physiological or pathological processes in the body, a clear relationship between compound concentrations in blood and in breath has to exist. For reasons of mass conservation, compound disappearance rates from the blood have to be equal to exhalation rates if compound concentrations in blood and in breath are determined simultaneously. Verifying this condition of instantaneous mass balance appears to be an easy and reliable method to test the consistency of data and to assess the effects of experimental errors in breath analysis.[104]

Biochemical pathways and exhalation kinetics have been investigated only for a small number of volatile compounds found in human breath.[2,15,17,18,20,32,33] Markers that are produced uniquely in the airways such as NO (see Ref. 5) cannot provide any information on processes occurring in other parts of the body. Exhaled compounds that are produced in the airways and in the rest of the body, such as CO (see Ref. 4), are difficult to interpret, since the fraction originating from one or the other compartment is impossible to assign. Investigations of environmental and occupational exposure by the Environmental Protection Agency, EPA,[101] have demonstrated that breath concentrations of compounds that are purely exogenous, such as methylated alkanes, depend on substance solubility, distribution in numerous compartments, duration of exposure, metabolic activity and on inhaled substance concentrations.[101] Using volatile substances as markers of healthy or diseased states without knowing their mode and site of generation carries the risk that interpretation of results may be erroneous and may be affected by chance happenings during the experiment.

4. Conclusions

Due to the large number of volatile markers found in exhaled breath, a great variety of physiological and pathological processes can be monitored via breath analysis. In contrast to NO, which is predominantly generated in the bronchial system, volatile organic compounds are mainly blood-borne and therefore enable monitoring of different processes occurring in the body. Then breath analysis can provide valuable information on a dynamically changing clinical status of a patient, especially in the critically ill. Breath analysis can provide information not only on healthy or diseased states but may also be used to assess lung physiology. Ventilation perfusion ratios of the lung can be calculated when endogenous markers are determined in blood and in breath. These data could then be employed to optimize respiratory control and mechanical ventilation in critically ill patients.

In order to exploit the potential of breath analysis in clinical practice, it is important to appreciate its limitations and the problems involved. The technical needs include reproducibility of sampling methods, fast and quantitative determination of volatile substances, and separation and simultaneous detection of all volatile markers. The impact of inhaled compound concentrations, physiological meaning and exhalation mechanisms of breath markers represent basic methodological issues. Considering the technical and scientific progress made during recent years, it can be expected that most of the technical problems can be solved in the near future. On-going development of real time analysis will further expand the potential of breath analysis in medicine.

More work is necessary to provide information on basic methodology. Biochemical pathways and exhalation kinetics have been investigated only for a small number of volatile compounds found in human breath. Special attention has to be paid to inhaled substances. Pathological conditions of the lung, for example, changes of ventilation and perfusion, may seriously affect exhalation mechanisms.

Fast and reliable diagnostic techniques play an important role in critical care. There still is an increasing need for new and non-invasive methods of monitoring and diagnosis. In principle, breath analysis can meet this need. It is without risk to the patient, even if repeated frequently, and can provide information far beyond conventional analyses of blood and urine.

References

1. Phillips M, Herrera J, Krishnan S, Zain M, Greenberg J, Cataneo RN. Variation in volatile organic compounds in the breath of normal humans. *J Chromatogr B Biomed Sci Appl* 1999; **729**: 75–88.
2. Gustafsson LE. Exhaled nitric oxide as a marker in asthma. *Eur Respir J Suppl* 1998; **26**: 49S–52S.
3. Yates DH. Role of exhaled nitric oxide in asthma. *Immunol Cell Biol* 2001; **79**: 178–190.
4. Chapman JT, Choi AM. Exhaled monoxides as a pulmonary function test: use of exhaled nitric oxide and carbon monoxide. *Clin Chest Med* 2001; **22**: 817–836.
5. Kharitonov SA, Barnes PJ. Biomarkers of some pulmonary diseases in exhaled breath. *Biomarkers* 2002; **7**: 1–32.
6. Riely CA, Cohen G, Lieberman M. Ethane evolution: a new index of lipid peroxidation. *Science* 1974; **183**: 208–210.
7. Frankel EN. Volatile lipid oxidation products. *Prog Lipid Res* 1983; **22**: 1–33.
8. Wade CR, van Rij AM. In vivo lipid peroxidation in man as measured by the respiratory excretion of ethane, pentane, and other low-molecular-weight hydrocarbons. *Anal Biochem* 1985; **150**: 1–7.
9. Weitz ZW, Birnbaum AJ, Sobotka PA, Zarling EJ, Skosey JL. High breath pentane concentrations during acute myocardial infarction. *Lancet* 1991; **337**: 933–935.
10. Miller ER, 3rd, Appel LJ, Jiang L, Risby TH. Association between cigarette smoking and lipid peroxidation in a controlled feeding study. *Circulation* 1997; **96**: 1097–1101.

11. Kazui M, Andreoni KA, Norris EJ, Klein AS, Burdick JF, Beattie C, Sehnert SS, Bell WR, Bulkley GB, Risby TH. Breath ethane: a specific indicator of free-radical-mediated lipid peroxidation following reperfusion of the ischemic liver. *Free Radic Biol Med* 1992; **13**: 509–515.

12. Kneepkens CM, Lepage G, Roy CC. The potential of the hydrocarbon breath test as a measure of lipid peroxidation. *Free Radic Biol Med* 1994; **17**: 127–160.

13. Aghdassi E, Wendland BE, Steinhart AH, Wolman SL, Jeejeebhoy K, Allard JP. Antioxidant vitamin supplementation in Crohn's disease decreases oxidative stress. A randomized controlled trial. *Am J Gastroenterol* 2003; **98**: 348–353.

14. Risby TH, Sehnert SS. Clinical application of breath biomarkers of oxidative stress status. *Free Radic Biol Med* 1999; **27**: 1182–1192.

15. Lebovitz HE. Diabetic ketoacidosis. *Lancet* 1995; **345**: 767–772.

16. Nelson N, Lagesson V, Nosratabadi AR, Ludvigsson J, Tagesson C. Exhaled isoprene and acetone in newborn infants and in children with diabetes mellitus. *Pediatr Res* 1998; **44**: 363–367.

17. Stone BG, Besse TJ, Duane WC, Evans CD, DeMaster EG. Effect of regulating cholesterol biosynthesis on breath isoprene excretion in men. *Lipids* 1993; **28**: 705–708.

18. Chen S, Zieve L, Mahadevan V. Mercaptans and dimethyl sulfide in the breath of patients with cirrhosis of the liver. Effect of feeding methionine. *J Lab Clin Med* 1970; **75**: 628–635.

19. Scislowski PW, Pickard K. The regulation of transaminative flux of methionine in rat liver mitochondria. *Arch Biochem Biophys* 1994; **314**: 412–416.

20. Simenhoff ML, Burke JF, Saukkonen JJ, Ordinario AT, Doty R. Biochemical profile or uremic breath. *N Engl J Med* 1977; **297**: 132–135.

21. Davies S, Španěl P, Smith D. Quantitative analysis of ammonia on the breath of patients in end-stage renal failure. *Kidney Int* 1997; **52**: 223–228.

22. Marczin N, Wright G, Yacoub M. Determinants of exhaled nitric oxide: Influence of ventilation and pulmonary blood flow., In: Marczin N, Kharitonov S, eds. *Lung Biology in Health and Disease Disease Markers in Exhaled Breath*, New York: Marcel Dekker, 2003: 91–113.

23. Gredilla R, Phaneuf S, Selman C, Kendaiah S, Leeuwenburgh C, Barja G. Short-term caloric restriction and sites of oxygen radical generation in kidney and skeletal muscle mitochondria. *Ann N Y Acad Sci* 2004; **1019**: 333–342.

24. Nohl H, Gille L, Kozlov A, Staniek K. Are mitochondria a spontaneous and permanent source of reactive oxygen species? *Redox Rep* 2003; **8**: 135–141.

25. Kobayashi T, Seguchi H. Novel insight into current models of NADPH oxidase regulation, assembly and localization in human polymorphonuclear leukocytes. *Histol Histopathol* 1999; **14**: 1295–1308.

26. Metodiewa D, Koska C. Reactive oxygen species and reactive nitrogen species: relevance to cyto(neuro)toxic events and neurologic disorders. An overview. *Neurotox Res* 2000; **1**: 197–233.

27. Hansen TK, Thiel S, Wouters PJ, Christiansen JS, Van den Berghe G. Intensive insulin therapy exerts antiinflammatory effects in critically ill patients and counteracts the adverse effect of low mannose-binding lectin levels. *J Clin Endocrinol Metab* 2003; **88**: 1082–1088.

28. Reilly PM, Schiller HJ, Bulkley GB. Pharmacologic approach to tissue injury mediated by free radicals and other reactive oxygen metabolites. *Am J Surg* 1991; **161**: 488–503.

29. Sun K, Kiss E, Bedke J, Stojanovic T, Li Y, Gwinner W, Grone HJ. Role of xanthine oxidoreductase in experimental acute renal-allograft rejection. *Transplantation* 2004; **77**: 1683–1692.

30. Izumi M, McDonald MC, Sharpe MA, Chatterjee PK, Thiemermann C. Superoxide dismutase mimetics with catalase activity reduce the organ injury in hemorrhagic shock. *Shock* 2002; **18**: 230–235.

31. Aghdassi E, Allard JP. Breath alkanes as a marker of oxidative stress in different clinical conditions. *Free Radic Biol Med* 2000; **28**: 880–886.

32. Evans C, List G, Doley A, McConel D, Hoffman R. Pentane from thermal decomposition of lipoxidase-derived products. *Lipids* 1967; **2**: 432–434.

33. Dumelin E, Tappel A. Hydrocarbon gases produced during in vitro peroxidation of polyunsaturated fatty acids and decomposition of preformed hydroperoxides. *Lipids* 1977; **12**: 894–900.

34. Kazui M, Andreoni KA, Williams GM, Perler BA, Bulkley GB, Beattie C, Donham RT, Sehnert SS, Burdick JF, Risby TH. Visceral lipid peroxidation occurs at reperfusion after supraceliac aortic cross-clamping. *J Vasc Surg* 1994; **19**: 473–477.

35. Mendis S, Sobotka PA, Leja FL, Euler DE. Breath pentane and plasma lipid peroxides in ischemic heart disease. *Free Radic Biol Med* 1995; **19**: 679–684.

36. Andreoni KA, Kazui M, Cameron DE, Nyhan D, Sehnert SS, Rohde CA, Bulkley GB, Risby TH. Ethane: a marker of lipid peroxidation during cardiopulmonary bypass in humans. *Free Radic Biol Med* 1999; **26**: 439–445.

37. Sobotka PA, Gupta DK, Lansky DM, Costanzo MR, Zarling EJ. Breath pentane is a marker of acute cardiac allograft rejection. *J Heart Lung Transplant* 1994; **13**: 224–229.

38. Scholpp J, Schubert JK, Miekisch W, Geiger K. Breath markers and soluble lipid peroxidation markers in critically ill patients. *Clin Chem Lab Med* 2002; **40**: 587–594.

39. Kohlmuller D, Kochen W. Is n-pentane really an index of lipid peroxidation in humans and animals? A methodological reevaluation. *Anal Biochem* 1993; **210**: 268–276.

40. Phillips M, Cataneo RN, Greenberg J, Grodman R, Gunawardena R, Naidu A. Effect of oxygen on breath markers of oxidative stress. *Eur Respir J* 2003; **21**: 48–51.

41. Phillips M, Cataneo RN, Greenberg J, Gunawardena R, Rahbari-Oskoui F. Increased oxidative stress in younger as well as in older humans. *Clin Chim Acta* 2003; **328**: 83–86.

42. Mitsui T, Kondo T. Inadequacy of theoretical basis of breath methylated alkane contour for assessing oxidative stress. *Clin Chim Acta* 2003; **333**: 91; author reply 93–94.

43. Paredi P, Kharitonov SA, Barnes PJ. Elevation of exhaled ethane concentration in asthma. *Am J Respir Crit Care Med* 2000; **162**: 1450–1454.

44. Olopade CO, Zakkar M, Swedler WI, Rubinstein I. Exhaled pentane levels in acute asthma. *Chest* 1997; **111**: 862–865.

45. Paredi P, Kharitonov SA, Leak D, Ward S, Cramer D, Barnes PJ. Exhaled ethane, a marker of lipid peroxidation, is elevated in chronic obstructive pulmonary disease. *Am J Respir Crit Care Med* 2000; **162**: 369–373.

46. Olopade CO, Christon JA, Zakkar M, Hua C, Swedler WI, Scheff PA, Rubinstein I. Exhaled pentane and nitric oxide levels in patients with obstructive sleep apnea. *Chest* 1997; **111**: 1500–1504.

47. Schubert JK, Muller WP, Benzing A, Geiger K. Application of a new method for analysis of exhaled gas in critically ill patients. *Intensive Care Med* 1998; **24**: 415–421.

48. Schubert J, Miekisch W, Geiger K. Exhaled breath markers in ARDS., In: Marczin N, Kharitonov S, eds. *Lung Biology in Health and Disease – Disease Markers in Exhaled Breath*, New York: Marcel Dekker, 2003: 363–380.

49. Kharitonov SA, Chung KF, Evans D, O'Connor BJ, Barnes PJ. Increased exhaled nitric oxide in asthma is mainly derived from the lower respiratory tract. *Am J Respir Crit Care Med* 1996; **153**: 1773–1780.

50. Szabó A, Kövesi T, Gál J, Royston D, Marczin N. Diagnostic aspects of exhaled nitric oxide in cardiothoracic anaesthesia. In: Amann A, Smith D, eds. *Breath Analysis for Clinical Diagnosis and Therapeutic Monitoring*, Singapore: World Scientific, 2005.

51. Dweik R. Nitric oxide in exhaled breath: a window on lung physiology and pulmonary disease. In: Amann A, Smith D, eds. *Breath Analysis for Clinical Diagnosis and Therapeutic Monitoring*, Singapore: World Scientific, 2005.

52. Foster WM, Jiang L, Stetkiewicz PT, Risby TH. Breath isoprene: temporal changes in respiratory output after exposure to ozone. *J Appl Physiol* 1996; **80**: 706–710.

53. Mendis S, Sobotka PA, Euler DE. Expired hydrocarbons in patients with acute myocardial infarction. *Free Radic Res* 1995; **23**: 117–122.

54. Mauriello G, Moio L, Moschetti G, Piombino P, Addeo F, Coppola S. Characterization of lactic acid bacteria strains on the basis of neutral volatile compounds produced in whey. *J Appl Microbiol* 2001; **90**: 928–942.

55. Claeson AS, Levin JO, Blomquist G, Sunesson AL. Volatile metabolites from microorganisms grown on humid building materials and synthetic media. *J Environ Monit* 2002; **4**: 667–672.

56. Smith D, Španěl P, Davies S. Trace gases in breath of healthy volunteers when fasting and after a protein-calorie meal: a preliminary study. *J Appl Physiol* 1999; **87**: 1584–1588.

57. Davis PL, Dal Cortivo LA, Maturo J. Endogenous isopropanol: forensic and biochemical implications. *J Anal Toxicol* 1984; **8**: 209–212.

58. Cope K, Risby T, Diehl AM. Increased gastrointestinal ethanol production in obese mice: implications for fatty liver disease pathogenesis. *Gastroenterology* 2000; **119**: 1340–1347.

59. Diskin AM, Španěl P, Smith D. Time variation of ammonia, acetone, isoprene and ethanol in breath: a quantitative SIFT-MS study over 30 days. *Physiol Meas* 2003; **24**: 107–119.

60. Sehnert SS, Jiang L, Burdick JF, Risby TH. Breath biomarkers for detection of human liver diseases: preliminary study. *Biomarkers* 2002; **7**: 174–187.

61. Holt DW, Johnston A, Ramsey JD. Breath pentane and heart rejection. *J Heart Lung Transplant* 1994; **13**: 1147–1148.

62. Studer SM, Orens JB, Rosas I, Krishnan JA, Cope KA, Yang S, Conte JV, Becker PB, Risby TH. Patterns and significance of exhaled-breath biomarkers in lung transplant recipients with acute allograft rejection. *J Heart Lung Transplant* 2001; **20**: 1158–1166.

63. West JB, Wagner PD. Pulmonary gas exchange. *Am J Respir Crit Care Med* 1998; **57**: S82–87.

64. Schutte H, Hermle G, Seeger W, Grimminger F. Vascular distension and continued ventilation are protective in lung ischemia/reperfusion. *Am J Respir Crit Care Med* 1998; **157**: 171–177.

65. Seeger W, Walmrath D, Grimminger F, Rosseau S, Schutte H, Kramer HJ, Ermert L, Kiss L. Adult respiratory distress syndrome: model systems using isolated perfused rabbit lungs. *Methods Enzymol* 1994; **233**: 549–584.

66. Hermle G, Schutte H, Walmrath D, Geiger K, Seeger W, Grimminger F. Ventilation–perfusion mismatch after lung ischemia–reperfusion. Protective effect of nitric oxide. *Am J Respir Crit Care Med* 1999; **160**: 1179–1187.

67. Walmrath D, Konig R, Ernst C, Bruckner H, Grimminger F, Seeger W. Ventilation–perfusion relationships in isolated blood-free perfused rabbit lungs. *J Appl Physiol* 1992; **72**: 374–382.

68. Dembinski R, Max M, Bensberg R, Bickenbach J, Kuhlen R, Rossaint R. High-frequency oscillatory ventilation in experimental lung injury: effects on gas exchange. *Intensive Care Med* 2002; **28**: 768–774.

69. Neumann P, Hedenstierna G. Ventilation–perfusion distributions in different porcine lung injury models. *Acta Anaesthesiol Scand* 2001; **45**: 78–86.

70. Feihl F, Eckert P, Brimioulle S, Jacobs O, Schaller MD, Melot C, Naeije R. Permissive hypercapnia impairs pulmonary gas exchange in the acute respiratory distress syndrome. *Am J Respir Crit Care Med* 2000; **162**: 209–215.

71. Wagner PD, Saltzman HA, West JB. Measurement of continuous distributions of ventilation–perfusion ratios: theory. *J Appl Physiol* 1974; **36**: 588–599.

72. Roca J, Wagner PD. Contribution of multiple inert gas elimination technique to pulmonary medicine. 1. Principles and information content of the multiple inert gas elimination technique. *Thorax* 1994; **49**: 815–824.

73. Wagner P, West J. Ventilation–perfusion relationships., In: West J, ed. *Pulmonary gas exchange*, New York: Academic press, 1980: 233–235.

74. Mols G, Hermle G, Schubert J, Miekisch W, Benzing A, Lichtwarck-Aschoff M, Geiger K, Walmrath D, Guttmann J. Volume-dependent compliance and ventilation–perfusion mismatch in surfactant-depleted isolated rabbit lungs. *Crit Care Med* 2001; **29**: 144–151.

75. Schubert JK, Spittler KH, Braun G, Geiger K, Guttmann J. CO_2-controlled sampling of alveolar gas in mechanically ventilated patients. *J Appl Physiol* 2001; **90**: 486–492.

76. Schubert JK, Esteban-Loos I, Geiger K, Guttmann J. In vivo evaluation of a new method for chemical analysis of volatile components in the respiratory gas of mechanically ventilated patients. *Technol Health Care* 1999; **7**: 29–37.

77. Pleil JD, Lindstrom AB. Measurement of volatile organic compounds in exhaled breath as collected in evacuated electropolished canisters. *J Chromatogr B Biomed Appl* 1995; **665**: 271–279.

78. Phillips M, Greenberg J. Ion-trap detection of volatile organic compounds in alveolar breath. *Clin Chem* 1992; **38**: 60–65.

79. Mueller W, Schubert J, Benzing A, Geiger K. Method for analysis of exhaled air by microwave energy desorption coupled with gas chromatography–flame ionization detection–mass spectrometry. *J Chromatogr B Biomed Sci Appl* 1998; **716**: 27–38.

80. Knutson MD, Viteri FE. Concentrating breath samples using liquid nitrogen: a reliable method for the simultaneous determination of ethane and pentane. *Anal Biochem* 1996; **242**: 129–135.

81. Grote C, Pawliszyn J. Solid-phase microextraction for the analysis of human breath. *Anal Chem* 1997; **69**: 587–596.

82. Miekisch W, Schubert JK, Vagts DA, Geiger K. Analysis of volatile disease markers in blood. *Clin Chem* 2001; **47**: 1053–1060.

83. Tangerman A, Meuwese-Arends MT, van Tongeren JH. New methods for the release of volatile sulfur compounds from human serum: its determination by Tenax trapping and gas chromatography and its application in liver diseases. *J Lab Clin Med* 1985; **106**: 175–182.

84. Risby T. Volatile organic compounds as markers in normal and deseased states., In: Marczin N, Yacoub M, eds. *Disease Markers in Exhaled Breath*, Amsterdam: IOS Press, 2002: 113–124.

85. Lärstad M, Loh C, Ljungkvist G, Olin AC, Toren K. Determination of ethane, pentane and isoprene in exhaled air using a multi-bed adsorbent and end-cut gas-solid chromatography. *Analyst* 2002; **127**: 1440–1445.

86. Lemoyne M, Van Gossum A, Kurian R, Jeejeebhoy KN. Plasma vitamin E and selenium and breath pentane in home parenteral nutrition patients. *Am J Clin Nutr* 1988; **48**: 1310–1315.

87. Španěl P, Davies S, Smith D. Quantification of breath isoprene using the selected ion flow tube mass spectrometric analytical method. *Rapid Commun Mass Spectrom* 1999; **13**: 1733–1738.

88. McGrath LT, Patrick R, Mallon P, Dowey L, Silke B, Norwood W, Elborn S. Breath isoprene during acute respiratory exacerbation in cystic fibrosis. *Eur Respir J* 2000; **16**: 1065–1069.

89. Lord H, Yu Y, Segal A, Pawliszyn J. Breath analysis and monitoring by membrane extraction with sorbent interface. *Anal Chem* 2002; **74**: 5650–5657.

90. Marchetti N, Felinger A, Pasti L, Pietrogrande M, Dondi F. Decoding two-dimensional complex multicomponent separations by autocovariance function. *Anal Chem* 2004; **76**: 3055–3068.

91. Bueno PJ, Seeley J. Flow-switching device for comprehensive two-dimensional gas chromatography. *J Chromatography A* 2004; **1027**: 3–10.

92. Dahnke H, Kleine D, Hering P, Mürtz M. Real-time monitoring of ethane in human breath using mid-infrared cavity leak-out spectroscopy. *J Appl Phys B* 2001; **72**: 971–975.

93. Smith D, Španěl P. Selected ion flow tube mass spectrometry, SIFT-MS, for on-line trace gas analysis of breath. In: Amann A, Smith D, eds. *Breath Analysis for Clinical Diagnosis and Therapeutic Monitoring*, Singapore: World Scientific, 2005.

94. Španěl P, Smith D. Selected ion flow tube: a technique for quantitative trace gas analysis of air and breath. *Med Biol Eng Comput* 1996; **34**: 409–419.

95. Amann A, Telser S, Hofer L, Schmid A, Hinterhuber H. Exhaled breath gas as a biochemical probe during sleep. In: Amann A, Smith D, eds. *Breath Analysis for Clinical Diagnosis and Therapeutic Monitoring*, Singapore: World Scientific, 2005.

96. Mohamed EI, Bruno E, Linder R, Alessandrini M, Di Girolamo A, Poppl SJ, Puija A, De Lorenzo A. A novel method for diagnosing chronic rhinosinusitis based on an electronic nose. *An Otorrinolaringol Ibero Am* 2003; **30**: 447–457.

97. Di Natale C, Macagnano A, Martinelli E, Paolesse R, D'Arcangelo G, Roscioni C, Finazzi-Agro A, D'Amico A. Lung cancer identification by the analysis of breath by means of an array of non-selective gas sensors. *Biosens Bioelectron* 2003; **18**: 1209–1218.

98. Baumbach JI, Vautz W, Ruzsanyi V, Freitag L. Metabolites in human breath: ion mobility spectrometers as diagnostic tools for lung diseases. In: Amann A, Smith D, eds. *Breath Analysis for Clinical Diagnosis and Therapeutic Monitoring*, Singapore: World Scientific, 2005.

99. Cope KA, Watson MT, Foster WM, Sehnert SS, Risby TH. Effects of ventilation on the collection of exhaled breath in humans. *J Appl Physiol* 2004; **96**: 1371–1379.

100. Phillips M. Method for the collection and assay of volatile organic compounds in breath. *Anal Biochem* 1997; **247**: 272–278.

101. Lindstrom AB, Pleil JD. A review of the USEPA's single breath canister (SBC) method for exhaled volatile organic biomarkers. *Biomarkers* 2002; **7**: 189–208.

102. Wallace LA, Nelson WC, Pellizzari ED, Raymer JH. Uptake and decay of volatile organic compounds at environmental concentrations: application of a four-compartment model to a chamber study of five human subjects. *J Expo Anal Environ Epidemiol* 1997; **7**: 141–163.

103. Phillips M, Cataneo RN, Cummin AR, Gagliardi AJ, Gleeson K, Greenberg J, Maxfield RA, Rom WN. Detection of lung cancer with volatile markers in the breath. *Chest* 2003; **123**: 2115–2123.

104. Schubert J, Miekisch W, Birken T, Geiger K, Nöldge-Schomburg G. Impact of inspired substance concentrations onto results of breath analysis in mechanically ventilated patients. *Biomarkers* 2005: in press.

HOW TO ANALYZE BREATH
AND MAKE SENSE OF THE DATA:
A PERSONAL VIEW

M. PHILLIPS

Menssana Research, Inc.,
1, Horizon Road, Suite 1415, Fort Lee, NJ 07024-6510, USA
and
Department of Medicine,
New York Medical College,
Valhalla, NY 10595, USA

1. Introduction

Experienced physicians routinely perform breath testing with their unaided noses. They learn to recognize patients with the "rotten apple" smell of diabetic , the urine-like aroma of renal failure, the sewer-like stench of a lung abscess, and the distinctive scent of fetor hepaticus that accompanies liver failure. The scientific study of breath testing was pioneered by Lavoisier in 1784, who found that carbon dioxide was excreted in human breath.[1] This was the first evidence for metabolic oxidation of foodstuffs, and it presents a very curious conundrum: Lavoisier established the importance of breath testing in biochemistry more than 200 years ago, so why has breath testing made so little progress since then? The major current applications of breath testing are remarkably limited (Table 1).

Once can only speculate why it has taken so long for breath testing to make a tentative return to the mainstream of medical research, and I

Table 1.   Breath testing at the dawn of the 21st century

Police	breath alcohol
Gastroenterologists	H_2, triolein breath tests — malabsorption ^{14}C and ^{13}C urea breath tests — *H. pylori*
Researchers	oxidative stress, markers of disease
Two breath tests recently approved by US FDA	NIOX test — nitric oxide in asthma Heartsbreath — heart transplant rejection

293

offer a completely personal and subjective explanation. First, the essential methodology has been slow to develop, because it is technically difficult. It is comparatively straightforward to collect a sample of a biological fluid such as blood, urine or sputum, and a vast number of chemical assays have been developed over the years to measure their complex contents. On the other hand, the technology required to collect and analyze gases such as breath is much more challenging, especially because most of the analytes of interest are present in very low concentrations. These difficulties have led to a curious evolution in the culture of breath testing: researchers have split into two cultures that I loosely term the "medics" and the "techies" (Table 2).

Table 2.   The world of breath testing: two cultures

	Medics	Techies
Start with ...	... a medical problem: breath test solution?	... a great breath test: medical application?
Technical ability	$+/-$	$+++$
Medical insight	$+++$	$+/-$
Resulting methods	useful seldom functional	functional seldom useful

The medics are investigators who, like Lavoisier, commence with a medical problem, and attempt to develop a breath test that will resolve the problem. The techies often start at the opposite end — they are investigators who are intrigued by the challenge of breath testing for its own sake. Both groups have their distinctive strengths and weaknesses. Medics are usually well informed about the medical and scientific needs for a breath test, but they tend to be clueless about technology. Consequently, they build instruments that are scientifically useful but technically inept. Techies are usually adept in the technology of constructing breath testing instruments, but they tend to be clueless about the medical and scientific requirements of the device. Consequently, they build instruments that are miracles of technology, but medically useless.

Admittedly, this is an exaggerated representation of two polar opposites, but it contains sufficient truth to highlight the realities of the situation. Another personal observation is that over the past several years, medics and techies have sometimes exhibited a curious failure to communicate with one another. As a result, both groups perpetuate the same old habits, year after year. The medical literature continues to abound with publications reporting *ad hoc* "home made" breath collectors from the medics that nobody else can emulate, while techies at trade shows continue to exhibit wondrously advanced breath analyzers that nobody needs or wants.

Breath tests are of two main kinds: load and no-load. In a load test, the patient is dosed beforehand with a drug *e.g.* radio-labeled urea, to test for radio-labeled CO_2 that is liberated in the presence of *H. pylori* infection. In a no-load test, no drug is administered beforehand; breath is tested either for expired breath condensate (EBC) or trace volatile inorganic compounds, such as NO and NH_3, and volatile organic compounds (VOCs). EBC, exhaled breath condensate is derived principally from the endobronchial tree — it is a condensed aerosol of interstitial fluid, and may contain high molecular weight compounds, such as proteins and interleukins. VOCs are derived from the alveolar breath, from low molecular weight compounds such as ethanol and acetone, which readily diffuse out of the pulmonary capillary blood. VOCs and EBC contain different information — VOCs generally reflect chemical changes in the systemic blood, while EBC composition varies with localized disease in the bronchial tree. Each contains unique information — they are complementary *not* competitive breath tests. The present discussion will focus principally on VOCs.

2. Breath Collecting Apparatus

A recent keyword search for volatile organic compounds in breath on the US National Library of Medicine PubMed website yielded 370 reports. A common theme that runs through many of these publications is the use of *ad hoc* "home made" methods that vary widely between investigators, and it is no surprise that their reported results vary widely as well. In recognition of this problem, my colleagues and I at Menssana Research developed a breath collection apparatus (BCA) with the objective of providing a standardized method of collecting breath VOCs outside the laboratory (Fig. 1).[2] This has made it possible to perform multi-center studies of breath VOCs for the first time. The BCA collects the VOCs in 1.0 L alveolar breath and 1.0 L room air on to two separate sorbent traps containing chemically clean activated carbon. These samples are then sent to the laboratory for analysis by conventional automated thermal desorption with gas chromatography and mass spectroscopy (ATD/GC-MS). A typical sample of human breath generally yields around 200 different VOCs. This technique has several advantages: it is patient-friendly, since it causes no discomfort, and it is also

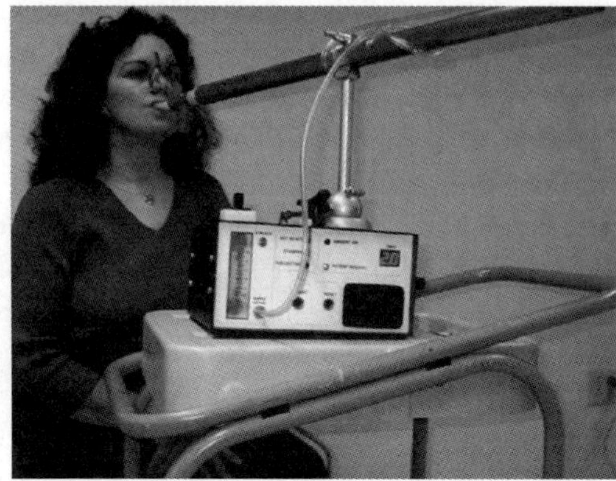

Fig. 1.   The breath collection apparatus (BCA) in use. The patient wears a nose clip and breathes in and out through a valved disposable mouthpiece into the BCA for 2.0 min. The patient inspires room air and expires into a breath reservoir which is open to room air at its distal end. There is virtually no resistance in the system, and breath samples may be readily collected even from elderly patients and those with respiratory disease. The breath reservoir separates alveolar from dead space breath, and alveolar breath is pumped from the reservoir through a sorbent trap, a stainless steel tube packed with two grades of activated carbon which capture the VOCs in 1.0 L breath. A 1.0 L sample of room is also collected onto a second trap. Every patient is given a clean new disposable valved mouthpiece, and there is no risk of cross infection.

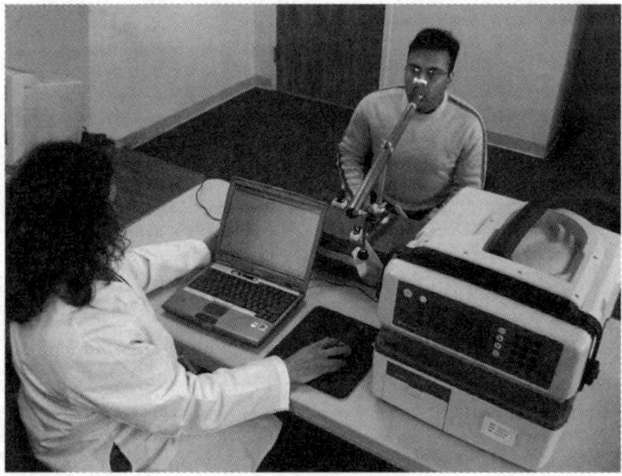

Fig. 2.   The Breathscanner 1.0 in use. The patient is shown respiring into a breath reservoir as in Figure 1. Alveolar breath is pumped from a sampling port (center, below end of breath reservoir) into an ATD/GC/MS instrument (bottom right). Analytic results are displayed on a computer screen (at left) within minutes. The MB-CAD is completely mobile and can function with no external power source by switching to an internal powerpack.

user-friendly because it is simple to operate. Also, the analysis employs "off-the-shelf" instruments that identify and quantify breath VOCs with picomolar sensitivity (10^{-12} mol/L).

We have subsequently developed a more advanced device, the Breathscanner 1.0, which interfaces the BCA with a mobile ATD/GC-MS system (Fig. 2). The advantage of this system is that it moves breath VOC analysis out of the laboratory to the point of care — for the first time.

These advanced instruments have generated an entirely new problem: researchers can easily find themselves overwhelmed by an avalanche of data! Gone are the days when breath data from a few major VOCs in a small number of subjects could be readily stored and analyzed on paper records. We have found it necessary to employ advanced relational databases in a linked network of computers in order to cope with the mass of data from large multicenter studies.

3. Some Problems Involved in Breath Analysis

Analysis of breath VOCs using advanced instruments has generated some other fascinating new problems and solutions.

3.1. *The Background Air Problem*

Some of the VOCs in alveolar breath are also present in room air in approximately similar concentrations.[3] A surprising number of investigators have elected to ignore this problem, and publications about breath VOCs continue to appear in the peer-reviewed literature in which VOCs in background air are not reported. The results of such studies are probably meaningless, since there is no way to distinguish the breath "signal" from the "noise" of ambient air contamination. This potential problem is discussed in several chapters in this book. We and others initially attempted to cope with this problem by supplying patients with ultra pure hydrocarbon-free air to breathe for a few minutes, in an attempt to flush out ambient air contamination from the lungs, before measuring the uncontaminated VOC signal in alveolar breath. These attempts failed, because we rapidly learned that even the purest (and most expensive) hydrocarbon-free air was only clean down to millimolar (10^{-3} mol/L) concentrations; when assayed at picomolar sensitivity (*i.e.* with nine orders-of-magnitude more sensitivity), heavy contamination was invariably encountered. We now routinely collect and analyze two VOC samples, one of alveolar breath and one of room air, and then subtract the air background from the breath signal (Fig. 3).

When we employ the convention of calculating the alveolar gradient (concentration of a VOC in alveolar breath minus its concentration in room air), it is apparent that some VOCs are present in greater concentrations in breath than in room air, and vice versa for others. If the alveolar gradient is positive then endogenous synthesis exceeds clearance, whereas if the alveolar gradient is negative, the room air VOCs are cleared from the body by metabolism or excretion more rapidly than it is synthesized.[4] It is interesting to note that humans are frequently vilified for polluting the environment, but seldom given credit for clearing VOCs from the environment with every breath!

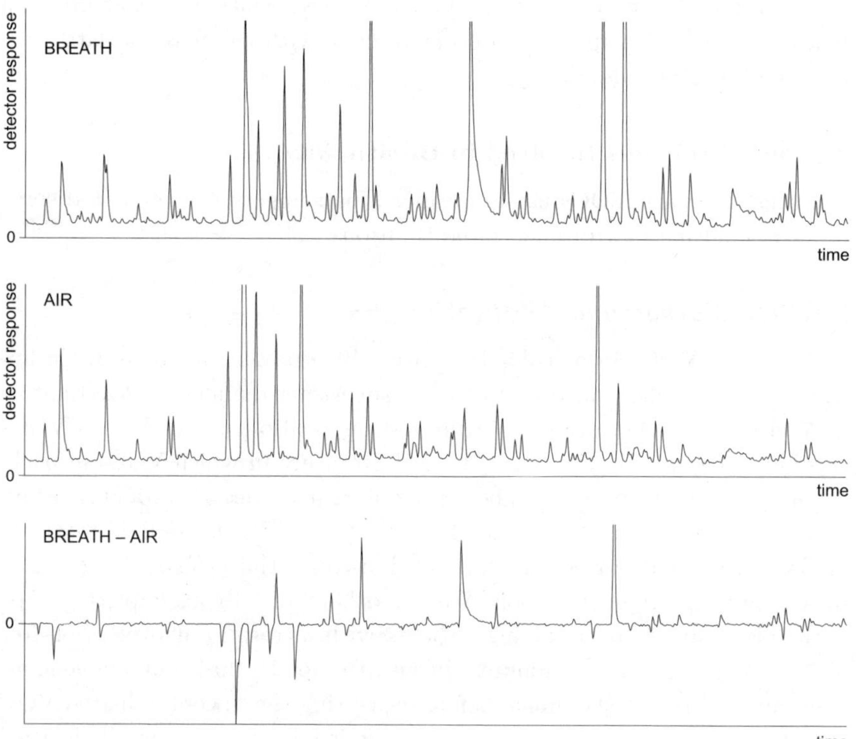

Fig. 3.   VOCs in alveolar air and breath: The upper panel displays a chromatogram of VOCs in a sample of normal human alveolar breath, and the middle panel displays a chromatogram of VOCs in room air collected immediately afterwards. The lower panel displays a subtraction chromatogram of alveolar breath minus room air. The positive peaks represent VOCs that are excreted in the breath in greater concentrations than in background room air, demonstrating endogenous synthesis. The negative peaks represent VOCs in room air that are cleared from the body by metabolism or excretion.

3.2. *Markers of Oxidative Stress*

One of the great strengths of breath testing has been its ability to identify biomarkers of oxidative stress.[5] Breath tests for lipid peroxidation products such as ethane and pentane have been employed for so long that it has hardened into a virtual orthodoxy that they are the sole definitive biomarkers of oxidative stress in breath. This is not the case. We have shown that advanced breath analysis technology can identify a much larger repertoire of biomarkers of oxidative stress in breath — the breath methylated alkane contour (BMAC), comprising up to 107 different C_4–C_{20} alkanes and their monomethylated derivatives[6] (Fig. 4). This has provided a powerful new

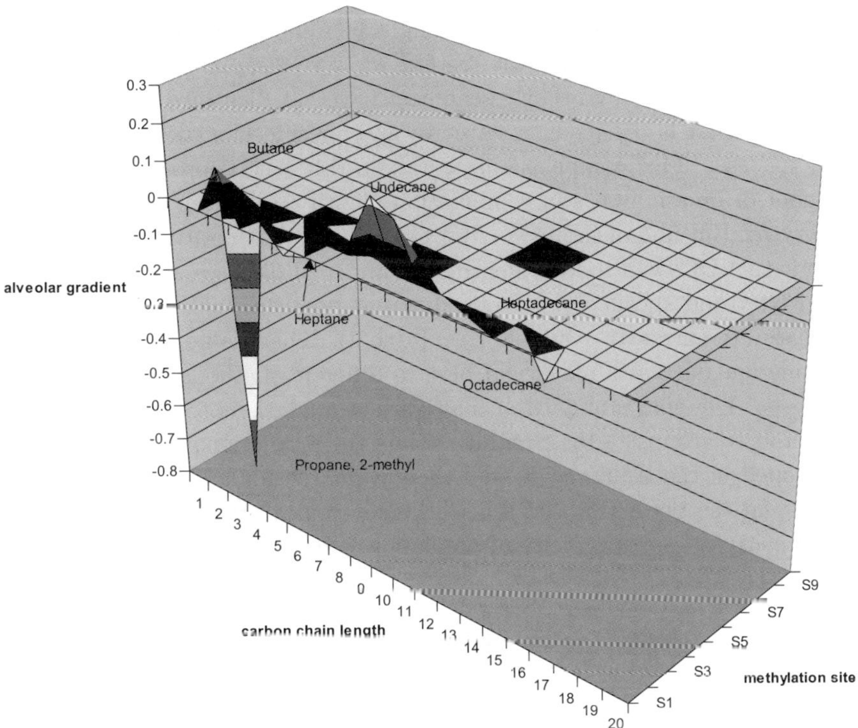

Fig. 4.   Breath methylated alkane contour (BMAC) in a healthy 30 year old female volunteer. The alkanes and the methylated alkanes in a breath VOC sample collected with the BCA were analyzed by gas chromatography and mass spectroscopy. The x-axis is the length of the carbon chain in the alkane or methylated alkane, the z-axis is the site of monomethylation, and the y-axis is the alveolar gradient (abundance in breath minus abundance in room air).

tool for the identification of breath markers of a diversity of diseases including heart transplant rejection,[7,8] lung cancer,[9,10] breast cancer,[11] pre-eclampsia of pregnancy,[12] and unstable angina,[13] as well as demonstrating increased oxidative stress in diabetes mellitus,[14] aging,[15] and oxygen breathing.[16]

3.3. *The Multiple Biomarker Problem*

The traditional diagnostic paradigm in clinical medicine has been one biomarker in the blood for one disease. Thus, diseases such as syphilis and HIV infection are routinely diagnosed with confidence based on the results of a single serological marker of infection. We and other researchers formerly entertained hopes that we might be able to repeat this diagnostic performance with a breath test. So far, we were disappointed in this hope — neither we nor any other researchers have yet identified a single VOC in breath that is, by itself, a sensitive and specific biomarker of a particular disease. This compelled us to take a different approach — could a number of breath VOCs in combination identify a disease? This has been a very fruitful line of inquiry — we have found that multivariate analysis of breath VOCs can indeed identify a number of diseases with remarkable sensitivity and specificity. Several different powerful tools of multivariate analysis are currently available (see Table 3). There is no single best tool — different data sets may yield best to different methods of multivariate analysis. The gold standard of multivariate analysis is to divide the data set into two groups — the training set and the prediction set. The model is developed in the training set, and then evaluated for its ability to predict disease in the prediction set, where the key indicators of performance are the sensitivity and specificity of prediction.

Table 3.   Candidate techniques for multivariate analysis of breath VOCs

Discriminant analysis	Statistica
Logistic regression	SPSS
Pattern recognition analysis	Pirouette
Data mining	PolyAnalyst
Fuzzy logic	IMD, Interrelation Miner

4. The Future of Breath Testing Technology

The best available breath testing instruments of today are heavy, bulky and expensive. This is probably unavoidable, because at this stage of our knowledge, sophisticated analytical instruments are indispensable in order to perform the research that is needed to identify the VOC profiles of disease. However, breath VOC analysis could probably be achieved using much smaller and more convenient devices. Only two requirements need to be fulfilled: first, it is necessary to identify a reduced universe of diagnostic marker VOCs. We do not need to routinely assay 200 breath VOCs with ATD/GC-MS if a diagnosis can be made with much smaller number of VOCs. We have shown with our studies of lung cancer and breast cancer that as few as 10 VOCs may be all that is needed. The next step is to develop detectors specific for these VOCs that are small, light, battery powered, inexpensive, and sufficiently sensitive. Detectors that fulfill these requirements are not yet available, but they are on the horizon. Candidate technologies include laser spectrophotometry on microchips and surface acoustic wave detectors. So if we dare to peer into the future, the next generation of breath testing may focus on hand-held devices that employ the diagnostic algorithms developed with present-day methods, but they will be applied using newer and more portable analytic technology. Perhaps the doctor of tomorrow will carry an advanced laboratory in her white coat pocket, along with a stethoscope (Fig. 5)?

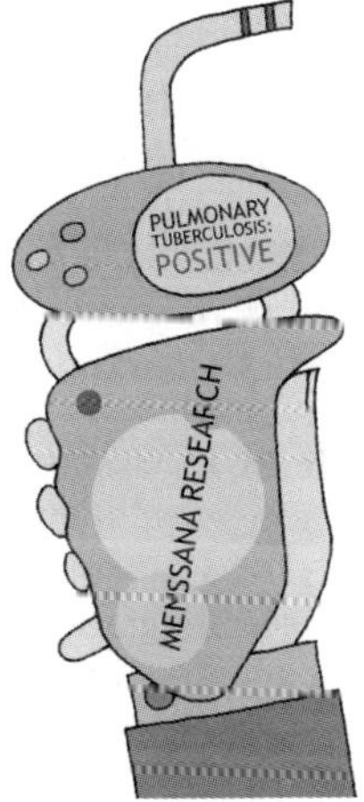

- Hand-held, battery powered
- Breath VOC detectors: laser spectrophotometers
- Picomolar sensitivity
- Diagnostic algorithms programmed on microchips
- Rapid, accurate diagnosis at point of care

Fig. 5.   The next-generation breath tester?

Acknowledgements

Research in this report was supported by SBIR award 5R44HL070411-03 from the National Heart Lung and Blood Institute of the National Institutes of Health. Michael Phillips is President and CEO of Menssana Research, Inc.

References

1. Phillips M. Breath tests in medicine. *Sci Am* 1992; **267**: 74–79.
2. Phillips M. Method for the collection and assay of volatile organic compounds in breath. *Anal Biochem* 1997; **247**: 272–278.
3. Phillips M, Greenberg J, Sabas M. Alveolar gradient of pentane in normal human breath. *Free Radic Res* 1994; **20**: 333–337.
4. Phillips M, Herrera J, Krishnan S, Zain M, Greenberg J, Cataneo RN. Variation in volatile organic compounds in the breath of normal humans. *J Chromatogr B Biomed Sci Appl* 1999; **729**: 75–88.
5. Kneepkens CM, Lepage G, Roy CC. The potential of the hydrocarbon breath test as a measure of lipid peroxidation. *Free Radic Biol Med* 1994; **17**: 127–160.
6. Phillips M, Cataneo RN, Greenberg J, Gunawardena R, Naidu A, Rahbari-Oskoui F. Effect of age on the breath methylated alkane contour, a display of apparent new markers of oxidative stress. *J Lab Clin Med* 2000; **136**: 243–249.
7. Phillips M, Boehmer JP, Cataneo RN, Cheema T, Eisen HJ, Fallon JT, Fisher PE, Gass A, Greenberg J, Kobashigawa J, Mancini D, Rayburn B, Zucker MJ. Heart Allograft Rejection: Detection with Breath Alkanes in Low Levels (the HARDBALL study). *The Journal of Heart and Lung Transplantation* 2004; **23**: 701–708.
8. Phillips M, Boehmer J, Cataneo R, Cheema T, Eisen H, Fallon J, Fisher P, Gass A, Greenberg J, Kobashigawa J, Mancini D, Rayburn B, Zucker M. Prediction of heart transplant rejection with a breath test for markers of oxidative stress. *Am J Cardiol* 2004; **94**: 1593–1594.
9. Phillips M, Gleeson K, Hughes JM, Greenberg J, Cataneo RN, Baker L, McVay WP. Volatile organic compounds in breath as markers of lung cancer: a cross-sectional study. *Lancet* 1999; **353**: 1930–1933.
10. Phillips M, Cataneo RN, Cummin AR, Gagliardi AJ, Gleeson K, Greenberg J, Maxfield RA, Rom WN. Detection of lung cancer with volatile markers in the breath. *Chest* 2003; **123**: 2115–2123.
11. Phillips M, Cataneo RN, Ditkoff BA, Fisher P, Greenberg J, Gunawardena R, Kwon CS, Rahbari-Oskoui F, Wong C. Volatile markers of breast cancer in the breath. *Breast J* 2003; **9**: 184–191.
12. Moretti M, Phillips M, Abouzeid A, Cataneo R, Greenberg J. Increased breath markers of oxidative stress in normal pregnancy and in preeclampsia. *American Journal of Obstetrics and Gynecology* 2004; **190**: 1184–1190.

13. Phillips M, Cataneo R, Greenberg J, Grodman R, Salazar M. Breath markers of oxidative stress in patients with unstable angina. *Heart Disease* 2003; **5**: 95–99.

14. Phillips M, Cataneo R, Cheema T, Greenberg J. Increased breath biomarkers of oxidative stress in diabetes mellitus. *Clinica Chimica Acta* 2004; **344**: 189–194.

15. Phillips M, Cataneo R, Greenberg J, Gunawardena R, Rahbari-Oskoui F. Increased oxidative stress in younger as well as in older humans. *Clinical Chimica Acta* 2003; **328**: 83–86.

16. Phillips M, Cataneo R, Greenberg J, Grodman R, Gunawardena R, Naidu A. Effects of oxygen on breath markers of oxidative stress. *European Respiratory Journal* 2003; **21**: 48–51.

EXHALED BREATH GAS
AS A BIOCHEMICAL PROBE DURING SLEEP

A. AMANN

Department of Anesthesia and General Intensive Care,
Innsbruck Medical University,
A-6020 Innsbruck, Austria
and
Department of Environmental Sciences,
Swiss Federal Institute of Technology,
ETH Hönggerberg, CH-8093 Zurich, Switzerland

S. TELSER AND L. HOFER

Department of Psychiatry, Sleep Laboratory,
Innsbruck Medical University,
A-6020 Innsbruck, Austria

A. SCHMID

Department of Anesthesia and General Intensive Care,
Innsbruck Medical University,
A-6020 Innsbruck, Austria
and
Department of Psychiatry, Sleep Laboratory,
Innsbruck Medical University,
A-6020 Innsbruck, Austria

H. HINTERHUBER

Department of Psychiatry, Sleep Laboratory,
Innsbruck Medical University,
A-6020 Innsbruck, Austria

1. Introduction

The physical, biochemical and molecular biological methods of medical diagnostics have been developed very rapidly in recent decades. The main focus has been on blood and urine diagnostics. The diagnostics based on exhaled human breath,[1-21] on the other hand, are much less developed and not yet widely utilized in clinical practice.

Volatile organic compounds, VOCs, in breath are produced by metabolic processes in the body, by bacteria in the gut,[22] or by both. Isoprene, for example, is a component which is (not necessarily exclusively) produced from dimethyl allyl pyrophosphate, an intermediate compound in the cholesterine synthesis pathway.[23] For a few substances, the biochemical origins are known. For most of the approximately 3000 substances apparently detected in different persons' breath,[24] biochemical background information is not available. Some of these substances result from inhalation of contaminants in room air, jet fuel[25] or gasoline.

An important and underestimated aspect concerns the sites of production of various endogenous compounds[26–29] and different blood–gas kinetics. Modeling of the influence of hemodynamics and lung mechanics (see Ref. 30, on page 361 of this book) on the concentration patterns of VOCs will therefore provide more information about the production and elimination rates of these compounds. This is of particular interest for isoprene, the concentration of which in exhaled breath depends considerably on both the heart rate and the breathing rate, as well as on breath volume. A more detailed knowledge of the behavior of other marker substances such as lipophilic hydrocarbons or aldehydes under different hemodynamic and respiratory conditions is surely required. The practical use of concentration patterns of such compounds for cancer screening, for example, could then be complemented by information about their variability due to changes in heart and breathing rates, as well as due to changes in breath volume.

On the other hand, substances in the breath, such as isoprene, could be used to estimate ventilation–perfusion ratios and their distribution[31] within the lung. At present, such estimates can only be given by injecting inert gases with different physicochemical properties (*e.g.* solubility in water and in lipophilic compartments) into the blood stream and measuring concentrations in exhaled breath. The celebrated multiple inert gas elimination technique (MIGET), developed by Wagner and West,[32–36] gives detailed information about the distribution of ventilation–perfusion ratios, but is not easily applicable in the clinical environment, especially in the intensive care unit, ICU. It may be worthwhile to make use of endogenous or ubiquitous exogenous substances to obtain at least part of the information supplied by MIGET technology. Hence, the scope for exploiting volatile compounds in breath might be much broader than previously envisaged.

Exhaled breath samples can be obtained essentially non-invasively by use of a bag, a mask or a catheter in the nasal cavity. Continuous sampling is possible, and on-line analysis of the samples by mass spectrometric or laser spectroscopic methods provides some valuable information on the biochemical status and its change during longer periods of time. This is of particular interest in the field of sleep medicine, where continuous sampling of blood or urine is not easy. In this context it is interesting to observe that nitric oxide has been suggested as one of the substances involved in the suppression or the support of sleep[37,38] or certain sleep stages.[39,40] Nevertheless, volatile compounds are only a small subsection of the biochemical metabolites. Non-volatile compounds such as interleukins, NFκB, prostaglandins, TNF-α, glucocorticoids, muramyl peptides,[41−44] which might be interesting in the context of sleep behaviour, do not appear in breath gas. Our ultimate goal, therefore, is certainly *not* to explain or model sleep generation and regulation and its disturbances in terms of volatile compounds only. It is much more important to keep an eye on *both* volatile and non-volatile compounds, exploit the non-invasive exhaled breath-based results for clinical applications as far as possible and include blood- or urine-based techniques where this is necessary.

Breath-gas analysis in the sleep laboratory is not necessarily restricted to sleep-related problems. For example, we are interested to learn about the (overnight) dynamics of the concentrations of those hydrocarbons and aldehydes, which have been proposed as candidates for the screening of lung or breast cancer.[1,2,45] Similarly, derived quantities (such as the quotient of the concentrations) suggested for identification of diseases might therefore be tested in such a setting. We therefore suggest that on-line analysis of VOCs in exhaled breath can provide insight into the metabolic processes, complement the information about brain activity obtained by polysomnography (PSG),[4] and serve as a "testbed" for exhaled breath-based disease markers.

In this chapter, preliminary results on the concentration time series of two compounds, methanol and isoprene, are presented. Thus, we focus on substances that can readily be detected by proton-transfer-reaction mass spectrometry (PTR MS), which are present in reasonable concentrations (close to 100 ppbv) and which are not usually present as exogenous contaminants in the sleep laboratory. We do not claim that these substances are particularly interesting for sleep research, but take them as test substances to show that interesting (overnight) dynamics occurs. In addition, breath isoprene is a substance of potential value for therapy control of dyslipidemias.

2. Methods

Our experimental setup consisting of a proton-transfer-reaction mass spectrometer (PTR-MS, Ionicon FDT-s) combined with polysomnography (PSG, Nihon-Kohden EEG 4317F), adapted for the simultaneous on-line monitoring of the exhaled breath of sleeping individuals and of electrophysiological sleep variables. Exhaled air was continuously sampled through a catheter in the nasal cavity and passed to the PTR-MS through perfluoro-alkoxy co-polymer tubing heated to 43 °C. The reported ionic mass-charge-ratios, m/z are those of the protonated neutral species (molecular mass + 1 u) according to the ionization process used in PTR-MS.[46,47] The concentration time series are partly smoothed using moving average techniques. Sleep stages were determined according to the rules of Rechtschaffen and Kales.[48] The breathing rate and pulse (heart) frequency were derived from the recorded thorax excursion and ECG data. All participating volunteers, 10 healthy men aged 20 to 28, spent 3 nights in the sleep laboratory. The first night was spent becoming familiar with the experimental setup (adaptation night). Subsequently, the volunteers were deprived of sleep for about 40 hours, *i.e.*, they did not sleep for one night, before returning to the laboratory to sleep (the night after sleep deprivation is called the recovery night). Thereafter, they underwent their daily routine. During the subsequent night, they returned again to the laboratory and slept there for the third and last time (normal night).

3. Observations and Results

Figures 1, 2 and 3 show the concentration time series for ionic masses 33 (tentatively methanol) and 69 (tentatively isoprene) during one particular night. In addition, the concentration of carbon dioxide (CO_2) is shown, which acts a control factor for the detection of any obvious artifacts (*e.g.*, to check if exhaled gas enters the analytical unit). These examples demonstrate that their can be considerable dynamical effects in the concentration time series for both ionic masses 33 and 69. Isoprene, in particular, fluctuates greatly, which is partly due to changes in the pulse and breathing rates (Fig. 4). In the example of Fig. 3, the progression of sleep stages is also shown. The isoprene concentration is influenced by the pulse frequency (see Fig. 4), breathing rate and breathing volume (not shown). It tends to increase during the night (Fig. 5). There is no obvious difference between normal nights and recovery nights. The methanol concentration decreases during normal nights (Fig. 6), whereas it stays rather constant during recovery nights (Fig. 7).

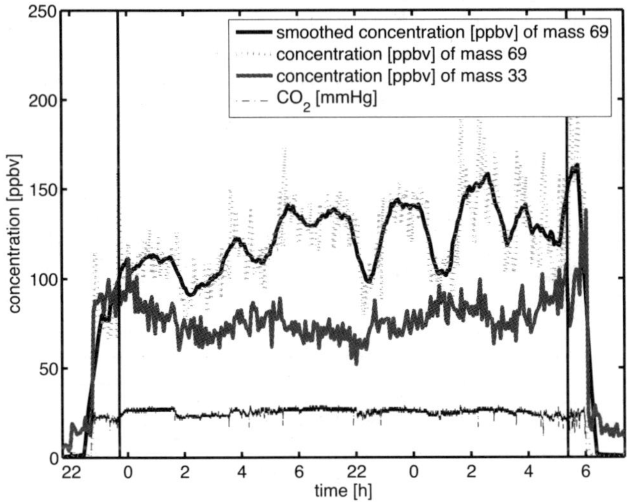

Fig. 1. Concentrations [ppbv] of ionic mass 33 (methanol) and ionic mass 69 (isoprene), and the concentration of CO_2 [mmHg] for one particular night. For isoprene, a smoothed version (moving average) is also shown.

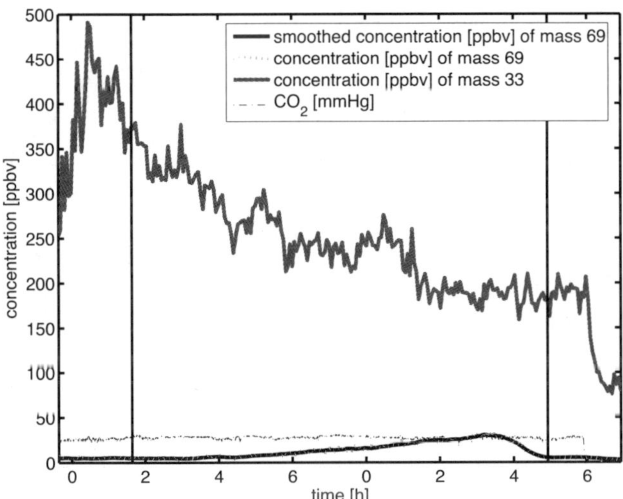

Fig. 2. Analogous to Fig. 1. The isoprene concentration is low, increases overnight until about 05.30 a.m. and then decreases during the morning hours. The volunteer in this case is a hobby marathon runner.

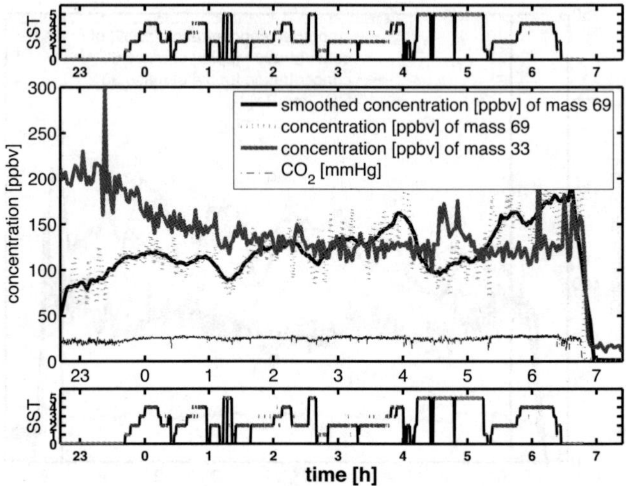

Fig. 3.   Analogous to Figs 1 and 2 (middle panel), but also showing the hypnogram of the particular proband (= progression of sleep stages; upper and lower panel)

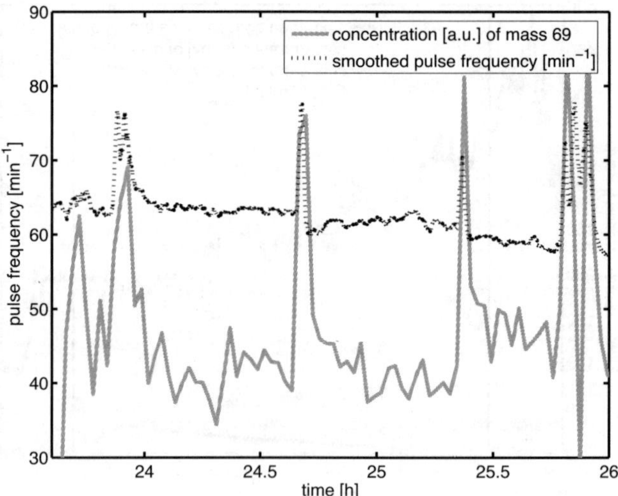

Fig. 4.   Variation of the breath concentration of isoprene (arbitrary units) with time (hours) and smoothed (moving average) pulse (heart) frequency (for one particular night).   The moving average of the pulse frequency has been made over 100 s; the isoprene concentration is sampled every 106 s.

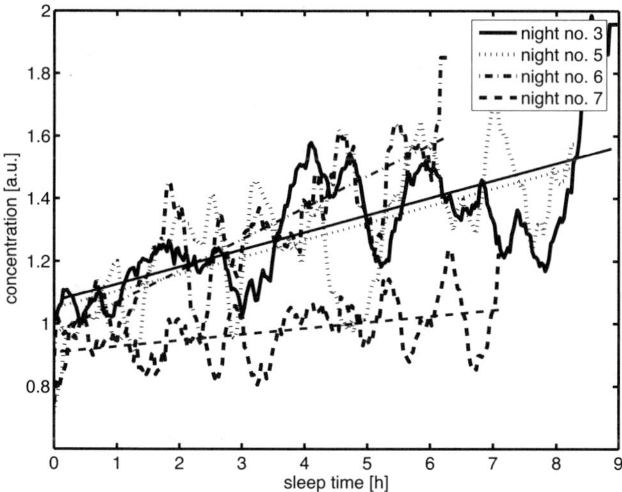

Fig. 5.   Normalized concentration for mass 69 (isoprene) for different volunteers during normal nights. Normalization of concentrations to 1 refers to $t_0 = 30$ min sleep time (*i.e.*, the concentration at $t_0 = 30$ min sleep time is arbitrarily set to 1). Four different representative nights have been chosen for illustration.

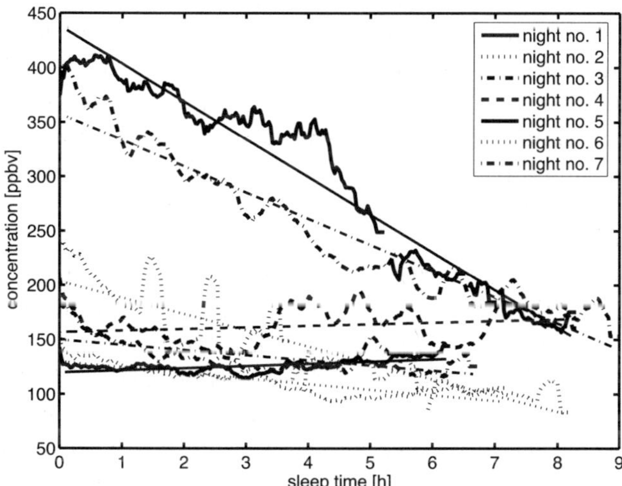

Fig. 6.   Concentration [ppbv] for mass 33 (methanol) for different volunteers during "normal" nights. If the concentration is high, it shows a tendency to decrease; if the concentration is low, it shows a tendency to remain constant.

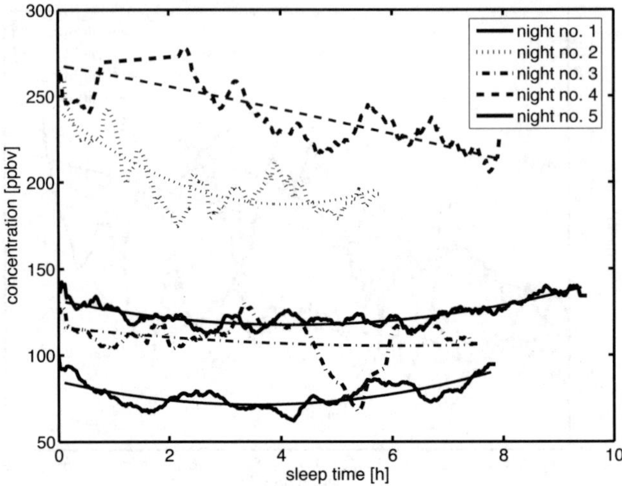

Fig. 7.　Concentration [ppbv] for mass 33 (methanol) for different volunteers in nights after sleep deprivation. Concentrations decrease slower than in normal nights or remain approximately constant.

4. Discussion

Breath gas analysis is non-invasive and offers the possibility of on-line measurements, such that (restricted) on-line information about the biochemical processes occurring during sleep can be obtained. Extensive quality control is still unavailable: room air contaminants, influences of the hemodynamics and lung mechanics, and measurement artefacts can lead to results which are easily misinterpreted. In addition, bacterial metabolization of food in the gut with the production of volatiles observed in breath has to be taken into account.

The evolving concentrations of VOCs, such as acetone, methanol, ethanol, acetaldehyde and isoprene, reflect biochemical processes. Sometimes it is more convenient to consider derived quantities: for example, the time evolution of the ratio of acetaldehyde to ethanol concentrations reflects the activity of alcohol dehydrogenase during the night. The variation of the breath isoprene concentration is special, since its concentration varies with pulse and breathing rates.

The results reported in this chapter may be spoiled by inaccurate concentration values, and are thus preliminary observations only. In fact, concentration measurements may be influenced by condensed water droplets selectively dissolving hydrophilic compounds, and the tubing between volunteers and the PTR-MS instrument may selectively absorb and desorb certain substances.

Breath gas analysis in sleeping individuals is non-invasive and enables us to monitor metabolic processes on-line, thus complementing the electrophysiological information obtained by polysomnography. Therefore, we believe that breath analysis has great potential as a source of information additional to the standard polysomnography.

Acknowledgement

We are grateful for the provision of a research grant by the "Medizinischer Forschungsfonds der TILAK" of the University Clinics of Innsbruck. In particular, we thank its Dir. Dr. Herbert Weissenböck for his continuous support. A. A. appreciates support by the Bernhard Lang research association. This work was supported in part by the "Jubiläumsfonds der Österreichischen Nationalbank" (project no. 9647).

References

1. Phillips M, Cataneo RN, Ditkoff BA, Fisher P, Greenberg J, Gunawardena R, Kwon CS, Rahbari-Oskoui F, Wong C. Volatile markers of breast cancer in the breath. *Breast J* 2003; **9**: 184–191.
2. Phillips M, Cataneo RN, Cummin AR, Gagliardi AJ, Gleeson K, Greenberg J, Maxfield RA, Rom WN. Detection of lung cancer with volatile markers in the breath. *Chest* 2003; **123**: 2115–2123.
3. Phillips M, Cataneo RN, Greenberg J, Grodman R, Gunawardena R, Naidu A. Effect of oxygen on breath markers of oxidative stress. *Eur Respir J* 2003; **21**: 48–51.
4. Amann A, Poupart G, Telser S, Ledochowski M, Schmid A, Mechtcheriakov S. Applications of breath gas analysis in medicine. *Int J Mass Spectrometry* 2004; **239**: 227–233.
5. Phillips M. Breath tests in medicine. *Sci Am* 1992; **267**: 74–79.
6. Cope KA, Watson MT, Foster M, Sehnert SS, Risby TH. Effects of Ventilation on the Collection of Exhaled Breath in Humans. *J Appl Physiol* 2003.
7. Risby TH, Jiang L, Stoll S, Ingram D, Spangler E, Heim J, Cutler R, Roth GS, Rifkind JM. Breath ethane as a marker of reactive oxygen species during manipulation of diet and oxygen tension in rats. *J Appl Physiol* 1999; **86**: 617–622.
8. Risby TH, Sehnert SS. Clinical application of breath biomarkers of oxidative stress status. *Free Radic Biol Med* 1999; **27**: 1182–1192.
9. Risby TH, Jiang L, Stoll S, Ingram D, Spangler E, Heim J, Cutler R, Roth GS, Rifkind JM. Breath ethane as a marker of reactive oxygen species during manipulation of diet and oxygen tension in rats. *J Appl Physiol* 1999; **86**: 617–622.

10. Risby TH. Volatile Organic Compounds as Markers in Normal and Diseased States. In: Marczin N, Yacoub MH, eds. *Disease Markers in Exhaled Breath*, IOS Press, 2002.

11. Andreoni KA, Kazui M, Cameron DE, Nyhan D, Sehnert SS, Rohde CA, Bulkley GB, Risby TH. Ethane: a marker of lipid peroxidation during cardiopulmonary bypass in humans. *Free Radic Biol Med* 1999; **26**: 439–445.

12. Scholpp J, Schubert JK, Miekisch W, Geiger K. Breath markers and soluble lipid peroxidation markers in critically ill patients. *Clin Chem Lab Med* 2002; **40**: 587–594.

13. Schubert JK, Noldge-Schomburg GF. Can the limits of intensive care management be defined? [in German] *Zentralbl Chir* 2001; **126**: 717–721.

14. Miekisch W, Schubert JK, Vagts DA, Geiger K. Analysis of volatile disease markers in blood. *Clin Chem* 2001; **47**: 1053–1060.

15. Schubert JK, Spittler KH, Braun G, Geiger K, Guttmann J. CO_2-controlled sampling of alveolar gas in mechanically ventilated patients. *J Appl Physiol* 2001; **90**: 486–492.

16. Schubert JK, Geiger K. Importance and perspectives of breath analysis. [in German] *Anasthesiol Intensivmed Notfallmed Schmerzther* 1999; **34**: 391–395.

17. Schubert JK, Esteban-Loos I, Geiger K, Guttmann J. *In vivo* evaluation of a new method for chemical analysis of volatile components in the respiratory gas of mechanically ventilated patients. *Technol Health Care* 1999; **7**: 29–37.

18. Diskin AM, Španěl P, Smith D. Time variation of ammonia, acetone, isoprene and ethanol in breath: a quantitative SIFT-MS study over 30 days. *Physiol Meas* 2003; **24**: 107–119.

19. Diskin AM, Španěl P, Smith D. Increase of acetone and ammonia in urine headspace and breath during ovulation quantified using selected ion flow tube mass spectrometry. *Physiol Meas* 2003; **24**: 191–199.

20. Smith D, Wang T, Španěl P. On-line, simultaneous quantification of ethanol, some metabolites and water vapour in breath following the ingestion of alcohol. *Physiol Meas* 2002; **23**: 477–489.

21. Smith D, Engel B, Diskin AM, Španěl P, Davies SJ. Comparative measurements of total body water in healthy volunteers by online breath deuterium measurement and other near-subject methods. *Am J Clin Nutr* 2002; **76**: 1295–1301.

22. Romagnuolo J, Schiller D, Bailey RJ. Using breath tests wisely in a gastroenterology practice: an evidence-based review of indications and pitfalls in interpretation. *Am J Gastroenterol* 2002; **97**: 1113–1126.

23. Sharkey TD. Isoprene synthesis by plants and animals. *Endeavour* 1996; **20**: 74–78.

24. Phillips M, Herrera J, Krishnan S, Zain M, Greenberg J, Cataneo RN. Variation in volatile organic compounds in the breath of normal humans. *J Chromatogr B Biomed Sci Appl* 1999; **729**: 75–88.

25. Tu RH, Mitchell CS, Kay GG, Risby TH. Human exposure to the jet fuel, JP-8. *Aviat Space Environ Med* 2004; **75**: 49–59.

26. Lundberg JO, Weitzberg E, Nordvall SL, Kuylenstierna R, Lundberg JM, Alving K. Primarily nasal origin of exhaled nitric oxide and absence in Kartagener's syndrome. *Eur Respir J* 1994; **7**: 1501–1504.

27. Lundberg JO, Farkas-Szallasi T, Weitzberg E, Rinder J, Lidholm J, Anggaard A, Hokfelt T, Lundberg JM, Alving K. High nitric oxide production in human paranasal sinuses. *Nat Med* 1995; **1**: 370–373.

28. Lundberg JO, Weitzberg E. Nasal nitric oxide in man. *Thorax* 1999; **54**: 947–952.

29. Lundberg JO, Maniscalco M, Sofia M, Lundblad L, Weitzberg E, Maniscalo M. Humming, nitric oxide, and paranasal sinus obstruction. *Jama* 2003; **289**: 302–303.

30. Teschl S, Batzel J, Kappel F. A model of the cardiovascular-respiratory control system with applications to excercise, sleep and congestive heart failure. In: Amann A, Smith D, eds. *Breath Analysis for Clinical Diagnosis and Therapeutic Monitoring,* Singapore: World Scientific, 2005.

31. Wagner PD. Estimation of distributions of ventilation/perfusion ratios. *Ann Biomed Eng* 1981; **9**: 543–556.

32. Wagner PD, Laravuso RB, Goldzimmer E, Naumann PF, West JB. Distribution of ventilation–perfusion ratios in dogs with normal and abnormal lungs. *J Appl Physiol* 1975; **38**: 1099–1109.

33. Wagner PD, Dantzker DR, Dueck R, Clausen JL, West JB. Ventilation–perfusion inequality in chronic obstructive pulmonary disease. *J Clin Invest* 1977; **59**: 203–216.

34. Wagner PD. Information content of inert gas elimination techniques. *Bull Eur Physiopathol Respir* 1982; **18**: 361–372.

35. Roca J, Wagner PD. Contribution of multiple inert gas elimination technique to pulmonary medicine. 1. Principles and information content of the multiple inert gas elimination technique. *Thorax* 1994; **49**: 815–824.

36. Rodriguez-Roisin R, Wagner PD. Clinical relevance of ventilation–perfusion inequality determined by inert gas elimination. *Eur Respir J* 1990; **3**: 469–482.

37. Kapas L, Shibata M, Kimura M, Krueger JM. Inhibition of nitric oxide synthesis suppresses sleep in rabbits. *Am J Physiol* 1994; **266**: R151–157.

38. Kapas L, Fang J, Krueger JM. Inhibition of nitric oxide synthesis inhibits rat sleep. *Brain Res* 1994; **664**: 189–196.

39. Chen Z, Gardi J, Kushikata T, Fang J, Krueger JM. Nuclear factor-kappaB-like activity increases in murine cerebral cortex after sleep deprivation. *Am J Physiol* 1999; **276**: R1812–1818.

40. Chen L, Taishi P, Majde JA, Peterfi Z, Obal F, Jr., Krueger JM. The role of nitric oxide synthases in the sleep responses to tumor necrosis factor-alpha. *Brain Behav Immun* 2004; **18**: 390–398.

41. Krueger JM, Fang J, Taishi P, Chen Z, Kushikata T, Gardi J. Sleep. A physiologic role for IL-1 beta and TNF-alpha. *Ann NY Acad Sci* 1998; **856**: 148–159.

42. Krueger JM, Majde JA. Microbial products and cytokines in sleep and fever regulation. *Crit Rev Immunol* 1994; **14**: 355–379.

43. Krueger JM, Obal FJ, Fang J, Kubota T, Taishi P. The role of cytokines in physiological sleep regulation. *Ann NY Acad Sci* 2001; **933**: 211–221.
44. Obal F, Jr., Krueger JM. Biochemical regulation of non-rapid-eye-movement sleep. *Front Biosci* 2003; **8**: d520–550.
45. Smith D, Wang T, Sule-Suso J, Španěl P, Haj AE. Quantification of acetaldehyde released by lung cancer cells *in vitro* using selected ion flow tube mass spectrometry. *Rapid Commun Mass Spectrom* 2003; **17**: 845–850.
46. Lindinger W, Hansel A, Jordan A. On-line monitoring of volatile organic compounds at pptv levels by means of proton-transfer-reaction mass spectrometry (PTR-MS) medical applications, food control and environmental research. *Int J Mass Spectrom Ion Processes* 1998; **173**: 191–241.
47. Hansel A, Jordan A, Holzinger R, Prazeller P, Vogel W, Lindinger W. Proton transfer reaction mass spectrometry: on-line trace gas analysis at the ppb level. *Int J Mass Spectrom Ion Processes* 1995; **149/150**: 609–619.
48. Rechtschaffen A, Kales A, eds. *A Manual of Standardized Terminology, Techniques, and Scoring System for Sleep Stages of Human Subjects*. Washington, D. C.: Public Health Service — US Government Printing Office, 1968.

ANALYSIS OF BREATH USING SIFT-MS: A COMPARISON OF THE BREATH COMPOSITION OF HEALTHY VOLUNTEERS AND SERIOUSLY-ILL ICU PATIENTS

C. TURNER AND S. WELCH

Silsoe Research Institute,
Wrest Park, Silsoe, Bedford, MK45 4HS, UK

G. BELLINGAN

Department of Critical Care,
Middlesex Hospital,
Mortimer Str., London, W1T 3AA, UK

M. SINGER

Dept of Medicine and Wolfson Institute of Biomedical Research,
University College London,
Middlesex Hospital, Jules Thorn Building, 5th Floor,
Mortimer Str., London W1T 3AA, UK

P. ŠPANĚL

V. Čermák Laboratory, J. Heyrovský Institute of Physical Chemistry,
Academy of Sciences of the Czech Republic,
Dolejškova 3, CZ-182 23 Prague 8, Czech Republic

D. SMITH

Institute of Science and Technology in Medicine,
Medical School, Keele University,
Thornburrow Drive, Hartshill, Stoke-on-Trent, ST4 7QB, UK

1. Introduction

Breath analysis has great potential as a rapid, non-invasive medical diagnostic tool. Selected ion flow tube mass spectrometry (SIFT-MS) is one method for monitoring breath volatile molecules and has previously been developed for the analysis of breath[1,2] and the headspace of body fluids of both healthy volunteers[3] and those with signs of clinical disease.[4] This study examines the use of SIFT-MS in analysing breath of healthy volunteers with a normal diet and under different dietary regimes, including fasting, which was looked at previously.[5] Breath spectra of several ventilated patients in intensive care units with a variety of medical conditions are also presented, and compared to those of the healthy volunteers.

2. Methods

There are two ways of introducing samples into the SIFT-MS instrument: either directly exhaled breath into the sample inlet, or by taking breath samples at a remote site in sampling bags, and then connecting the sampling bags to the sample inlet. In this preliminary study, healthy volunteers provided direct breath samples; ventilated patients provided bag samples. Both sets of samples were taken using the three precursor ions: H_3O^+, NO^+, and O_2^+ to facilitate compound identification.

2.1. *Healthy Volunteers*

Breath samples from healthy volunteers were obtained by asking them to breathe through a disposable mouthpiece directly past the capillary at the entrance to the SIFT-MS instrument, thus displacing the air and ensuring that alveolar breath could be analysed.[1] Three sets of data were obtained. Firstly, samples were taken of three healthy volunteers following a normal dietary regime. Secondly, breath spectra were taken of two volunteers who had fasted for 40 hours, and thirdly, of two volunteers who had followed exactly the same dietary regime for 4 days.

2.2. *Seriously Ill Ventilated Patients*

Bag samples of breath were taken from a number of seriously-ill ventilated patients with a variety of medical conditions in several visits to the intensive care unit (ICU) of Middlesex Hospital, London, UK. Breath samples were taken from some patients on more than one day. The bags were constructed from Nalophan, a polymer of polyethyleneterephthalate, each with a polypropylene and stainless steel fitting to allow ready attachment to the SIFT-MS, which were disposed of after a single use. After taking samples of the exhaled breath from the ventilators, the samples were transported to the laboratory, after which they were incubated at 40 °C for at least 30 minutes and then analysed within 4 hours of acquisition. Control samples were taken while healthy volunteers breathed through the ventilator.

The same subjects also breathed directly into a sample bag and some also provided breath directly into the SIFT-MS instrument at the time of analysis to provide controls. The main difficulty in obtaining breath spectra from ventilated patients is probably not in the use of breath bags, but in obtaining breath from the ventilator exhaust, with the exhaled breath having passed through the HME filters and all ventilator tubing and pipework etc., all of which may either "lose" many trace gases (either through chemical adsorption or condensation of volatile species), or release other trace gases. In the latter case, use of appropriate controls may assist; however, in the case of adsorption or condensation, erroneously low values may be obtained.

3. Results

3.1. *Healthy Volunteers*

Any evaluation of the volatiles present in the breath of patients with clinical conditions should be compared to the range of volatiles present in apparently healthy individuals under various conditions, *e.g.* fasting, feeding, smoking etc. Firstly, mid-morning breath samples were taken from three healthy volunteers and the common breath metabolites present are shown in Table 1 This shows the presence of a various metabolites at normal levels.[6] A compound not included in the table is acetonitrile, which would be expected in the breath of a smoker,[7] and was indeed found in the breath of volunteer 3. However, volunteer 2 is a non-smoker and there is significant acetonitrile present in this breath sample from volunteer 2 and in other breath samples from this volunteer. The reason for this is not clear; it is currently being investigated as to whether any use of acetronitrile in a neighbouring laboratory is responsible for this.

Table 1. Concentrations of common breath metabolites, in parts-per-billion (ppb) in breath samples from three healthy volunteers. Volunteer 3 is a smoker.

Compound	Volunteer 1	Volunteer 2	Volunteer 3
Acetone	330	580	450
Ammonia	560	250	150
Methanol	420	380	70
Ethanol	120	320	125
Propanol	130	50	400
Isoprene	250	110	150

Several breath samples were given and analysed during the 40-hour fast by the two healthy volunteers, which were done at different times, so there were different breath sampling times throughout the fast. Figures 1 and 2 compares the concentrations of some key breath metabolites observed during the 40 hours period. As expected, acetone rises to a high level in the breath of both volunteers during this fasting period, although the maximum values obtained were markedly different. However, it can be seen that in volunteer 1, propanol peaks soon after resuming eating before declining,

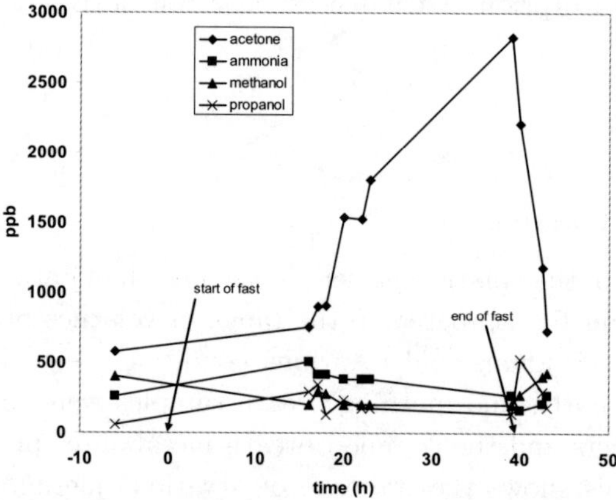

Fig. 1.   Concentrations of acetone, ammonia, methanol and propanol in breath samples before, during and after fasting of volunteer 1 in parts-per-billion (ppb)

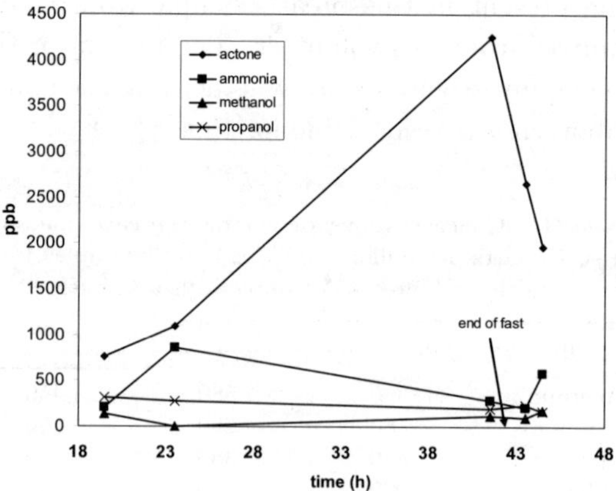

Fig. 2.   Concentrations of acetone, ammonia, methanol and propanol in breath samples during and after fasting of volunteer 2 in parts-per-billion (ppb)

while ammonia and methanol appear to increase after feeding begins. In volunteer 2, only ammonia seems to increase after the end of the fast. The reason for this is not yet known.

The final experiment was to look at the breath of two healthy female volunteers who consumed exactly the same "normal" diet for 4 days, *i.e.* eating the same food at the same time. The only difference in dietary intake was that the consumption of tea (without sugar) was not controlled, and volunteer 1 was a smoker and 2 a non-smoker. The purpose of this experiment was to identify the underlying differences in breath metabolites while excluding the effect of diet. Figures 3 and 4 give the concentrations of common metabolites in the breath volunteers 1 and 2. It can clearly be

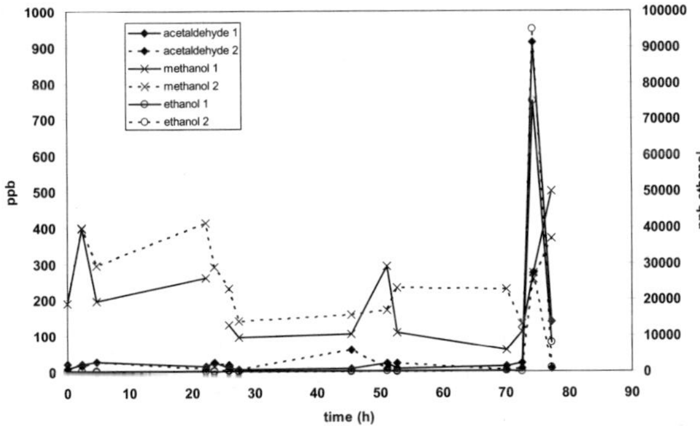

Fig. 3. Concentrations in ppb of ethanol, acetaldehyde, methanol in breath samples from volunteers 1 and 2 after eating the same diet of "normal food" for 77 hours

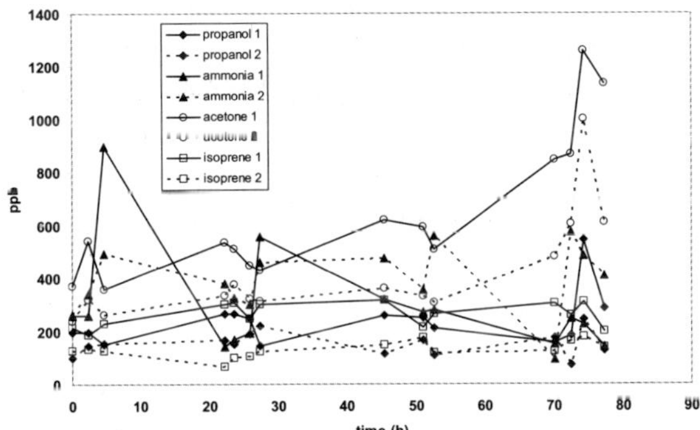

Fig. 4. Concentrations in ppb of propanol, ammonia, acetone and isoprene in breath samples from volunteers 1 and 2 after eating the same diet of "normal food" for 77 hours

seen that volunteer 1 consistently has higher levels of acetone and isoprene, whereas volunteer 2 has consistently higher levels of propanol, and generally higher levels of ammonia. After approximately 40 hours, 2 units of alcohol were consumed by each person; however the levels of ethanol present in the breath of the volunteers were different, as were the levels of acetaldehyde (Fig. 3).

3.2. *ICU Patients*

Several trips were made to the ICU unit in London. Results from the initial visits are presented in Table 2, including analysis of breath taken from a healthy volunteer coupled to a ventilator, the breath of the same volunteer sampled into a bag and sampled directly into the SIFT-MS instrument, and a bag filled with dry air from a compressed air cylinder. Notable findings from this preliminary study are that trace compounds such as acetone and ammonia appear to be present in lower concentrations when sampled through the ventilator. This is probably due to adsorption and condensation within the ventilator which is kept at a temperature of about 25 °C; this is considerably colder than body temperature. On the other hand, formaldehyde and acetaldehyde levels are high, especially in the case of healthy volunteers breathing through the ventilator. Other data (not shown) indicate that the HME filter and tubing emit these aldehydes, especially when new, but their levels decline over time, with only very little acetaldehyde being present after three hours. Formaldehyde persists for longer; still being present after 12 hours albeit at much lower levels. Other notable findings from this study are the surprisingly high levels of ethanol present in patients 7, 9 and 15, and the high levels of propanol in patients 7, 8 and 18. The reason is not immediately obvious, although it is possible that the ethanol has its origin from bacterial infection. Patient 7 suffered duodenitis and liver disease; patient 9 with severe blood loss following AAA (abdominal aortic aneurism) repair; patient 15 with pneumonia; patient 8 with bronchopneumonia and patient 18 with myocardial infarction and pulmonary oedema.

A second set of data was obtained by sampling the breath of all ventilated patients at the ICU over the course of a week. Again, high propanol was measured in the breath of a number of patients: MK (suffering pancreatitis); JR suffering heart failure; RA following AAA repair; and HC following cardiac arrest. Higher than expected levels of acetone were also found in the breath of two patients: MM, who was being fed parenterally,

Table 2. Concentrations of breath compounds in ppb of ill patients and healthy volunteers from an initial visit to the ICU unit in Middlesex hospital. "HV": healthy volunteer; "DB": direct breath into SIFT-MS; "vent": sample taken from volunteer on ventilator; "bag": bag filled with dry air

	Formaldehyde ppb	Acetaldehyde ppb	Acetone ppb	Propanol ppb	Isoprene ppb	Methanol ppb	Ethanol ppb	Ammonia ppb
Bag	0	12	6	9	0	111	0	0
HV in bag	0	0	204	91	0	538	0	978
HV DB	0	0	294	120	48	250	191	487
HV vent	505	764	152	79	65	186	82	1614
Bed No. 15	3	60	167	150	0	48	3694	1
Bed No. 9	618	203	48	92	97	361	9136	17
Bed No. 18	0	72	5	788	0	0	518	15
Bed No. 8	376	128	240	691	0	173	689	108
Bed No. 14	376	74	190	136	72	82	69	55
Bed No. 7	0	0	163	2176	0	98	1915	24
Bed No. 17	816	276	137	270	174	170	71	24

suffering from peritonitis and septic shock and another patient, PC, who suffered AIDS-related acute respiratory distress syndrome. PC was very ill, and his decline was also marked by a sudden, rapid increase in isoprene concentration indicating oxidative stress. Isoprene in breath originates mostly from the decomposition of dimethylallyldiphosphate, a precursor of cholesterol and other isoprenoids.[8]

3.2.1. *Nitric oxide, nitrogen dioxide, and nitrous acid*

Samples were taken on three successive days from patient PC, suffering ARDS, who was prescribed nitric oxide (NO) — a selective pulmonary vasodilator. He was given NO at a concentration of 20 ppm in 100% oxygen on the first two sampling days; when the third sample was taken on day 3, the NO had been reduced to 11 ppm. SIFT-MS analysis of breath samples shows the presence of NO_2 in the ventilator exhaust at levels of 18 ppm, 25 ppm and 4 ppm on each of the three days respectively. In addition, high levels of HNO_2 (nitrous acid) were found to be present in the sample bags of exhaled breath. The presence of NO_2 is expected, and is produced very quickly in the body and ventilator circuit from the reaction of NO with oxygen.[9,10] NO_2 is toxic, and the levels should be closely monitored. The production of HNO_2 is less understood. Some conversion from NO to NO_2 and also some conversion to HNO_2 is due to reactions occurring in the breath bags in the three hours between sampling and analysis during sample transport. It is also possible that the HNO_2 could have arisen in breath because the blood pH was lower than the optimal pH of 7.4, having dropped to between 7.04 and 7.19 on the days of sampling.

HNO_2 was also found to have present in the sample bag containing the breath of another patient, GA, who sustained severe neurological damage following head trauma. He was ventilated with 30% oxygen, and was prescribed antibiotics due to an elevated temperature of 38.6 °C during the 3 successive days of sampling. However, the patient was not believed to be in sepsis, with the prescribed antibiotics being precautionary. Air contamination from NO or NO_2 from other patients in the ICU has been ruled out due to the ventilated gas mixtures being produced outside the unit, and the air handling system installed within the ICU. The origin of this HNO_2 has not yet been discovered.

4. Conclusions

Direct breath samples from healthy volunteers and bag samples of breath from seriously-ill ICU patients have been analysed. Direct breath sampling is more sensitive; however, this is currently impractical in monitoring ICU patients, so trace amounts of some compounds may not be detected. In spite of this, it has still been possible to identify abnormal concentrations of certain molecular species, and identify some unexpected species, such as nitrous acid. Further work involves more intensive monitoring of ICU patients over time, and in obtaining exhaled breath from the ventilator line as close to the patient as possible. A modification to the ventilator circuits is currently being investigated to reduce both the contamination of samples by compounds produced in the ventilator circuitry and the adsorption and condensation of breath compounds.

Acknowledgement

This work was funded through SRI's core strategic grant from the Biotechnology and Biological Sciences Research Council (BBSRC) UK.

References

1. Španěl P, Smith D. Selected ion flow tube: a technique for quantitative trace gas analysis of air and breath. *Med Biol Eng Comput* 1996; **34**: 409–419.
2. Smith D, Španěl P. On-line measurement of the absolute humidity of air, breath and liquid headspace samples by selected ion flow tube mass spectrometry. *Rapid Commun Mass Spectrom* 2001; **15**: 563–569.
3. Smith D, Španěl P, Holland TA, al Singari W, Elder JB. Selected ion flow tube mass spectrometry of urine headspace. *Rapid Commun Mass Spectrom* 1999; **13**: 724–729.
4. Španěl P, Smith D, Holland TA, Al Singary W, Elder JB. Analysis of formaldehyde in the headspace of urine from bladder and prostate cancer patients using selected ion flow tube spectrometry. *Rapid Commun Mass Spectrom* 1999; **13**: 1354–1359.
5. Smith D, Španěl P, Davies S. Trace gases in breath of healthy volunteers when fasting and after a protein-calorie meal: a preliminary study. *J Appl Physiol* 1999; **87**: 1584–1588.
6. Diskin AM, Španěl P, Smith D. Time variation of ammonia, acetone, isoprene and ethanol in breath: a quantitative SIFT-MS study over 30 days. *Physiol Meas* 2003; **24**: 107–119.
7. Smith D Španěl P. Application of ion chemistry and the SIFT technique to the quantitative analysis of trace gases in air and on breath. *Int Reviews Phys Chem* 1996; **15**: 231–271.

8. Hyspler R, Crhova S, Zadak Z, Gasparic J. Breath isoprene as a measure of the depression in cholesterol synthesis in intensive care patients. *Atherosclerosis Supplements* 2001; **2**: 102.

9. Losa M, Tibballs J, Carter B, Holt MP. Generation of nitrogen dioxide during nitric oxide therapy and mechanical ventilation of children with a Servo 900C ventilator. *Intensive Care Med* 1997; **23**: 450–455.

10. Qureshi MA, Shah NJ, Hemmen CW, Thill MC, Kruse JA. Exposure of intensive care unit nurses to nitric oxide and nitrogen dioxide during therapeutic use of inhaled nitric oxide in adults with acute respiratory distress syndrome. *Am J Crit Care* 2003; **12**: 147–153.

BREATH GAS ANALYSIS
AND VECTOR-BORNE DISEASE DIAGNOSIS:
THE CASE OF MALARIA

B. G. J. KNOLS

Laboratory of Entomology,
Wageningen University and Research Centre,
PO Box 8031, NL-6700EH Wageningen, The Netherlands
and
Entomology Unit, Agency's Laboratories Seibersdorf,
International Atomic Energy Agency (IAEA),
A-2444 Seibersdorf, Austria

1. Introduction

In spite of increased global efforts to combat malarial disease, its impact on human health remains intolerably high. It is estimated that malaria causes three million deaths and half-a-billion episodes *per annum*, 90 % of which occur in sub-Saharan Africa.[1] Malaria slows economic growth in Africa by 1.3 % per year.[2] The disease is most severe in young children (less than 5 years of age) and pregnant women. Its control is facing difficulties due to increased drug[3] and insecticide resistance.[4] New candidate vaccines are being tested,[5] but it may take another decade before a safe and effective product becomes widely and commercially available. Molecular and genomic approaches may deliver novel targets for drug and insecticide development, yet the full exploitation of genomic information of *P. falciparum* and the main malaria vector *Anopheles gambiae*[6] is still in its infancy.

Thus, whilst anticipating an extension of the arsenal of tools to control malaria, efforts to prevent and/or cure disease with contemporary tools remain critical. The four pillars of malaria control are to: (1) provide early diagnosis and prompt treatment, (2) plan and implement selective and sustainable preventive measures, including vector control, (3) detect early, contain and/or prevent epidemics and (4) strengthen local capacity in basic and applied research.[7] Further information about malaria and its control is available online (see for instance `mosquito.who.int/malariacontrol`).

The remainder of this article focuses on one of these key strategies, namely the timely and accurate diagnosis of malarial disease.

2. Diagnosis of Malaria

Prompt and accurate diagnosis of malaria is a key element of effective case management. However, widespread mis-diagnosis of malaria is the cause of significant morbidity and mortality and often leads to inappropriate medication and irrational use of (expensive) drugs.[8] A variety of diagnostic procedures and tools are in use to detect malarial parasites in humans, each posing its own advantages and limitations and applicability in (rural and peripheral) health care systems. These are:[9]

2.1. *Clinical Diagnosis*

Clinical diagnosis is the most commonly used method, particularly in areas of high endemicity where resource limitations prevent laboratory diagnosis. The most commonly used indicator for malaria is fever, often accompanied by chills, headaches, vomiting etc. Clinical diagnosis is inexpensive, does not require special equipment, yet suffers from non-specificity because symptoms overlap with a myriad of other (febrile) illnesses.[10] As a stand-alone tool for disease management it is unjustifiable, except in areas of high prevalence where case definition is more intricate.

2.2. *Microscopy*

Conventional light microscopy remains the most widely accepted and utilised method for actual detection of parasites. Examination of (Giemsa-stained) peripheral blood (from a finger prick) on a blood slide is both sensitive (trained microscopists can detect as few as 5–10 parasites per μL of blood) and informative (it provides details about parasite species, parasite stage and density). Moreover, it is fairly inexpensive (ca. 0.4 US$ per slide) and provides a permanent record (the slide) that can be stored and examined by others at a later date. It has three main disadvantages: it is labour-intensive and requires about an hour from collection of blood to result; requires well-maintained equipment, reagents, and well-trained laboratory staff (often absent in rural areas); it creates a time lag between test result and (often urgently needed) treatment. In settings where microscopy is available, improvements in test accuracy can be obtained through training programmes,[11] yet absence of this facility (in many parts of rural Africa and the topics at large) remains a major concern.

2.3. *Rapid Diagnostic Tests (RDTs)*

Immunochromatographic methods that detect malaria parasite antigens (*e.g.* histidine-rich protein II (HRPII) or parasite lactate dehydrogenase (pLDH)) are increasingly used in malaria case management, particularly when microscopy is not available.[12] Though such 'dipstick' products are useful assets in case management, easy to use by non-specialists and more 'mobile', they are more expensive than blood slide examination (depending on the specificity of the test, purchase quantity and manufacturer these are ca. 1 US\$ per test). Further difficulties relate to sensitivity (this is 90 % at densities of 100 parasites per μL of blood but drops sharply at lower densities), absence of information on parasite density, and false positives due to circulating antigen after parasite clearance. Nevertheless, in spite of these and other problems,[13] it is expected that RDTs will gain popularity due to ease of use and the possibility of self-diagnosis (*e.g.* by travellers).

2.4. *Other Techniques*

Additional methods for malaria parasite detection are available, *i.e.* microscopy using fluorochromes (*e.g.* acridine orange),[14] polymerase chain reaction (PCR)[15] or antibody detection by serology.[16] Recently, direct laser desorption mass spectrometry has been developed for detection of heme (iron protoporphyrin) as a unique molecular biomarker for malaria.[17] Though highly sensitive, none of these methods is currently suitable for wide-scale and routine diagnosis under field conditions.

Clearly, each of the above diagnostic tools present technical, logistic or financial challenges or combinations thereof, but additional problems are present: both microscopy and RDTs require collection of blood samples, which particularly for young children in developing countries can be stressful. Maintenance of microscopes is often inadequate and hindered further by absence of electricity in remote areas. Peripheral health facilities often lack drugs, which stops people from visiting them even if diagnostic facilities are present. Worst of all, many regions lack both, leaving clinical diagnosis as the only remaining alternative and often involve long hours of travel to seek appropriate health care.[18]

3. Breath and Mosquito Olfaction

It has long been noted that humans may produce specific olfactory signals when infected by certain diseases,[19] including mosquito-borne diseases such as yellow fever.[20] Modern science is developing technology to use such signals for diagnostic purposes.[21] To date, however, no research into the use of malaria-related olfactory signals for diagnostic purposes has been undertaken. In contrast, many studies have been conducted to elucidate the nature of human volatiles used by mosquito vectors to locate its blood host.[22] The findings of these studies, important for the main discussion of this article, are listed below:

1. Humans vary in their attractiveness to African malaria vectors.[23–26]
2. This differential attractiveness to mosquitoes can be attributed to variations in olfactory profiles of human hosts[26] and may be related to skin micro-organisms and *Plasmodium* infection status.[27]
3. Human breath has been incriminated as having an allomonal effect on mosquitoes — *i.e.* favourable to the emitter (human), unfavourable for the receiver (mosquito) — and causes differential attractiveness.[28]
4. Human breath has been shown to influence short-range behaviour (*i.e.* the selection of biting sites on humans) during the host-seeking process.[29,30]
5. Several breath components have been shown to affect African mosquito behaviour, such as carbon dioxide,[31,32] acetone and 1-octen-3-ol,[22] various fatty acids,[22] and ammonia.[33]

Although the above studies clearly demonstrate an olfactory basis for mosquito-human interactions, the link between malarial disease and change in the olfactory signature of humans remains speculative. Mukabana *et al.* (unpublished data, 2002) observed a marked decline in attractiveness to *Anopheles gambiae* of two of their test persons during the onset of clinical malaria (confirmed by blood slides). Moreover, this phenomenon has been clearly demonstrated in mice infected with rodent malaria, where the onset of gametocytaemia (*i.e.* the stage of the parasite infectious to mosquitoes) led to marked increase of mosquito feeding over non-infected mice.[34] There is evidence that this effect is governed by olfactory cues (H. Hurd, personal communication, 2002). Nevertheless, a field study in Kenya, in which the attractiveness of a pair of identical twins to malaria vectors was compared daily for over 100 days, failed to demonstrate altered attractiveness during times when gametocytes circulated in the peripheral blood of either of the twins.[35]

However, in spite of the absence of solid evidence to link human olfactory cues to the presence of malaria parasites, there are good arguments to support further research in this area. First, a recent report argues that increased mosquito feeding leads to increased infectiousness of the human reservoir.[36] Second, and perhaps more importantly, it can be argued that an increase in human attractiveness to mosquito vectors at the time when parasites are infectious to mosquitoes will enhance parasite fitness. Any parasite that succeeds in rendering its host more vulnerable to mosquito bites will increase its transmission potential and hence its reproductive rate. This hypothesis would be invalid if all parasite-infected humans were carrying infectious stages at all times, if gametocytes were present in most of the human population, or if mosquito biting was intense and continuous both in space and time. Neither of these arguments is true: gametocyte prevalence is highest in children below 10 yrs of age, gametocytes are not always present, and transmission is often focal and restricted to few individuals in a low-density mosquito biting setting.[37–40] Two additional points act against the parasite. First, African malaria vectors prefer biting adults to children.[41] Second, parasite infection affects mosquito fitness negatively[42] and the force of evolution therefore acts against the parasite. This impasse may either lead to an increase in parasite virulence or the development of alternative ways to increase its transmission potential (*e.g.* by increasing the attractiveness of human hosts).

4. Breath and Malaria

The above argument draws on parasite-human-vector interactions in a multi-facetted context, but this may not be important in terms of malarial disease diagnosis. What matters is whether or not parasite infection alters breath to an extent that it can (*i*) be measured, (*ii*) be indicative of the level of infection, and (*iii*) provide information on the stages of parasite in circulation.

4.1. *Parasite Invasion*

It seems unlikely that sporozoites (the stage of parasite injected into the human host during mosquito bloodfeeding) can be detected in breath. First, the number of sporozoites injected is generally low.[43] Second, invasion of liver hepatocytes occurs rapidly after sporozoites enter the bloodstream.[44] Thus, even if present, the detection of an olfactory signal using breath gas analysis would be highly unlikely.

4.1.1. *Liver and blood stages*

It is not known if the development of sporozoites in the liver (into thousands of merozoites) produces volatile organic compounds. However, the subsequent release of merozoites and invasion of red blood cells is a more dramatic event (that often leads to the onset of clinical malaria symptoms). The erythrocytic cycle that follows may present the best target for signal detection, as parasites are present in large numbers (often millions), metabolic activity is high, and parasite presence in the bloodstream more continuous.[45]

4.1.2. *Sexual parasites*

Beyond the possible detection of blood stages of *Plasmodium*, the possibility that sexual parasites produce specific signals to render the host more attractive to mosquitoes has been discussed above. Differentiation of asexual parasites into gametocytes remains poorly understood and this part of parasite biology has received less attention than the pathogenic asexual blood stages.[46] Gametocyte density is far lower than asexual parasite density,[40] which may affect the production of a specific and detectable signal negatively.

5. Prospects

Given the above discussion, would diagnosis of malaria by breath gas analysis be feasible? It is tempting to speculate on the impact a simple portable device, analogous to an alcohol breathalyzer, could have on early disease diagnosis in rural parts of the tropics, yet this would be premature. However, given the rapid advances in breath gas analysis for disease diagnosis (this book), rigorous analysis of volatile organic compounds from breath of humans infected with various densities, species and different stages of *Plasmodium* seems justifiable. Malaria control has never focused on the selective targeting of gametocytes in humans, as daily blood sample analysis is impractical. However, the availability of a non-invasive, rapid diagnostic tool could provide an entirely new way of transmission control through selective chemotherapy or protection against mosquito bites of only those children that are actively passing on parasites to mosquitoes.

Depending on the success of breath gas analysis as a diagnostic tool for malaria, and the ultimate availability of a commercial product that is equal or better in performance to existing diagnostic tools, a variety of end-users can be identified. First and foremost, such a device should serve to attain the goals of global malaria control, *i.e.* to provide more rapid and reliable diagnosis in disease-endemic settings to aid case management. Second, like the use of RDTs, the travelers' market may be targeted.[47]

Third, considering ever expanding operations in malaria-endemic regions, self-diagnosis by military personnel can be envisaged. Other uses, like in travel clinics, are foreseen.

The development of breath gas analysis as a diagnostic tool for malaria will require close collaboration between malariologists and those working on breath gas analysis for other diseases like lung cancer, breast cancer, tuberculosis and other ailments (this book). It will encompass research in tropical settings, will provide a whole new array of challenges, but should be viewed as an undertaking with huge potential to alleviate the burden of one of the world's most debilitating diseases. "Mal' aria" means "bad air." Perhaps this is truer than previously thought?

Acknowledgement

I thank Dr. Hervé Bossin for critically reviewing the manuscript.

References

1. Breman JG, Alilio MS, Mills A. Conquering the intolerable burden of malaria: what's new, what's needed: a summary. *Am J Trop Med Hyg* 2004; **71**: 1–15.
2. Sachs J, Malaney P. The economic and social burden of malaria. *Nature* 2002; **415**: 680–685.
3. Wernsdorfer G, Wernsdorfer WH. Malaria at the turn from the 2nd to the 3rd millenium. *Wien Klin Wochenschr* 2003; **115** Suppl 3: 2–9.
4. Hemingway J, Field L, Vontas J. An overview of insecticide resistance. *Science* 2002; **298**: 96–97.
5. Alonso PL, Sacarlal J, Aponte JJ, Leach A, Macete E, Milman J, Mandomando I, Spiessens B, Guinovart C, Espasa M, Bassat Q, Aide P, Ofori-Anyinam O, Navia MM, Corachan S, Ceuppens M, Dubois MC, Demoitie MA, Dubovsky F, Menendez C, Tornieporth N, Ballou WR, Thompson R, Cohen J. Efficacy of the RTS,S/AS02A vaccine against *Plasmodium falciparum* infection and disease in young African children: randomised controlled trial. *Lancet* 2004; **364**: 1411–1420.
6. Mongin E, Louis C, Holt RA, Birney E, Collins FH. The *Anopheles gambiae* genome: an update. *Trends Parasitol* 2004; **20**: 49–52.
7. Implementation of the global malaria control strategy. *World Health Organ Tech Rep Ser* 1993; **893**.
8. Amexo M, Tolhurst R, Barnish G, Bates I. Malaria misdiagnosis: effects on the poor and vulnerable. *Lancet* 2004; **364**: 1896–1898.
9. *Malaria Diagnosis: New Perspectives. Report of a Joint WHO/USAID Informal Consultation*, WHO/CDS/RBM 2000.14.
10. Kallander K, Nsungwa Sabiiti J, Peterson S. Symptom overlap for malaria and pneumonia — policy implications for home management strategies. *Acta Trop* 2004; **90**: 211–214.

11. Bates I, Bekoe V, Asamoa-Adu A. Improving the accuracy of malaria-related laboratory tests in Ghana. *Malar J* 2004; **3**: 38.

12. *The Use of Malaria Rapid Diagnostic Tests. Report of a Joint WHO/USAID Informal Consultation,* 2004, WHO/CDS/RBM 2000.14.

13. Trachsler M, Schlagenhauf P, Steffen R. Feasibility of a rapid dipstick antigen-capture assay for self-testing of travellers' malaria. *Trop Med Int Health* 1999; **4**: 442–447.

14. Kawamoto F. Rapid diagnosis of malaria by fluorescence microscopy with light microscope and interference filter. *Lancet* 1991; **337**: 200–202.

15. Snounou G, Viriyakosol S, Zhu XP, Jarra W, Pinheiro L, do Rosario VE, Thaithong S, Brown KN. High sensitivity of detection of human malaria parasites by the use of nested polymerase chain reaction. *Mol Biochem Parasitol* 1993; **61**: 315–320.

16. Sulzer AJ, Wilson M. The fluorescent antibody test for malaria. *CRC Crit Rev Clin Lab Sci* 1971; **2**: 601–619.

17. Demirev PA. Mass spectrometry for malaria diagnosis. *Expert Rev Mol Diagn* 2004; **4**: 821–829.

18. McCombie SC. Treatment seeking for malaria: a review of recent research. *Soc Sci Med* 1996; **43**: 933–945.

19. Stoddart D. *The Scented Ape: The Biology and Culture of Human Odour.* Cambridge: Cambridge University Press, 1990.

20. Liddell K. Smell as a diagnostic marker. *Postgrad Med J* 1976; **52**: 136–138.

21. Turner AP, Magan N. Electronic noses and disease diagnostics. *Nat Rev Microbiol* 2004; **2**: 161–166.

22. Takken W, Knols BGJ. Odor-mediated behavior of Afrotropical malaria mosquitoes. *Annu Rev Entomol* 1999; **44**: 131–157.

23. Lindsay SW, Adiamah JH, Miller JE, Pleass RJ, Armstrong JR. Variation in attractiveness of human subjects to malaria mosquitoes (Diptera: Culicidae) in The Gambia. *J Med Entomol* 1993; **30**: 368–373.

24. Knols BGJ, de Jong R, Takken W. Differential attractiveness of isolated humans to mosquitoes in Tanzania. *Trans R Soc Trop Med Hyg* 1995; **89**: 604–606.

25. Kelly DW. Why are some people bitten more than others? *Trends Parasitol* 2001; **17**: 578–581.

26. Mukabana WR, Takken W, Coe R, Knols BGJ. Host-specific cues cause differential attractiveness of Kenyan men to the African malaria vector *Anopheles gambiae. Malar J* 2002; **1**: 17.

27. Braks MA, Anderson RA, Knols BGJ. Infochemicals in mosquito host selection: human skin microflora and *Plasmodium* parasites. *Parasitol Today* 1999; **15**: 409–413.

28. Mukabana WR, Takken W, Killeen GF, Knols BGJ. Allomonal effect of breath contributes to differential attractiveness of humans to the African malaria vector *Anopheles gambiae. Malar J* 2004; **3**: 1.

29. Knols BGJ, Takken W, de Jong R. Influence of human breath on selection of biting sites by *Anopheles albimanus. J Am Mosq Control Assoc* 1994; **10**: 423–426.

30. De Jong R, Knols BGJ. Selection of biting sites on man by two malaria mosquito species. *Experientia* 1995; **51**: 80–84.

31. Knols BGJ, de Jong R, Takken W. Trapping system for testing olfactory responses of the malaria mosquito *Anopheles gambiae* in a wind tunnel. *Med Vet Entomol* 1994; **8**: 386–388.

32. Mboera LEG, Knols BGJ, Braks MAH, Takken W. Comparison of carbon dioxide-baited trapping systems for sampling outdoor mosquito populations in Tanzania. *Med Vet Entomol* 2000; **14**: 257–263.

33. Meijerink J, Braks MA, Van Loon JJ. Olfactory receptors on the antennae of the malaria mosquito *Anopheles gambiae* are sensitive to ammonia and other sweat-borne components. *J Insect Physiol* 2001; **47**: 455–464.

34. Day JF, Edman JD. Malaria renders mice susceptible to mosquito feeding when gametocytes are most infective. *J Parasitol* 1983; **69**: 163–170.

35. Mukabana W. *Differential Attractiveness of Humans to the African Malaria Vector* Anopheles Gambiae*: Effects of Host Characteristics and Parasite Infection.* Wageningen University and Research Centre, 2002.

36. Paul RE, Diallo M, Brey PT. Mosquitoes and transmission of malaria parasites — not just vectors. *Malar J* 2004; **3**: 39.

37. Akim NI, Drakeley C, Kingo T, Simon B, Senkoro K, Sauerwein RW. Dynamics of *P. falciparum* gametocytemia in symptomatic patients in an area of intense perennial transmission in Tanzania. *Am J Trop Med Hyg* 2000; **63**: 199–203.

38. Abdel-Wahab A, Abdel-Muhsin AM, Ali E, Suleiman S, Ahmed S, Walliker D, Babiker HA. Dynamics of gametocytes among *Plasmodium falciparum* clones in natural infections in an area of highly seasonal transmission. *J Infect Dis* 2002; **185**: 1838–1842.

39. van der Kolk M, Tebo AE, Nimpaye H, Ndombol DN, Sauerwein RW, Eling WM. Transmission of *Plasmodium falciparum* in urban Yaounde, Cameroon, is seasonal and age-dependent. *Trans R Soc Trop Med Hyg* 2003; **97**: 375–379.

40. Bousema JT, Gouagna LC, Drakeley CJ, Meutstege AM, Okech BA, Akim IN, Beier JC, Githure JI, Sauerwein RW. *Plasmodium falciparum* gametocyte carriage in asymptomatic children in western Kenya. *Malar J* 2004; **3**: 18.

41. Carnevale P, Frezil JL, Bosseno MF, Le Pont F, Lancien J. The aggressiveness of *Anopheles gambiae A* in relation to the age and sex of the human subjects. *Bull World Health Organ* 1978; **56**: 147–154.

42. Hurd H. Manipulation of medically important insect vectors by their parasites. *Annu Rev Entomol* 2003; **48**: 141–161.

43. Kabiru EW, Mbogo CM, Muiruri SK, Ouma JH, Githure JI, Beier JC. Sporozoite loads of naturally infected *Anopheles* in Kilifi District, Kenya. *J Am Mosq Control Assoc* 1997; **13**: 259–262.

44. Frevert U. Sneaking in through the back entrance: the biology of malaria liver stages. *Trends Parasitol* 2004; **20**: 417–424.

45. Becker K, Kirk K. Of malaria, metabolism and membrane transport. *Trends Parasitol* 2004; **20**: 590–596.

46. Talman AM, Domarle O, McKenzie FE, Ariey F, Robert V. Gametocytogenesis: the puberty of *Plasmodium falciparum*. *Malar J* 2004; **3**: 24.
47. Zuckerman JN. Preventing malaria in UK travellers. *Bmj* 2004; **329**: 305–306.

RECENT DEVELOPMENTS
IN EXHALED BREATH ANALYSIS
AND HUMAN EXPOSURE RESEARCH*

A. B. LINDSTROM

Methods Development and Applications Branch,
National Exposure Research Laboratory,
U. S. Environmental Protection Agency,
Research Triangle Park, NC 27711, USA

1. Introduction

Exhaled breath collection and analysis has historically been used in environmental research studies to help characterize exposures to volatile organic compounds (VOCs). The use of this approach is based on the fact that xenobiotic compounds present in the blood are reflected in the breath, thus providing a non-invasive means of demonstrating exposure, establishing conclusive links between specific activities and corresponding body burdens, characterizing uptake and elimination kinetics, and illuminating relevant pathways of exposure.[1] While this research has been extremely valuable in this regard, it has tended to only provide information about what has already happened to an individual after exposure has occurred. As this field has advanced in recent years, it has now become possible to use exhaled breath in a more predictive manner to help characterize biological responses and possibly give what might be the earliest indications of the onset of disease. In this paper we briefly review some of the historical uses of exhaled breath analysis and then proceed to examine some of the most interesting recent applications of this technique in the field of environmental exposure research.

2. Methods

While exhaled breath analysis has been used in various forms for many years as an aid to medical diagnostics and occupational medicine, its application in the field of environmental exposure assessment has been a relatively recent development. One of the best examples of its use came about in the 1980's when the United States Environmental Protection Agency (USEPA) conducted a series of investigations known as the Total Exposure Assessment Methodology (TEAM) studies to help determine some of the most basic aspects of how humans are exposed to environmental pollutants (see review by Wallace *et al.*, Ref. 2). In these studies, approximately 750 people from a variety of locations across the USA (*e.g.* urban, suburban, rural) were monitored for two consecutive 12 hour periods with samples of ambient air, indoor air, personal air, and water collected and analyzed for over 25 target VOC analytes. Personal activity patterns, including job type and duration, transportation use, and leisure time activities were also recorded. Exhaled breath analysis was chosen as the means to determine body burdens of the target compounds in favor of a traditional blood-based sampling approach due to the relatively low detection limits possible with breath (typically in the parts-per-trillion, ppt, range) and the widespread acceptance of this non-invasive procedure among study subjects.

One of the most interesting initial findings of these studies was the fact that average outdoor air VOC levels were generally 2–5 times lower than measurements made indoors or with personal monitors (portable monitors that the study subjects carried with them). This, coupled with the fact that most subjects spent the vast majority of their time indoors, led to the realization that large ambient point sources (*e.g.* power plants, chemical production facilities) were far less important in influencing exposure than an individual's personal activities.

Among the personal activities that were found to be most important in influencing exhaled breath measurements was cigarette smoking. It was determined that smokers had 6–10 times more benzene in their breath (and therefore blood) than non-smokers. These findings made it immediately clear that for 50 million Americans cigarette smoke was the single most important source of exposure to this carcinogen. Other personal activities that were associated with potentially significant exposures included the use of chlorinated water supplies and chloroform, motor vehicle use and benzene and other aromatics, and various hobbies which were associated with a variety of solvent compounds (from paints, thinners, and adhesives).

Also significant was the finding that food was generally not a source of exposure to VOCs. While chloroform was found to be associated with some dairy products, and the consumption of citrus fruits contributed to limonene exposure, food in general was determined to be a relatively minor pathway of exposure to VOCs.

Data from the TEAM studies and other more recent investigations using similar techniques have provided critical pharmacokinetic data that have helped to provide a more detailed understanding of how particular compounds are distributed and retained in the human body. Each compound has its own specific uptake and elimination constants which can be used to determine how much an individual will have in his or her body and the length of time it will take before this material is eliminated or reaches a steady state.[3]

3. Results and Discussion

While exposure research continues to depend on these types of traditional approaches to evaluate the basic nature of specific exposures, improvements in our understanding of the pathophysiology and metabolism of some of our most important air pollutants have now helped increase the utility of exhaled breath analysis. Now, instead of merely reflecting an absorbed dose, in some cases we are beginning to be able to use exhaled breath as a sensitive indicator of a specific physiological response to an exposure, thus providing the potential for exhaled breath to be used in a truly predictive manner. As outlined below, these new markers may indicate an adaptive response, a specific toxic endpoint, or even an individual's particular vulnerability or resistance to a pollutant. In particular, many of these new applications involve a better appreciation of the importance of oxidative stress as a fundamental indicator and cause of disease.

3.1. *Ozone and Oxidative Stress*

One of the most important pollutants affecting public health is tropospheric ozone (O_3), which is a potent oxidant formed by complex reactions between sunlight, hydrocarbons, and nitrogen oxides. The USEPA's current 8 hour standard for ozone is 80 ppb, but many urban areas are regularly out of attainment with this standard, and short-term excursions in the range 100 200 ppb are quite common during hot summer months in many congested urban areas. The public health impact of ozone is thought to be enormous. It has been estimated that for every 50 ppb increase in ozone concentration hospital admissions increase by almost 10 percent. The American Lung Association estimates that high ozone levels are responsible for approximately 10,000 to 15,000 extra hospital admissions and 30,000 to 50,000 additional emergency room visits in the U.S. each year.[4] A specific and noninvasive measure of ozone exposure indicating the subtle signs of stress or incipient damage would be extremely valuable for helping to protect susceptible subpopulations and for designing therapeutic approaches to manage illness related to exposure.

Previous studies clearly show that ozone causes lung inflammation[5] with an influx and activation of neutrophils, ultimately leading to the production of a number of reactive oxygen species (ROS, *e.g.* superoxide, H_2O_2) that are part of the normal host defense process. However, if left unchecked, these ROS can lead to lipid peroxidation and the destruction of essential cell membranes, modification and deactivation of proteins, and irreversible damage to DNA. Ultimately this oxidative stress gives rise to a number of small molecules including non-volatiles like malondialdehyde and 8-isoprostane, which have been measured in bronchoalveolar lavage fluid (BALF)[5] and induced sputum.[6] Great benefit could be derived from a noninvasive measure of ozone induced oxidative damage as discussed below.

In an early study, Foster *et al.*[7] examined exhaled isoprene as a potential indicator of the oxidative damage associated with ozone exposure. Ten subjects were exposed to ozone (ramped from 150–350 parts-per-billion [ppb]) during a 130 minute period that included intervals of light exercise and rest. Immediately after the exposure period, breath isoprene was found to be lower, possibly due to a washout effect previously observed with the increased respiration rates associated with exercise. But for the 6 individuals who were tested 19 hours after the end exposure period, all had significant increases in isoprene (over and above the normal diurnal fluctuation that had been previously noted). To explain this observation, the authors suggested that the airways might have been damaged by the direct oxidative effects of ozone and (potentially) by secondary oxidative damage due to the influx and activation of inflammatory cells. Because isoprene is a normal byproduct of cholesterol metabolism,[8] and repair of cell membranes and other cellular constituents damaged by lipid peroxidation would require more cholesterol, a delayed increase in isoprene would be expected as repair was initiated. Interestingly, however, Foster *et al.*[7] found no evidence of increased ethane or 1-pentene in this experiment, despite the fact that these compounds have been associated with reperfusion of ischemic tissues, vascular surgery, ionizing radiation, and other conditions known to induce lipid peroxidation.[9] While these results indicate that production of isoprene might be useful as an early indicator of ozone exposure and respiratory damage, no follow up of this study has been reported to date.

In a more recent study employing exhaled breath condensate (EBC), Montuschi *et al.*[10] exposed healthy subjects ($n = 9$) to relatively high levels of ozone (400 ppb) while they were performing intermittent moderate exercise during a 2 hour period. These subjects had significant increases in 8-isoprostane measured in EBC within 4 hours after exposure terminated. Pretreatment with the inhaled corticosteroid (ICS) Budesonide did not affect increases in 8-isoprostane associated with the exposure. 8-Isoprostane had previously been shown to be present in EBC from patients with inflammatory airway diseases such as asthma, chronic obstructive pulmonary disease (COPD), and cystic fibrosis (CF), but this was the first indication that EBC could be useful in assessing healthy individuals' exposures to ozone. Isoprostanes are known to be specifically produced by free radical peroxidation of arachidonic acid and they have biological activities that may be involved with the development of lung disease. Aside from the one tentative study involving isoprene cited above, no other noninvasive markers of oxidative stress (NO, CO, nitrate) had ever been measured after similar ozone exposures. And while 400 ppb is a fairly high exposure level, these results suggest that EBC could potentially be useful as a noninvasive monitor of ozone exposure and resulting inflammation.

In another study involving EBC biomarkers and lung inflammation, Corradi *et al.*[11] exposed 22 healthy volunteers to 100 ppb of ozone for 2 hours during moderate exercise. They found that individuals with the wild genotype for NAD(P)H:quinone oxidoreductase (NQO1) and the null genotype for glutathione-S-transferase M1 (GSTM1) had significant increases in 8-isoprostane, TBARS (thiobarbituric acid reactive substances), and LTB_4 (PMN chemotactic mediator leukotriene B4) after exposure. Complementary measurements of these same parameters in blood were noted to be less sensitive to these changes, and traditional measures of lung function (FEV_1, FVC, and FEF) showed no discernable change with exposure. Interestingly, the increase in 8-isoprostane was observed immediately whereas increases in TBARS and LTB_4 were observed 18 hours after exposure. These findings are consistent with other studies that show similar results with BALF, but this approach offers the benefit of being completely non-invasive. In is notable that this study may be the first to show how exhaled breath markers can be useful in identifying specific genetic vulnerabilities to environmental pollutants.

3.2. *Particulates and Exhaled NO*

One of the most interesting developments in environmental health over recent years is the discovery that relatively small changes in ambient particulate concentration are responsible for substantial increases in morbidity and mortality. When considered on an individual basis, small changes in ambient particulate level seem trivial, but when dealing with large populations, the number of individuals with critical vulnerabilities becomes quite significant. In one of the largest studies of the situation to date[12] it was estimated that for a long-term increase in PM 2.5 (particulate matter 2.5 microns or smaller in mean aerodynamic diameter) of only 10 $\mu g/m^3$ one would expect to see significant increases in general mortality (4%), cardiopulmonary mortality (6%), and lung cancer mortality (8%) in an affected area.

In recent years exhaled nitric oxide (eNO) has been used as a sub-clinical marker to gauge the severity and progress of a number of deleterious inflammatory airway conditions. These studies have shown that with inflammation there is an influx of cytokines that appear to stimulate inducible nitric oxide synthase (iNOS), which in turn leads to elevated levels of eNO observed in asthma, COPD, and other diseases. Other research has shown that particulate-mediated airway inflammation may be an important factor in inducing the deleterious cardiovascular effects that have been associated with high pollution episodes.[13] Together, these observations suggest that eNO might prove to be a useful early indicator of exposure to the air pollutants that are responsible for the adverse health outcomes noted in large population-based studies.

In the first study to relate eNO with relatively small changes in ambient air pollutants, Van Amsterdam *et al.*[14] monitored 16 non-smoking ($n = 16$) subjects and local air pollution levels for 14 days. A positive association between eNO and CO ($r = 0.85$), NO ($r = 0.81$), PM_{10} (particulate matter 10 microns or smaller in mean aerodynamic diameter) ($r = 0.52$) and NO_2 ($r = 0.49$) was observed, suggesting for the first time that a non-invasive test could be used to gauge the severity of inflammatory responses related to ambient air pollution. Because all of the pollutants that were monitored were also correlated with each other, the authors suspected that ambient CO and NO may not have been the true causative factors, but instead these compounds were surrogates for high pollution in general. They noted that the specific cause of increased airway inflammation and elevated eNO could have been any single pollutant or combination of pollutants the study group was exposed to. However, because *in vitro* studies have shown that airborne particulate matter causes an increase in iNOS production, the authors suggested that the PM_{10} may have been responsible for the rise in eNO levels observed in their study.

In a similar study Steerenberg *et al.*[15] measured the pulmonary and inflammatory responses of 38 children living in a relatively polluted urban area and contrasted these results with those from 44 children living in a less heavily impacted suburban setting in Holland. Urban children were found to have increased peak expiratory flow (PEF), higher eNO, and (in nasal lavage fluids) more uric acid, urea, and nitric acid metabolites per unit increase of air pollutants than their suburban counterparts. In mixed linear-regression analysis, urban children had significant increases in eNO following increased exposures to PM_{10}, black smoke, NO_2, and NO. In general, children living in an urban setting had increased levels of inflammatory nasal markers, increased response in peak expiratory flow (PEF), and higher eNO associated with elevated air pollution relative to their suburban counterparts.

To see if eNOS could provide a more sensitive means of assessing respiratory health than standard lung function tests, Fischer *et al.*[16] measured respiratory complaints, lung function, and eNO, in a group of 68 children (aged 10–11) for 7 weeks. Ambient air pollution levels were also monitored in the study area during this period. They founds that levels of eNO, and not standard lung function measures (*e.g.* spirometry, FVC, FEV_1), were correlated with increased ambient pollution (PM_{10}, black smoke, NO, NO_2, CO). Moreover, self-reported respiratory symptoms (*e.g.* sore throat, cold) were found to be significantly correlated with eNO measurements made the following week. They concluded that eNO may be a more sensitive indicator of respiratory health than the more traditional pulmonary measures.

In a study involving 19 asthmatic children between 6–13 years of age (9 of whom were being treated with ICS), Koenig *et al.*[17] measured eNO and related it to $PM_{2.5}$ collected from outdoor, indoor, personal, and regional samplers. A linear mixed-effects model was used to test for associations between eNO and $PM_{2.5}$. eNO from all subjects was found to be significantly associated with all $PM_{2.5}$ measures and no differences were noted between the various $PM_{2.5}$ collection sites and eNO. This study suggests while $PM_{2.5}$ was clearly related to eNO levels in these asthmatics, regional scale monitoring was sufficient to assess exposure. In addition, ICS use was found to be significantly associated with eNO, providing further evidence of the inflammatory effect of fine particulate matter in this group of susceptible individuals. These results suggest that eNO can be used as an early sensitive marker of airway inflammation and that $PM_{2.5}$ may be responsible for inflammation associated with elevated morbidity and mortality.

Most recently, Adamkiewicz *et al.*[18] conducted a study where eNO was measured weekly in a group of elderly non-smoking individuals ($n = 29$, mean age = 70.7 years) over a 3 month period while various ambient pollutants were also measured. An increase in the average 24 hour $PM_{2.5}$ of 17.7 $\mu g/m^3$ was associated with a 1.95 ppb (15 %) increase in eNO in this population. The association between $PM_{2.5}$ and eNO was found to be most significant for individuals with COPD. Ambient 24 hour NO levels were also significantly correlated with eNO in one of the models, but the effect was not as great as for $PM_{2.5}$ (0.73 ppb eNO for one inter-quartile range increase in ambient NO). These data show that increases in ambient particulates can lead to elevated eNO and airway inflammation, which may underlie particulate-based disease and mortality.

4. Conclusions

Together, these recent studies illustrate how exhaled breath analysis has matured to the point that it is now being used to indicate early biological responses to exposures, help identify potential vulnerabilities of susceptible sub-populations, and generally provide a more thorough understanding of the basic mechanisms of the diseases associated with some of our most important public health threats. It is interesting to note that good biomarkers are thought to be intimately associated with both the relevant exposure and the early physiological manifestations of disease.[19] The more closely the biomarker is related to the adverse outcome, the more likely it will have predictive value that will be useful in an epidemiological context. Exhaled breath biomarkers have truly come much closer to this ideal in the past few years. As our understanding of pollutant-induced disease increases we can anticipate much more use of exhaled breath analysis in the future.

Acknowledgements

I thank Myriam Medina-Vera and Joachim D. Pleil for their consistent support of this research. The United States Environmental Protection Agency through its Office of Research and Development funded and managed the research described here. It has been subjected to Agency's administrative review and approved for publication as an EPA document.

References

1. Lindstrom AB, Pleil JD. A review of the USEPA's single breath canister (SBC) method for exhaled volatile organic biomarkers. *Biomarkers* 2002; **7** (3): 189–208.
2. Wallace L, Buckley T, Pellizzari E, Gordon S. Breath measurements as volatile organic compound biomarkers. *Environ Health Perspect* 1996; **104** Suppl 5: 861–869.
3. Wallace L, Pellizzari E, Gordon S. A linear model relating breath concentrations to environmental exposures: application to a chamber study of four volunteers exposed to volatile organic chemicals. *J Expo Anal Environ Epidemiol* 1993; **3** (1): 75–102.
4. Özkaynak H. *Ambient Ozone Exposure and Emergency Hospital Admissions and Emergency Room Visits for Respiratory Problems in 13 U.S. Cities.* Washington, D.C.: American Lung Association, 1996.
5. Koren HS, Devlin RB, Graham DE, Mann R, McGee MP, Horstman DH, Kozumbo WJ, Becker S, House DE, McDonnell WF. Ozone-induced inflammation in the lower airways of human subjects. *Am Rev Respir Dis* 1989; **139** (2): 407–415.
6. Fahy JV, Wong HH, Liu JT, Boushey HA. Analysis of induced sputum after air and ozone exposures in healthy subjects. *Environ Res* 1995; **70** (2): 77–83.
7. Foster WM, Jiang L, Stetkiewicz PT, Risby TH. Breath isoprene: temporal changes in respiratory output after exposure to ozone. *J Appl Physiol* 1996; **80** (2): 706–710.
8. Stone BG, Besse TJ, Duane WC, Evans CD, DeMaster EG. Effect of regulating cholesterol biosynthesis on breath isoprene excretion in men. *Lipids* 1993; **28** (8): 705–708.
9. Risby TH, Sehnert SS. Clinical application of breath biomarkers of oxidative stress status. *Free Radic Biol Med* 1999; **27** (11-12): 1182–1192.
10. Montuschi P, Nightingale JA, Kharitonov SA, Barnes PJ. Ozone-induced increase in exhaled 8-isoprostane in healthy subjects is resistant to inhaled budesonide. *Free Radic Biol Med* 2002; **33** (10): 1403–1408.
11. Corradi M, Alinovi R, Goldoni M, Vettori M, Folesani G, Mozzoni P, Cavazzini S, Bergamaschi E, Rossi L, Mutti A. Biomarkers of oxidative stress after controlled human exposure to ozone. *Toxicol Lett* 2002; **134** (1–3): 219–225.
12. Pope CA, 3rd, Burnett RT, Thun MJ, Calle EE, Krewski D, Ito K, Thurston GD. Lung cancer, cardiopulmonary mortality, and long-term exposure to fine particulate air pollution. *Jama* 2002; **287** (9): 1132–1141.
13. Brook RD, Brook JR, Urch B, Vincent R, Rajagopalan S, Silverman F. Inhalation of fine particulate air pollution and ozone causes acute arterial vasoconstriction in healthy adults. *Circulation* 2002; **105** (13): 1534–1536.
14. Van Amsterdam JG, Verlaan VP, Van Loveren H, Elzakker BG, Vos SG, Opperhuizen A, Steerenborg PA. Air pollution is associated with increased level of exhaled nitric oxide in nonsmoking healthy subjects. *Arch Environ Health* 1999; **54** (5): 331–335.

15. Steerenberg PA, Nierkens S, Fischer PH, van Loveren H, Opperhuizen A, Vos JG, van Amsterdam JG. Traffic-related air pollution affects peak expiratory flow, exhaled nitric oxide, and inflammatory nasal markers. *Arch Environ Health* 2001; **56** (2): 167–174.

16. Fischer PH, Steerenberg PA, Snelder JD, van Loveren H, van Amsterdam JG. Association between exhaled nitric oxide, ambient air pollution and respiratory health in school children. *Int Arch Occup Environ Health* 2002; **75** (5): 348–353.

17. Koenig JQ, Jansen K, Mar TF, Lumley T, Kaufman J, Trenga CA, Sullivan J, Liu LJ, Shapiro GG, Larson TV. Measurement of offline exhaled nitric oxide in a study of community exposure to air pollution. *Environ Health Perspect* 2003; **111** (13): 1625–1629.

18. Adamkiewicz G, Ebelt S, Syring M, Slater J, Speizer FE, Schwartz J, Suh H, Gold DR. Association between air pollution exposure and exhaled nitric oxide in an elderly population. *Thorax* 2004; **59** (3): 204–209.

19. Schulte PA, Talaska G. Validity criteria for the use of biological markers of exposure to chemical agents in environmental epidemiology. *Toxicology* 1995; **101** (1–2): 73–88.

THE UNIQUE VALUE OF BREATH BIOMARKERS FOR ESTIMATING PHARMACOKINETIC RATE CONSTANTS AND BODY BURDEN FROM ENVIRONMENTAL EXPOSURES*

J. D. PLEIL

*Human Exposure and Atmospheric Sciences Division,
National Exposure Research Laboratory, Office of Research and Development,
U. S. Environmental Protection Agency,
Mail Drop D205-05, Research Triangle Park, NC 27711, USA
and
Department of Environmental Sciences and Engineering,
School of Public Health, University of North Carolina at Chapel Hill,
Chapel Hill, NC 27599, USA*

D. KIM

*Department of Environmental Sciences and Engineering,
School of Public Health, University of North Carolina at Chapel Hill,
Chapel Hill, NC 27599, USA*

J. D. PRAH

*Human Studies Division,
National Health and Environmental Effects Research Laboratory,
Office of Research and Development, U. S. Environmental Protection Agency,
58B USEPA Mailroom, Research Triangle Park, NC 27711, USA*

D. L. ASHLEY

*Division of Laboratory Sciences, National Center for Environmental Health,
Centers for Disease Control and Prevention,
Chamblee, GA 30341, USA*

S. M. RAPPAPORT

*Department of Environmental Sciences and Engineering,
School of Public Health, University of North Carolina at Chapel Hill,
Chapel Hill, NC 27599, USA*

1. Introduction

1.1. *Use of Biomarkers*

Biomarkers are generally defined as chemicals measured in biological media; these include native compounds and their metabolic products. Biomarker measurements are used in three ways: (1) evaluating the time course and distribution of a chemical in the body, (2) estimating previous exposure or dose, and (3) assessing disease state. Blood and urine measurements are the primary methods employed. Of late, it has been recognized that collecting exhaled breath is an attractive alternative to blood and urine sampling because it is less invasive and is not restricted by sample volume or time frame. The ensuing discussions are restricted to the first two biomarker applications, time course and dose estimation.

For the purposes of deducing time course and distribution of a chemical in the body, we require a series of time dependent data points, a conceptual model, and knowledge of the exposure route and dose profile. Certainly, urine sampling is a poor choice for time frames shorter than a few hours as sample volume and collection frequency are limited. Blood can be sampled quite effectively even with short time scale resolution, but is invasive, is restricted in total volume, and requires trained medical personnel. Breath volume and frequency of sampling are essentially unlimited; the subject never runs out of sample and one can collect even adjacent breaths with existing technology. Furthermore, there is a fundamental difference between blood and breath measurement in that blood levels report the *status quo* at the time of collection, whereas exhaled breath is reflective of current blood levels as well as an elimination mechanism allowing calculation of real time removal rates. Therefore, from a mathematical standpoint, the time courses of blood and breath are interpreted differently and give complementary information.

1.2. *Specific Example — Methyl Tertiary Butyl Ether*

The advantages of breath biomarkers can be illustrated using the example of methyl tertiary butyl ether (MTBE) exposure and environmental classical pharmacokinetics (PK). MTBE exposure is ubiquitous in the U. S. and has been linked to toxicity and cancer in animal studies. It was originally introduced to replace lead in gasoline as an octane enhancer and comprises 1 to 5 % of automotive fuel. More recently, it has become the most common "oxygenate" added to fuel to reduce vehicular carbon monoxide emissions in cold climates.[1-3] MTBE is a volatile, flammable and colorless liquid that readily evaporates and dissolves easily in water; it has a very distinctive odor and (unpleasant) taste at very low levels.[4] Fuel spills, atmospheric deposition, leaking underground storage tanks, and fuel transmission pipe leaks have introduced MTBE into drinking water supplies; evaporative emissions from auto refueling add vapor phase MTBE to the ambient air.[5,6] MTBE has one major metabolite, tertiary butyl alcohol (TBA), which is easily measured in human breath, blood and urine.[7] In a recent EPA study of controlled human exposures, native MTBE and the metabolite TBA were measured during uptake and elimination in blood and breath. Time dependent data were collected for inhalation, ingestion and dermal exposure routes.[8]

1.3. *Classical vs. Biologically Based Pharmacokinetic Modeling*

Estimating uptake (or production), distribution, target organ dose, metabolism, and elimination of an endogenous or exogenous chemical generally requires detailed knowledge of many physical, chemical, and biological parameters. These parameters are measured or estimated from *in vitro* laboratory studies, animal models, and controlled human studies. Subsequently, the results are interpreted to deduce potential mechanisms, diffusion constants and tissue transfer rates that are then incorporated into a complex physiologically based pharmacokinetic (PPBK) model. Such models may incorporate more than 40 distinct accumulation points for individual organs, body fluids, and tissues. If, however, we are only interested in assessing average exposures, dose, basic rates of uptake, metabolism, and elimination, then simple classical pharmacokinetic (PK) models suffice. PK models are empirical; the body is treated as a few theoretical compartments without a detailed physiological relationship (*e.g.* highly, moderately, and poorly perfused tissues rather than brain, lung, fat, blood, muscle, etc.). PK models can be developed and validated using simple measurements of a few compounds in blood, urine, and breath. For this work, we rely on the classical PK model and follow the approach and the general principles invoked in standard texts (*e.g.* Ref. 9).

1.4. *Uptake and Volume of Distribution*

In any dosing or exposure scenario, one of the most important parameters is the total mass of chemical administered and made biologically available. Given a concentration measurement of a particular compound in units of mass/volume in blood, one would assume that the total burden could be quickly calculated by multiplying by the known volume of blood. This is only accurate in the absence of tissue adsorption and other temporary sinks of the analyte in the body. In classical PK, the conversion of concentration to body burden is performed with an empirically determined parameter called volume of distribution (V_d). This parameter is used for calculation purposes and is generally not well characterized biologically; it can vary depending upon exposure route and metabolic activity. V_d is important, however, to determine the uptake rate of analyte from the environment into the body and also the "mass/time" elimination rate through various mechanisms. To the best of our knowledge, these values are not available in the literature for MTBE or TBA.

1.5. *Exploitation of Breath Data*

The primary goal of this work is to demonstrate the value of breath measurement as complementary to other measurements. Through the MTBE example and a simple PK model, we employ breath data to help determine the rate constants of transfer of analyte among theoretical compartments using controlled experiments. We estimate uptake rates and V_d's using the exhaled breath concentration during inhalation exposure. We further demonstrate how breath measurements are similar in character to their corresponding blood measurements; some differences are presented as well with respect to time dependence, and we provide guidance for the calculation of blood/breath concentration ratios.

2. Methods

2.1. *Available Data*

From previous work, we have available sets of data "building blocks" of MTBE and TBA in blood and breath from separate controlled ingestion, inhalation, and dermal exposures. These time series data follow the uptake and elimination for 24 hours from short term (1 hour dermal and inhalation exposure, bolus ingestion exposure). The methods and results of these experiments have been described in detail and published elsewhere;[8] for clarity, we provide a brief description of the inhalation experiments:

Inhalation exposure was studied through collection of blood samples from 14 individual male subjects; breath samples were co-collected for a subset of seven subjects due to resource constraints. Volunteers were exposed to 3 ppmv (10.93 μg/L) MTBE in air for one hour. Blood and breath samples were collected periodically before, during, and after the exposures on a timing pattern chosen to properly describe the temporal behavior ending about 23 h post exposure.[10] About 16 samples per subject were collected for each experiment; in addition to pre-exposure controls, samples were collected at 0, 15, 30, 45, 60 minutes during the exposures, and at 0, 5, 15, 30, 60, 120, 180, 360, and approximately 1320 minutes post exposure. Blood samples were assayed for MTBE and TBA at the Centers for Disease Control Laboratories in Atlanta, Georgia using their specific GC-MS methods;[11] breath samples were assayed for MTBE and TBA at the Environmental Protection Agency Laboratories in Research Triangle Park, North Carolina using sampling and analytical methods developed by Pleil and Lindstrom.[10,12–14]

2.2. *Classical Pharmacokinetic Model*

Figure 1 shows a simple PK model for the disposition of MTBE and TBA in the body. The central compartment represents the circulating blood and other fluids in equilibrium with the blood. We consider only one peripheral compartment to serve as an empirical representation of the moderately and poorly perfused tissues. This model assumes that once MTBE is absorbed into the central compartment (blood), the rate constants for exchange with the peripheral compartment, elimination via breath, and

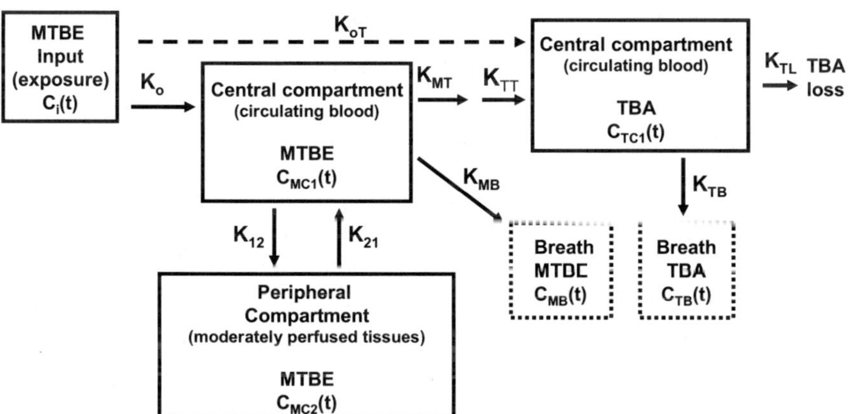

Fig. 1. Simple classical pharmacokinetic diagram of disposition of absorbed MTBE among compartments, metabolite, and excretion; the K's are first-order rate constants except for K_0 which is zeroth order for inhalation and dermal exposures. K_{0T} represents direct conversion of MTBE to TBA.

conversion to metabolite are first order. We also allow for direct conversion of MTBE to TBA in the lung via cytochrome P450 enzymes as indicated by the dashed path and the rate constant K_{0T} in Fig. 1. Furthermore, we assume that MTBE is entirely eliminated via breath or metabolized to TBA; we do not consider any other loss mechanisms. The breath compartments for MTBE and TBA are not considered as standard accumulation points and are thus represented with dashed lines.

2.3. *Mass Balance Equations*

From Fig. 1, the concentrations (mass/volume) in the represented model boxes are defined as follows:

$C_i(t)$:   exposure input concentration at time t
$C_{MC1}(t)$: blood concentration of MTBE in central compartment at time t
$C_{MC2}(t)$: blood concentration of MTBE in peripheral compartment at time t
$C_{TC1}(t)$ blood concentration of TBA in central compartment at time t
$C_{MB}(t)$:   breath concentration of MTBE at time t
$C_{TB}(t)$:   breath concentration of TBA at time t

K_0 is in units of mass/time and the other various K's are all first-order rate constants in units of 1/time. The conversion of MTBE to TBA is adjusted by a change from K_{MT} to K_{TT}. For the accumulation compartments for blood levels, the differential equations are:

$$\frac{d}{dt}C_{MC1}(t) = K_0\, k_a\, C_i(t) + K_{21}\, k_b\, C_{MC2}(t) - K_{12}\, C_{MC1}(t)$$
$$- (K_{MT} + K_{MB})\, C_{MC1}(t) \tag{1}$$

$$\frac{d}{dt}C_{MC2}(t) = K_{12}\, k_c\, C_{MC1}(t) - K_{21}\, C_{MC2}(t) \tag{2}$$

$$\frac{d}{dt}C_{TC1}(t) = K_{MT}\, k_d\, C_{MC1}(t) - (K_{TL} + K_{TB})\, C_{TC}(t)$$
$$+ K_{0T}\, k_e\, C_i(t) \tag{3}$$

Lower case $k_a \ldots k_e$ represent adjustment for concentration units, volume of distribution, and analyte molecular weight. The term $K_{0T}\, k_e\, C_i(t)$ in Eq. (3) is only invoked if there is evidence for direct pulmonary metabolism of MTBE to TBA. Furthermore, the rate constant for TBA appearance in the model is related to the loss of MTBE as $K_{TT} \approx K_{MT}\, k_d$.

The conventional method for relating exhaled alveolar breath levels to alveolar blood levels is to use simple multiplicative constants:

$$C_{MB}(t) = A_{pMB0}\, C_{MC1}(t), \tag{4}$$
$$C_{TB}(t) = A_{pTB0}\, C_{TC1}(t). \tag{5}$$

A_{pMB0} and A_{pTB0} are experimentally determined, often from *in vitro* experiments. Because we actually measure venous blood from the antecubital vein (arm) and not the alveolar blood in the lung, we have to allow for the venous blood to mix and to reach the alveoli. To adjust for this disparity, we use a simple empirical function that incorporates current exposure status in conjunction with current blood levels:

$$C_{\mathrm{MB}}(t) = [A_{\mathrm{pMB0}} + A_{\mathrm{pMB1}}C_{\mathrm{i}}(t)]\, C_{\mathrm{MC1}}(t), \tag{6}$$

$$C_{\mathrm{TB}}(t) = [A_{\mathrm{pTB0}} + A_{\mathrm{pTB1}}C_{\mathrm{i}}(t)]\, C_{\mathrm{TC1}}(t). \tag{7}$$

Note that as the exposure term $C_{\mathrm{i}}(t)$ decreases, we expect the blood concentrations to be closer to uniformity throughout the body and these equations reduce to the functional forms expressed in eqs. (4) and (5).

2.4. *Exposure Profile Demonstrations*

We utilize the inhalation exposure data from Prah *et al.*[8] controlled exposure experiments, which are comprised of a single 1 hour exposure followed by an approximately 22 hour elimination period. We fit the means of empirical data to the simple model presented in Fig. 1 as described by eqs. (1)–(3), (6), and (7) above to estimate the various rate constants. All modeling and rate constant optimization calculations were performed using acslXtreme (Xcellon, Austin, TX); statistical results were calculated and graphed using GraphPad Prism (GraphPad Software Inc., San Diego, CA).

3. Results and Discussions

In the following discussions, any mention of empirical data, or blood and breath measurements, refers to raw data for all subjects from the aforementioned Prah *et al.*[8] article. These data are presented graphically as means with 95 % confidence interval flags in Figs. 2 and 3. Any empirical calculations mentioned heretofore are performed using measurement means of all subjects.

3.1. *Elimination Pathways for MTBE*

Figure 1 indicates that following the exposure period ($K_{\mathrm{U}} = 0$) and before the slower peripheral compartment absorbs appreciable amounts of analyte, only K_{MT} and K_{MB} are influential in changing the blood concentration. Therefore, we can estimate the total rate $K_{\mathrm{MT}} + K_{\mathrm{MB}}$ of elimination from

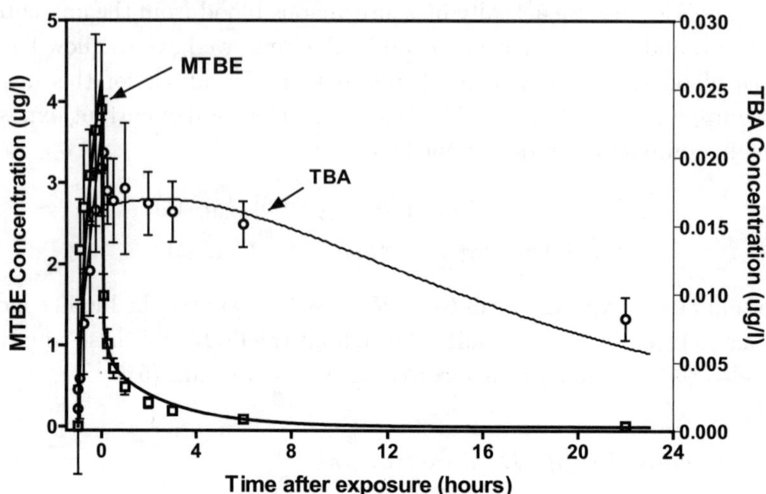

Fig. 2.   Breath measurements and classical PK model calculations for native compound and biomarker from inhalation exposure to MTBE

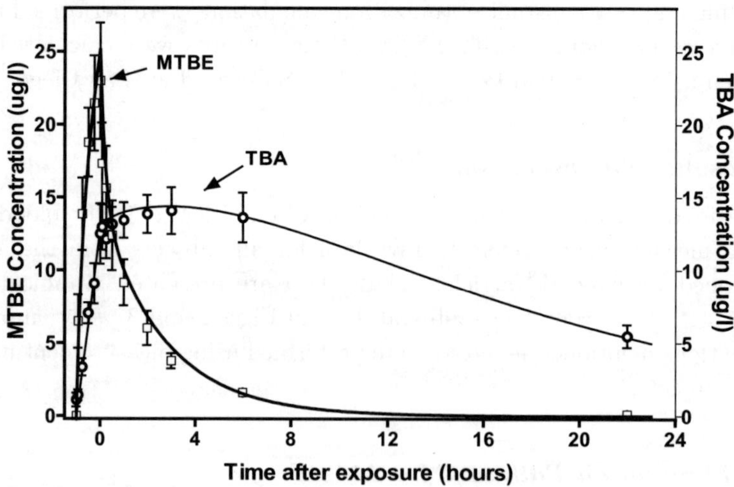

Fig. 3.   Blood measurements and classical PK model calculations for native compound and biomarker from inhalation exposure to MTBE

blood using a reduced version of Eq. (1):

$$\frac{d}{dt}C_{\mathrm{MC1}}(t) \approx -(K_{\mathrm{MT}} + K_{\mathrm{MB}})\,C_{\mathrm{MC1}}(t) \tag{8}$$

for the time period for $0 < t <$ ca. 1 h which has the empirical solution using measured blood levels:

$$\begin{aligned}
C_{\mathrm{MC1}}(t) &\approx A_{\mathrm{MC1}}\ \exp[-(K_{\mathrm{MT}} + K_{\mathrm{MB}})\,t] \\
&= 21.34\ (\mu\mathrm{g/L})\ \exp[-(1.203/\mathrm{h})\,t]
\end{aligned} \tag{9}$$

Therefore, we estimate $K_{\mathrm{MT}} + K\mathrm{MB} \approx 1.20/\mathrm{h}$. We have disregarded other excretion pathways because previous work has shown that urinary excretion of MTBE is minor and that essentially all metabolized MTBE goes through the TBA pathway.[7,15,16]

To determine the metabolic conversion rate K_{MT} separately, we employ breath measurements during the uptake period of the inhalation exposure. We calculate parameters for exhaled breath with experimental data and a simple exponential uptake model:

$$C_{\mathrm{MB}}(t) = A(1 - e^{-\alpha t}) = 3.49\ \mu\mathrm{g/L}\left(1 - \exp[-(9.006/\mathrm{h})\,t]\right) \tag{10}$$

3.49 μg/L represents the steady state value in breath. From this, we see that for an infinitely long exposure, $3.49/10.9 = 32\,\%$ of the MTBE body burden is excreted via breath and $68\,\%$ is metabolized to TBA. Therefore, we estimate that the metabolic conversion rate constant is about $K_{\mathrm{MT}} \approx 0.68 \times 1.20/\mathrm{h} \approx 0.82/\mathrm{h}$, and that the breath excretion rate constant is $K_{\mathrm{MB}} \approx 0.38/\mathrm{h}$.

3.2. *MTBE Uptake and Volumes of Distribution Calculations*

The integral of Eq. (10) over the 1 h exposure time period represents the mass/volume of MTBE eliminated in one hour which is 3.10 μg/L. The controlled inhalation exposure was 10.9 μg/L for the same hour so we find that 72 % of the MTBE entering the alveolar space was actually absorbed. Given that the average resting alveolar ventilation rate is about 4.2 L/min, we calculate the total MTBE mass absorbed as 1.98 mg; also, from empirical measurements, the blood level at the end of the exposure is approxmately 23 μg/L. Therefore, we find that the hypothctical volume of distribution for MTBE is

$$V_{\mathrm{d}} \approx \frac{1.98\ \mathrm{mg}}{23\ \mu\mathrm{g/L}} \times 1000\ \mu\mathrm{g/mg} \approx 86\ \mathrm{L}.$$

Furthermore, a similar calculation using the plateau value of blood TBA concentration (14 μg/L) and the assumed total conversion of 1.98 mg MTBE to 2.45 mg TBA yields the hypothetical volume of distribution for TBA as $V_d \approx 175$ L.

3.3. *Elimination Pathways for TBA*

From the above results, we can estimate the TBA distribution rates to exhaled breath (K_{TB}) and to metabolic and other loss mechanisms (K_{TL}). During the time period $t \geq 6$ h, conversion of new TBA is negligible because $K_{MT}\, C_{MC1}(t) \approx 0$, and so we model the experimental blood data as a simple exponential decay:

$$C_{TC1}(t) = A\, e^{-\alpha t} = 19.14 \ \mu\text{g/L} \ \exp[-(0.0568/\text{h})\, t] \qquad (11)$$

0.0568/h represents ($K_{TB} + K_{Tl}$). Using the empirical breath data, we estimate the total amount of TBA eliminated by breath using numerical integration as approximately 0.052 (μg/L) h which results in 0.052 (μg/L) h $\times$ 4.2 L/min $\times$ 60 min/h = 13.1 μg TBA. We have previously estimated that a total of 2.45 mg TBA was created, so the breath elimination pathway represents about 0.53 % of the total removal of TBA. Therefore, we estimate $K_{TL} \approx 0.0565/\text{h}$ and $K_{TB} \approx 0.00028/\text{h}$.

3.4. *Breath Models*

The breath models are not amenable to a differential form; breath values can be calculated directly from blood concentrations based on ratio parameters that depend only on current exposure status. For the case of inhalation exposure in eqs. (6) and (7), we estimate the steady state post exposure values as $A_{pMB0} = 0.0592$ and $A_{pTB0} = 0.00118$ for MTBE and TBA respectively. From simple curve fitting, we find the adjustment parameters to be $A_{pMB1} = 0.010$ and $A_{pTB1} = 0.00009$, respectively.

3.5. *Full PK Model Implementation*

The basic PK model (Fig. 1) was implemented using Eqs. (1)–(3), (6), and (7), and estimates for the various parameters were used as initial conditions. The model was processed through the acslXreme software package and adjustable parameters were optimized to fit means of empirical blood and breath data. The classical PK model derived for MTBE using Eqs. (1), (2), and (6) was found to predict the empirical data very well. For the

TBA profiles, we needed to invoke direct conversion of MTBE to TBA in the lungs via the additional parameter K_{0T} as shown in Eq. (3); the appearance of TBA is much faster than predicted with hepatic metabolism alone. This suggests that there is indeed pulmonary metabolism during inhalation exposure and the optimized value for the rate was estimated to be $K_{0T} \approx 1.038/h$. Based on previous estimates of TBA volume of distribution (175 L), alveolar ventilation rate (252 L/h), mass ratio (73/59) and the empirical data, we estimate that about 0.022 mg of TBA appears in the first hour from direct pulmonary conversion from inhaled MTBE. We recall from Section 3.2 that the total amount of TBA created was estimated as 2.45 mg thus about 0.8 % is attributed to pulmonary metabolism during the exposure period.

We found that the model converged rapidly suggesting that the functional forms are appropriate. Figures 2 (breath) and 3 (blood) present the PK models plotted with the empirical data for MTBE and TBA. The final optimized constants for the PK model as represented in μg/L units concentrations, 1/h time constants, and adjusted for volumes of distribution in eqs. (1)–(7) are:

$$
\begin{aligned}
K_0\, k_a &= 6.85 & K_{MT} &= 0.820 & A_{pMB0} &= 0.0592 \\
K_{21} &= 0.938 & K_{MB} &= 0.380 & A_{pTB0} &= 0.00118 \\
K_{21}\, k_L &= 5.12 & K_{MT}\, k_d &- 0.165 & A_{pMB1} &= 0.0101 \\
K_{12} &= 3.12 & K_{0T}\, k_e &= 0.901 & A_{pTB1} &= 0.000090 \\
K_{12}\, k_c &= 0.530 & K_{TL} &= 0.0594 \\
& & K_{TB} &= 0.000317
\end{aligned}
$$

The functional form of the simple PK model and the associated differential equations reproduce the character of the measured data well suggesting that the model assumptions are reasonable and that the uptake and elimination kinetics are linear. It also reinforces the conjecture that the model could be generalized to multiple and intermittent exposures.

3.6. *Equilibrium Ratios Relating Blood, Breath, and Inhalation Exposure Levels*

Given a stable, known inhalation exposure, the expected equilibrium MTBE and TBA levels in the circulating blood can be calculated using the established classical PK model. The relative response factors with respect to actual blood or breath measurements can then be used to infer previous mean exposures as follows:

$$
\begin{aligned}
\text{Mean MTBE exposure (air)} &= (\text{MTBE in breath}) \times 1.23 \\
&= (\text{TBA in breath}) \times 16.3 \\
&= (\text{MTBE in blood}) \times 0.209 \\
&= (\text{TBA in blood}) \times 0.0353
\end{aligned}
$$

We note that the TBA concentrations are more stable with respect to variability in exposure (see Figs. 2 and 3) so a blood or breath measurement of the metabolite is likely more reflective of average MTBE exposure. Although this concept is not developed here, the concentration relationships among ambient exposure, native compound blood levels, and biological damping of metabolites expressed in blood levels have been discussed in the literature.[17,18]

4. Conclusions

In this demonstration, we used complementary blood and breath data to estimate pharmacokinetic parameters necessary for predicting the disposition of MTBE and TBA in the human body. The breath measurements furnished key information about elimination without which there is no direct access to mass balance of exposure compounds and metabolite concentrations. The kinetics at typical exposure levels appear linear so the classical PK model would presumably allow prediction of MTBE (parent compound) and its metabolite (TBA) at any time for other exposure scenarios. As such, we could presumably generalize to any hypothetical input function $C_i(t)$ and determine the expected time progression of MTBE and TBA in the blood. Because the breath and blood levels have similar temporal response, we can exploit this relationship to predict circulating blood levels from only non-invasive breath measurements. The use of a simple PK model developed from empirical blood and breath data is a powerful tool for predicting internal dose, or conversely, estimating previous exposure from current biological measurements.

References

1. USGS, Clawges R, Rowe R, Zogorski J. *National Survey of MTBE and other VOCs in Community Drinking Water Sources.* USGS FS-064-01, Oct 2001.
2. USGS, Personal communication: John S. Zogorsky, David A. Bender, VOC National Synthesis, U. S. Geological Survey, 2004.
3. EPA. *Methyl Tertiary Butyl Ether,* www.epa.gov/mtbe, 2001.

4. Prah J, Goldstein G, Devlin R, Otto D, Ashley D, House D, Willingham F, Cohen K, Gerrity T. Sensory, symptomatic, inflammatory, and ocular responses to and the metabolism of methyl tertiary butyl ether in a controlled human exposure. *Inhalation Toxicology* 1994; **6**: 521–538.
5. McCarthy J, Tiernan M. MTBE in Gasoline: Clean Air and Drinking Water Issues. *Congressional Research Service, The Library of Congress* 2001: OC 98-290 ENR.
6. ATSDR, Agency for Toxic Substances and Disease Registry, `www.atsdr.cdc.gov/toxprofiles/tp91.html`, 1996.
7. Dekant W, Bernauer U, Rosner E, Amberg A. Toxicokinetics of ethers used as fuel oxygenates. *Toxicology Letters* 2001; **124**: 37–45.
8. Prah J, Ashley D, Blount B, Case M, Leavens T, Pleil J, Cardinali F. Dermal, oral, and inhalation pharmacokinetics of methyl tertiary butyl ether (MTBE) in human volunteers. *Toxicol Sci* 2004; **77**: 195-205.
9. Boroujerdi M. *Pharmacokinetics: Principle and Applications.* New York: Mc-Graw Hill, 2002.
10. Pleil J, Lindstrom A. Sample timing and mathematical considerations for modeling breath elimination of volatile organic compounds. *Risk Analysis* 1998; **18**: 585–602.
11. Ashley DL, Bonin MA, Cardinali FL, McCraw JM, Holler JS, Needham LL, Patterson DG, Jr. Determining volatile organic compounds in human blood from a large sample population by using purge and trap gas chromatography/mass spectrometry. *Anal Chem* 1992; **64**: 1021–1029.
12. Pleil J, Lindstrom A. Collection of a Single Alveolar Exhaled Breath for Volatile Organic Compounds Analysis. *Journal of Industrial Medicine* 1995; **28**: 109–121.
13. Pleil J, Lindstrom A. Measurement of Volatile Organic Compounds in Exhaled Breath as Collected in SUMMA Canisters. *Journal of Chromatography B, Biomedical Applications* 1995; **665**: 271–279.
14. Lindstrom A, JD Pleil J. Alveolar breath sampling and analysis to assess exposures to methyl tertiary butyl ether (MTBE) during motor vehicle refueling. *J Air Waste Manage Assoc* 1996; **46**: 676–682.
15. Nihlen A, Lof A, Johanson G. Liquid/air partition coefficients of methyl and ethyl *t*-butyl ethers, *t*-amyl methyl ether, and *t*-butyl alcohol. *Journal of Exposure Analysis and Environmental Epidemiology* 1995; **5**: 573–582.
16. Nihlen A, Lof A, G Johanson G. Experimental exposure to methyl tertiary-butyl ether: Toxicokinetics in humans. *Toxicol Appl Pharm* 1998; **148**: 274–280.
17. Rappaport SM. Smoothing of exposure variability at the receptor: implications for health standards. *Ann Occup Hyg* 1985; **29**: 201–214.
18. Rappaport SM, Symanski E, Yager JW, Kupper LL. The relationship between environmental monitoring and biological markers in exposure assessment. *Environ Health Perspect* 1995; **103** Suppl 3: 49–53.

A MODEL OF THE CARDIOVASCULAR–RESPIRATORY CONTROL SYSTEM WITH APPLICATIONS TO EXERCISE, SLEEP, AND CONGESTIVE HEART FAILURE

S. TESCHL

University of Applied Sciences Technikum Wien,
Höchstädtplatz 5, A-1200, Vienna, Austria

J. BATZEL AND F. KAPPEL

Institute of Mathematics,
Karl Franzens University of Graz,
Heinrichstraße 36, A-8010 Graz, Austria

1. Introduction

Models of the human circulatory and respiratory system have a long history. However, in the past both systems have usually been studied independently. The purpose of this article is to summarize recent work[1] which applies a combined model of the human cardiovascular–respiratory system to simulating the transition from rest to exercise and from quiet awake to stage 4 (NREM) sleep, respectively. The equations describing the state of the system are developed following the ideas in Refs. 2 and 3. Cardiovascular and respiratory control is implemented via an optimal control approach which specifies heart rate and ventilation. This modeling approach was previously applied in Refs. 4 and 5. We include one and two transport delays in the state equations of the respiratory system and consider as an application the congestive heart condition where these transport delays are increased due to the reduced cardiac output.

2. The Model

2.1. *Model Equations*

The model consists of two respiratory compartments and four cardiovascular compartments. It is represented by Fig. 1 and is mathematically described by the system of nonlinear ordinary differential equations (1)–(13) in Table 1.

The respiratory component is based on a model developed in Ref. 2. It consists of two compartments which are connected by the circulating blood: a single homogeneous alveolar (lung) compartment and a single homogeneous tissue compartment. For each compartment mass balance equations for CO_2 and O_2 are derived. They are represented by equations (1)–(4). We assume that the lung compartment is ventilated by a continuous, unidirectional stream of gas and we neglect the events of the respiratory circle. Furthermore, the alveolar blood gas levels are assumed to be instantly equilibrated with the arterial blood gas levels. Analogously, we assume that

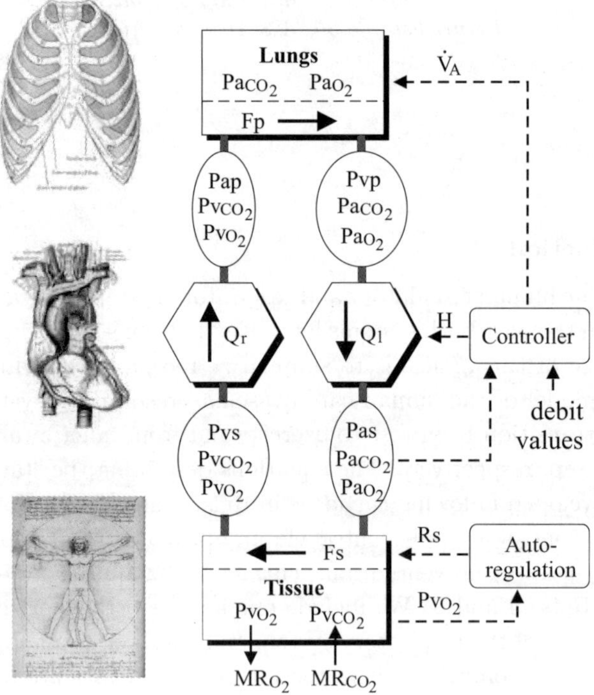

Fig. 1.   The model

Table 1. The model equations. The indices correspond to the following abbreviations: a: arterial, v: venous, A: alveolar, T: tissue, s: systemic, p: pulmonary, I: inspiratory, l: left, r: right

$$V_{A\,CO_2}\dot{P}_{v\,CO_2}(t) = 863\,F_p(t)\left[C_{v\,CO_2}(t) - C_{a\,CO_2}(t)\right] + \dot{V}_A(t)\left[P_{I\,CO_2} - P_{a\,CO_2}(t)\right] \quad (1)$$

$$V_{A\,O_2}\,\dot{P}_{v\,O_2}(t) = 863\,F_p(t)\left[C_{v\,O_2}(t) - C_{a\,O_2}(t)\right] + \dot{V}_A(t)\left[P_{I\,O_2} - P_{a\,O_2}(t)\right] \quad (2)$$

$$V_{T\,CO_2}\dot{C}_{v\,CO_2}(t) = \mathrm{MR}_{CO_2} + F_s(t)\left[C_{a\,CO_2}(t) - C_{v\,CO_2}(t)\right] \quad (3)$$

$$V_{T\,O_2}\,\dot{C}_{v\,O_2}(t) = -\mathrm{MR}_{O_2} + F_s(t)\left[C_{a\,O_2}(t) - C_{v\,O_2}(t)\right] \quad (4)$$

$$c_{as}\,\dot{P}_{as}(t) = Q_l(t) - F_s(t) \quad (5)$$

$$c_{vs}\,\dot{P}_{vs}(t) = F_s(t) - Q_r(t) \quad (6)$$

$$c_{vp}\dot{P}_{vp}(t) = F_p(t) - Q_l(t) \quad (7)$$

$$\dot{S}_l(t) = \sigma_l(t) \quad (8)$$

$$\dot{S}_r(t) = \sigma_r(t) \quad (9)$$

$$\dot{\sigma}_l(t) = -\gamma_l\,\sigma_l(t) - \alpha_l\,S_l(t) + \beta_l\,H(t) \quad (10)$$

$$\dot{\sigma}_r(t) = -\gamma_r\,\sigma_r(t) - \alpha_r\,S_r(t) + \beta_r\,H(t) \quad (11)$$

$$\dot{H}(t) = u_1(t) \quad (12)$$

$$\ddot{V}_A(t) = u_2(t) \quad (13)$$

the gas concentrations in the tissues are at every instant equal to the gas concentrations in the mixed venous blood returning to the lungs. Partial pressures and gas volumes are related by the ideal gas law and dissociation relationships describe the dependencies of total blood gas concentrations on the corresponding partial pressures.

The cardiovascular part of the model is based on the ideas in Refs. 3 and 4 and is described by equations (5)–(11). This component consists of two circuits (pulmonary and systemic) which are arranged in series, and two pumps (left and right ventricle). Each circuit contains a single elastic artery, a single elastic vein and a single resistance vessel (where the gas exchange occurs). Cardiac output is modeled for both left and right hearts. Blood flow is assumed to be unidirectional and non pulsatile. Thus, blood flow and blood pressure are to be interpreted as mean values over the length of a pulse. A fixed blood volume is distributed among the systemic artery and vein and the pulmonary artery and vein. Continuity equations for the blood volume in each of these four compartments are derived.

Equations (1)–(4) include expressions for the partial pressures of arterial carbon dioxide and oxygen ($P_{a\,CO_2}$ and $P_{a\,O_2}$), and venous CO_2 and O_2 concentrations ($C_{v\,CO_2}$ and $C_{v\,O_2}$). $V_{A\,CO_2}$, $V_{A\,O_2}$, $V_{T\,CO_2}$, and $V_{T\,O_2}$ denote the effective lung and tissue storage volumes for CO_2 and O_2, respectively. MR_{CO_2} and MR_{O_2} are the metabolic rates of CO_2 and O_2 production, respectively, in the tissue compartment. Equations (5)–(7) are mass balance equations expressed with the help of left and right cardiac outputs (Q_l and Q_r) and systemic and pulmonary blood flows (F_s and F_p). The left hand sides of these mass balance equations involve arterial and venous systemic pressures (P_{as} and P_{vs}), venous pulmonary pressure P_{vp}, and the compliance of the respective artery or vein (c_{as}, c_{vs}, and c_{vp}). Arterial pulmonary pressure P_{ap} is found using these pressures assuming constant blood volume.

Equations (8)-(11) describe a relation assuming a second order delay between heart rate H and contractility S (Bowditch effect) for the left and right heart. They involve constants α, β, and γ which need to be determined by parameter identification. To obtain differential equations of first order the abbreviation $\sigma = \dot{S}$ has been introduced.

Equations (12)–(13) include the controls u_1 and u_2 determining the rate of change of the heart rate H and the ventilation rate $\dot{V}_A$.

Additional equations relate systemic and pulmonary blood flows (F_s and F_p) to systemic and pulmonary resistances (R_s and R_p), respectively (Ohm's Law). Further, a relationship between stroke volume V_{str}, contractility S, and blood pressure based on the Frank–Starling mechanism is given. A relation between R_s and venous oxygen concentration C_{vO_2} describes the local metabolic control of systemic resistance. All other control features are subsumed under the action of the control equations which describe an optimal control process. This mechanism is discussed in section 2.2. We refer the reader to Refs. 4 and 5 for further details.

2.2. *Cardiovascular and Respiratory Control*

We model the complex cardiovascular and respiratory control mechanism via an optimal stabilizing feedback control derived from control theory. This is motivated by the fact that many physiologists assume that optimization is a basic concept in the evolution of biological systems.[6,7] Hence, the controlling instances of the organism ("central command") are lumped into one controller. Variation of the heart rate $\dot{H}$ and variation of alveolar ventilation $\dot{V}_A$ are the outputs of the controller. Input to the controller is information about mean blood pressure and blood gas concentrations. The control is optimal in the sense that (i) deviations of these variables from their debit values during the transient phase are as small as possible and (ii) heart rate and alveolar ventilation must not change too fast (*i.e.* control effort must stay within certain bounds).

The design of an optimal control mathematically determines the control functions u_1 and u_2 that transfer the system from a steady initial condition (rest/quiet awake, respectively) to an equilibrium state (ES) (exercise/ NREM sleep, respectively) such that the cost functional

$$\int_0^\infty \Big(q_{as} \left[P_{as}(t) - P_{as}^{ES} \right]^2 + q_{CO_2} \left[P_{a\,CO_2}(t) - P_{a\,CO_2}^{ES} \right]^2$$

$$+ q_{O_2} \left[P_{a\,O_2}(t) - P_{a\,O_2}^{ES} \right]^2 + q_1\, u_1(t)^2 + q_2\, u_2(t)^2 \Big)\, dt \quad (14)$$

is minimized subject to the constraints given by the model equations (1)–(13). The cost functional measures deviations in P_{as}, $P_{a\,CO_2}$, $P_{a\,O_2}$, as well as deviations in the controls u_1 and u_2. The corresponding positive weighing coefficients q_{as}, q_{CO_2}, q_{O_2}, q_1 and q_2 determine the relative importance of each term of the integrand. Delay in the optimal control is not included. States (rest/quiet awake, respectively) and (exercise/NREM sleep, respectively) are determined by parameters. For further details please refer to Ref. 8.

2.3. *Application to Simulating Exercise*

We model exercise (*e.g.* a bicycle ergometer test) below the anaerobic threshold. In this case the model predicts an increase in heart rate, alveolar ventilation (see Fig. 2), cardiac output, contractility, stroke volume and a decreased systemic resistance. Figures 3 and 4 show the dynamics of mean arterial blood pressure and arterial concentrations of CO_2 and O_2 which are regulated towards their debit values. The simulation dynamics show qualitatively and quantitatively reasonable behavior.[5] For a more precise statement empirical dynamical data for a parameter identification will be needed.

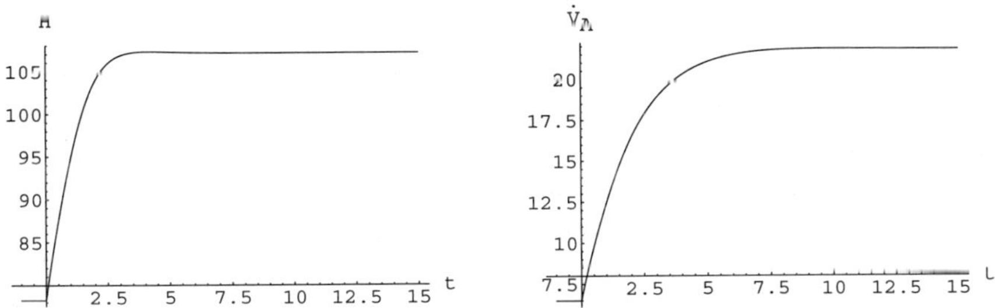

Fig. 2.   Transition to exercise equilibrium with constant workload: Dynamics of heart rate and alveolar ventilation

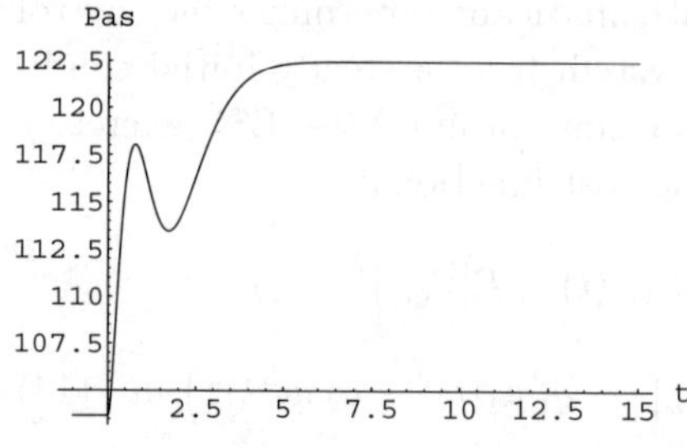
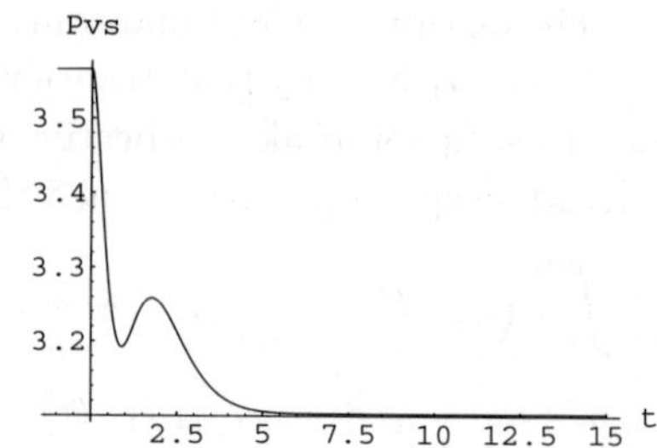

Fig. 3.   Transition to exercise equilibrium with constant workload: Dynamics of mean arterial and venous blood pressure

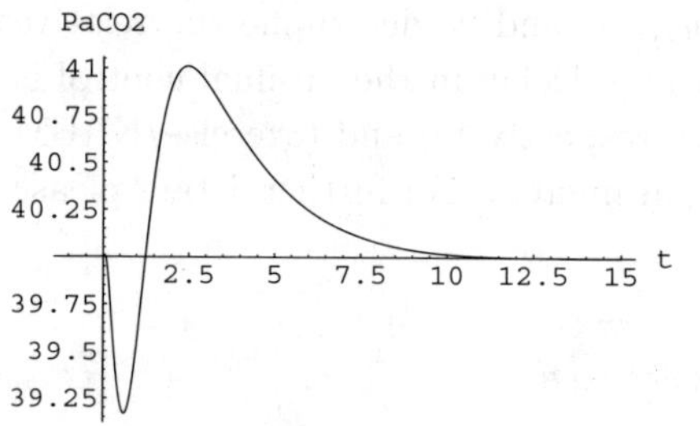
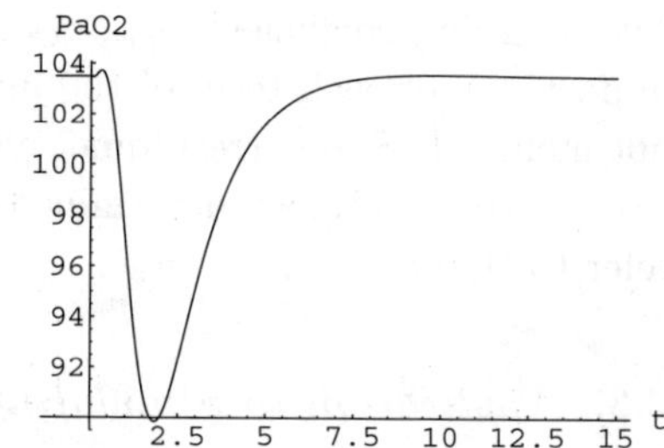

Fig. 4.   Transition to exercise equilibrium with constant workload: Dynamics of arterial partial pressures of CO_2 and O_2

3. Introducing Delay into the Model

The model was modified by including delays into the state equations of the respiratory component.[1]

$$V_{A\,CO_2}\dot{P}_{v\,CO_2}(t) = 863 F_p(t)\big[C_{v\,CO_2}(t-\tau_V)-C_{a\,CO_2}(t)\big] + \dot{V}_A(t)\big[P_{I\,CO_2}-P_{a\,CO_2}(t)\big] \quad (1')$$

$$V_{A\,O_2}\ \dot{P}_{v\,O_2}\ (t) = 863 F_p(t)\big[C_{v\,O_2}\ (t-\tau_V)-C_{a\,O_2}\ (t)\big] + \dot{V}_A(t)\big[P_{I\,O_2}\ -P_{a\,O_2}\ (t)\big] \quad (2')$$

$$V_{T\,CO_2}\dot{C}_{v\,CO_2}(t) = \quad MR_{CO_2} + F_s(t)\big[C_{a\,CO_2}(t-\tau_T) - C_{v\,CO_2}(t)\big] \quad\quad\quad\quad (3')$$

$$V_{T\,O_2}\ \dot{C}_{v\,O_2}\ (t) = -MR_{O_2}\ + F_s(t)\big[C_{a\,O_2}\ (t-\tau_T) - C_{v\,O_2}\ (t)\big] \quad\quad\quad\quad (4')$$

Delays occur because it takes time for the blood to transfer the blood gases from the lungs to the tissue compartment (τ_T) and to return from the tissue to lungs (τ_V). We assume that the delays τ_V and τ_T are equal. As an alternative to the optimal control approach we consider an empirical representation of ventilatory control given in Ref. 9,

$$\dot{V}_A(t) = G_p\, e^{-0.05 P_{a\,O_2}(t-\tau_p)}\big[P_{a\,CO_2}(t-\tau_p) - I_p\big]$$

$$+ G_c\left[P_{B\,CO_2}(t) - \frac{MR_{B\,CO_2}}{K_{CO_2}\,F_B}\,I_c\right]. \tag{15}$$

In this equation the first term describes the effect of the blood gases O_2 and CO_2 as measured by the peripheral sensors located in the carotid artery. The second term represents the central control and describes the effect of the brain CO_2 level. $P_{B\,CO_2}$ denotes the partial pressure of CO_2 and $MR_{B\,CO_2}$ the metabolic rate of CO_2 production in the brain tissue. K_{CO_2} is the slope of the physiological CO_2 dissociation curve , F_B is the blood flow perfusing the brain, G_p and G_c are control gains and I_p and I_c are cutoff thresholds. The delay τ_p is the transport delay from the lungs to peripheral control. Due to this delay ventilation is at time t adjusted according to the arterial blood gas levels which have been sensored at time $t - \tau_p$ by the peripheral sensor.

One way the cardiovascular and respiratory systems interact is through cardiac output determination of the transport delay τ_p in the respiratory feedback control loop. This can effect the stability of the control (see, *e.g.*, Ref. 10 and the next section).

3.1. *Application to Simulating Congestive Heart Failure*

As an application of this model we consider the transition from "quiet awake" to "stage 4 (NREM) sleep" for normal individuals and for patients suffering from congestive heart problems, where the transport delays are larger than normal due to the reduced cardiac output.

Heart failure (HF) refers to the clinical condition of reduced heart pumping efficiency. When left forward failure occurs excess blood accumulates in the pulmonary venous system because the left heart cannot effectively push blood to the systemic arterial system. This can result in fluid congestion in the lungs — hence the term congestive heart failure.

Cheyne–Stokes respiration (CSR) is common in heart failure patients during sleep. CSR is an unstable breathing pattern which is non-voluntary and oscillates between rising and falling breath volumes interspersed with apneas. CSR is an important clinical condition because it contributes to the progressive deterioration in heart function seen in heart failure. Among a number of possible contributing factors to CSR is the increased delay in the respiratory control loop which affects feedback loop efficiency. This is due to the increased time needed for blood gases to move from the site where these blood gas levels are adjusted (the lungs) to the sensory sites where these levels are measured. Another factor may be increased control sensitivity to CO_2.

In the first simulation depicted in Fig. 5 we use an optimal control defining both $\dot{V}_A$ and H and the system transition from quiet awake to stage 4 sleep in case of acute left heart failure. Table 2 gives the corresponding parameters and computed steady states.

Only one delay τ_T occurs in the lung to tissue transport loop. Compared with parameter values for normal adults,[1] acute heart failure is modeled by reducing the parameters β_l and β_r which affect contractility, by increasing the systemic resistance parameter A_{pesk}, by an increased heart rate H and by an increased transport delay τ_T. No change is assumed in pulmonary resistance R_p, in $P_{a\,CO_2}$ or in total blood volume V_0.

In the second simulation defined by Table 3 we modify the model by taking $\dot{V}_A$ out of the optimal control and define $\dot{V}_A$ via the empirical equation (15). By doing this we introduce a second delay τ_p in the state equations and implement a delay in the respiratory control loop. For the change of ventilation during the transition to sleep we use a model given in Ref. 9,

$$\dot{V}_{sleep}(t) = G_s(t)\,\max\left[0, \dot{V}_{awake}(t) - K_{shift}(t)\right]. \tag{16}$$

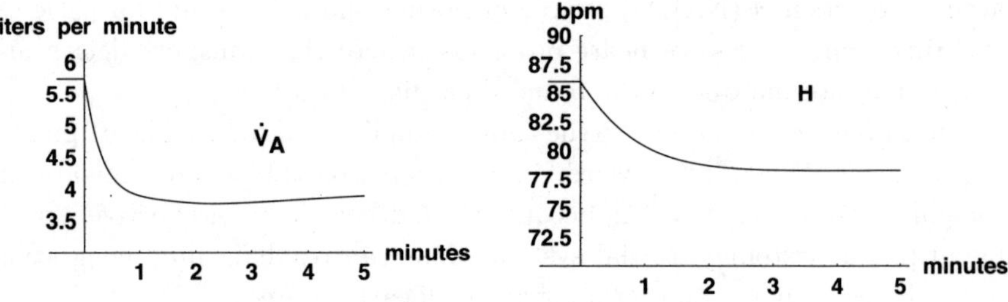

Fig. 5.   Acute heart failure transition to NREM sleep: $\dot{V}_A$ implemented via optimal control without delay

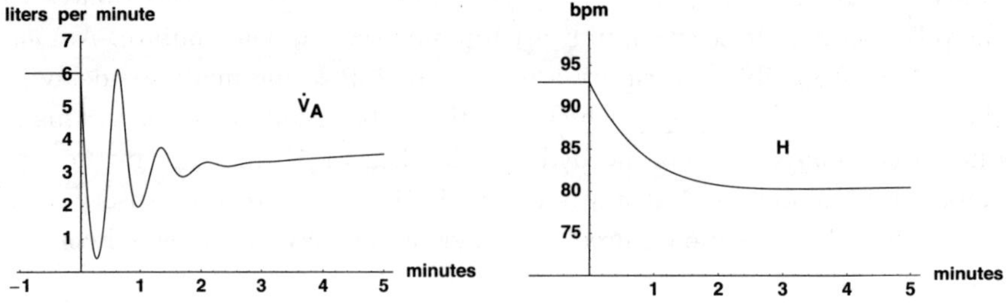

Fig. 6.   Chronic heart failure transition to NREM sleep: $\dot{V}_A$ implemented via an empirical formula with delay

The factor $G_s(t)$ and the shift $K_{shift}(t)$ are modeled by exponential functions which change smoothly through the various sleep stages. The transit time from awake to stage 4 sleep is denoted by $S_{4\,transit}$.

We now model chronic congestive heart failure by reducing contractilities via a decrease of β_l and β_r, by increasing the systemic resistance parameter A_{pesk}, by increasing pulmonary resistance R_p, by an increased heart rate H, increased transport delays τ_T and τ_p and an increased total blood volume V_0. We assume a fast transition to sleep by decreasing

Table 2. Optimal control parameters and steady states: acute left heart failure sleep transition

Parameter	Awake	Sleep
A_{pesk}	198.7	188.7
β_l	25.8	23.19
β_r	1.77	1.59
R_p	1.965	1.965
V_0	5.0	5.0
H	86.02	78.02
$P_{a\,CO_2}$	40.0	44.5
τ_T	32.0	32.0

Steady State	Awake	Sleep
H	86.02	78.02
P_{as}	86.6	74.08
P_{ap}	19.24	18.30
P_{vs}	2.77	3.02
P_{vp}	11.97	11.96
$P_{a\,CO_2}$	40.0	44.5
$P_{a\,O_2}$	103.38	98.35
$P_{v\,CO_2}$	51.06	55.17
$P_{v\,O_2}$	28.12	28.83
$Q_l,\ Q_r$	3.70	3.23
R_s	22.64	22.00
S_l	24.77	20.22
S_r	5.35	4.37
$\dot{V}_A$	5.739	4.34
$V_{str,l},\ V_{str,r}$	0.0430	0.0414

Table 3. Empirical control parameters and steady states: chronic left and right heart failure sleep transition

Parameter	Awake	Sleep
A_{pesk}	250.17	237.7
β_l	12.88	11.60
β_r	1.46	1.31
R_p	2.16	2.16
V_0	6.9	6.9
H	93.02	80.02
I_c	35.5	35.5
I_p	35.5	35.5
G_s	1.60	0.480
K_{shift}	0.	5.2
τ_p	11.6	11.6
τ_T	36.0	36.0
$S_{4,transit}$	—	2 min

Steady State	Awake	Sleep
H	93.00	80.02
P_{as}	92.08	72.78
P_{ap}	26.80	25.17
P_{vs}	3.57	4.05
P_{vp}	19.58	19.14
$P_{a\,CO_2}$	37.87	44.15
$P_{a\,O_2}$	105.86	98.76
$P_{v\,CO_2}$	50.08	56.51
$P_{v\,O_2}$	25.92	25.49
$P_{B\,CO_2}$	45.95	51.81
$Q_l,\ Q_r$	3.35	2.79
R_s	26.40	24.67
S_l	13.39	10.37
S_r	4.76	3.69
$\dot{V}_A$	6.06	4.38
$V_{str,l},\ V_{str,r}$	0.036	0.035

$S_{4\,\mathrm{transit}}$, increasing the awake gain G_{s} (which in effect increases CO_2 sensitivity), and by decreasing the corresponding sleep gain G_{s}. For a detailed discussion of the parameter changes see Ref. 1. Under these conditions the respiratory function is driven to CSR-like instability as the dynamics in Fig. 6 show.

4. Discussion

Our model describes the interactions of the cardiovascular and the respiratory system in a rather satisfactory way. In case of a congestive heart condition the transport delays in the state equations of the respiratory system are increased due to the reduced cardiac output. As a consequence the efficiency of the feedback loop of ventilatory control is reduced which induces instabilities in our simulation of alveolar ventilation.

As a next step empirical data need to be gained for the situations we consider in order to validate the model. In particular, measurements of cardiovascular and respiratory quantities and a subsequent parameter identification will allow to compare the predictions of the model with real life situations.

The model can be adapted to simulate other situations, such as short-term regulatory mechanisms (*e.g.* following hemorrhage or transfusion), consequences of a suddenly increased systemic resistance (*e.g.* after infusion of a vasoconstrictor substance). Also, the inclusion of long term control mechanisms (such as control of blood volume by the kidneys) to simulate the hemodynamics and gas concentrations during a dialysis process can be an issue of future research.

Furthermore, mass balance equations for other substances (*e.g.* isoprene) can be included in order to investigate the interrelationships between this substance and other state variables. This is of particular importance for breath gas analysis where breath gas concentrations need to be linked to blood gas concentrations. The importance of this interrelationship is *e.g.* pointed out in Ref. 11.

Acknowledgement

This project was supported by the Austrian Science Fund (FWF) under grant F310 as a subproject of the Special Research Center F003 "Optimization and Control."

References

1. Batzel JJ, Teschl (née Timischl) S, Kappel F. A cardiovascular-respiratory control system model including state delay with application to congestive heart failure in humans. *J Math Biol*; to appear.
2. Khoo MC, Kronauer RE, Strohl KP, Slutsky AS. Factors inducing periodic breathing in humans: a general model. *J Appl Physiol Respirat Environ Exercise Physiol* 1982; **53** (3): 644–659.
3. Grodins FS. Integrative cardiovascular physiology: a mathematical model synthesis of cardiac and blood vessel hemodynamics. *Q Rev Biol* 1959; **34** (2): 93–116.
4. Kappel F, Peer RO. A mathematical model for fundamental regulation processes in the cardiovascular model. *J Math Biol* 1993; **31**: 611–631.
5. Teschl (née Timischl) S. *A Global Model of the Cardiovascular and Respiratory System*. PhD thesis, Karl-Franzens-University Graz, 1998.
6. Kenner T. Physical and mathematical modeling in cardiovascular systems. In: Hwang NHC, Gross ER, Patel DJ, ed. *Clinical and Research Applications of Engineering Principles*, Baltimore: University Park Press, 1979: 41–109.
7. Swan GW. *Applications of Optimal Control Theory in Biomedicine*. New York, Marcel Dekker Inc., 1984.
8. Teschl (née Timischl) S, Batzel JJ, Kappel F. Modeling the human cardiovascular-respiratory control system: an optimal control application to the transition to NREM sleep. Technical Report 2000; 190. SFB F-003, Mathematics Dept., Karl-Franzens-University Graz.
9. Khoo MCK, Gottschalk A, Pack AI. Sleep-induced periodic breathing and apnea: a theoretical study. *J Appl Physiol* 1991; **70** (5): 2014–2024.
10. Batzel JJ, Tran HT. Stability of the human respiratory control system. Part 2: Analysis of a three dimensional delay state-space model. *J Math Biol* 2000; **41**: 80–102.
11. Karl T, Prazeller P, Mayr D, Jordan A, Rieder J, Fall R, Lindinger W. Human breath isoprene and its relation to blood cholesterol levels: new measurements and modeling. *J Appl Physiol* 2001; **91**: 762–770.

PART D

FOCUSED STUDIES

BREATH GAS ANALYSIS IN PATIENTS WITH CARBOHYDRATE-MALABSORPTION SYNDROME

M. LEDOCHOWSKI

Department of Clinical Nutrition,
University Hospital Innsbruck,
Innrain 66a, A-6020 Innsbruck, Austria

A. AMANN

Department of Anesthesia and General Intensive Care,
Innsbruck Medical University,
A-6020 Innsbruck, Austria
and
Department of Environmental Sciences,
Swiss Federal Institute of Technology,
ETH Hönggerberg, CH-8093 Zurich, Switzerland

D. FUCHS

Division of Biological Chemistry, Biocentre,
Innsbruck Medical University,
A-6020 Innsbruck, Austria

1. Introduction

Carbohydrate malabsorption syndromes are characterized by either a defect of the intestinal transport system for the affected sugar molecule (such as in fructose malabsorption) or by an enzyme deficiency that is needed for the cleavage of disaccharides or polysaccharides.[1,2] In the present contribution we report some of our studies concerning patients with fructose malabsorption (FM) and lactose maldigestion.

Fructose malabsorption is a well-characterised gastrointestinal disorder[3-5] that was described some years ago. It is characterized by a defect of the fructose-related GLUT5 transport system, which is responsible for the duodenal uptake of the monosaccharide fructose (see Fig. 1).[6,7] Hence, patients are unable to sufficiently absorb the ingested monosaccharide. As a result, fructose reaches the colon where it is broken down by colon bacteria into short-chain fatty acids (SCFA), carbon dioxide (CO_2), methane (CH_4), lactic acid and hydrogen (H_2) (Table 1).

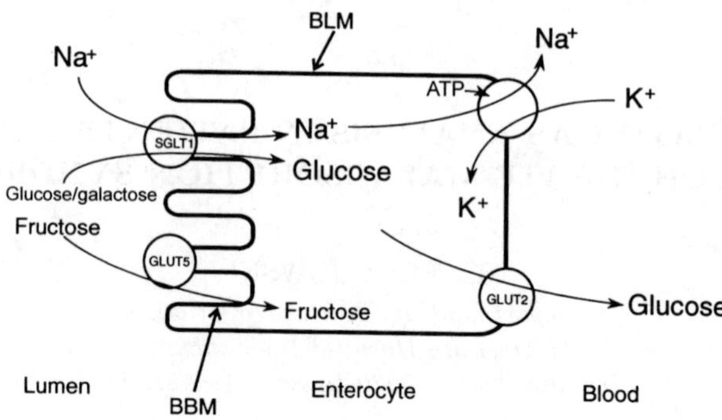

Fig. 1.   The fructose related GLUT5 transport system[38]

According to the present state of knowledge, the following classification of carbohydrate malabsorption syndromes can be made:

- Fructose malabsorption
- Lactose intolerance and lactose maldigestion
- Intolerance of sugar alcohols (sorbitol or xylitol intolerance)
- Amylase deficiency and partial pancreas deficiency
- Functional carbohydrate malabsorptions caused by food processing and food preparation

Carbon dioxide and methane usually lead to the symptoms "bloating" and "flatulence," while SCFA and lactic acid usually induce abdominal discomfort and osmotic diarrhoea. The hydrogen produced during the fermentation process in the colon passes through the wall of the colon and reaches the lung via the blood stream where it is exhaled and can be measured as "breath hydrogen." The kind and extent of gastrointestinal discomfort largely depends on the kind of colonic bacterial activity.[8] In turn, these factors depend on various circumstances like the kind of food, speed of eating,

Table 1.   Some SCFA, aldehydes and alcohols produced by anaerobic fermentation of gut bacteria

Short chain fatty acids (SCFA)	Aldehydes	Alcohols
Formic acid	Formaldehyde	Methanol
Acetic acid	Acetaldehyde	Ethanol
Propionic acid	Propanal	Propanol
Butyric acid	Butanal	Butanol
Valeric acid	Pentanal	Pentanol

Table 2. Description of different carbohydrates that usually cannot be absorbed

Carbohydrates that normally cannot be absorbed	Lactulose (Fru-Gal)	Synthetic sugar
	Raffinose (Gal-Glu-Fru)	"dietary fibre"
	Verbascose (Gal-Gal-Glu-Fru)	"dietary fibre"
	Stachyose (Gal-Gal-Glu-Fru)	"dietary fibre"
Carbohydrates that cannot be absorbed by a large percentage of persons	Fructose (Fru)	Fructose malabsorption
	Lactose (Gal-Glu)	Lactose intolerance

stress, age, phase of the female cycle, season of the year, cultural differences in cooking and the contemporary occurrence of other illnesses, especially hormonal or psychological disorders. It is believed that up to 36% of the European population suffers from fructose malabsorption to a greater-or-less degree, and about half of them are symptomatic. Withdrawal of dietary fructose can reverse these effects and does not only ameliorate gastrointestinal symptoms, but also diminishes the symptoms of depression.

Another better known carbohydrate malabsorption syndrome is hypolactasia or lactose intolerance, which is characterized by intestinal lactase deficiency. In patients with lactase deficiency, undigested lactose reaches the colon where it is fermented to the same substances as listed above (see Table 1). The diagnosis of fructose malabsorption or lactose intolerance can easily be made by measuring the hydrogen (H_2) concentration in the exhaled breath after an oral load of fructose or lactose respectively.[9–11] We indicated earlier that fructose malabsorption[12] and lactose malabsorption[13] were associated with signs of mental depression and that these signs were ameliorated by a fructose- and sorbitol-reduced diet.[14] The data available to date suggest that abnormalities of tryptophan availability could be involved in the development of fructose malabsorption-associated depression. Some other malabsorbed carbohydrates are listed in Table 2.

2. Patients and Methods

Three case studies were carried out. In all three studies breath H_2 was measured using a Bedfont gastrolizer (Bedfont Ltd., Kent, ME9 7HN, UK), which has been validated by several authors.[15–17] After an overnight fast (at least 12 hours), a baseline breath H_2 was measured. After an oral dose of 50 g fructose given in 250 mL of tap water, the H_2 concentration in the exhaled breath was monitored in 30 minute intervals for at least 2 hours. Examinations started between 8.00 to 8.30 a.m. Maximum breath H_2 concentrations were registered (H_2-max) and the differences from baseline values were calculated (ΔH_2). In the first study another H_2-breath test was performed with an oral dose of 50 g lactose given in 250 mL of tap water at least one week later.

3. Case Studies

3.1. *First Study*

3.1.1. *Patients*

One hundred eleven otherwise healthy outpatients aged from 17 to 81 years (mean 45.6±13.3 S.D.) who visited the physician's office for a medical health check-up and who complained about meteorism were included in this study. The group comprised 30 males aged from 23 to 72 years (mean ± S.D. 42.9 ± 12.8 years) and 81 female patients aged 17 to 81 years (46.5 ± 13.5). None of these patients showed signs of inflammatory bowel disease, any other chronic disease or infectious diseases. None were taking medication except for oral contraceptives by some of the females. All patients filled out a Beck's depression inventory-questionnaire at the time of examination.[8-10] Body weight and height were measured at the beginning of the trials and the body mass index (BMI) was calculated for all individuals.

3.1.2. *Data analysis*

A threshold breath H_2 concentrations greater than 20 parts-per-million, ppm, above baseline after the fructose or lactose load was defined for the diagnosis of lactose malabsorption.[18,19] Subjects with an increase of breath H_2 concentrations equal to or less than 20 ppm above baseline were considered to be normal fructose or lactose absorbers. Subjects that showed neither fructose nor lactose malabsorption were classified as "normals" (group 1); subjects that showed isolated fructose malabsorption were classified as fructose malabsorbers (group 2); subjects that showed isolated lactose malabsorption were classified as lactose malabsorbers only (group 3); subjects that showed both fructose and lactose malabsorption were classified as fructose and lactose malabsorbers (group 4). For group comparisons the Kruskal–Wallis-test was performed. For further statistical analysis, the *t*-test for independent samples was employed using a standard PC statistical program (STATISTICA for Windows version 5.0).[20] In addition, nonparametric tests (Mann–Whitney *U*-test and Spearman rank correlation analysis) have been performed for confirmation and the results were in good agreement.

3.1.3. *Results*

Twenty-five subjects [22.5 %] (5 males [16.7 %] and 20 females [24.7 %]) were neither fructose nor lactose malabsorbers and where therefore classified as "normals" (group 1). Sixty-nine subjects [62.2 %], (21 males [70.0 %] and 48 females [59.3%]) were isolated fructose malabsorbers (group 2) and 4 subjects [3.6 %] (1 male [3.3 %] and 3 females [3.7 %]) were isolated lactose malabsorbers (group 3). The remaining 13 subjects [11.7 %], (3 males [10 %] and 10 females [12.3 %]) showed signs of both fructose and lactose malabsorption (group 4). Their average BMI was 23.98 (S.D. ±4.7) and there were no significant differences between normals and malabsorbers, which remained so when the group was separated into two groups differentiated by sex. No significant differences were found between the 4 groups regarding the Beck's score when the whole set of data was analyzed. However, when individuals were differentiated by sex, in females the differences within the four groups in Beck's inventory depression scores were significant ($p < 0.003$ Kruskal–Wallis-Test). However, there was no such difference in males ($p = 0.16$), so they were excluded from further statistical analysis. In females, the Beck's inventory depression score was significantly higher ($p < 0.026$) in fructose malabsorbers (group 1) with a mean score of 11.4 (S.D. ±7.3) than in normals with a mean score of 7.5 (S.D. ±3.7) and the depression score was also significantly higher ($p < 0.004$) in fructose/lactose malabsorbers (group 4) with a mean score of 14.6 (S.D. ±8.7) (see Fig. 2). There was no significant difference between normals and isolated lactose malabsorbers (group 3).

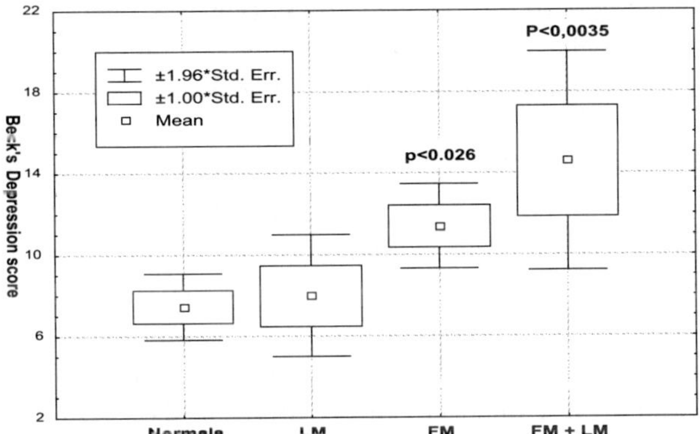

Fig. 2. Beck's depression scores in fructose and lactose malabsorption syndromes in females (LM: lactose malabsorbers, FM: fructose malabsorbers, FM+LM: fructose and lactose malabsorbers)[39]

3.2. Second Study

3.2.1. Patients

All adult outpatients who visited the physician's office between November 1997 and March 1998 for a medical health check and complained of gastrointestinal discomfort were considered for inclusion into this study. Subjects were included if they presented with any of the following symptoms: stool irregularities, bloating, abdominal cramps, diarrhoea, constipation or nausea. The 50 patients (16 men, 34 women) were aged from 16 to 72 years (mean 43.3 years) and were otherwise healthy. Physical examination and routine laboratory assessment did not reveal abnormalities. None of the patients showed signs of inflammatory bowel disease, any other chronic disease or infectious diseases and were not taking medication, except for oral contraceptives in some cases. Body weight and height were measured, and blood samples were taken after an overnight fast for plasma tryptophan and kynurenine measurements before breath hydrogen testing was performed. Patients with breath hydrogen concentrations higher than 10 ppm during fasting were excluded from the study. During the times between breath H_2 monitoring, all the patients filled out a Beck's depression inventory-questionnaire.

Tryptophan in the blood was measured simultaneously with kynurenine, a metabolite of the tryptophan catabolism, by high performance liquid chromatography (HPLC) according to a recently established method.[21] In brief, 100 μL serum was diluted with 100 μL of buffer solution (pH $= 6.4$) containing 10 μM of 3-nitro-L-tyrosine as an internal standard. Protein was then precipitated with 25 μL trichloroacetic acid (2-molar). The specimens were centrifuged and 100 μL of the supernatant was injected in the HPLC column. A Lichrochart RP-18 reversed phase column (grain size 5 μm; Merck, Darmstadt, Germany) was used. The elution buffer was a 15 mM phosphate buffer (pH $= 6.4$). The pump and the data system were obtained from Varian (Palo Alto, CA, USA). Tryptophan was detected by its natural fluorescence (excitation: 285 nm, emission: 365 nm) with a HP 1046A fluorescence detector (Hewlett Packard, Vienna, Austria). Kynurenine and nitrotyrosine were detected by UV absorption at 360 nm with a UV detector (UV 975, Jasco, Tokyo, Japan). External calibration was carried outdone using an albumin-based standard containing 10 μM kynurenine, 50 μM tryptophan and 10 μM nitrotyrosine. All chemicals used (Merck) were of high analytical grade.

3.2.2. *Data analysis*

The cut-off point for the diagnosis of fructose malabsorption was breath H_2 concentrations greater than 20 ppm above baseline.[18,19] Subjects showing an increase of breath H_2 concentration equal or less than 20 ppm above baseline were considered to be normal fructose absorbers. For comparison of groups, the Mann–Whitney U-test was employed using a standard PC statistical program (STATISTICA for Windows);[20] for correlation analyses, Spearman rank correlation coefficients were calculated and frequencies were compared using Fisher's exact test.

3.2.3. *Results*

In 35 patients breath H_2-concentrations increased by more than 20 ppm over basal fasting values. They were classified as fructose malabsorbers. The remaining 15 subjects with lower breath H_2 were classified as normal fructose absorbers. The two groups of individuals showed were not significantly different in age. There was only a trend towards higher Beck's inventory depression scores in fructose malabsorbers (9.47 ± 7.35) than in normal fructose absorbers (7.07 ± 4.62), but no significant difference was observed between the two groups of individuals. When subjects were split into two groups by gender, the Beck's inventory depression scores were higher in female fructose malabsorbers (12.30 ± 7.10) than in females with normal fructose absorption (6.66 ± 5.50; $p = 0.02$). No such difference was observed in males. Mean plasma tryptophan concentrations were significantly lower in fructose malabsorbers than in normal fructose absorbers ($p = 0.02$). Plasma kynurenine concentrations and tryptophan per kynurenine quotients were within the normal range of healthy controls in most individuals (4 out of 50 had kynurenine concentrations higher than 3 μM, 4 out of 50 individuals presented with a kynurenine per tryptophan quotient higher than 40) and they did not significantly differ between the two groups. When patients were divided into two groups by sex, serum tryptophan concentrations were lower in individuals with fructose malabsorption compared to normals only in females (fructose malabsorbers: 61.3 ± 14.0 μM, normals: 74.7 ± 16.5 μM, $p = 0.03$), but not in males (fructose malabsorbers: 70.3 ± 10.4 μM, normals: 76.4 ± 12.5 μM, not significant). Kynurenine concentrations (females, fructose malabsorbers: 1.81 ± 0.58 μM, normals: 1.98 ± 0.64 μM; males, fructose malabsorbers: 2.12 ± 0.46 μM, normals: 1.93 ± 0.30 μM) and kynurenine per tryptophan ratios (females, fructose malabsorbers: 30±9 mM/M, normals: 27±10 mM/M; males, fructose malabsorbers: 31 ± 8 mM/M, normals: 26 ± 3 mM/M) did not differ between the groups.

When comparing tryptophan concentrations with the Beck's depression inventory scores, there was no significant correlation in the whole group of individuals ($n = 50$; $r_s = -0.182$, not significant). There was also no significant correlation when groups were separated by gender. However, individuals with tryptophan concentrations lower than the median (67.0 μM) more often presented with a Beck's depression inventory score above the median value of 6 ($p = 0.036$; Fisher's exact test). When analyses were restricted to female fructose malabsorbers, a significant inverse correlation between tryptophan concentrations and the Beck's score was found for the whole group of individuals ($n = 35$; $r_s = -0.348$, $p = 0.043$) and for females ($n = 24$; $r_s = -0.503$, $p = 0.014$). There was no such correlation between the Beck's score and serum tryptophan levels in male fructose malabsorbers ($n = 11$; $r_s = 0.205$, not significant).

3.3. *Third Study*

3.3.1. *Patients*

From one hundred patients who presented at our office for a medical health check-up, 53 individuals with gastrointestinal complaints were chosen to participate in this follow-up study on the basis of the H_2-breath test results. Sigmoideoscopy had been performed previously in most of these patients, because of chronic gastrointestinal complaints, and negative results were one of the reasons for a further check-up in our office. For those who had not had sigmoideoscopy, this examination was prescribed to rule out inflammatory bowel diseases. The otherwise healthy outpatients, aged from 17 to 75 years (mean 44.8 ± 14.5 standard deviation), gave informed consent to participate in the clinical trial with fructose-reduced diet, which was approved by the local ethics committee. There were 12 male (range 23 to 75 years; mean 42.3 ± 14.6) and 41 female patients (17 to 73 years; 45.6 ± 14.6). Gastrointestinal infections were excluded by stool culture examination for pathogenic *Clostridia, Yersinia, Campylobacter, Salmonella, Shigella*, and *Candida*. Routine blood examination showed no signs of systemic inflammatory or infectious diseases. None of these patients was taking medication, except for oral contraceptives in some females.

Diagnosis of fructose malabsorption was established by the H_2-breath test. From the patient's first visit to the beginning of the therapeutic intervention, 4–6 weeks passed in which extended medical and laboratory diagnostic examinations were completed. At the end of this pre-intervention period when fructose malabsorption was diagnosed and confirmed, all patients were asked to complete the following 4 tests: (*i*) Beck's depression inventory-questionnaire (BDI) for quantifying clinical signs of mental depression, (*ii*) estimate their grade of meteorism on an arbitrary analogue scale ranging from 0 (no meteorism complaints) to 10 (major complaints), (*iii*) stool frequency ranging from -5 (stool frequency less than once every fifth day) to $+10$ (stool frequency 10 and more each day) and (*iv*) their subjective feeling of well-being on an arbitrary analogous scale ranging from 0 (no complaints) to 10 (major complaints). Following these tests there was the dietary consultation scheduled. After 4 weeks of the dietary change, the patients were asked again to retrospectively complete the aforementioned tests.

3.3.2. *Diet*

The patients were instructed to maintain a diet intended to exclude or reduce the intake of fructose and sorbitol. For this purpose they were told to avoid fruits (with the exception of bananas, honey melons, and tangerines), all kinds of dried fruits, fruit juices, soft drinks, honey and all kinds of sorbitol-containing food such as sugarless chewing gums and sugarless sweets. The patients were told that saccharose containing 50 % fructose should be supplemented with 2 parts of regular sugar to 1 part of glucose, which is commonly available as dextropur^{TM}. In some cases, those patients with severe complaints were told to avoid stachyose- and verbascose-containing foods (oligosaccharides) such as onions, beans and cauliflower. In those patients who did not know whether a certain vegetable was of a high stachyose- or verbascose-content, they were told to avoid this vegetable, at least for the duration of the study. They were allowed to eat any other kind of carbohydrate-containing food (*e.g.* cereals, wheat, corn, potatoes), rich protein- (fish, meat, dairy products) and fat-containing foods. Mean dietary fructose (as a monosaccharide) and sorbitol intake up to the dietary consultation was assessed by an additional questionnaire, and the amount of fructose and sorbitol intake after consultation during the time of study was controlled by a patient's diary.

3.3.3. *Data analysis*

Individuals with ΔH_2 higher than 20 ppm after the fructose load were classified as fructose malabsorber. Subjects with ΔH_2 equal or less than

20 ppm were considered as normal fructose absorbers and were therefore excluded from the study. Statistical analysis was performed using the paired t-test with the standard statistic software STATISTICA 5.0.[20]

3.3.4. *Results*

The mean dietary fructose intake (as a monosaccharide) was about 20 g/day during the 4 weeks before the dietary observation period and about 5 g/day during this period. On an arbitrary scale for the measurement of meteorism, the mean score before intervention was 7.5 ± 1.8 (mean $\pm$ standard deviation) and fell to 4.8 ± 1.9 ($t > 1000$; $p < 0.0001$) 4 weeks after the beginning of the dietary intervention (Fig. 3a). For women, the mean score for meteorism fell from 7.6 ± 1.4 to 4.8 ± 1.7 ($t > 1000$; $p < 0.0001$) and for males it fell from 7.0 ± 2.6 to 4.6 ± 2.5 ($t = 2.867$; $p < 0.005$). The score for general well-being during the 4 weeks before dietary intervention was 6.4 ± 2.3 and fell to 4.9 ± 2.0 during the intervention period ($t = 4.407$; $p < 0.0001$). For women the score dropped from 6.6 ± 2.3 to 5.2 ± 1.9 ($t = 4.275$; $p < 0.001$) and for men it dropped from 5.4 ± 2.4 to 3.9 ± 2.1 ($t = 1.480$, not significant). The mean stool frequency score was 2.1 ± 1.3 per day before and 1.5 ± 1.0 per day during dietary intervention ($t = 3.374$; $p < 0.01$; see Fig. 3b). For women, the average score was 2.2 ± 1.3 before and 1.6 ± 1.1 during intervention ($t = 2.916$; $p < 0.01$; see Fig. 3b). For men, the scores were 1.8 ± 1.1 before and 1.2 ± 0.3 during dietary intervention, $t = 1.621$; not significant. The majority of the subjects studied showed mild-to-moderate mood disturbances before dietary intervention. The average Beck's depression score was 13.8 ± 9.3 during the 4 weeks before dietary intervention. After 4 weeks of dietary change the BDI score fell to 9.1 ± 7.7 on average ($t = 5.290$; $p < 0.0001$; see Fig. 3c), which means a

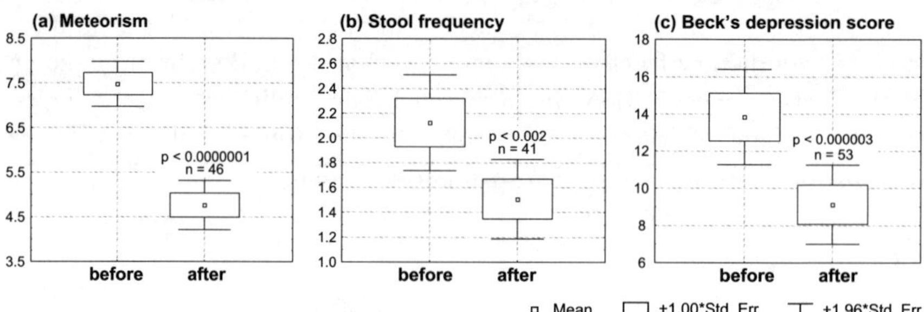

Fig. 3.   (a) Meteorism, (b) stool frequency, and (c) Beck's depression score before and after fructose reduced diet

reduction by 65.2% related to the whole cohort. Separated by gender, the mean BDI scores for women were 15.1 ± 10.0 before and 9.9 ± 8.3 during the dietary intervention ($t = 4.880$; $p < 0.0001$), and for men the mean BDI score was 9.3 ± 3.1 before intervention and fell to 6.5 ± 4.2 4 weeks after the dietary change ($t = 2.243$; $p < 0.05$).

4. Discussion

Carbohydrate malabsorption syndromes such as fructose malabsorption and lactose maldigestion can easily be diagnosed by hydrogen breath testing. The data in the presented case studies show that isolated fructose malabsorption and combined fructose/lactose malabsorption is associated with a significantly higher score for mental depression in females as compared to subjects with no signs of carbohydrate malabsorption. In earlier studies we showed that both fructose malabsorption[12] and lactose malabsorption[13] were associated with early signs of mental depression. The extended study described in this chapter confirms that isolated fructose malabsorbers show significantly higher depression scores than normals. This association is apparently amplified by the concomitant presence of lactose malabsorption, whereas isolated lactose malabsorbers do not show increased Beck's scores (see Fig. 2). In the majority of the study population lactose malabsorption co-existed with fructose malabsorption, because fructose malabsorption is a very common finding in the Central European population. In fact, we found that only 4 out of 17 individuals with lactose malabsorption suffered from isolated lactose malabsorption (3 females and 1 male among 111 tested subjects). A re-examination of a previously investigated population with fructose malabsorption also showed that a large proportion had lactose malabsorption in addition. Thus, the conclusion has to be made, that lactose malabsorption itself has only little, if any, association with a higher Beck's score. However, the limited number of individuals with isolated lactose malabsorption studied so far does not allow a definite conclusion, although all of them had a Beck's depression score less than 10 (see Fig. 2).

As suggested earlier, abnormal tryptophan metabolism could be involved in the development of depression[22-25] and also the pre-menstrual syndrome.[26,27] Since the development of signs of mental depression found in our patients may be related with impaired 5-hydroxytryptamin (serotonin) metabolism,[28] the data suggest that fructose malabsorption interferes with the L-tryptophan availability.[22] Indeed, our data in the second study show significantly lower serum-tryptophan concentrations in fructose malabsorbers compared to healthy controls[29] and show inverse correlation with breath hydrogen concentrations (see Fig. 4). Another explanation for the development of depressive signs could be the formation of toxic bacterial degradation products that may be formed when aminoacids and carbohydrate compounds reach the colon and possibly interfere with neurotransmitter metabolism. Interestingly the association of fructose malabsorption with mental depression is only significant in females ($p < 0.002$). We did not find such an association in men. This goes along with findings by several authors of gender differences in mood responses to acute tryptophan depletion,[27,30] and may serve as a further argument that fructose malabsorption interferes with L-tryptophan metabolism. In females, the normal range of serum L-tryptophan concentrations was found to be lower than in males.[22] This might be due to a higher activity of the hepatic tryptophan-2,3-dioxygenase (= tryptophan pyrrolase) which is up-regulated by estrogen.[31] If baseline tryptophan concentrations are lower, an additional influence of fructose malabsorption may more rapidly contribute to a pathologically low tryptophan level, leading to the development of depression. Carbohydrate consumption increases the availability of the amino acid L-tryptophan in the central nervous system, which in turn increases brain 5-hydroxytryptamin (serotonin) levels.[32]

Since modern food processing involves the replacement of regular sugar in sweet foods with fructose and/or lactose, the hunger for (sweet) carbohydrates may lead to a vicious circle of worsened fructose/lactose malabsorption and accelerate L-tryptophan depletion. From our first case study

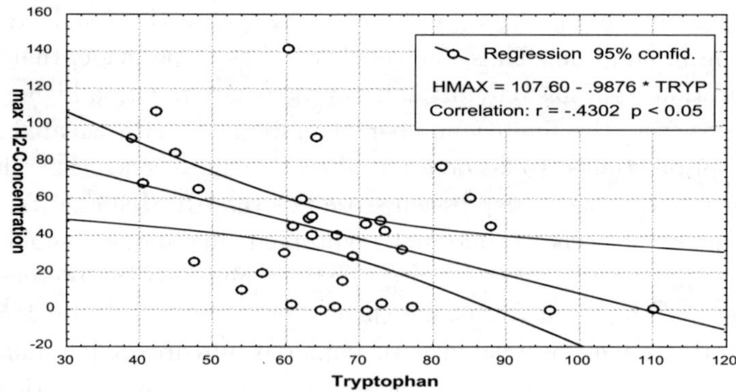

Fig. 4.   Serum tryptophan concentration (μmol/L) versus breath hydrogen concentration (ppm)[29]

(Section 3.1) it seems that lactose malabsorption alone does not have an effect; however, it amplifies the effect of fructose malabsorption in the development of signs of depression. This amplifying effect of additional lactose malabsorption might be due to a reduced oro-caecal transit time in these subjects, thus decreasing the mucosal contact time of tryptophan and also of other nutrients. Consequently, tryptophan availability further diminishes. In addition, micronutrient deficiencies (*e.g.* zinc and folic acid) may further deteriorate the signs of mental depression. The associations between fructose malabsorption, lactose malabsorption and depression do not necessarily reflect a cause-effect relationship, and both conditions may result from another yet unknown cause. However, the data suggest fructose may possibly interfere with L-tryptophan metabolism and lactose intolerance may worsen this effect. Another mechanism that may aggravate the depressive disorders in patients with FM may be a change in tryptophan metabolism due to chronic TH1-immune stimulation. TH1-immune stimulation leads to an increase production of interferon-γ which stimulates the enzyme indoleamine-(2,3)-dioxygenase (IDO) as it is shown in Fig. 5). As a consequence tryptophan metabolism is shifted towards the

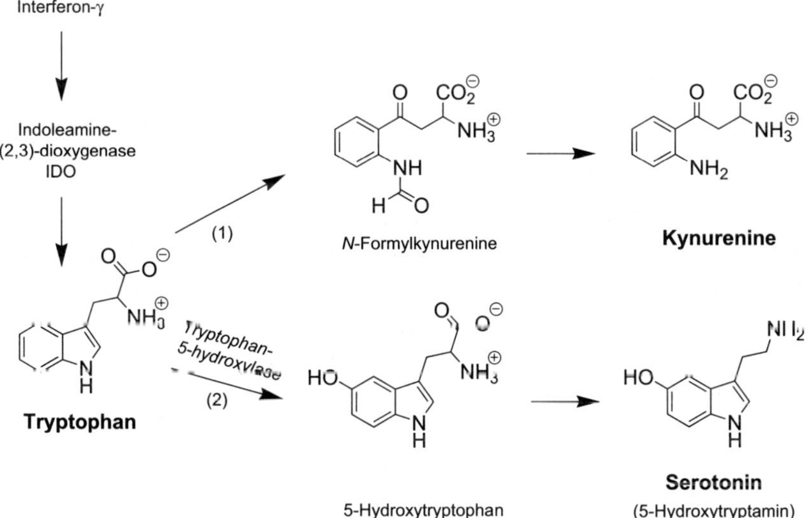

Fig. 5. TH1-immunestimulation and tryptophan metabolism. Interferon-γ stimulates Indoleamine-(2,3)-dioxygenase shifting the tryptophan metabolism towards the kynurenine pathway. Therefore TH1-type immune stimulation leads to a decrease in serotonin-production.

kynurenine-pathway with a decrease in serotonin-production. Carbohydrate malabsorption should be considered in patients with mental depression, pre-menstrual syndrome and other serotonin-deficiency syndromes. In our third case study (Section 3.3), we were able to show that a fructose-reduced diet improves clinical and psychopathological symptoms of fructose malabsorption. Stool frequency and meteorism also were significantly reduced (see Fig. 3). Since there was a highly significant improvement of BDI, this study further supports the notion that fructose malabsorption is involved in the development of the early signs of depression. Also, sorbitol intake usually leads to gastrointestinal symptoms in fructose malabasorption; therefore sorbitol, in particular, has to be avoided within the scope of a fructose malabsorption diet.

In these studies, no control groups could be included, because most of the subjects studied had gastrointestinal complaints, and we could not avoid dietary interventions for ethical reasons. Thus, it cannot fully be excluded, that a placebo effect could have contributed to the observed amelioration of symptoms, *e.g.* the improvement of BDI after dietary change. However, the first set of data was obtained at the end of the pre-intervention period, and the patients were asked to retrospectively estimate the interesting parameters of gastrointestinal symptoms using an arbitrary scale. During this period it is unlikely that the individuals changed their dietary behaviour; therefore one can consider the present study as a preliminary follow-up investigation that outlines the consequences of a fructose-reduced diet. Furthermore, a dietary observation period of 4 weeks may compensate for a potential bias due to instantaneous amelioration of symptoms. Because all scores were measured exactly 4 weeks apart, it can be ruled out that the menstrual cycle has a major influence on the outcome of depression scores or meteorism scores. Our own observations indicate that for the majority of subjects irritable bowel syndrome is due to a carbohydrate malabsorption syndrome, such as fructose malabsorption, sorbitol malabsorption, lactose maldigestion or xylitol malabsorption (unpublished data).

Patients with fructose malabsorption often have a clear history of post-infective onset of their symptoms as has been shown for patients with irritable bowel syndrome.[33] However, during the pre-intervention period it was confirmed that all our subjects were free of infectious symptoms. We have previously shown that fructose malabsorption is associated with early signs of mental depression[12] and decreased serum tryptophan concentrations.[29] Earlier studies imply that disturbances of L-tryptophan metabolism induce depression[22-25] and the pre-menstrual syndrome.[26,27] In fructose malabsorbers, the resorption of L-tryptophan seems to be disturbed.[34] Reduction of non-absorbable intestinal fructose would probably normalize tryptophan resorption by the intestinal mucosa, resulting in a higher availability of tryptophan and possibly also of other essential amino acids, thus reducing development of signs of depression. It is well known that carbohydrate consumption increases the transport of the amino acid L-tryptophan via the blood-brain-barrier so that, in turn, brain 5-hydroxytryptamin (serotonin) levels increase.[35] This seems to be the reason for the clinically well-known phenomenon of hunger for sweets in patients with depression.[36] Since fructose malabsorbers have a higher risk for the development of mood disturbances they are prone to develop an appetite for carbohydrates and especially for sweets. Fructose is the monosaccharide with the most intensive sweetness and is inexpensively produced. Therefore, modern food processing increasingly involves the replacement of regular sugar in sweet foods by fructose (see Fig. 6).[37] Depressive patients with fructose malabsorption and appetite for sweets arc thcrcforo at a high risk of ending up with reduced tryptophan availability. As a result, a vicious circle may develop of craving for sugar leading to a short-lived improvement of depressive symptoms, but leading to prolonged tryptophan depletion also, thus accelerating both the development of mental depression and gastrointestinal disturbances in fructose malabsorbers. At this point, dietary restriction of fructose seems therefore to be the only means to avoid this vicious cyclc in thcoc pationts.

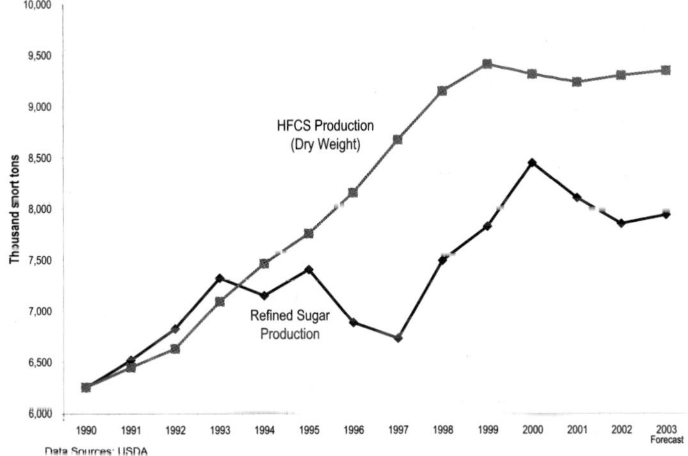

Fig. 6. U.S. refined sugar and high fructose corn syrup (HFCS) production from 1990 to 2003 (**www.sugaralliance.org/library/2004/25-us_sugar_hfcs_prod.pdf**)

5. Conclusions

Carbohydrate malabsorption syndromes can be diagnosed by hydrogen breath testing. Fructose malabsorption is associated with signs of depression, especially in females. Co-existing lactose maldigestion seems to worsen depressive symptoms in patients with fructose malabsorption. Interference of the non-absorbed sugar with the amino acid tryptophan may lead to tryptophan depletion that is seen more frequently in subjects with fructose malabsorption. This might be an explanation for the pathophysiology of fructose malabsorption-associated depression. Depressive symptoms and gastrointestinal disturbances in patients with fructose malabsorption significantly improve by a 4 week period on a fructose-reduced diet.

Acknowledgement

We thank Ernst Ellmerer for drawing Fig 5.

References

1. Gudmand-Hoyer E. The clinical significance of disaccharide maldigestion. *Am J Clin Nutr* 1994; **59** (3 Suppl): 735S–741S.
2. Gudmand-Hoyer E,, Skovbjerg H. Disaccharide digestion and maldigestion. *Scand J Gastroenterol Suppl* 1996; **216**: 111–121.
3. Evans PR, Piesse C, Bak YT, Kellow JE. Fructose-sorbitol malabsorption and symptom provocation in irritable bowel syndrome: relationship to enteric hypersensitivity and dysmotility. *Scand J Gastroenterol* 1998; **33**: 1158–1163.
4. Fernandez-Banares F, Esteve-Pardo M, de Leon R, Humbert P, Cabre E, Llovet JM, Gassull MA. Sugar malabsorption in functional bowel disease: clinical implications. *Am J Gastroenterol* 1993; **88**: 2044–2050.
5. Wales JK, Primhak RA, Rattenbury J, Taylor CJ. Isolated fructose malabsorption. *Arch Dis Child* 1990; **65**: 227–229.
6. Wasserman D, Hoekstra JH, Tolia V, Taylor CJ, Kirschner BS, Takeda J, Bell GI, Taub R, Rand EB. Molecular analysis of the fructose transporter gene (GLUT5) in isolated fructose malabsorption. *J Clin Invest* 1996; **98** (10): 2398–2402.
7. Wright EM, Martin MG, Turk E. Intestinal absorption in health and disease — sugars. *Best Pract Res Clin Gastroenterol* 2003; **17** (6): 943–956.
8. Born P, Zech J, Lehn H, Classen M, Lorenz R. Colonic bacterial activity determines the symptoms in people with fructose-malabsorption. *Hepatogastroenterology* 1995; **42**: 778–785.
9. Hoekstra JH, van Kempen AA, Bijl SB, Kneepkens CM. Fructose breath hydrogen tests. *Arch Dis Child* 1993; **68**: 136–138.
10. Hoekstra JH. Fructose breath hydrogen tests in infants with chronic nonspecific diarrhoea. *Eur J Pediatr* 1995; **154**: 362–364.

11. Romagnuolo J, Schiller D, Bailey RJ. Using breath tests wisely in a gastroenterology practice: an evidence-based review of indications and pitfalls in interpretation. *Am J Gastroenterol* 2002; **97** (5): 1113–1126.

12. Ledochowski M, Sperner-Unterweger B, Widner B, Fuchs D. Fructose malabsorption is associated with early signs of mental depression. *Eur J Med Res* 1998; **3**: 295–298.

13. Ledochowski M, Sperner-Unterweger B, Fuchs D. Lactose malabsorption is associated with early signs of mental depression in females: a preliminary report. *Dig Dis Sci* 1998; **43**: 2513–2517.

14. Ledochowski M, Widner B, Bair H, Probst T, Fuchs D. Fructose- and sorbitol-reduced diet improves mood and gastrointestinal disturbances in fructose malabsorbers. *Scand J Gastroenterol* 2000; **35** (10): 1048–1052.

15. Braden B, Braden CP, Klutz M, Lembcke B. Analysis of breath hydrogen (H_2) in diagnosis of gastrointestinal function: validation of a pocket breath H_2 test analyzer. *Z Gastroenterol* 1993; **31**: 242–245.

16. Fernandez-Banares F, Gassull MA. Accuracy of breath H_2 criteria to detect carbohydrate malabsorption [letter; comment]. *Gastroenterology* 1994; **107**: 323–324.

17. Lee WS, Davidson GP, Moore DJ, Butler RN. Analysis of the breath hydrogen test for carbohydrate malabsorption: validation of a pocket-sized breath test analyser. *J Paediatr Child Health* 2000; **36** (4): 340–342.

18. Veligati LN, Treem WR, Sullivan B, Burke G, Hyams JS. Delta 10 ppm versus delta 20 ppm: a reappraisal of diagnostic criteria for breath hydrogen testing in children. *Am J Gastroenterol* 1994; **89**: 758–761.

19. Karcher RE, Truding RM, Stawick LE. Using a cutoff of < 10 ppm for breath hydrogen testing: a review of five years' experience. *Ann Clin Lab Sci* 1999; **29** (1): 1–8.

20. *STATISTICA for Windows* [Computer program manual]. Tulsa, OK: StatSoft, Inc., 1995.

21. Widner B, Werner ER, Schennach H, Wachter H, Fuchs D. Simultaneous measurement of serum tryptophan and kynurenine by HPLC. *Clin Chem* 1997; **43**: 2424–2426.

22. Ledochowski M, Widner B, Murr C, Sperner-Unterweger B, Fuchs D. Fructose malabsorption is associated with decreased plasma tryptophan. *Scand J Gastroenterol* 2001; **36** (4): 367–371

23. Widner B, Laich A, Sperner-Unterweger B, Ledochowski M, Fuchs D. Neopterin production, tryptophan degradation, and mental depression — What is the link? *Brain Behav Immun* 2002; **16** (5): 590–595.

24. Benkelfat C, Ellenbogen MA, Dean P, Palmour RM, Young SN. Mood-lowering effect of tryptophan depletion. Enhanced susceptibility in young men at genetic risk for major affective disorders. *Arch Gen Psychiatry* 1994; **51**: 687–697.

25. Moroni F. Tryptophan metabolism and brain function: focus on kynurenine and other indole metabolites [In Process Citation]. *Eur J Pharmacol* 1999; **375**: 87–100.

26. Menkes DB, Coates DC, Fawcett JP. Acute tryptophan depletion aggravates premenstrual syndrome. *J Affect Disord* 1994; **32**: 37–44.

27. Rapkin AJ. The role of serotonin in premenstrual syndrome. *Clin Obstet Gynecol* 1992; **35**: 629–636.

28. Delgado PL, Price LH, Miller HL, Salomon RM, Aghajanian GK, Heninger GR, Charney DS. Serotonin and the neurobiology of depression. Effects of tryptophan depletion in drug-free depressed patients. *Arch Gen Psychiatry* 1994; **51**: 865–874.

29. Ledochowski M, Widner B, Fuchs D. Fructose malabsorption and the decrease of serum tryptophan concentration. In: Huether G, Kochen W, Simat TJ, Steinhart H, eds. *ISTRY 98 Proceedings: Tryptophan, Serotonin, Melatonin — Basic Aspects and Applications*. New York: Plenum Press, 1999: 73–78.

30. Ellenbogen MA, Young SN, Dean P, Palmour RM, Benkelfat C. Mood response to acute tryptophan depletion in healthy volunteers: sex differences and temporal stability. *Neuropsychopharmacology* 1996; **15**: 465–474.

31. Nemeth S. Development and significance of estrogen-induced increase in the activity of several liver enzymes. *Z Gesamte Inn Med* 1988; **43** (15): 418–420.

32. Young SN. The use of diet and dietary components in the study of factors controlling affect in humans: a review. *J Psychiatry Neurosci* 1993; **18**: 235–244.

33. Spiller RC. Postinfectious irritable bowel syndrome. *Gastroenterology* 2003; **124** (6): 1662–1671.

34. Ledochowski M, Widner B, Propst-Braunsteiner T, Vogel W, Sperner-Unterweger B, Fuchs D. Fructose malabsorption is associated with decreased plasma tryptophan. *Adv Exp Med Biol* 1999; **467**: 73–78.

35. Wurtman RJ. Nutrients that modify brain function. *Sci Am* 1982; **246**: 50–59.

36. Wurtman RJ, Wurtman JJ. Brain Serotonin, Carbohydrate-craving, obesity and depression. *Adv Exp Med Biol* 1996; **398**: 35–41.

37. Kumar A, Rawlings RD, Beaman DC. The mystery ingredients: sweeteners, flavorings, dyes, and preservatives in analgesic/antipyretic, antihistamine/decongestant, cough and cold, antidiarrheal, and liquid theophylline preparations. *Pediatrics* 1993; **91**: 927–933.

38. Scriver CR, Beaudet AM, Sly WS, Valle D. eds. *The Metabolic and Molecular Bases of Inherited Disease*, Vol. 3, 8th ed. New York: McGraw-Hill, 2001.

39. Ledochowski M, Widner B, Sperner-Unterweger B, Propst T, Vogel W, Fuchs D. Carbohydrate malabsorption syndromes and early signs of mental depression in females. *Dig Dis Sci* 2000; **45** (7): 1255–1259.

DETECTION OF *H. PYLORI* INFECTION BY BREATH AMMONIA FOLLOWING UREA INGESTION*

C. PENAULT

The Medical House PLC,
199 Newhall Road, Attercliffe, Sheffield, S9 2QJ, UK

P. ŠPANĚL

V. Čermák Laboratory, J. Heyrovský Institute of Physical Chemistry,
Academy of Sciences of the Czech Republic,
Dolejškova 3, CZ-182 23 Prague 8, Czech Republic
and
Trans Spectra Limited,
9, The Elms, Porthill, Newcastle-under-Lyme, Staffs., ST5 8RP, UK

D. SMITH

Institute of Science and Technology in Medicine,
Medical School, Keele University,
Thornburrow Drive, Hartshill, Stoke-on-Trent, ST4 7QB, UK
and
Trans Spectra Limited,
9, The Elms, Porthill, Newcastle-under-Lyme, Staffs., ST5 8RP, UK

1. Introduction

In 1983, Marshall and Warren reported the presence of a spiral, microaerophilic, gram-negative bacterium — now known as *Helicobacter pylori* — in the mucous lining of the stomach of patients with chronic gastritis.[1] Strong evidence now exists that *H. pylori* causes chronic active gastritis[2] and ulcers in the stomach and duodenum.[3] While infection is asymptomatic in most cases, it is a very common infection found in up to 50 % of the world's population,[4] the prevalence being much higher in developing countries. Infection with *H. pylori* accounts for 95 % of duodenal ulcers and the majority of gastric ulcers (60–80 %).[5] It also plays a

---

*The Medical House PLC, UK, is the rightful owner of this contribution. World Scientific is granted the permission to publish the contribution as part of this collective work.

role in the development of stomach cancer.[6] Several diagnostic tests are now available, and range from endoscopy of the stomach with biopsies and rapid urease tests, histology, tissue culture, to serological tests (antibodies detection) and ^{13}C or ^{14}C urea breath testing.[7] However, each available test has its own significant limitations (invasive, discomforting, time-consuming and/or inaccurate) with variable cost and the need for complex and time-consuming strategy for the detection of CO_2, with no immediate results.

Most current non-invasive tests for *H. pylori* depend on the conversion of labelled (^{13}C or ^{14}C) urea (administrated as part of the test) to labelled carbon dioxide ($^{13}CO_2$ or $^{14}CO_2$) and ammonium ions (NH_4^+) by the bacterium's urease enzyme system, with the labelled CO_2 being detected in exhaled air. A variation on such methods is the detection in urine of ^{15}N from the bacterial metabolism of ^{15}N-urea.[8]

Despite suggestions going back over a number of years, the alternative possibility, of using NH_4^+ — in the form of gaseous ammonia, NH_3, as the test parameter, has received little attention. It is known that the liver and the kidney are partly active in removing any ammonia from the bloodstream because of its relative toxicity, but a portion of the ammonia produced by the bacteria in the stomach is expected to be absorbed into the blood stream without being removed by the liver, passing the alveoli system of the lung and being delivered to the expired air.

In 1996, D. Smith and P. Španěl developed selected ion flow tube mass spectrometry, SIFT-MS,[9] with which breath metabolites, including ammonia, can be measured in real time, with exhalations directly sampled into the instrument with immediate result. Their previous studies[9–11] indicate that ammonia was found in all human breath within a wide range of concentration between individuals (200–3000 ppb). The level of ammonia was found to be elevated after a protein meal and at high levels in the breath of patients suffering form end-stage renal failure and in the uraemic state.[12] They then reported measurement of elevated breath ammonia in an *H. pylori* positive volunteer following the ingestion of 2 g of normal (unlabelled) urea.[9] Consequently, they were the first to demonstrate that ammonia measurement in breath following ingestion of normal urea can be used to differentiate *H. pylori* positive from *H. pylori* negative subjects. However, it is recognised that subjects will also need to avoid food intake before the test to minimise interferences. This SIFT-MS study has recently been extended in association with The Medical House, PLC, which aims to develop a simple, convenient breath test for the detection of *H. pylori*.

In this short paper we present the results obtained from these two studies, indicating an increase in breath ammonia for *H. pylori* positive volunteers following the ingestion of normal urea, but no significant change for *H. pylori* negative volunteers.

2. Material and Methods

2.1. *The SIFT-MS Technique*

A description of the SIFT-MS analytical technique has been previously given in some research papers and reviews (*e.g.*, see Ref. 9 and the chapter by Smith and Španěl[13] on page 3 of this book). In only single breath exhalations, metabolites such as ethanol, acetaldehyde, ammonia, acetone, isoprene and routinely water vapour, can be accurately and simultaneously measured at the part per billion (ppb) level. Breath exhalations are directly sampled into the instrument and results are available immediately in real time. The technique is sensitive and quantitative and uses chemical ionisation of the sample trace gases by selected precursor positive ions (*viz*: H_3O^+, NO^+, O_2^+), during a well-defined time period in an inert carrier gas (usually helium) in a flow tube. These precursor ions do not react with the major components of air but do react with most volatile organic molecules and many inorganic molecules that are present in an air/breath sample producing characteristic product ions. The precursor and product ions are then sampled from the carrier gas by a downstream pinhole orifice, mass analysed and counted by a differentially-pumped quadrupole mass spectrometer/detection system. Several trace gas components of the sample can be analysed by switching between the three precursor ions and by utilizing the ion-molecule kinetics database that has been constructed for SIFT-MS analyses.[9-12] A major advantage of SIFT-MS is that regular calibration is unnecessary to obtain accurate analyses.

2.2. *The Test Procedure*

The breath ammonia analyses were carried out by direct sampling into the SIFT-MS instrument. Subjects were asked to fast overnight. The *H. pylori* positive and negative subjects were asked to gently exhale through a cardboard disposable mouthpiece at the sample entry port of the SIFT-MS for about 10 seconds. Three consecutive exhalations were analysed every 3 to 4 minutes for about 70 minutes. Measurements were made for about 10 minutes before urea ingestion; then a solution of 2 g of urea in approximately 50 mL of water was briskly administrated. Subjects then rapidly rinsed their mouth with water and then the breath samples were taken and analysed for ammonia.

3. Results and Discussion

The results of the latest study are shown in Fig. 1. The initial ammonia levels for both subjects were the same, within the measurement uncertainties. Following urea ingestion (time 0), there was a pronounced "mouth effect" in the case of the positive subject, but only a slight effect for the negative subject. The sharp rise in the breath ammonia presumably represents the immediate hydrolysis of urea by the urease-associated bacteria of mouth flora. However, it is possible that part of the large "mouth effect" for the positive subject is associated with the presence of *H. pylori* in the mouth. Some evidence for the presence of *H. pylori* in dental plaque of individuals suffering from *H. pylori*-associated gastric disease have been reported.[14,15]

The mean breath ammonia level for the negative subject did not change significantly over the 60 minutes duration, although a slow increase with time may be discernible. In the case of the positive subject, following the large "mouth peak" the breath ammonia falls rapidly initially then relatively slowly, indicative of a combination of ammonia production, by *H. pylori*, and its loss by normal metabolic processes. There is a dis-

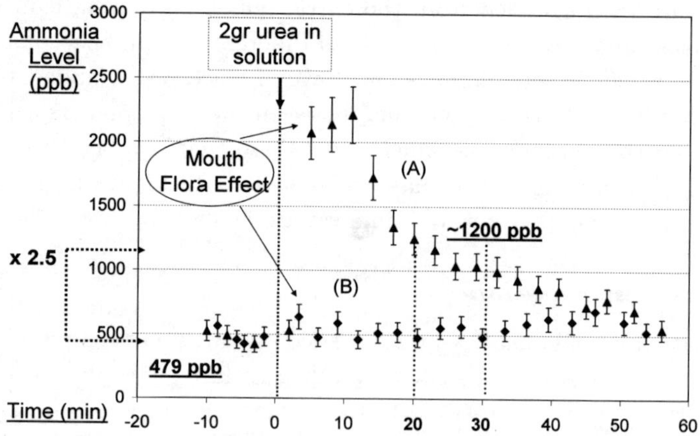

Fig. 1. Time dependence of the partial pressures of breath ammonia after the consumption of 2 g of urea by two subjects. The values of the partial pressures were obtained by analysing breath directly exhaled into the SIFT-MS apparatus. (A) Breath from a volunteer known to be infected by *H. pylori*. (B) Breath from a volunteer known not to be infected by *H. pylori*.

cernible plateau at 20–30 minutes after urea ingestion, with the breath ammonia concentration about 2.5 times greater than the pre-dose level; after 60 minutes it had returned close to the pre-dose level.

Referring to the results of the much earlier SIFT-MS study[9] (see Fig. 2), although the initial breath ammonia levels in *H. pylori* positive and negative volunteers were different (around 1.8 ppm and 1 ppm respectively), the results are similar to those in Fig. 1, namely minor changes for the negative volunteer and a sharp rise due to the "mouth effect" for the positive volunteer, followed by a drop and then a plateau, which indicates a level of ammonia approximately 2.5 times greater than initial ammonia values prior to urea ingestion. The 20–30 minutes increase of breath ammonia for the positive subject following urea ingestion is readily recognised.

The peak breath ammonia concentration following urea ingestion is likely to depend on the degree of *H. pylori* infection, the gastric emptying rate and the rate of loss of ammonia from the blood stream by metabolic processes. As is often used in the ^{13}C urea breath test, orange juice could be administrated before the urea ingestion to slow down gastric emptying. Clearly, these parameters will vary for different individuals, which could explain the differences in detail of the two *H. pylori* positive subjects from which the data in Fig. 1 and Fig. 2 were obtained.

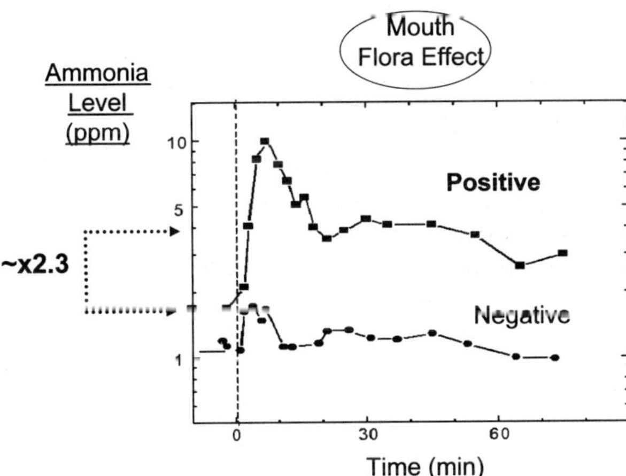

Fig. 2.　Time dependence of the partial pressures of breath ammonia after the consumption of 2 g of urea by two subjects, one known to be infected with *H. pylori* ("Positive") and one known not to be infected with *H. pylori* ("Negative"). The values of the partial pressures were obtained by analysing breath directly exhaled into the SIFT-MS apparatus.

4. Concluding Remarks

While the ^{13}C urea breath test aims to detect changes in labelled breath CO_2 following carbon labelled urea, we aimed to detect changes in breath ammonia following the ingestion of non-labelled urea. The results of our previous SIFT-MS study, confirmed by our present study, show that breath ammonia analysis can be used to detect the presence of *H. pylori* infection and therefore provide the basis for a diagnostic breath test for *H. pylori*. This is now being explored by The Medical House PLC, using a highly sensitive chemiresistive sensor to detect very low ammonia concentrations.[16-20] The Medical House aims to develop a point-of-care test for the detection of *H. pylori* infection using a simple, disposable device to be used as a primary care diagnostic and/or screening tool by general practitioners and practice nurses and also after eradication treatment to assess the effectiveness of the therapeutic regime. The SIFT-MS research involving a greater patient cohort is also on-going.

Acknowledgements

We are grateful to Mick Williams for participating in this study.

References

1. Marshall BJ, Warren JR. Unidentified curved bacilli in the stomach of patients with gastritis and peptic ulceration. *Lancet* 1984; **1**: 1311–1315.
2. Marshall BJ, McGechie DB, Rogers PA, Glancy RJ. Pyloric Campylobacter infection and gastroduodenal disease. *Med J Aust* 1985; **142**: 439–444.
3. Labenz J, Borsch G. Evidence for the essential role of *Helicobacter pylori* in gastric ulcer disease. *Gut* 1994; **35**: 19–22.
4. Pounder RE, Ng D. The prevalence of *Helicobacter pylori* infection in different countries. *Aliment Pharmacol Ther* 1995; **9** Suppl 2: 33–39.
5. NIH Consensus Conference. *Helicobacter pylori* in peptic ulcer disease. NIH Consensus Development Panel on *Helicobacter pylori* in Peptic Ulcer Disease. *Jama* 1994; **272**: 65–69.
6. Parsonnet J, Friedman GD, Vandersteen DP, Chang Y, Vogelman JH, Orentreich N, Sibley RK. *Helicobacter pylori* infection and the risk of gastric carcinoma. *N Engl J Med* 1991; **325**: 1127–1131.
7. Mitchell H, Megraud F. Epidemiology and diagnosis of *Helicobacter pylori* infection. *Helicobacter* 2002; **7** Suppl 1: 8–16.
8. Krumbiegel P, Herbarth O, Kiess W, Muller DM, Richter T. Diagnosis of *Helicobacter pylori* infection in children: is the ^{15}N urine test more reliable than the ^{13}C breath test? *Scand J Gastroenterol* 2000; **35**: 353–358.

9. Smith D, Španěl P. The novel selected-ion flow tube approach to trace gas analysis of air and breath. *Rapid Commun Mass Spectrom* 1996; **10**: 1183–1198.

10. Diskin AM, Španěl P, Smith D. Time variation of ammonia, acetone, isoprene and ethanol in breath: a quantitative SIFT-MS study over 30 days. *Physiol Meas* 2003; **24**: 107–119.

11. Smith D, Španěl P, Davies S. Trace gases in breath of healthy volunteers when fasting and after a protein-calorie meal: a preliminary study. *J Appl Physiol* 1999; **87**: 1584–1588.

12. Davies S, Španěl P, Smith D. Quantitative analysis of ammonia on the breath of patients in end-stage renal failure. *Kidney Int* 1997; **52**: 223–228.

13. Smith D, Španěl P. Selected ion flow tube mass spectrometry, SIFT-MS, for on-line trace gas analysis of breath. In: Amann A, Smith D, eds. *Breath Analysis for Clinical Diagnosis and Therapeutic Monitoring,* Singapore: World Scientific, 2005.

14. Siddiq M, Haseeb ur R, Mahmood A. Evidence of *Helicobacter pylori* infection in dental plaque and gastric mucosa. *J Coll Physicians Surg Pak* 2004; **14**: 205–207.

15. Karczewska E, Konturek JE, Konturek PC, Czcsnikiowicz M, Sito E, Bielanski W, Kwiecien N, Obtulowicz W, Ziemniak W, Majka J, Hahn EG, Konturek SJ. Oral cavity as a potential source of gastric reinfection by *Helicobacter pylori*. *Dig Dis Sci* 2002; **47**: 978–986.

16. Ratcliffe N. Poly(pyrrole)-based sensor for hydrazine and ammonia. *Anal Chim Acta* 1990; **239**: 257–262.

17. Ratcliffe N. The simple preparation of a conducting and transparent poly(pyrrole) film. *Synth Metals* 1990; **38**: 87–92.

18. Cowell D, Dunn CDR, Greenman J, Ratcliffe N, Teare C, Black M, Penault C, Spence R. *The non-invasive detection of* Helicobacter pylori *using a polypyrrole sensor*. Gas Analysis and Sensing Group, St Bartholomew's Hospital, London, 7th December 2000.

19. Dunn C, Cowell D, Penault C, Spence R, Ratcliffe N, Teare C, Black M. Ammonia in mouth 'air' as a diagnostic marker for infection with *Helicobacter pylori*: preliminary 'proof of principle' pharmacological investigations. *British Journal of Biomedical Science* 2001; **58**: 66–75.

20. Ratcliffe NM, Teare C, Dunn C, Cowell DC, Black M, Chambers P, Penault C. Detection of *Helicobacter pylori* and apparatus therefore. UK Patent Application No. GB2364778, 2002-02-06.

BREATH GAS ANALYSIS IN PATIENTS SUFFERING FROM PROPIONIC ACIDAEMIA

U. JANOVSKY, S. SCHOLL-BÜRGI, AND D. KARALL

Clinical Department of General Paediatrics,
Innsbruck Medical University,
Anichstraße 35, A-6020 Innsbruck, Austria

J. BEAUCHAMP AND A. HANSEL

Institute of Ion Physics,
Leopold-Franzens University Innsbruck,
Technikerstraße 25, A-6020 Innsbruck, Austria

G. POUPART AND A. SCHMID

Department of Anesthesia and General Intensive Care,
Innsbruck Medical University,
A-6020 Innsbruck, Austria

A. AMANN

Department of Anesthesia and General Intensive Care,
Innsbruck Medical University,
A-6020 Innsbruck, Austria
and
Department of Environmental Sciences,
Swiss Federal Institute of Technology,
ETH Hönggerberg, CH-8093 Zurich, Switzerland

1. Introduction

Propionyl-CoA carboxylase (PCC, E.C. 6.4.1.3) catalyzes the carboxylation of propionyl-CoA to D-methylmalonyl-CoA (Fig. 1). PCC is a heteropolymeric enzyme composed of α and β subunits, which are encoded by the *PCCA* and *PCCB* genes, respectively. The *PCCA* gene is located on chromosome 13q32, the *PCCB* gene on chromosome 3q13.3-q22.[1-3]

Propionic acidaemia (PA), an autosomal recessive inborn error of metabolism, is caused by a deficiency of this biotin-dependent, mitochondrial enzyme and characterized by greatly increased concentrations of propionyl-CoA in the body fluids. The metabolically highly reactive

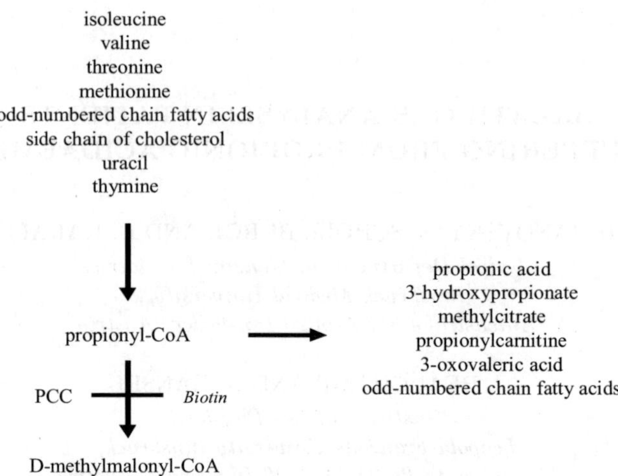

Fig. 1.   Reactions catalyzed by the enzyme propionyl-CoA carboxylase and secondary metabolites formed in patients suffering from propionic acidaemia

propionyl-CoA is metabolised into various substances like the organic acids methylcitric acid, 3-oxovaleric acid or 3-hydroxypropionic acid (Fig. 1). Propionyl-CoA arises in the metabolism of the aminoacids methionine, isoleucine, threonine and valine, the odd-numbered chain fatty acids, the pyrimidines thymine and uracil and cholesterol side chains (Fig. 1). The quantitative production of propionyl-CoA is estimated as follows: 50 % amino acid metabolism, 25 % odd-numbered chain fatty acid metabolism and 25 % via propionic acid of gut bacteria.[4]

Beside elevated excretion of organic acids, Menkes reported that the urine of PA patients contained large amounts of butanone, a by-product of isoleucine catabolism, as well as 2-pentanone and 2-hexanone.[5] Unusual ketones are likely to be formed by non-enzymatic degradation of the thermolabile 3-oxoacids.[6] Nevertheless, in contrast to Menkes, Lehnert *et al.* could not detect 2-pentanone and 2-hexanone.[7]

PA is clinically very heterogeneous. Metabolic derangements with ketoacidosis, seizures, vomiting, lethargy and hypotonia, caused by excessive ingestion of proteins, obstipation or catabolic situations like infections with degradation of endogenously-produced protein are frequently observed.[8] PA patients further suffer from feeding problems, neurological symptoms like muscular hypotonia and convulsions, respiratory problems and other symptoms.[7] Today, PA therapy includes a protein-defined nutrition, substitution of essential amino acids, vitamins, carnitine and treatment of complications, *i.e.* seizures.

Although several parameters like amino acids, organic acids, acylcarnitines and odd-numbered long-chain fatty acids (OLCFA) have been studied, there are presently no satisfactory parameters available to quantify the patients' condition.[9] Hence, to assess the metabolic state one is still limited to the clinical picture. Monitoring the concentrations of aminoacids, especially glycine, alanine, glutamine and acylcarnitine, is mainly used to detect an inadequate intake of these substances, but does not serve as a quantitative assessment of the patients' condition. So far, no breath gas analysis has been performed in PA patients to check for unusual metabolites or to monitor therapy.

2. Methods

Breath gas was collected into 3-L Tedlar® (polyvinylfluoride) bags; the reference ambient air inhaled by the patients and healthy controls was collected into 1-litre glass bottles. The samples were analysed at 40 °C using proton-transfer-reaction mass spectrometry (PTR-MS, Ionicon FDT-s) by scanning the analytical mass spectrometer over the mass-to-charge ratio, m/z, range from 20 u to 230 u. The reported ionic masses are those of the respective protonated ions (molecular mass + 1 u) as detected by the PTR-MS instrument. Additionally, 2 samples of patient breath gas were further investigated using gas chromatography with mass spectrometric detection (GC-MS, Agilent 6890N-5973N) to identify breath air components of interest.

2.1. *Patients*

Two breath gas samples per patient (1 exception) were taken at an interval of about 1 hour from 4 PA patients, and 2 of them were re-examined on a second occasion giving a sample total of $N = 11$. The ages as well as the physical and mental development of each of the 4 investigated PA patients are reported in Tables 1 and 2.

The clinical diagnosis of their PA was confirmed by enzymatic and molecular-genetic tests. Two patients showed a mutation in the *PCCA* gene, the other two, brother and sister, a mutation in the *PCCB* gene. All underwent a standard therapy supervised by general paediatricians. In addition, 44 healthy children aged 6–10 (mean 8 years, SD 2 years) recruited from local schools produced 2 breath gas samples each for reference, providing a control collective of $N = 88$ samples. The study was approved by the local ethics board for human studies. Informed consent was obtained from all patients, controls and their parents.

Table 1. Age, weight, height and BMI of the PA patients on the examination day (percentiles determined as described in Ref. 10)

Patient	Sex	Age [a]	Weight [kg] (percentile)	Height [m] (percentile)	BMI [kg/m^2] (percentile)
1	female	18.5	47.3 (5)	1.60 (10)	18.5 (10)
2	male	5.8	17.6 (19)	1.12 (8)	13.8 (10)
3	male	14.1	35.8 (1)	1.49 (2)	16.1 (6)
3	male	14.3	36.0 (1)	1.50 (1)	16.0 (5)
4	female	17.6	46.0 (3)	1.61 (16)	17.7 (6)
4	female	17.8	45.7 (2)	1.62 (19)	17.3 (3)

Table 2. Clinical course and therapy on the examination day (AS: amino acid mixture free of isoleucine, valine, threonine and methionine, VIT: vitamin and trace element preparation)

Patient	Symptom on-set at age of	Diagnosis at age of	Compli-cations	Cognitive abilities	Therapy
1	1 month	2 months	seizures, long QT-time	subnormal	AS, valproate, clobazam, carnitine
2	5 days	5 days	none	normal	AS, VIT, carnitine
3	1 week	2 weeks	seizures, long QT-time	subnormal	AS, VIT, valproate, atenolol, carnitine
4	1 month	4 months	seizures, long QT-time	subnormal	VIT, valproate, carnitine

3. Results

All mass concentration profiles recorded by PTR-MS were screened in terms of the concentration differences between exhaled and inhaled (expiratory–inspiratory) air. For ionic mass 73 u (molecular mass 72 daltons) and ionic mass 115 u (molecular mass 114 daltons), these differences are found to be significantly higher in the PA patients than in the control subjects. Our PTR-MS findings are summarised in Table 3 and depicted in Fig. 2.

Two breath gas samples taken from the PA patients were further investigated using GC-MS in an attempt to identify the components detected by the PTR-MS analysis. Using diluted gaseous mixtures in nitrogen of butanone, a possible candidate for molecular mass 72 daltons, it was shown that this compound was not present in the breath samples at concentrations above the detection limit; other candidate compounds such as butanal have not yet been identified. In contrast, GC-MS analysis of the breath gas samples specified above revealed the presence of 3-heptanone having molecular mass 114 daltons, established using diluted gaseous solutions of 3-heptanone in nitrogen.

Table 3. Expiratory-inspiratory concentrations of compounds in breath samples from PA patients that produce ions at m/z values of 115 u and mass 73 u as determined by PTR-MS (number of patients $n = 4$, number of control children $n = 44$)

		Number of measure-ments	Mean conc. [ppbv]	Median conc. [ppbv]	SD [ppbv]	Min. [ppbv]	Max. [ppbv]
Ionic mass	patients	11	8.5	8.9	5.5	−0.02	19.7
115 u	controls	88	0.2	0.2	0.2	−0.3	0.7
Ionic mass	patients	11	14.0	12.8	4.0	6.7	20.2
73 u	controls	88	−1.7	−1.4	3.1	−12.9	6.2

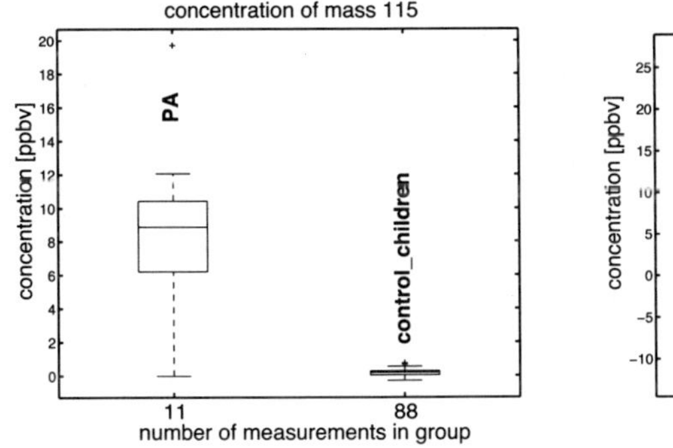

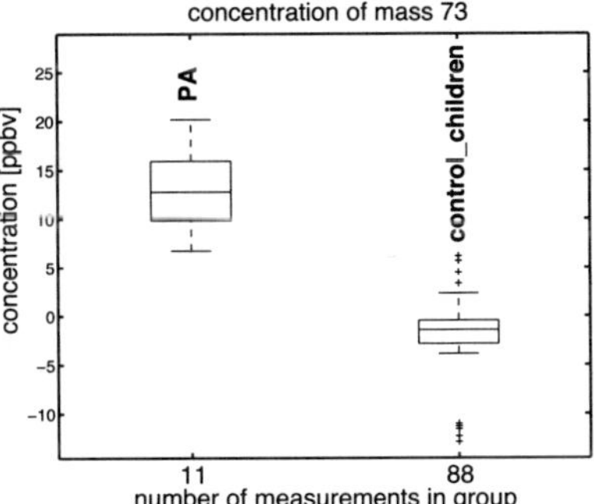

Fig. 2. Expiratory–inspiratory concentrations of compounds in breath samples from PA patients that produce ions at m/z values of 115 u and mass 73 u in box plot representation (median value, 25- and 75-percentiles)

4. Discussion

At present, we still do not have an experimentally-supported[11] proposal for the compound that leads to the ion at m/z value of 73 u. The precise interplay between substances in urine[7] and breath, and the influence of CoA-depletion in PA-patients is not clear either. The presence of 3-heptanone may be understood by the pathway via valeryl-CoA presented in Fig. 3. The methylmalonyl-CoA in this pathway could be provided by the methylmalonyl CoA mutase (MCM), which is responsible for the isomerization between methylmalonylCoA and succinylCoA.[12] It should, nevertheless, be noted that MCC provides the (R)-epimere of methylmalonyl-CoA which has to be equilibrated with the (S) epimere by the respective methylmalonyl-CoA epimerase,[13] before it can be used for the synthesis of carboxylic acids. Perhaps this epimerization even determines the rate of heptanone production. This pathway for 3-heptanone corroborates our

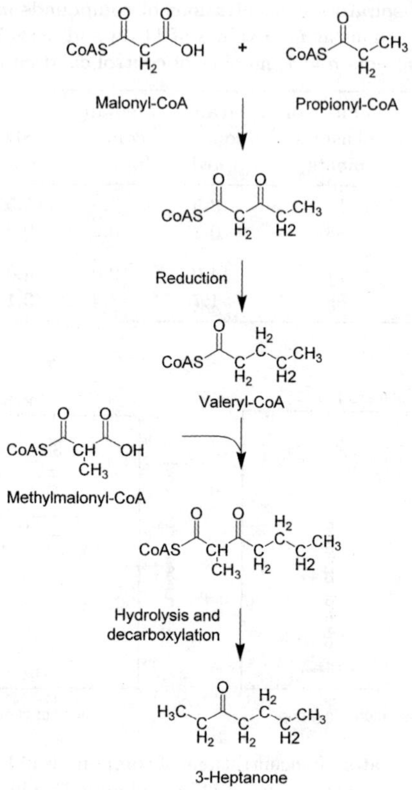

Fig. 3.   Possible pathway for the biochemical synthesis of 3-heptanone

previous conjecture based on a search in the MS library Wiley7n (quality factor up to 93).[14] Should this single experimental observation be reproduced, enhanced unusual ketone exhalation through the lungs would add to the known increased urinary excretion as a PA diagnostic. This justifies the speculations that breath gas analysis may become a useful diagnostic tool for the long-term supervision of PA patients.

Acknowledgements

A. A. thanks Duilio Arigoni for suggesting a biochemical pathway for 3-heptanone, and Ernst Ellmerer for drawing Fig 3. We are grateful for a research grant from the "Medizinischer Forschungsfonds der TILAK" of the University Clinics of Innsbruck. We thank the University Clinics of Innsbruck (TILAK) and its Dir. Dr. Herbert Weissenböck for continuous support. A. A. appreciates the support of the Bernhard Lang Research Association.

References

1. Lamhonwah AM, Barankiewicz TJ, Willard HF, Mahuran DJ, Quan F, Gravel RA. Isolation of cDNA clones coding for the alpha and beta chains of human propionyl-CoA carboxylase: chromosomal assignments and DNA polymorphisms associated with PCCA and PCCB genes. *Proc Natl Acad Sci USA* 1986; **83**: 4864–4868.
2. Kennerknecht I, Suormala T, Barbi G, Baumgartner ER. The gene coding for the alpha-chain of human propionyl-CoA carboxylase maps to chromosome band 13q32. *Hum Genet* 1990; **86**: 238–240.
3. Kraus JP, Williamson CL, Firgaira FA, Yang-Feng TL, Munke M, Francke U, Rosenberg LE. Cloning and screening with nanogram amounts of immunopurified mRNAs: cDNA cloning and chromosomal mapping of cystathionine beta-synthase and the beta subunit of propionyl-CoA carboxylase. *Proc Natl Acad Sci USA* 1986; **83**: 2047–2051.
4. Leonard JV. Stable isotope studies in propionic and methylmalonic acidaemia. *Eur J Pediatr* 1997; **156** Suppl 1: S67–69.
5. Menkes JH. Idiopathic hyperglycinemia: isolation and identification of three previously undescribed urinary ketones. *J Pediatr* 1966; **69**: 413–421.
6. Lehnert W, Schuchmann L, Urbanek R, Niederhoff H, Bohm N. Excretion of 2-methyl-3-oxovaleric acid in propionic acidemia. *Eur J Pediatr* 1978; **128**: 197–205.
7. Lehnert W, Sperl W, Suormala T, Baumgartner ER. Propionic acidaemia: clinical, biochemical and therapeutic aspects. Experience in 30 patients. *Eur J Pediatr* 1994; **153**: S68–80.
8. Wolf B, Hsia YE, Sweetman L, Gravel R, Harris DJ, Nyhan WL. Propionic acidemia: a clinical update. *J Pediatr* 1981; **99**: 835–846.
9. Sperl W, Lehnert W. Metabolic disorders of branched-chain amino acids: most common forms of organic aciduria in the neonatal period [in German]. *Klin Pädiatr* 1990; **202**: 334–339.
10. Kromeyer-Hausschield K, Wabitsch M, Kunze D, Hebebrand J. Perzentile für den Body-mass-Index für das Kindes- und Jugendalter unter Heranziehung verschiedener deutscher Stichproben. *Monatsschrift Kinderheilkunde* 2001; **149**: 807.
11. Doderer, H. *Die Merowinger oder Die totale Familie*. Munich: Biederstein, 1962: p. 142
12. Mancia F, Evans PR. Conformational changes on substrate binding to methylmalonyl CoA mutase and new insights into the free radical mechanism. *Structure* 1998; **15**: 711-720.
13. Mancia F, Evans PR. On the mechanism of action of methylmalonyl-CoA mutase. Change of the steric course on isotope substitution. *European Journal of Biochemistry* 1986; **156**: 545-554.
14. McLafferty FW. *Wiley Registry of Mass Spectral Data, 7th Edition*. New York: John Wiley and Sons, 2000.

APPLICATIONS OF SELECTED ION FLOW TUBE MASS SPECTROMETRY, SIFT-MS, IN ADDICTION RESEARCH

R. BLOOR

Academic Psychiatry Unit, Medical School,
Keele University, Academic Suite, Harplands Hospital,
Hilton Road, Harpfields. ST4 6TH, UK

T. S. WANG

Institute of Science and Technology in Medicine,
Medical School, Keele University,
Thornburrow Drive, Hartshill, Stoke-on-Trent, ST4 7QB, UK

P. ŠPANĚL

V. Čermák Laboratory, J. Heyrovský Institute of Physical Chemistry,
Academy of Sciences of the Czech Republic,
Dolejškova 3, CZ-182 23 Prague 8, Czech Republic

D. SMITH

Institute of Science and Technology in Medicine,
Medical School, Keele University,
Thornburrow Drive, Hartshill, Stoke-on-Trent, ST4 7QB, UK

1. Introduction

1.1. *SIFT-MS Technology*

Trace gas analysis of exhaled air and liquid headspace using selected ion flow tube mass spectrometry (SIFT-MS) has been developed at Keele University[1] and has resulted in the development of clinical applications of the technique.[2,3] SIFT-MS is unique in that it provides real time, online analysis of breath and of liquid headspace and is non-invasive.[4]

The SIFT-MS technique uses precursor ions H_3O^+, NO^+, and O_2^+, which are generated in a discharge ion source, mass selected by a quadrupole mass filter and then injected as selected ionic species into a fast-flowing helium gas carrier. The sample gas to be analysed is introduced to the flow tube through an inlet port where the trace gases react with the chosen precursor ion species. The precursor ions and the product ions of the reactions are then detected and counted by a downstream quadrupole mass spectrometer.

1.2. *SIFT-MS Applications in Addiction Psychiatry*

The use of breath analysis in addiction studies has been limited apart from the detection of alcohol.[5] The diagnostic potential of breath sampling was described[6] in 1983 and it has attracted a considerable amount of scientific and clinical interest during the last two decades (see Ref. 7, on page 251 of this book, and Ref. 8). There have, however, been limited practical applications in addiction. Verstraete[9] describes the potential for detection of cannabis on the breath but acknowledges that most studies have been hampered by problems with techniques, which require complex analytical methods on prepared stored samples. The application of SIFT-MS with its ability to detect trace gases at concentrations down to parts per billion (ppb) in real time may overcome these issues and lead to the development of non-invasive diagnostic techniques for use in addiction treatment and research. Several areas of addiction psychiatry would appear to be appropriate areas for SIFT-MS research including:

- Breath detection of drug use,
- Breath detection of markers of related and comorbid diseases,
- Investigation of the chemical composition of smoked drugs of abuse.

We describe initial investigations into breath detection of drug use and preliminary work towards developing a methodology for detection of markers of comorbid and related disease. The potential for SIFT-MS research into the chemical composition of smoked drugs of abuse is also discussed.

2. Detection of Breath Markers of Drug Use

The development of applications of SIFT-MS to the detection of breath markers of drug use consist of a series of stages of investigation:

1. Investigation of the feasibility of individual detection and quantification of compounds resulting from drug use,
2. Identification of suitable marker ions in the headspace above drug samples,
3. Identification of suitable marker ions from samples during pyrolysis,

4. Analysis of urine headspace of subjects using the target drug,
5. Analysis of breath samples of subjects using the target drug.

A series of preliminary studies into the application of SIFT-MS technology to the detection of breath markers of drug use have been undertaken. These are part of the first stages of a programme of research focusing on the development of a methodology for the detection of drugs through breath sampling. Studies of two drugs, cannabis and γ-hydroxybutyric acid, have been the focus of the current research.

2.1. *Cannabis*

Concentrated plant extracts of *Cannabis sativa* for use in the development of standardised medications for clinical trials in the UK are now available.[10] The headspace volatiles of unprocessed *Cannabis sativa* have previously been analysed[11] and shown to be a complex mixture of compounds. The variations in the composition of unprocessed *Cannabis sativa* have been studied and analysis of headspace volatiles of marijuana using gas chromatography has shown that profiling of the volatile compounds can be used to relate samples to a common source.[12]

The family of chemicals isolated from *Cannabis sativa* are classified as cannabinoids and are analogues of the parent compound Cannabinol that is a fusion product of a terpene and a substituted resorcinol. Two cannabinoids, tetrahydrocannabinol (THC), which is psychoactive, and cannabidiol (CBD), which is non-psychoactive, are shown in Figures 1 and 2. They have been selected for use in their pure form in clinical trials for a variety of conditions.[13]

The mass-to-charge ratio, m/z, of the parent ions of THC and CBD molecules are beyond the range of the current SIFT-MS detection system

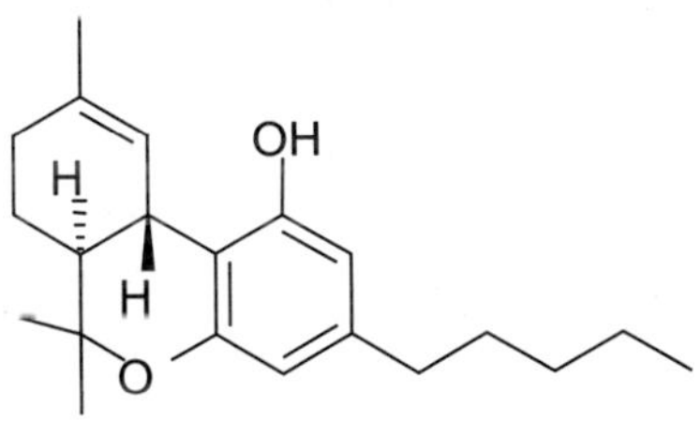

Fig. 1. Δ^1-Δ^9-tetrahydrocannabinol (THC), $C_{21}H_{30}O_2$, MW 314.46

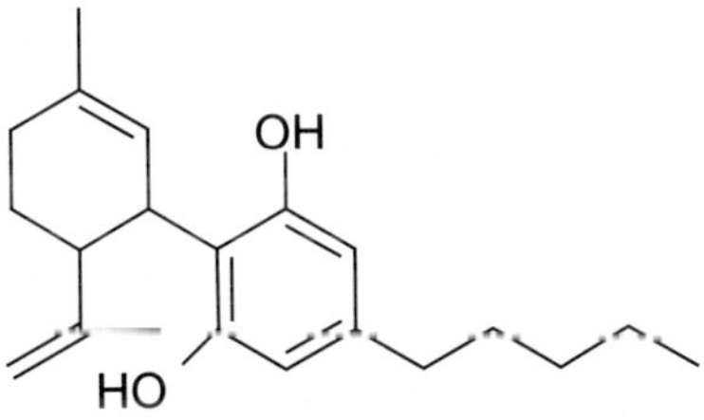

Fig. 2.   Cannabidiol (CBD), $C_{21}H_{30}O_2$, MW 314.46

and this study explores identification of marker ions of lower m/z resulting from fragmentation in the analytical ion-molecule reactions.

Two experiments have been conducted using samples of cannabinoids. The first involves the analysis of the volatile compounds in the air above prepared concentrated samples of THC and CBD. These samples were provided by GW Pharmaceuticals and stored under a Home Office License. The second study investigated the vapour produced by heating these samples in a commercially available "drug vaporizer" commonly used for inhalation of cannabis fumes. A major objective of the reported study is to investigate whether or not these compounds are amenable to individual identification and quantification using SIFT-MS.

Experiment 1 — Analysis of the headspace above samples containing THC and CBD at room temperature

Monitor ions of lower m/z than those of the protonated or ionized parent compounds were identified in the air above THC and CBD at room temperature. The monitor ions for THC were identified as (m/z 231, and 244) and for CBD (m/z 231, 244, and 246). Previous studies of cannabinoids have reported these as the major ions in the 70 eV electron ionization spectra.[14]

The estimated concentrations of THC in the air above the THC sample was 80 ppb using O_2^+ precursor ions, the estimated concentration of ethanol using H_3O^+ precursor ions was 230 ppm and that of terpene was 3 ppm using H_3O^+ precursor ions.

The corresponding data for the CBD were as follows, the CBD concentration was 140 ppb using O_2^+ precursor ions, the ethanol concentration was 110 ppm using H_3O^+ precursor ions and the terpene concentration was 8 ppm using H_3O^+ precursor ions.

Experiment 2 — Analysis of pyrolysis products of samples of THC and CBD

A sample of the THC/CBD preparation was placed on the heating plate of the "vaporizer" which was then sealed within a glass enclosure. The heating plate was activated and the resulting vaporised products were introduced to the SIFT-MS apparatus by connecting the "vaporiser" outlet to the SIFT-MS inlet port.

Three phases of the pyrolysis of the THC and CBD samples are identified in Figure 3.

Phase 1 occurs when the low boiling points/low molecular compounds vaporise. In this phase, the compounds that have low boiling points (usually having low molecular weights, *e.g.* ethanol), leave the resin at relatively low temperatures and react with the precursor ion and reduce the total ion signals significantly (halved over 100 seconds as shown in Figure 3. The spectrum of the ions during this phase is shown in Figure 4. The major species emitted are ethanol, acetaldehyde and acetone.

Phase 2 occurs when the higher boiling points/high molecular weight compounds vaporise.

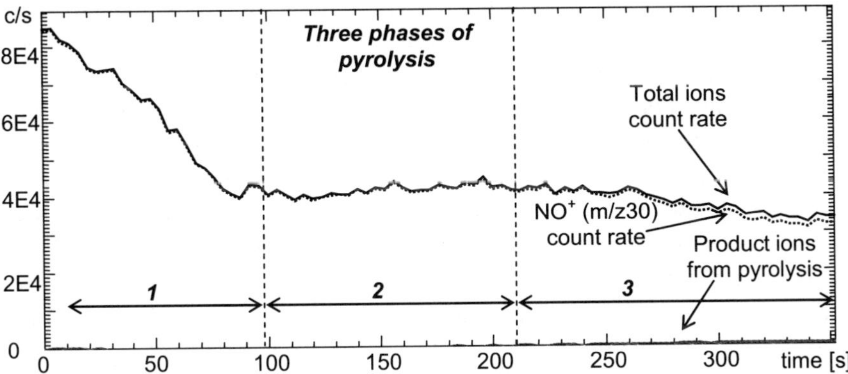

Fig. 3.   The change of the count rate with time of the NO$^+$ precursor ions during the heating process which identifies the three phases

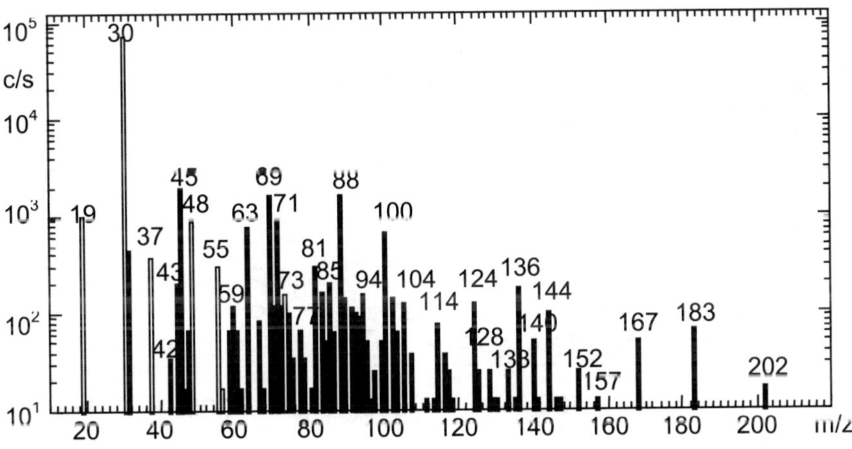

Fig. 4.   Mass spectrum of a Phase 1 sample

Phase 3 is the vaporising/pyrolysing phase. In Phase 3, the highest molecular weight compounds begin to vaporise and also probably partially pyrolyse as the temperature approaches 200 °C. The ions observed at m/z of 104 and 204 using NO^+ precursor ions in this phase (Figure 5) are either due to the presence of molecules of molecular weight 104 and 204 formed by pyrolysis or are formed from larger molecules by the dissociation that can sometimes occur in the analytical ion-molecule reactions.

These results show that SIFT-MS is able to detect markers for THC and CBD in both the headspace above drug samples and in the volatile phases of pyrolysis. The ability to detect markers of cannabis use on the breath will depend on the retention time of these markers following cannabis use. THC has previously been detected from breath samples of human subjects by gas chromatography/mass spectrometry (GC/MS) up to twelve minutes after smoking marijuana.[15] Using chemical detection methods, cannabinoids have been reported to be detectable on breath samples up to 2 hours after smoking cannabis, but with many false positive results from a variety of other substances.[16] The current project will continue by analysing urine headspace of subjects smoking cannabis to attempt to identify additional lower m/z monitor ions. Breath samples will then be obtained from subjects using cannabis that will be analysed by SIFT-MS techniques. Ethical approval has been granted by the Local Research Ethics Committee for analysis of breath and urine samples from patients attending for treatment of drug addiction.

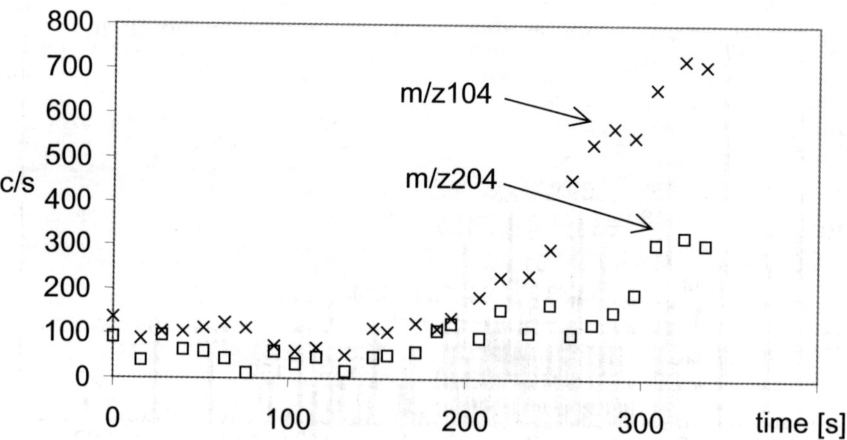

Fig. 5.   The increasing count rate of the ions at m/z 104 and m/z 204 with time during the heating process. (NO^+ as precursor ions)

2.2. *γ-Hydroxybutyric Acid (GHB)*

γ-butyrolactone (GBL) is a precursor of γ-hydroxybutyric acid (GHB) — both are misused as sedative-hypnotics with a high risk of dependence[17] and are shown in Figures 6 and 7. GHB is a short-chain fatty acid neuromodulator that occurs naturally in the brain. The endogenous nature of γ-hydroxybutyric acid (GHB) causes difficulty in detection of exogenous GHB. At low levels, using gas chromatography with mass spectrometry (GC-MS) it is not possible to determine whether any GHB detected is endogenous or exogenous in nature.[18] The short detection window exacerbates this problem for GHB. Following oral administration, even at doses up to 60 mg/kg, the drug is cleared from the blood within 6 hours and is excreted in urine in small amounts in the free form within 10–12 hours after ingestion.[19]

The potential for the use of SIFT-MS technology in the measurement of markers of GHB use in urine headspace was explored with a view to developing a methodology for body fluid or breath detection. This study was conducted as follows:

1. A sample of commercially available GBL was used to investigate the feasibility of detection of these compounds. The samples were acetone free nail polish remover pads, which are used as a source of GBL by drug users.
2. Following informed consent, a sample of the GHB solution used by a patient with GHB dependence was obtained and stored at −70 °C for later analysis.
3. A urine sample was obtained from the same patient; the sample was taken during a prolonged continuous period of GHB use. The sample was frozen at −70 °C for later analysis

Analysis of headspace over the nail polish remover pads using SIFT MS detected GBL and 2-butoxy-1-ethanol. The ratio was 80 % GBL and 20 % 2-butoxy-1-ethanol. This is consistent with the known formulation of this product.

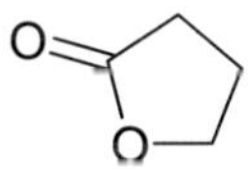

Fig. 6.   γ-butyrolactone (GBL), $C_4H_6O_2$, MW 86.09

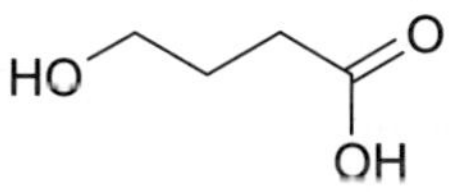

Fig. 7.   γ-hydroxybutyric acid (GHB), $C_4H_8O_3$, MW 104.10

The sample of GHB solution prepared for use by a patient being treated for GHB addiction showed ions of m/z 87 and m/z 105 using H_3O^+ precursor ions. The headspace concentration above the urine from a user of GBL is at about 100 ppb level by using m/z 105 in the analysis. The origin of the product ion at m/z 105 may be either 2- or 3-pentanone,[20,21] 3-methyl-2-butanone or γ-butyrolactone (GBL).[22] However, an ion at m/z 105 is also detected at similar ppb levels in the headspace of control normal urine samples.

Having used SIFT-MS technology to demonstrate the ability to detect markers ions for both GBH and GBL in liquid sample headspace, it is proposed to move to the analysis of breath samples with a view to exploring breath markers of GHB use in dependent patients.

3. Breath Detection of Markers of Related and Comorbid Diseases

There is a high prevalence of psychiatric disease in patient with addiction problems, 37 % of alcohol abusers and 53 % of drug abusers also have at least one serious mental illness. Of all people diagnosed with schizophrenia, up to 50 % have a coexisting drug or alcohol problem.[23] There is increasing evidence that abnormalities of fatty acid and membrane phospholipid metabolism are a factor in the aetiology of neurodevelopmental and psychiatric disorders such as schizophrenia.[24] These abnormalities are likely to be associated with well-characterised genes involved in eicosanoid synthesis and metabolism of the products of oxidative stress and lipid peroxidation[25,26] and it is possible to detect markers of oxidative stress and lipid peroxidation in breath samples.[27]

A research programme for the investigation of breath analysis of volatile markers for oxidative stress as biomarkers in a study of gene targets for vulnerability to neurodevelopmental and psychiatric disorders using SIFT-MS technology has been devised and funding is being sought. The evidence for altered phospholipid dependent signal transduction (PDST) in patients with schizophrenia is, in part, derived from investigations of the niacin challenge test.[28] Niacin dilates cutaneous blood vessels, resulting in a pronounced skin flush in most people. The flush response to niacin is attenuated in some patients with schizophrenia. This is believed to be related to altered PDST mechanisms. The heterogeneous nature of groups of patients with schizophrenia has produced inconsistencies in previous research. The use of the Niacin challenge test to select a subset of patients is a key element of the proposed study. The quantification and physiological mechanism of the niacin challenge test have not been described in detail and the effect of a Niacin flush test on breath trace gases has not been reported. As part of the preliminary work for this research programme we have investigated the effect of a Niacin flush test on breath trace gases in healthy subjects.

Two healthy volunteers undertook a Niacin flush test following a standardised protocol.[28] Subjects were aware of the protocol and possible reactions to niacin. They took nothing by mouth overnight before the challenge. Baseline breath gas analysis using standard SIFT-MS procedures was undertaken. The subjects then self-administered a 200 mg dose of niacin as nicotinic acid tablets with 200 mL of water. Breath gas analysis was then performed several times over the period of the niacin flush reaction. The niacin flush was monitored by visual inspection.

Both subjects were observed to experience a niacin flush. Breath analysis showed steady isoprene and acetone levels but with a significant rise in breath ammonia over the analysis period of some 80 minutes. The results are shown in Figure 8.

Ammonia is notoriously difficult to quantify in moist air at low partial pressure.[29] SIFT-MS studies have enabled the establishment of normal reference values of breath metabolites and the ability to measure on line, real time changes. This preliminary finding of changes in ammonia levels following a Niacin flush test demonstrates the values of SIFT-MS in such studies. The significance of the increase in ammonia levels is to be investigated through planned work on the measurement of breath gases following varied doses of niacin and niacinamide in healthy subjects. This work is in support of the wider planned research on breath markers in schizophrenia and patients with dual diagnosis.

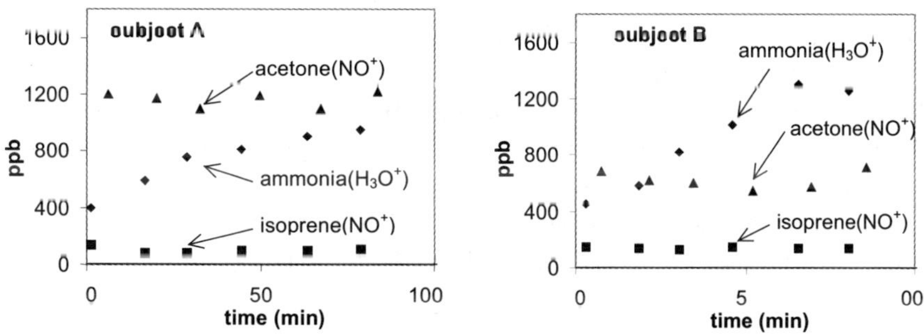

Fig. 8.   Niacin challenge test results for two healthy volunteers

4. Investigation of the Chemical Composition of Smoked Drugs of Abuse

Research on the products resulting from the burning or pyrolysis of drugs of abuse is a key priority for the National Institute on Drug Abuse (NIDA). Research that will further the understanding of the chemical composition of smoked drugs of abuse, and the resulting pharmacological and toxicological effects associated with such exposure is encouraged.[30] SIFT-MS has been applied to analysis of volatile organic compounds resulting from cigarette smoking.[1] Studies have examined volatile organic substances, isoprene, acetone, ammonia and ethanol in breath before and after smoking a cigarette in addition to volatile compounds produced by unburned cigarettes.[31] This important area of addiction research is one where the application of SIFT-MS techniques could overcome some of the limitations of other analytical methods.

5. Conclusions

These preliminary investigations into applications of SIFT-MS in addiction research has shown that real time breath analysis technique can overcome the limitations of those techniques which require complex analytical methods on prepared stored samples. The planned research programme will focus on the development of practical applications of breath analysis in addiction research and clinical practice. The strong multidisciplinary SIFT-MS research grouping based at the University of Keele is well placed to develop the numerous potential applications of SIFT-MS in the field of addiction psychiatry.

Acknowledgements

We are grateful to Edward Hall for his help with the experimental work.

We gratefully acknowledge financial support by the North Staffordshire Medical Institute, The North Staffordshire Research and Development Consortium and the Grant Agency of the Czech Republic (project numbers 202/03/0827 and 203/02/0737.

We also acknowledge the support of GW Pharmaceuticals who gave us access to the samples of THC and CBD Botanical Drug Substances.

References

1. Španěl P, Rolfe P, Rajan B, Smith D. The selected ion flow tube (SIFT) — a novel technique for biological monitoring. *Ann Occup Hyg* 1996; **40**: 615–626.
2. Smith D, Španěl P, Davies S. Trace gases in breath of healthy volunteers when fasting and after a protein-calorie meal: a preliminary study. *J Appl Physiol* 1999; **87**: 1584–1588.
3. Davies S, Španěl P, and Smith D. Quantitative analysis of ammonia on the breath of patients in end-stage renal failure. *Kidney Int* 1997; **52**: 223–228.
4. Smith D and Španěl P. SIFT applications in mass spectrometry., In: Lindon J, Trantner G, Holmes J, eds. *Encyclopedia of spectroscopy and Spectrometry, Mass Spectrometry*, London: Academic Press, 1999: 2092–2105.
5. Wang TS, Španěl P, Smith D. A comparative study of breath ethanol and HDO using SIFT-MS and FA-MS, ethanol metabolism and total body water. Abstract in the booklet of the conference *Breath Gas Analysis for Medical Diagnostics*, Dornbirn, 2004.
6. Manolis A. The diagnostic potential of breath analysis. *Clin Chem* 1983; **29**: 5–15.
7. Risby TH. Current status of clinical breath analysis. In: Amann A, Smith D, eds. *Breath Analysis for Clinical Diagnosis and Therapeutic Monitoring*, Singapore: World Scientific, 2005.
8. Miekisch W, Schubert JK, Noeldge-Schomburg GF. Diagnostic potential of breath analysis — focus on volatile organic compounds. *Clin Chim Acta* 2004; **347**: 25–39.
9. Verstraete A. Perspectives for detection of cannabis in breath , In: *Proceedings of 15th International Conference on Alcohol, Drugs, and Traffic Safety wwwvvse/trafsak/t2000*. Stockholm, 2000.
10. *Cannabis-based medicines–GW pharmaceuticals: high CBD, high THC, medicinal cannabis-GW pharmaceuticals, THC:CBD*, In: *Drugs R D* 2003: 306–309.
11. Hood LV, Dames ME, Barry GT. Headspace volatiles of marijuana. *Nature* 1973; **242**: 402–403.
12. Hood LV Barry GT. Headspace volatiles of marihuana and hashish: gas chromatographic analysis of samples of different geographic origin. *J Chromatogr* 1978; **100**: 499–506.
13. Smith PF. GW-1000. GW Pharmaceuticals. *Curr Opin Investing Drugs* 2004; **5**: 748–754.
14. Baptista MJ, Monsanto PV, Pinho Marques EG, Bermejo A, Avila S, Castanheira AM, Margalho C, Barroso M, Vieira DN. Hair analysis for delta(9)-THC, delta(9)-THC-COOH, CBN and CBD, by GC/MS-EI. Comparison with GC/MS-NCI for delta(9)-THC-COOH. *Forensic Sci Int* 2002; **128**: 66–78.
15. Manolis A, McBurney LJ, Bobbie BA. The detection of delta-9-tetrahydrocannabinol in the breath of human subjects. *Clin Biochem* 1983; **16**: 229–233.

16. McCarthy T, Van Zyle J. Breath analysis of cannabis smokers. *J Pharm Pharmac* 1971; **24**: 489.

17. Wong CG, Chan KF, Gibson KM, Snead OC. γ-hydroxybutyric acid: neurobiology and toxicology of a recreational drug. *Toxicol Rev* 2004; **23**: 3–20.

18. Elliott SP. Gamma hydroxybutyric acid (GHB) concentrations in humans and factors affecting endogenous production. *Forensic Sci Int* 2003; **133**: 9–16.

19. Villain M, Cirimele V, Ludes B, Kintz P. Ultra-rapid procedure to test for γ-hydroxybutyric acid in blood and urine by gas chromatography-mass spectrometry. *J Chromatogr B Analyt Technol Biomed Life Sci* 2003; **792**: 83–87.

20. Španěl P, Ji Y, Smith D. SIFT studies of the reactions of H_3O^+, NO^+, and O_2^+ with a series of aldehydes and ketones. *Int J Mass Spectrom Ion Processes* 1997; **165**: 25–37.

21. Smith D, Wang TS, Španěl P. Analysis of ketones by selected ion flow tube mass spectrometry. *Rapid Commun Mass Spectrom* 2003; **17**: 2655–2660.

22. Wang TS, Španěl P, Smith D. A selected ion flow tube, SIFT, study of the reactions of H_3O^+, NO^+, and O_2^+ ions with several N- and O-containing heterocyclic compounds in support of SIFT-MS. *International Journal of Mass Spectrometry* 2004; **237**: 167–174.

23. Dixon L. Dual diagnosis of substance abuse in schizophrenia: prevalence and impact on outcomes. *Schizophr Res* 1999; **35** Suppl: S93–100.

24. Richardson AJ, Ross MA. Fatty acid metabolism in neurodevelopmental disorder: a new perspective on associations between attention-deficit/hyperactivity disorder, dyslexia, dyspraxia and the autistic spectrum. *Prostaglandins Leukot Essent Fatty Acids* 2000; **63**: 1–9.

25. Ross MA. Could oxidative stress be a factor in neurodevelopmental disorders? *Prostaglandins, Leukotrienes and Essential Fatty Acids* 2000; **63**: 61–63.

26. Bennett CN, Horrobin DF. Gene targets related to phospholipid and fatty acid metabolism in schizophrenia and other psychiatric disorders: an update. *Prostaglandins, Leukotrienes and Essential Fatty Acids* 2000; **63**: 47–59.

27. Kovaleva ES, Orlov ON, Tsutsu'lkovskaia M, Vladimirova TV, Beliaev BS. Lipid peroxidation processes in patients with schizophrenia. *Zh Nevropatol Psikhiatr Im S S Korsakova* 1989; **89**: 108–110.

28. Hudson CJ, Lin A, Cogan S, Cashman F, Warsh JJ. The Niacin Challenge Test: Clinical Manifestation of Altered Transmembrane Signal Transduction in Schizophrenia? *Biological Psychiatry* 1997; **41**: 507–513.

29. Španěl P, Davies S, Smith D. Quantification of ammonia in human breath by the selected ion flow tube analytical method using H_3O^+ and O_2^+ precursor ions. *Rapid Commun Mass Spectrom* 1998; **12**: 763–766.

30. National Institute on Drug Abuse. *Chemistry, Pharmacology, and Toxicology of Smoked Drugs of Abuse* 2002: PA-02-095.

31. Senthilmohan ST, McEwan MJ, Wilson PF, Milligan DB, Freeman CG. Real time analysis of breath volatiles using SIFT-MS in cigarette smoking. *Redox Rep* 2001; **6**: 185–187.

EXHALED BREATH CONDENSATE (EBC): AN ALTERNATIVE OR ADDITIONAL DIAGNOSTIC?

G. BECHER, M. ROTHE, AND M. DECKER

FILT Lungen- und Thoraxdiagnostik GmbH,
Robert-Rössle-Straße 10, D-13125 Berlin, Germany

1. Introduction

Chronic inflammatory airway diseases such as COPD, asthma and cystic fibrosis are important diseases in relation to human healthcare. Furthermore, the early detection of acute respiratory failure requires diagnostic methods of high sensitivity and accuracy. Traditional pulmonary function tests (PFT) provide information about the mechanical properties of the respiratory system, *i.e.* about static or dynamic lung volumes, and expiratory and inspiratory flow rates, respectively. Using rapid gas analyzers, additional information is available about gas exchange and distribution of ventilation. Although conventional pulmonary function tests are able to demonstrate the therapeutic effect of anti-obstructive agents and the reaction to bronchial challenge tests, none of the traditional PFT's is able to provide primary information about the reasons for lung disturbances. In other words, diagnostic procedures for inflammatory airway diseases are inadequate. From the diagnostic point of view, airway inflammation is still the domain of invasive and semi-invasive diagnostic methods (like bronchoalveolar lavage and induced sputum).

Except for anti-obstructive agents, anti-inflammatory treatment become more and more important for therapeutic strategies. However, there is a gap between available routine diagnostic methods and the molecular and cellular approach to therapeutic intervention. Qualified healthcare in respiratory medicine needs more non-invasive diagnostic methods that should be repeatable, sensitive, specific and available everywhere (and applicable to all kinds of patients). Analysis of exhaled breath condensate (EBC) may become such a method.

Several non-volatile components have been found in EBC. These components are thought to be released into the exhaled breath either as vapour or as aerosols from deeper airways. A major fraction of the EBC components may be inflammatory markers because they are well known from *in-vitro* experiments and studies of bronchoalveolar lavage fluids and sputum. A variety of markers is known to be either specific or non-specific for the activation of different cell types (for example macrophages, neutrophils, monocytes, eosinophils and other cells located in the alveolar and bronchial lumen). In comparison to traditional lung function tests, EBC may provide additional information related to pathophysiological processes in the airways. In comparison to similar to bronchoalveolar lavage and sputum, EBC collection has the advantage that it is completely non-invasive and frequently repeatable.

2. Methods

2.1. *Collection of Exhaled Breath Condensate (EBC)*

Exhaled breath condensate offers the opportunity to collect a specimen from the deeper airways in a non-invasive way.[1] Collection is performed by exhalation via a non-re-breathing valve into a cooled sampling system. In humans, 1.5 to 2.5 mL of condensate can be sampled within 10 minutes of tidal breathing, *i.e.* approximately 100 litres exhaled air. EBC contains many different non-volatile substances like proteins, leukotrienes, prostaglandins, nitrite and nitrate, ammonium, interleukins related to certain pathophysiological stages of airway cell activation.[1,2]

Breath condensate must be collected and stored at $-80\,^\circ$C and biological inert materials must be used for collection and storage. For each marker to be measured biochemically, a standard addition trial should be carried out to check the data obtained for the particular vials that are used. In general, the samples should not be stored at $-80\,^\circ$C for more than 10–12 weeks. General recommendations for collection and analyses of EBC are given in a special issue of the JAEGER-Info.[9]

2.2. *Measurement of Markers in EBC*

The analysis of biomarkers in EBC is still a highly sophisticated procedure. Concentrations of markers are usually lower than 1/1000 of known concentrations in other biological specimens, *e.g.* serum. Consequently, particular analytical procedures must be developed to analyse the cell-free and nearly protein-free EBC-solution.

Measurement of arachidonic acid metabolites (*e.g.* leukotriene B4, leukotriene CDE4, 8-isoprostane, prostacyclines) is possible using sensitive immunoassays. Certain non-protein containing markers of fatty acid metabolism are measurable using LC-MS. Protein in EBC is measurable using the Micro BCA-Method. Nitrate/nitrite can be measured by the Griess method. Ammonium is measurable using according to the Berthelot principle with photometry. The measurement of pH demands special pH-electrodes because of the low conductivities of the samples and because the dependence on pH of some of the compounds is not defined. How the ingredients of the EBC determine the pH is still incomplete because of the very low ion concentration in EBC, so the pH measurement remains very challenging.

A new approach has been developed for the measurement of H_2O_2 in EBC. The newly introduced biosensor measuring system for H_2O_2 — ECoCheck[TM] — is much more sensitive than spectrophotometry or fluorometric methods.[4] This biosensor has a detection limit of 30 nmol/L. The ECoCheck system enables the immediate analysis of fresh EBC samples. The measurement of H_2O_2 in EBC provides non-specific but sensitive information about airway inflammation. Concentrations below 500 nmol/L seem to be normal while values above 1000 nmol/L indicate severe airway inflammation. A sensitive differentiation between healthy and borderline inflammation and severe exacerbation seems to be possible.

3. Results

Comparing different studies, the range of absolute concentrations obtained for biomarkers measured in EBC seems to be dependent on the different analytic methods used. Nevertheless, relative trends and comparisons between healthy volunteers, untreated patients and patients on different treatments are quite clear. Some markers in EBC are measurable even in healthy volunteers. For example, LTB_4 has been detected in healthy non-smokers. However, a significant increase of LTB_4 was measured in hairdressers in comparison to office-workers with no history of lung and airway diseases.[6] It seems that LTB_4 in EBC is a sensitive marker of low-dose airway sensitivity to inhaled irritants. Interestingly, there was no correlation between results of pulmonary function tests (FEV_1, FVC, MEF_{50}, PEF and oscillatory resistance R_{os}) and the concentration of various markers measured in EBC.

In another controlled study, patients with allergic asthma underwent an inhalative challenge test with a specific allergen.[7] A low allergen dosage was chosen to induce only a small decrease in FEV_1 (lower than 20 %).

In none of the patients, clinical symptoms or any other indications of a late response were found. FEV_1 was normalized within 2–3 hours after the challenge. A significant increase of $LTCDE_4$ and LTB_4 was seen within 30 minutes after the challenge test. While $LTCDE_4$ was normalized within 3–6 hours, LTB_4 remained at high levels (100% increase) compared to the initial level for more than 24 hours. Following this, the specific inhalative allergen challenge induced a short-term bronchial constriction, but a long-lasting increase of LTB_4, which is an indicator of neutrophilic activation! The LTB_4 levels in EBC were correlated to clinical asthma scores but not to the results of conventional lung function test.[7]

The aim of the present study was to test the reproducibility of H_2O_2 levels within several days or within one day in order to investigate a possible circadian rhythm. In 8 healthy volunteers, stable concentration of H_2O_2 were found in EBC for 2 weeks. Overall, 80 samples were analysed, leading to a mean concentration of 569 ± 29.7 nmol/L (mean $\pm$ SEM)and a standard deviation of ±109 nmol/L. The individual trends within ten days for H_2O_2 are shown in Fig. 1. Significant trends were not detected within 10 days.

In 11 patients with acute exacerbations of asthma and COPD, the concentration of H_2O_2 was increased 5–10 fold compared to healthy controls. The mean was 3970 ± 868 (Mean $\pm$ SEM), the maximum was 8778, the minimum was 873, and the median was 1929 nmol/L. Because all healthy volunteers had a H_2O_2-level below the minimum level of the patients, these results indicate a clear differentiation between healthy volunteers and non-treated exacerbated patients with COPD and asthma.

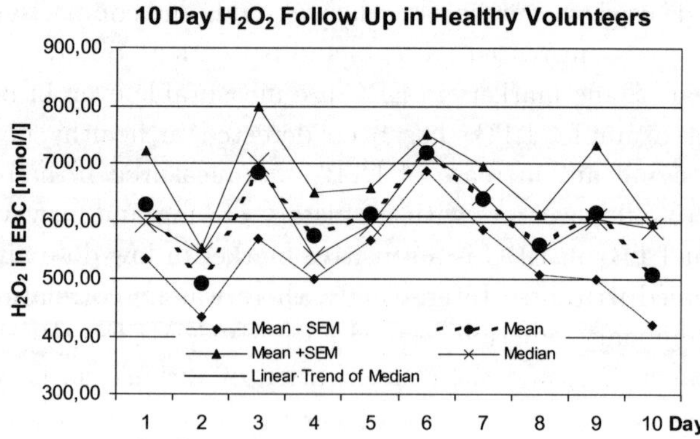

Fig. 1.   The concentration of hydrogen peroxide (H_2O_2) [nmol/L] measured once per day in EBC from 9 healthy volunteers over a 10-day period. The results show a linear trend of the median value.

There was no indication of a circadian rhythm of the H_2O_2 in EBC. Between 8:00 a.m. and 04:00 p.m., the mean concentration was found to be between 620 and 660 nmol/L with a standard error of the mean (SEM) between approximately 50 and 70 nmol/L.

Comparing different individuals, a marked inter-individual variability of the H_2O_2-concentration in EBC was observed that was much larger than intra-individual variability.

Within one day, there were only a few subjects showing significant differences of the H_2O_2-concentration in EBC, visible in Fig. 2. In general, the daily mean trend did show not any significant changes in relation to daytime (Fig. 3). Compared to the mean values over 10 days mentioned above, the mean value of all measurements was 658 ± 55 (mean $\pm$ SEM).

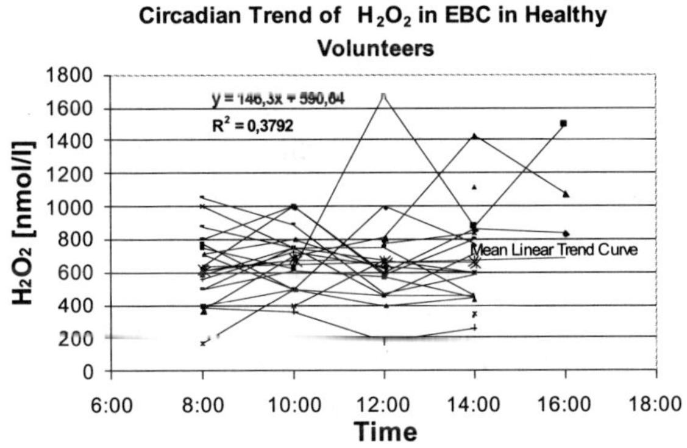

Fig. 2. H_2O_2 in 21 circadian measurement cycles on different days in healthy volunteers (individual tracings)

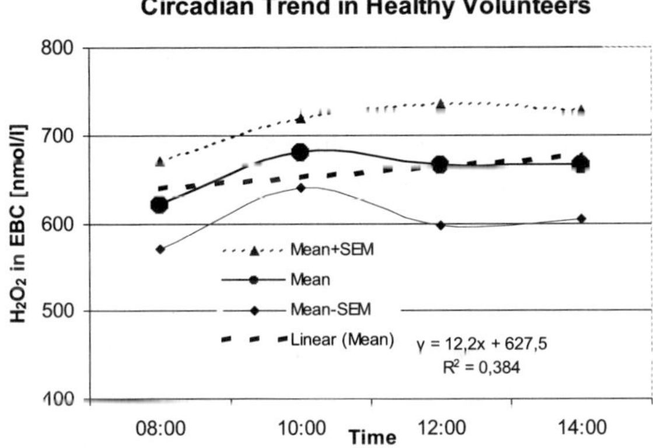

Fig. 3. H_2O_2 in circadian measurement cycles on different days in healthy volunteers (mean $\pm$ SEM) and linear trend

4. Discussion

In the international literature, there is an increasing number of papers that report significant correlations between markers of inflammation measured in EBC (leukotriene, 8-isoprostane, hydrogen peroxide) and airway inflammation processes. In certain studies[5,8,10] the strong correlation between the number of neutrophils in bronchial lavage fluid or sputum and the concentration of hydrogen peroxide in EBC ($r^2 > 0.8$) is reported. Consequently, hydrogen peroxide seems to be a clear surrogate marker of the neutrophilic inflammation in the airways.

Different *in-vitro* studies have been able to demonstrate the pathophysiological significance of several markers in relation to cellular inflammation and airway diseases.[2] Other studies in occupational[6] and pulmonary medicine[3,5,7] have showed the value of EBC for diagnosing airway inflammation.

Markers of inflammation measurable in EBC are more informative provide a better description of airway inflammation than traditional lung function tests. Thus, the identification of different markers combined with the calculation of the abundance ratios of several markers may offer the opportunity to distinguish between certain cell activities in the airways.

In conclusion, exhaled breath condensate can be recommended as a useful diagnostic tool in ambulant medicine, occupational medicine and in the intensive care unit (ICU). Further studies are needed to establish reference values for the concentration of EBC-components, as well as to monitor therapy for various lung diseases.

References

1. Becher G, Winsel K, Beck E, Stresemann E. Leukotriene B_4 in breathing condensate of patients with bronchopulmonary diseases and in normal patients. *Appl Cardiopulm Pathophysiol* 1995; **5**: 215–219.
2. Barnes PJ, Chung KF, Page CP. Inflammatory Mediators of asthma: an update. *Pharmacological Reviews* 1998; **50** (4): 517–596.
3. Rosias PPR *et al.* Exhaled breath condensate in children: Pearls and pitfalls. *Pediatr Allergy Immunol* 2004; **15**: 4–19.
4. Lehmann C, Rothe M, Becher G. Empfindliche Wasserstoffperoxid-Messung. *LABO* 2004; **35** (2): 31–32.
5. Kostikas K, Papatheodorou G, Psathakis K, Panagou P, Loukides S. Oxidative stress in expired breath condensate of patients with COPD. *Chest* 2003; **124**: 1373–1380.

6. Becher G, Stresemann E, Beck E, Neubauer G, Rothe M, Falck K. *Die Bestimmung von Entzündungsmediatoren im Atemkondensat zur Früherkennung von Folgen einer irritativen inhalativen Belastung im Friseurgewerbe.* Bundesanstalt für Arbeitsmedizin und Arbeitsschutz, Fb 788. Bremerhaven: Wirtschaftsverlag NW, 1998, ISBN 3-89701-091-7.

7. Becher G, Beck E, Schuette W, Rothe M, Tacke A, Georgi G, Stresemann E. Erste klinische Erfahrungen mit der Messung von Leukotrienen- und Eosinophilen-Parametern im Atemkondensat. *Pneumologie* 1997; **51** Suppl 2: 456–945.

8. Loukides S, Bouros D, Papatheodorou G, Lachanis S, Panagou P, Siafakas NM. Exhaled H_2O_2 in steady-state bronchiectasis — relationship with cellular composition in induced sputum, spirometry, and extent and severity of disease. *Chest* 2002; **121** (1): 81–87.

9. *JAEGER Info. Special Edition "Breath Condensate."* Würzburg 2001, Item No. 791764.

10. Deaton CM, Marlin DJ, Smith NC, Smith KC, Newton RJ, Gower SM, Cade SM , Roberts CA, Harris PA, Schroter RC, Kelly FJ. Breath condensate hydrogen peroxide correlates with both airway cytology and epithelial lining fluid ascorbic acid concentration in the horse. *Free Radical Research* 2004; **38** (2): 201–208.

RAPID DIAGNOSIS
OF GASTRO-INTESTINAL INFECTION
USING FAECAL ODOUR

R. EWEN, B. DE LACY COSTELLO, C. GARNER,
N. M. RATCLIFFE, AND S. SMITH

Faculty of Applied Sciences,
Centre for Research in Analytical, Material and Sensor Sciences,
University of the West of England,
Coldharbour Lane, Bristol, BS16 1QY, UK

S. J. PROBERT

Department of Medicine, Bristol Royal Infirmary,
Marlborough Street, Bristol, BS2 8HW, UK

1. Introduction

Diarrhoea due to infection is a major cause of morbidity and mortality In the United States, the major disease vector is *Clostridium difficile* with about 3 million patients suffering from *Clostridium difficile* associated diarrhoea and colitis (CDAD) each year.[1] In 1989, it was reported that 10 % of patients hospitalized for more than 2 days suffer from CDAD.[2] In England and Wales, there are approximately 15,000 cases of *Clostridium difficile* infection *per annum*, but this is dwarfed by the 55,000 cases of *Campylobacter* infection. However, viral infections of the gastrointestinal tract are also a major problem: in England and Wales, there are 16,000 cases of *Rotavirus* infection *per annum* and in the United States *Rotavirus* infection accounts for 56,000 hospitalizations per year and 48 % of viral gastroenteritis in the US.[3] In developing countries *Rotavirus* accounts for 600,000 deaths per year.[4] Whilst there remain few appropriate anti-viral agents for these disorders, isolation of infected individuals would limit epidemics.

Despite the development of ELISAs and molecular techniques, in most cases there is a delay of several days between the collection of a stool sample and a microbiological diagnosis. The delay is, in part, due to shipping of the samples to an appropriate laboratory, but mainly due to the time required to complete the diagnostic techniques in common use. The limited availability of expensive microbiological techniques in developing countries compounds the problem. Depending on the patient's circumstance, the results of a diagnostic delay is likely to range from lost productivity to prolonged hospitalization or death. There is a pressing need to make a rapid, accurate diagnosis in all patients. Diarrhoea has a wide variety of physical characteristics that have been used to try to determine its aetiology, with limited success. The flatus that accompanies diarrhoea can be particularly unpleasant for patients; however, neither the use of such gases for diagnostic purposes nor the characteristics of the volatiles from stool samples has received any detailed attention. We studied volatiles from stool samples of patients with diarrhoea and from healthy volunteers to ascertain their respective vapor profiles. In the case of potato tuber diseases, we have previously shown[5,6] that use of gas chromatography/mass spectroscopy vapor analysis can be successfully used for identification of the disease state of vegetables. This paper discusses the combination of the recently developed advances in solid state micro extraction with the novel approach of volatile profile analyses from stool samples in order to diagnose diseased states of the gastro-intestinal tract.

2. Methods

Flatus was obtained from stool samples from 38 subjects with diarrhoea and from 6 healthy controls. 10 samples were donated from a healthy individual over a 4 week period in intervals of about 3 days. For each subject, the aetiology of the diarrhoea was determined by routine microbiological assessment ($n = 35$). Three of the subjects had an exacerbation of inflammatory bowel disease involving the colon. Diarrhoea samples (ca. 0.75 g) were portioned into sealed headspace vials (Supelco, 10 mL) designed for solid phase microextraction (SPME). Samples were equilibrated in a water bath (37 °C) and their volatile compounds entrained from the headspace onto SPME fibre (Supelco, 85 μm carboxen/polydimethylsiloxane), 12 hours and 30 minutes for the 10 samples from the normal individual. Any samples not extracted within 1 hour of collection were stored in the vials at -18 °C. Sample volatile compounds were desorbed from the fibre thermally via splitless injection (HP 5890 II, 1.5 min, 25 °C) onto a thick film column (Supelco, SPB-1 Sulfur, 30 m $\times$ 30 m $\times$ 0.32 mm). Volatile compounds were eluted from the column (35 °C (5 min) $\times$ 10 °C/min to 250 °C (2 min), 1 mL/min) directly into a quadrupole mass spectrometer

(HP 5971) full scan (positive mode, 15–60 amu 2 min, 19–350 amu until 28.5 min). Compounds identification was performed by spectral analysis undertaken using proprietary Hewlett Packard software (G1034C, V1.05) running the NBS75K library, and also by their elution order.

3. Discussion

Volatiles were successfully concentrated onto short SPME fibres. Thermal desorption and analysis were undertaken via a small bench top gas chromatography-mass spectrometry system. The composition of the VOCs emitted by stools from normal subjects showed many similarities; however, in patients with various types of diarrhoea the distribution of VOCs was consistently different and characteristic changes in the volatile pattern occurred with specific types of diarrhoea.

The volatiles present in the flatus of normal subjects were remarkably similar. The predominant class of volatile was the phenols, which accounted for 20–50 % of the measured volatiles. In each subject, 4-methylphenol was the by far the most prevalent. Indole and 3-methylindole were also abundant (5–25 %) in the volatiles from stool samples of normal subjects, as were a group of volatiles classified, without detailed differentiation, as monoterpenes and hydrocarbons (10–20 %). The principle volatile components of normal flatus were. 4-methylphenol, indole, 3 methylindole and limonene. Benzaldehyde was ubiquitous though less abundant, and sulfides and fatty acids were common species in varying degrees. Table 1 shows the main compounds present in the faeces analysed from 10 samples over 30 days from one subject. There is consistency to the data. All the acids from ethanoic to octanoic acid were found as were the aldehydes from ethanal to octanal and the alcohols from methanol to heptanol. A series of methyl ketones from acetone to nonan-2-one were found. The branched aliphatics also showed a pattern with 2 methylpontanol, and the corresponding aldehyde, 2-methylpentanal, and 2-methylpentanoic acid present.

It is well known that carbohydrates (di-, oligo- and polysaccharides) are broken down to monosaccharides and then to short-chain fatty acids, (ethanoic – hexanoic acids), by bacterial fermentation in the large colon. The branched fatty acids, however, always originate from amino acids derived from protein hydrolysis. Short chain fatty acids (SCFAs) can also originate from amino acids and *Clostridium propionicum* can produce propionic and butyric acid from threonine *via* oxidation or reduction of the ketobutyrate intermediate respectively. *Clostridium saccharobutyricum* can

Table 1.   Principal compounds found in 10 faecal samples from a normal subject

Acids	Aldehydes	Primary alcohols	Secondary alcohols	Hydrocarbons
$CH_3(CH_2)_nCO_2H$ $n = 0$ to 6	$CH_3(CH_2)_nC{\overset{H}{\underset{O}{}}}$ $n = 0$ to 6	$CH_3(CH_2)_nOH$ $n = 1$ to 6		Dodecane Undecane

Methyl ketones	Branched aliphatics	Esters	Sulphur compounds
$CH_3(CH_2)_n$ $n = 0$ to 6, 8, and 10	CH_2OH CHO CO_2H CHO CO_2H		NCS (mustard) (garlic) SH SH $S=C=S$

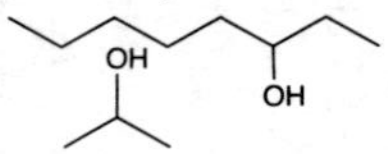

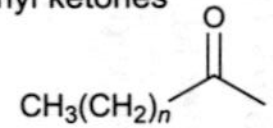

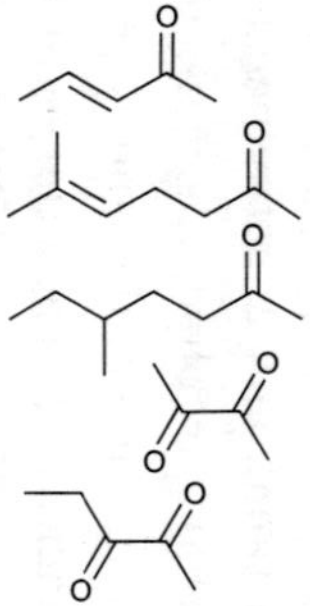

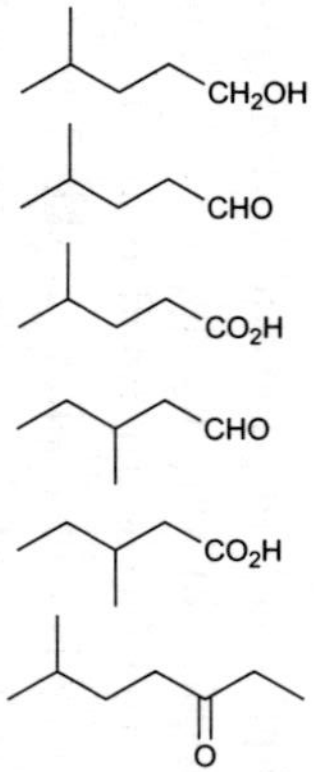

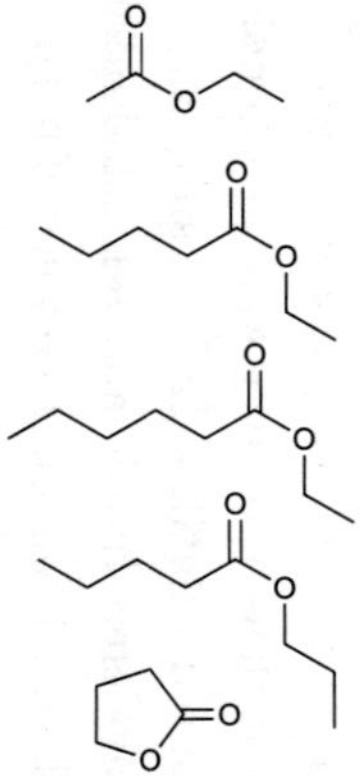

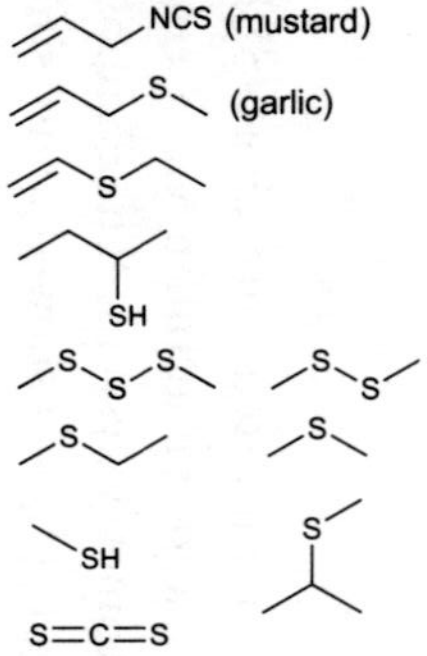

Phenolics 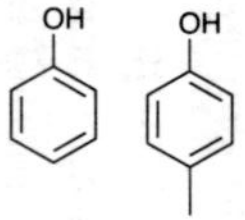	Aromatics (alkyl mono-substituted) 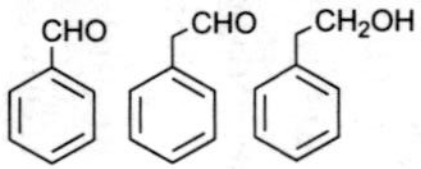	Indoles 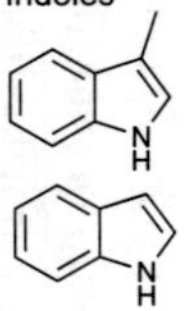	Terpenes 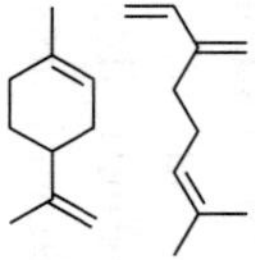	Other 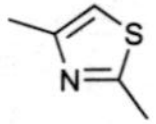
OH OH	CHO CHO CH_2OH			

produce ethanoic, propionic and butanoic acid from the amino acids, glutamate, aspartate and alanine. Detection and monitoring of SCFAs could be important in assessing body energy intake, as it is estimated that 5–10 % of human energy needs come from these species and in ruminants, such as rabbits, horses, etc., it is estimated at 70–80 %. There is also some evidence that there is less butyrate in ulcerative colitis patients. We observed a homologous series of 2-ketones and we have not found a report of a series of 2-ketones from gut bacteria, although volatiles from the headspace from *E. coli* produce 2-tridecanone, 2-undecanone and 2-nonanone and 2-ketones are known to be volatile metabolites from many bacteria and fungi. We have monitored the diet of the individual, who ate plentiful amounts of cheddar cheese. 2-propanone, 2-butanone and 2-heptanone are known to be to be present in cheddar cheese, so we cannot discount dietary effects.

Indoles are ubiquitous in normal stool and in most patients with diarrhoea. Their occurrence is related to the metabolism of tryptophan by *Escherichia coli*. and a simple laboratory test for *E. coli* based on the detection of indoles has been in clinical use since 1963.[7] Broad spectrum antibiotics suppress the growth of *E. coli* allowing the overgrowth of *C. difficile*. The reduced production or absence of indoles in patients being prescribed antibiotics with *C. difficile* infection is likely to be a result of the disruption of metabolism by *E. coli*. This explanation for the vapor profile of the stool samples is supported by the fact that *C. difficile* does not produce indole from tryptophan.[8]

In flatus from patients with diarrhoea due to *Clostridium difficile*, furans (principally 2-furan carboxaldehyde and 5-methyl-2-furan carboxaldehyde) were particularly prevalent (25–55 % of the measured volatiles). Furans are not found in the flatus of normal subjects or that from the majority of patients with other forms of infectious diarrhoea. Furans are likely to be related to bacterial metabolism of furanose from dietary fructose.

The absence of 3-methylindole in the presence of high levels of 2-furancarboxaldehyde occurred exclusively among patients with *Clostridium difficile*. However, even without quantification, the presence of these furans in the absence of 3-methylindole may be used to diagnose *Clostridium difficile*. Many *Clostridia* species are capable of fermenting sugars and amino acids. Efforts were made to rapidly identify *C. difficile* in cultures by the presence of p-cresol and caproic acid.[9,10] However, this approach was not widely used and, unlike our approach, requires the organism to be cultured before it can be identified. Multiple enzyme immunoassays do provide a rapid test for *C. difficile*.[11] However, ELISAs have a sensitivity of 70–90 % and specificity of 99 %.[12] As quick as they may be, they are not used for near-patient-testing and still are dependent on transport to a microbiology laboratory.

Ethyl dodecanoate was common to the volatiles of stools from patients with *Rotavirus*; one of the samples from a patient with enteritis due to *Adenovirus* infection also contained this. It is also of interest that dodecanoic acid was also detected in 4 out of 5 of the *Rotavirus* samples and absent from all but one of the remaining samples. Ethyl dodecanoate has not been previously reported, although a relative increase in propionic and butyric acids have been reported in the stool of patients with *Rotavirus*.[13] We found that, while the amount of short chain (C_3 to C_5) fatty acids appeared greatest in the flatus of patients with *Rotavirus*, there were also significant amounts in patients with *Campylobacter* and *Clostridium difficile*. Hence, diagnoses of a single vector type cannot be made based on the presence of short chain carboxylic acids.

Patients with *Campylobacter* each produced flatus which was quite similar to normal stool. Phenols were abundant (10-40 % of measured volatiles) as were indoles (20–30 %). Moreover, patients with *Campylobacter* infection produced flatus containing more volatile organic acids (30–35 % of measured volatiles) than any other group of patient. However, patients in this group produced flatus that contained no volatile compound belonging to the terpenes/hydrocarbon group. Every other sample analysed contained VOCs belonging to this group.

These chemical fingerprints could be used to rapidly determine the aetiology of acute or chronic diarrhea. However, the need is often most urgent in the immuno-compromised patient – the bone marrow recipient, the HIV/AIDS patient as well as the very young or old. We are undertaking more analyses to build up a large library correlating volatile composition with disease state of the gastro-intestinal tract. On the hardware side, a relatively unsophisticated small bench top GC-MS system with pattern recognition software would be the next step forward, although further research to target sensors to the key volatiles identified in our work would be potentially very useful in order to produce an electronic nose with a sensor array with a minimal number of sensors. Such an array would be the key component of an inexpensive electronic nose system capable for near-patient testing. We are actively pursuing these goals.[14]

In the future it might be possible to diagnose bowel conditions from volatiles found on the breath. If key volatiles can be found from faeces they could be looked for in the breath. The concentrations would be expected to be much lower, however if they could be detected it might be a more socially acceptable way forward for disease diagnoses.

Acknowledgements

The authors would like to thank Peter Jones, Cardinal Health, UK, for his assistance in this work.

References

1. Mylonakis E, Ryan ET, Calderwood SB. Clostridium difficile–associated diarrhea: A review. *Arch Intern Med* 2001; **161**: 525–533.
2. McFarland LV, Mulligan ME, Kwok RY, Stamm WE. Nosocomial acquisition of Clostridium difficile infection. *N Engl J Med* 1989; **320**: 204–210.
3. Lew JF, Glass RI, Petric M, Lebaron CW, Hammond GW, Miller SE, Robinson C, Boutilier J, Riepenhoff-Talty M, Payne CM, *et al.* Six-year retrospective surveillance of gastroenteritis viruses identified at ten electron microscopy centers in the United States and Canada. *Pediatr Infect Dis J* 1990; **9**: 709–714.
4. Ciarlet M, Estes MK. Interactions between rotavirus and gastrointestinal cells. *Curr Opin Microbiol* 2001; **4**: 435–441.
5. De Lacy Costello BP, Ewen R, Gunson H, Ratcliffe N, Spencer-Phillips P. The development of a sensor system for the early detection of soft rot in stored potato tubers. *Measurement Science and Technology* 2000; **11**: 1685–1691.
6. De Lacy Costello B, Evans P, Ewen R, Gunson H, Ratcliffe N, Spencer-Phillips P. GC-MS analyses of volatile organic compounds from potato tubers inoculated with Phytophthora infestans or Fusarium coeruleum. *Plant Pathology* 2001; **50**: 489–496.
7. Vracko R, Sherris JC. Indole-spot test in bacteriology. *Tech Bull Regist Med Technol* 1963; **33**: 47–50.
8. Cowan S, Steel K. *Cowan and Steel's Manual for the Identification of Medical Bacteria.* 3rd ed., Cambridge: Cambridge University Press, 1993.
9. Johnson LL, McFarland LV, Dearing P, Raisys V, Schoenknecht FD. Identification of Clostridium difficile in stool specimens by culture-enhanced gas liquid chromatography. *J Clin Microbiol* 1989; **27**: 2218–2221.
10. Nonhoff C, Struelens MJ, Serruys E. Evaluation of gas-liquid chromatography (GLC) for rapid detection of Clostridium difficile in fecal specimens. *Acta Clin Belg* 1995; **50**: 76–80.
11. Delmee M. Laboratory diagnosis of Clostridium difficile disease. *Clin Microbiol Infect* 2001; **7**: 411–416.
12. Gerding DN, Johnson S, Peterson LR, Mulligan ME, Silva J, Jr Clostridium difficile-associated diarrhea and colitis. *Infect Control Hosp Epidemiol* 1995; **16**: 459–477.
13. Brooks JB. Review of frequency-pulsed electron-capture gas-liquid chromatography studies of diarrheal diseases caused by members of the fam-

ily Enterobacteriaceae, Clostridium difficile, and rotavirus. *J Clin Microbiol* 1986; **24**: 687–691.

14. Probert CS, Jones PR, Ratcliffe NM. A novel method for rapidly diagnosing the causes of diarrhoea. *Gut* 2004; **53**: 58–61.

PART E

USE OF ISOTOPES

FLOWING AFTERGLOW MASS SPECTROMETRY (FA-MS) FOR THE DETERMINATION OF THE DEUTERIUM ABUNDANCE IN BREATH WATER VAPOUR AND AQUEOUS LIQUID HEADSPACE

P. ŠPANĚL

*V. Čermák Laboratory, J. Heyrovský Institute of Physical Chemistry,
Academy of Sciences of the Czech Republic,
Dolejškova 3, CZ-182 23 Prague 8, Czech Republic*

D. SMITH

*Institute of Science and Technology in Medicine,
Medical School, Keele University,
Thornburrow Drive, Hartshill, Stoke-on-Trent, ST4 7QB, UK*

1. Introduction

The chemical element hydrogen, H, is a mixture of two stable isotopes: hydrogen, ^{1}H, and deuterium, ^{2}H or D. Both of these isotopes are naturally present in water; in one million terrestrial water molecules, there is typically 999,700 ^{1}H$_2$O molecules and 300 HDO (or ^{1}H^{2}HO) molecules. The probability of finding a single D$_2$O molecule in this water is very low. The deuterium abundance is conventionally determined in liquid water, urine, saliva and blood samples by first equilibrating a sample of these media with gaseous hydrogen in the presence of a catalyst, thus producing hydrogen gas above the liquid. Then, conventional mass spectrometry, sometimes coupled with gas chromatography, GC-MS,[1] is used to analyse the isotopic composition of this gas.[2,3] However, this approach requires long-term sample preparation and relatively laborious analysis. Thus, several days pass from sample acquisition to analytical results. The value of a method that would provide immediate results is obvious. In particular, it became clear during our contacts with renal physicians that a rapid, non-invasive method to determine total body water in patients suffering from end-stage renal failure would have great value if it could be used directly in the clinical environment. A potential approach to this was presented to us during our development of the SIFT-MS trace gas analytical techniques for the determination of trace gas metabolites in breath for clinical diagnosis and therapeutic monitoring (see the chapter by Smith and Španěl[4] on page 3 of this book). When injecting hydronium ions, H_3O^+ (mass-to-charge ratio, m/z, value of 19), into helium carrier gas containing water vapour, we observed that ions of m/z values of 20 and 21 were present. These are undoubtedly the isotopomers (H_2DO^+ and $H_3{}^{17}O^+$) and $H_3{}^{18}O^+$ respectively. Further to these, the hydrated hydronium cluster ions at m/z values of 35, 36 and 37; 55, 56 and 57; and 73, 74 and 75; were formed. It is these observations that led us to the development of flowing afterglow mass spectrometry, FA-MS,[5] a new analytical approach that offers a route to on-line, real-time deuterium abundance measurements in water vapour in breath and above aqueous liquids, including urine and serum. This method involves the production and flow of thermalised hydrated hydronium cluster ions in inert helium or argon carrier gas along a flow tube following the introduction of a humid air sample. These ions react in multiple collisions with water molecules, their isotopic compositions reach equilibrium and the relative magnitudes of their isotopomers are measured by a mass spectrometer located downstream. Such measurements provide the required abundance of deuterium in the air/water vapour sample.

2. The FA-MS Method

2.1. *FA-MS Instrumentation*

A weak microwave discharge is created in helium or argon carrier gas flowing through a narrow glass tube connected to a stainless steel flow tube. Thus, flowing afterglow plasma is formed in the steel flow tube (see Fig. 1). The gas phase ion chemistry initiated by He^+ or Ar^+ ions reacting with trace amounts of H_2O molecules results in the formation of H_3O^+ ions in the carrier gas. (Note that here H here tacitly assumes the presence of both isotopes ${}^1H$ and ${}^2H$). The sample of air/water vapour mixture to be analyzed is introduced at a known flow rate into the carrier gas and its composite water molecules react with the H_3O^+ ions to form the $H_3O^+(H_2O)^+_{1,2,3}$ cluster ions and their analogous ${}^2H$, ${}^{17}O$ and ${}^{18}O$ isotopic variants, as referred to above. The mixture of ions are sampled from the flowing swarm via a pinhole orifice (about 0.3 mm diameter) located at the downstream end of the flow tube and they are mass analyzed by a differentially pumped quadrupole mass spectrometer (pressure less than 10^{-4} Torr) with a single channel multiplier ion counting detector. A typical mass spectrum obtained using the FA-MS method is shown in Fig. 2a. Clearly, there is information in these mass spectra on the isotopic composition of the water present in the carrier gas. Specifically, the deuterium content of a water vapour sample introduced into the helium carrier gas can be determined from such spectra if the ^{17}O and ^{18}O content of the ions is known. To properly understand how the analysis is achieved, we need to distinguish between the isotopic composition of the following three "phases": the liquid water sample (designated by the subscript "liq"), the water vapour transferred from an aqueous sample headspace into the helium carrier gas (designated by the subscript "vap") and the $H_3O^+(H_2O)_{0,1,2,3}$ ions and their isotopomers that comprise the ion swarm created in the carrier gas (designated by the subscript "ion").

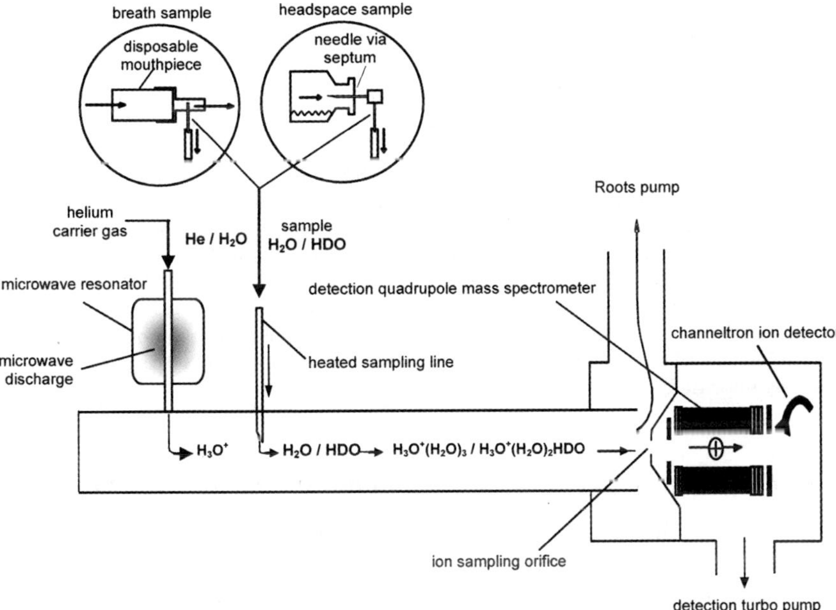

Fig. 1. A schematic of the FA-MS instrumental configuration. The reagent ions are created in the carrier gas by a microwave discharge, thus producing a weak flowing afterglow along the flow tube. Direct samplings of breath and liquid headspace are achieved as shown in the insets.

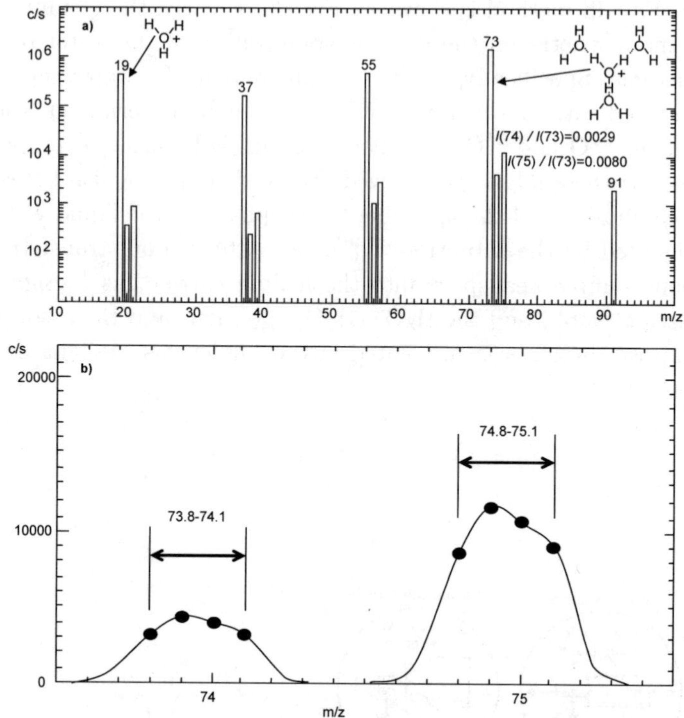

Fig. 2.   A spectrum obtained by FA-MS plotted on a semi-logarithmic scale as counts per second (c/s) versus mass to charge ratio (m/z). **a)** A spectral scan over the m/z range 10 to 100 when H_3O^+ ions ($m/z = 19$) are produced in the carrier gas upstream and water vapour is added downstream. Note the production of the three hydrates $H_3O^+(H_2O)_{1,2,3}$ at m/z values 37, 55 and 73 and the appearance of their D, ^{17}O, and ^{18}O isotopomers. **b)** A spectral scan from m/z 73.5 to 75.5 for tap water. Note the clear separation of the mass peaks at m/z 74 and 75. Mean count rates of the ions were obtained for each m/z value by recording and averaging the count rates at four mass settings around each peak, as indicated.[9]

2.2. *Partition of HDO Between Liquid Water and Its Vapour*

In water containing a low abundance of deuterium almost all the deuterium is contained in ^1HDO molecules. Therefore, in order to determine the deuterium isotope abundance ratio in a liquid water sample, $R_{1\text{liq}} = D/(^1H + D)$, by analysing its vapour, the partition of ^1HDO between the liquid and vapour phases needs to be addressed. A difference arises because ^1HDO has a lower saturated vapour pressure than ^1H_2O at sub-boiling temperatures. The ratio $K_1 = R_{1\text{vap}}/R_{1\text{liq}}$ of the deuterium abundance in the headspace vapour, $R_{1\mathrm{vap}}$, to that in liquid, $R_{1\mathrm{liq}}$, has been accurately determined for a range of temperatures.[6-8] Also, the isotope abundance ratios of ^{17}O in the water vapour, $R_{2\mathrm{vap}} = {}^{17}O/({}^{16}O+{}^{17}O+{}^{18}O)$, and that of ^{18}O, $R_{3\mathrm{vap}} = {}^{18}O/({}^{16}O+{}^{17}O+{}^{18}O)$, are proportional to their corresponding abundances in the liquid, $R_{2\mathrm{liq}}$ and $R_{3\mathrm{liq}}$, and their partition coefficients $K_2 = R_{2\mathrm{vap}}/R_{2\mathrm{liq}}$ and $K_3 = R_{3\mathrm{vap}}/R_{3\mathrm{liq}}$ that are accurately known.[6-8]

2.3. *Direct Sampling of Breath*

In FA-MS, air or breath is sampled directly into the flow tube via a heated, calibrated capillary tube coupled to the flow tube via heated stainless steel tubing. The tip of the capillary extends into a stainless steel coupling positioned perpendicularly to the capillary axis (Fig. 1). Exhaled breath is introduced into the coupling via a standard disposable cardboard mouthpiece (about 15 mm diameter). This arrangement is patient friendly, offering a suitable resistance to the flow of breath such that a steady exhalation can be made over a few seconds. The exhaled breath totally displaces the ambient air from the entrance to the sampling capillary and so a sample of breath enters the capillary and immediately expands into the coupling tubing and enters the flow tube/carrier gas (pressure of about 1 Torr).[9] The entrance to the capillary is again exposed to the ambient air upon oral inhalation. By suitable choice of the dimensions of the calibrated capillary, the flow rate of the sampled air/breath is sufficient to establish a concentration of H_2O molecules in the carrier gas that converts the majority of the ions in the ion swarm into the $H_3O^+(H_2O)_3$, *i.e.* $H_9O_4^+$ ions, at m/z 73 and its isotopomers at 74 and 75. The carrier gas is flowing rapidly, the flow time through the flow tube being typically 3 milliseconds, and so the net response time of a FA-MS instrument is about 20 ms. A typical breath exhalation is about 5 s, so time profiles of the individual ion signals can be defined. Typical time profiles of the $m/z - 74$ and 75 ions are shown in Fig. 3a for three breath exhalation/inhalation cycles. It is imperative to heat the capillary and the coupling lines to minimise the condensation of water, and thus to eliminate "memory" effects.

2.4. *Sampling Liquid Headspace*

FA-MS can be used very effectively to accurately determine deuterium (HDO) in the headspace above water and aqueous media such as urine, dialysate or serum. In a typical analysis, about 10 mL of fluid is placed in

200 mL glass bottle sealed with a septum-sealed. The bottle is then placed in a temperature controlled water bath and the headspace is allowed to develop for about 10 min. A sampling needle connected directly to the input line of the FA-MS instrument (Fig. 1) then punctures the septum and headspace vapour is drawn into the carrier gas by the existing pressure differential (initially from atmosphere down to the flow tube pressure). Again, the sampling lines are held at about 100 °C to inhibit the condensation of water vapour and other condensable vapours.

2.5. *Ion Molecule Reactions; Equilibrium Between Ions and Water Vapour Molecules in the Gas Phase*

To determine the deuterium abundance using FA-MS, it is essential to understand the ion chemistry that establishes the distributions between the isotopomers of the cluster ions. The following three-body association reactions occur to form these cluster ions:

$$^{1,2}H_3O^+ + {}^{1,2}H_2O + M \rightarrow {}^{1,2}H_5O_2^+ + M \tag{1a}$$

$$^{1,2}H_5O_2^+ + {}^{1,2}H_2O + M \rightarrow {}^{1,2}H_7O_3^+ + M \tag{1b}$$

$$^{1,2}H_7O_3^+ + {}^{1,2}H_2O + M \rightarrow {}^{1,2}H_9O_4^+ + M \tag{1c}$$

Here, M is a carrier gas atom, either He or Ar. As result of this sequence, $^{1,2}H_3O^+({}^{1,2}H_2O)_3$ ions become the dominant ionic species in the carrier gas at sufficiently large water molecule concentrations, since further association to produce $H_{11}O_5^+$ ions is inhibited due to the lower stability of this larger cluster ion. Thus, $^{1,2}H_3O^+({}^{1,2}H_2O)_3$ cluster ions reach isotopic equilibrium with water vapour molecules. The following forward and backward reactions establish the equilibrium:

$$^{1}H_9O_4^+ + {}^{1}HDO \rightleftharpoons {}^{1}H_8DO_4^+ + {}^{1}H_2O. \tag{2}$$

These reactions proceed via isotope exchange and ligand switching reactions, involving efficient mixing of H and D atoms within the intermediate reaction complex ion $(H_{10}DO_5^+)^*$ (see Ref 10). The enthalpy change, ΔH, in reaction (2) is close to zero, the translational and rotational entropy changes are also relatively small and thus the entropy change, ΔS, is entirely described by statistical factors.[8] Therefore, when equilibrium is established in reactions (2), the deuterium abundance ratio in the $H_3O^+(H_2O)_3$ cluster ion swarm, $R_{1\text{ion}}$, will be equal to that in the water vapour, $R_{1\text{vap}}$. Note that isotope exchange and ligand switching reactions analogous to reaction (2) also ensure that the abundances of the ^{17}O and ^{18}O isotopes is the same in the swarm of ions as it is in the sample water vapour molecules. This chemistry has been experimentally validated under both SIFT-MS[8] and FA-MS[11] conditions using standard deuterium enriched water. The speed of approach to equilibrium in these reactive systems depends on the number density of water molecules in the carrier gas. Thus, for FA-MS deuterium analyses the number density of water molecules in the carrier gas should be more than 10^{13} cm^{-3}, in order to establish equilibrium in about a millisecond.[8]

2.6. *Ion Signals and Isotopomer Overlap*

The final important issue to be addressed is the relationship of $R_{1\text{vap}}$ to the observed ion signals. The equilibrium distribution of the various isotopomer ions (and hence their count rates at the detector; see Fig. 2) can be expressed using the binomial distribution.[1] Thus, it is seen[8] that the ratio of ion signals counted at mass to charge ratios, m/z, 74 and 73, *i.e.* $I(74)$ and $I(73)$ is:

$$\frac{I(74)}{I(73)} = \frac{[\mathrm{H_8D^{16}O_4^+}]}{[\mathrm{H_9{}^{16}O_4^+}]} + \frac{[\mathrm{H_9{}^{17}O_4^+}]}{[\mathrm{H_9{}^{16}O_4^+}]} = \frac{9R_{1\text{vap}}}{1 - R_{1\text{vap}}} + \frac{4R_{2\text{vap}}}{1 - R_{2\text{vap}}}. \tag{3}$$

Note that the deuterium abundance in these cluster ions is amplified by a factor of about 9 relative to water vapour molecules and that the abundance of ^{17}O is amplified about four times.

Using this FA-MS arrangement,[9] very large count rates at m/z of 73, $I(73)$ are seen, typically several millions per second. Such large count rates cannot be counted sufficiently accurately by a conventional counting system.[12] Instead, $I(74)$ and $I(75)$ are used (see Fig. 2b) to determine the deuterium content of the water vapour sample (*e.g.* in breath). The ion at $m/z = 75$ (^{18}O isotopomer of the $\mathrm{H_9O_4^+}$) will have a signal level given by:

$$\frac{I(75)}{I(73)} = \frac{[\mathrm{H_9{}^{16}O_3{}^{17}O^+}]}{[\mathrm{H_9{}^{16}O_4^+}]} = \frac{4R_{3\text{vap}}}{1 - R_{3\text{vap}}}. \tag{4}$$

Note that it has been shown[8,9] that when $R_1 < 10^{-3}$ the contribution of doubly deuterated $\mathrm{H_7D_2O_4^+}$ ions to $I(75)$ is negligible (less than 3×10^{-5} representing less than 0.15 % of a typical R_3 value of 0.02). Thus, from an accurate measurement of the ion count rate ratio, $Q = I(74)/I(75)$, $R_{1\text{vap}}$, is determined by combining Eqs. (3) and (4) and considering all $R_{1\text{vap}}$, $R_{2\text{vap}}$, $R_{3\text{vap}}$ are much less than unity. Then:

$$R_{1\text{vap}} = \tfrac{4}{9}(Q\,R_{3\text{vap}} - R_{2\text{vap}}). \tag{5}$$

The Q value obtained for normal water is typically 0.35. Thus, the actual measurements involve ion count rates at m/z of 74 and 75 that are not very different (in this case by a factor of 3; see Fig. 2b), which is inherently more accurate than attempting to measure count rates that are vastly different. When the signals of both m/z 74 and 75 ions are within the range 10,000 to 30,000 counts per second, optimum accuracy and precision can be achieved. In practice, it is also important to ensure that the abundance sensitivity of the analytical mass spectrometer (separation between masses) is better than 10^{-5} and mass discrimination between the m/z 74 and 75 ions is less than 0.1 %.[5]

In the commercially available instrumentation (Trans Spectra Limited, UK) all numerical analysis using equations (5) and the appropriate K_1 partition coefficient are performed on-line by data acquisition software, thus providing an instantaneous readout of the Q, $R_{1\text{vap}}$ and $R_{1\text{liq}}$ values.

2.7. *Accuracy and Precision*

The accuracy of the measured $R_{1\text{vap}}$ also depends on the accuracy of the adopted values of $R_{2\text{vap}}$ and $R_{3\text{vap}}$. Unless the accurate local water values of the last two parameters are available, the generic natural abundances of $R_{2\text{liq}} = 0.000379$ and $R_{3\text{liq}} = 0.002006$ can be used.[13,14] When breath is analysed for deuterium, values of K_1 corresponding to the alveolar interface temperatures must be used, which can range from 34 to 37 °C.[15] This spread in temperature results in a variation of K_1 that is less than 0.3 %.[5]

The measurement precision is dominated by the Poisson distribution of the total numbers of ions counted within the sampling time interval. The standard error in R_1 calculated using equation (5) is thus:

$$\Delta R_1 = \tfrac{4}{9} R_3 \left(\frac{\sqrt{N(74)}}{N(74)} + \frac{\sqrt{N(75)}}{N(75)} \right). \tag{6}$$

In this case, $N(74)$ and $N(75)$ represent the *total* numbers of ions counted at $m/z = 74$ and 75 *not* the ion count rates as used previously. Equation (6) can be routinely evaluated on-line providing an immediate estimate of the measurement precision. Validation of the SIFT-MS and FA-MS methods for deuterium analyses, carried out using standard mixtures, demonstrates that both accuracy and precision (reproducibility) are typically 1 % for headspace sampling when using the experimental procedure described above.[8,11] A precision better than 1 % can be achieved for breath deuterium analysis when the average value for three consecutive exhalations is taken (see Section 2.3).

3. Examples of Clinically Relevant FA-MS Studies

3.1. *Measurements of Total Body Water*

Total body water (TBW)[16] is a fundamental component of body composition, which is influenced by many physiological and patho-physiological states. These conditions include oedematous conditions, such as cirrhosis and the nephrotic syndrome.[17,18] In renal failure, soluble uraemic toxins are distributed in the TBW volume and so knowledge of the TBW is critical in determining the dialysis dose.[19] Therefore, there are a number of situations in which a precise but simple and rapid measurement of TBW would be beneficial. Bioimpedance analysis (BIA) is currently used for rapid assessments of body fluid status,[20] but the conversion of tissue reactance and resistance into absolute measures of body water,[21] particularly in diseased states, is difficult, since formulae derived from the normal (healthy) population may not apply.[22] The standard methods used to measure TBW, which employ isotopic dilution, provide well-validated results, but sample analysis is expensive and time-consuming.[23] Indeed, multiple sample acquisition, such as is required to analyse deuterium dispersal kinetics (see below), is not practical by blood sampling. Consequently, isotopic methods to measure TBW have remained research tools, with clinicians resorting to equations (*e.g.* the formula by Watson *et al.*[24]) derived from normal population data. Whilst this approach works reasonably well for individuals with close to normal body composition, this cannot be said for malnourished, obese or fluid-loaded patients. For such cases, FA-MS can be used as a rapid, non-invasive method to determine the deuterium abundance in breath water, which when combined with conventional oral loading of D_2O may be used to determine total body water.[14,16] Additionally, using this approach, the dispersal kinetics of deuterium throughout the body can be studied.[16]

3.1.1. *Protocol for TBW measurement*

A baseline deuterium abundance in the breath of the subject should first be obtained by direct breath sampling (see Section 2.1). Several consecutive exhalations (typically three) should be recorded by the FA-MS instrument. The subjects then drink an accurately weighted amount of 99.9 % pure D_2O in 200 mL of regular drinking water. The dose of D_2O should be approximately 0.3 g/kg body weight. Such a dose is somewhat higher than that conventionally used in measuring TBW by isotope ratio mass spectrometry.[23] This higher dose is desirable to ensure that accurate measurements can be obtained from single breath exhalations. It is, however, well within safe limits.[25] Following the dose, the subjects immediately drink an additional 200 mL of water, in order to minimise the deuterium in the mouth mucosa, saliva and gullet. When the dispersal kinetics of HDO following ingestions is to be studied, breath samples are analysed by FA-MS at approximately 3 minute intervals until equilibration in the breath deuterium is reached (usually within 2 hours; see Fig. 3b). When just the TBW is required, it is sufficient to analyse the breath deuterium abundance 2 hours after ingestion.[23,26]

3.1.2. *Kinetics of dispersal of HDO in the body*

Typical breath time profiles of the isotopic variant hydrated ions (m/z values of 74 and 75) before the oral D_2O ingestion are shown in Fig. 3a. Exhalations are easily identified by the rapid increases in the count rates of the ions as the water vapour in the helium carrier gas increases, followed by a relatively constant level during the alveolar portion of the breath exhalation. The abundance of deuterium in breath can be calculated for each exhalation as it is shown in Figure 3a.

A typical time variation of breath deuterium abundance during the two hours following ingestion of isotopically labelled water (HDO) is shown in Fig. 3b. Three phases can be seen in these data: an immediate and short increased level due to deuterium still present within the oral cavity: a rise to a second peak, which is usually reached 20 to 50 minutes following ingestion, due to the passage of HDO from the stomach and upper intestine into the blood stream: finally, decay towards an equilibrium value as the HDO disperses into the TBW. It is possible, therefore, using this FA-MS method, to track the equilibration of deuterium between three distinct body compartments, the gastro-intestinal tract, the blood compartment and the TBW. A number of factors will determine the rates at which HDO will equilibrate in each case, including the rate of gastric emptying, the blood volume and the delivery of HDO to the tissues. The transport of HDO can be modelled mathematically by considering diffusion (permeation) through the idealised interfaces between these model body compartments.[16] Finally, it should be noted that water in ingested food and drink and even in inhaled humid air will dilute the HDO in the TBW. For one subject with a TBW of 50 litres, we observed a slow decay of the residual HDO in the body over 5 days and estimated an assumed exponential time constant of about 12 days, corresponding to a total water intake of about 3 litres per day.

The difference ΔR_{1liq} (see Fig. 3b) between the baseline deuterium abundance prior to ingestion and the asymptotic level of the final phase can be used to calculate the total body water (TBW) volume:

$$\text{TBW} = \frac{V(\text{D}_2\text{O})}{\Delta R_{1\text{liq}}}. \tag{7}$$

Here, $V(\text{D}_2\text{O})$ is the volume of the ingested D_2O. Note that $1\ \text{cm}^3$ of D_2O is 0.05535 mol whilst $1\ \text{cm}^3$ of H_2O is 0.05555 mol. Thus, the simple equation (6) is valid within $0.36\,\%$ if the difference between the molar volumes of H_2O and D_2O is ignored.

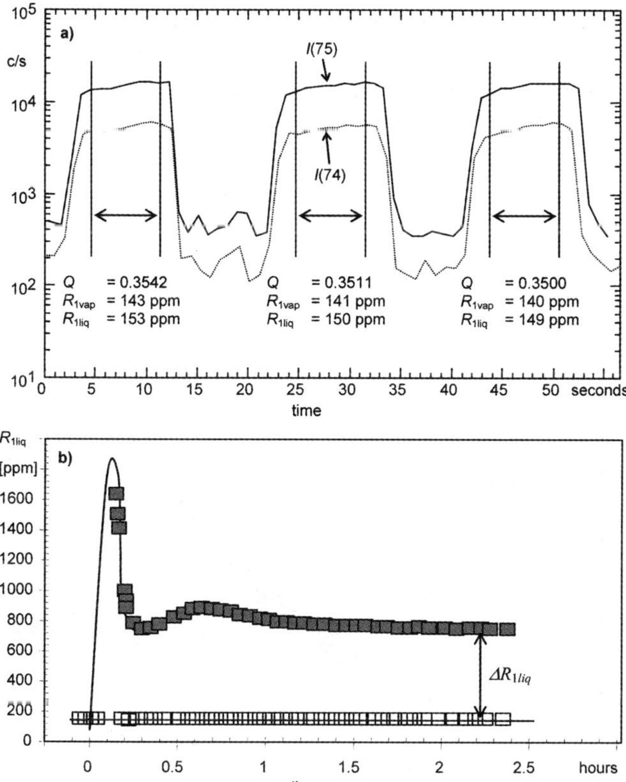

Fig. 3. **a)** Mean values of the FA-MS ion count rates (c/s, obtained at the four mass settings as described in the caption to Fig. 2) for m/z values of 74 and 75, as three breath exhalations are directly sampled. The mean values of the ion count rate ratios, Q, over the alveolar breath intervals indicated are used to calculate the values of $R_{1\text{vap}}$ (and then $R_{1\text{liq}}$), the last values being given in ppm for each exhalation (data from Ref. 9). **b)** An example of a typical long time variation of $R_{1\text{liq}}$ determined for breath HDO following oral ingestion of 18.7 g of D_2O by a volunteer (filled squares). The open squares are simultaneous measurements for a control who has not ingested D_2O (data from Ref. 9). The TBW is obtained from the value of $\Delta R_{1\text{liq}}$ as described in the text.

3.1.3. *Comparison of FA-MS with population equations and BIA*

The TBW values obtained using our FA-MS method for 24 healthy subjects have been compared with the results obtained using parallel multifrequency bioimpedance analyses (BIA) and the available population-based regression equations.[26] The TBW values obtained by the isotope dilution method using FA-MS were within 2% of those published for age-matched controls. TBW determined by FA-MS and those estimated by BIA correlated well, ($r = 0.97$, $P < 0.001$), although BIA tended to underestimate TBW in smaller female subjects (see Fig. 4). When these FA-MS data were compared to the values derived using the older regression equations of Watson *et al.*[24] and the more recent regression equations of Chumlea *et al.*,[27] better agreement was observed with the more recent equations, especially in male subjects.[26]

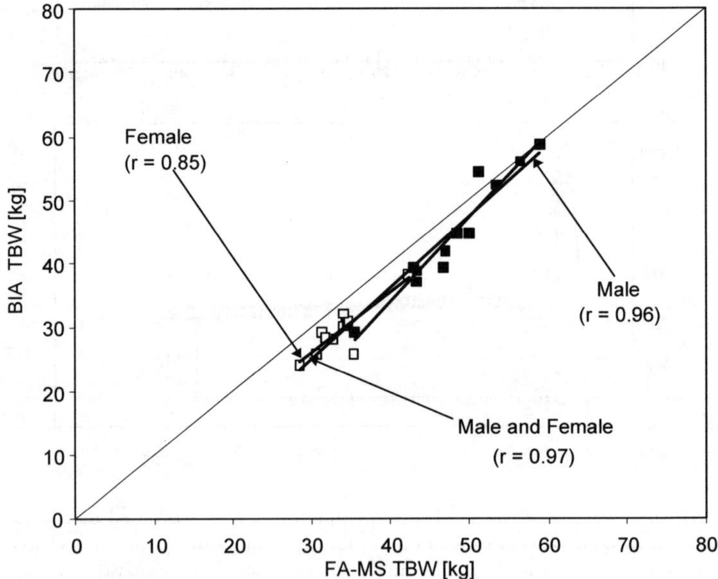

Fig. 4.   Correlation of the bioimpedance analysis, BIA, estimates of total body water, TBW, with the FA-MS measurements of TBW for 12 male and 12 female healthy volunteers (data from Ref. 26). The values of correlation coefficients are given in brackets as *r*.

3.2. *Measurements of Water Transport Across the Peritoneal Membrane*

We have recently begun to study the transport properties of the peritoneal membrane of patients being treated by continuous ambulatory peritoneal dialysis (CAPD) in collaboration with our renal physician colleague Simon Davies. Thus we have used deuterium labelling in combination with FA-MS headspace analyses to characterise the transport properties of the membrane for water (see papers by Asghar *et al.*[28,29]). In CAPD treatment, the peritoneal cavity of the patient is loaded with a solution of the dialysing liquid (dialysate),[30] which causes the flow of water and unwanted toxins from the blood to the dialysate. To study water flow across the membrane using deuterium labelling, either D_2O can be administered orally or the dialysate can be "spiked" with D_2O. The breath analysis is performed in the usual way, as described above. The dialysate analysis is performed by sampling a few millilitres of the dialysate, the headspace of which was then analysed by FA-MS, as indicated previously in Section 2.4. Typical data are shown in Fig. 5, the form of the curves being explained in the caption.

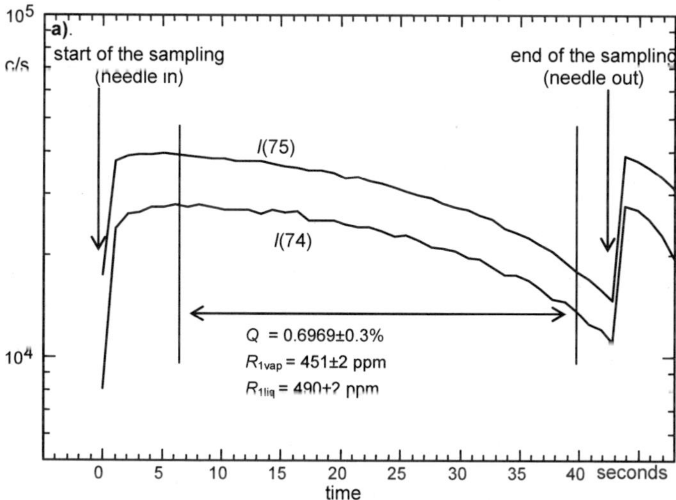

Fig. 5.   Mean values of FA-MS ion count rates at $m/z = 74$ and 75, accumulated as the headspace from a sealed bottle containing dialysate fluid at 37 °C flows into the carrier gas. The decrease with time of the count rates for each ion is due to the decrease in the water vapour/air pressure in the sealed bottle during sampling. The mean ion count rate ratio, Q, is used to calculate R_{1vap} (and then R_{1liq})

Figure 6a shows the increase with time of the HDO abundance in dialysate fluid in the peritoneal cavity following a regular dialysate exchange by a CAPD patient who four hours previously had orally ingested a small quantity of D_2O.[28,29] Note the well-defined increase of the deuterium content from which the transport rate of water across the membrane can be accurately determined. Conclusions can then be drawn concerning the mechanisms of transport of water through the system of pores that connect the capillary blood vessels with the peritoneal membrane.[29] In the comple-

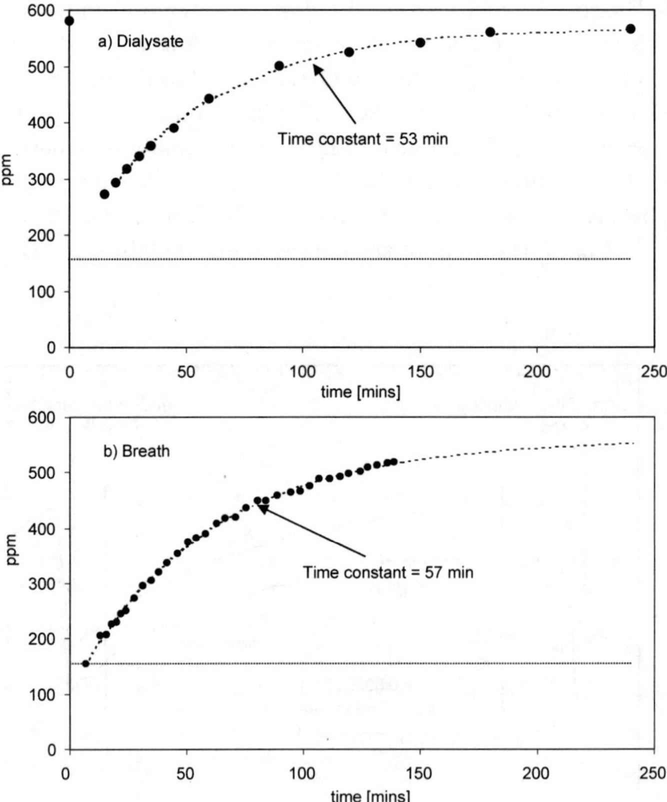

Fig. 6.   **a)** Time profile of R_{1liq} (in ppm) for dialysate samples taken during a CAPD (continuous ambulatory peritoneal dialysis) session using 1.36 % physioneal dialysate following a dialysate exchange at time $= 0$. The patient (weight $= 77.4$ kg) ingested 19.76 g of D_2O four hours prior to time $= 0$. **b)** Time profile of $R1liq$ for breath samples (in ppm) taken during a CAPD session using 1.36 % physioneal dialysate liquid labelled with 20.11 g D_2O for the same patient several month later. The baseline deuterium abundances are indicated by the horizontal dotted lines.

mentary experiment, in which the dialysate water is labelled with a known quantity of D_2O, the breath HDO is monitored with time following the dialysate exchange. The data obtained for the same patient are shown in Fig. 6b. Note the many more sampling points that can be obtained using breath analysis, which can be carried out every minute or so. This very well defines the breath/blood increase of deuterium with time and provides even more accurate transport rates. With such data the renal physician is assisted in determining the appropriate dialysis regime for the particular CAPD patient.

4. Some Concluding Remarks

The novel FA-MS technique uniquely provides on-line, real time analysis of the deuterium abundance in the water vapour of single exhalations of breath. It is painless and non-invasive. Currently, instrumentation is available ("FA-MS system 50" isotope flow tube analyser developed by Trans Spectra Limited, UK) that can conveniently be used in the clinical environment. It can also be used to provide real time analyses of the deuterium content of the headspace of aqueous liquids, including blood, urine and dialysate fluid, seriously reducing the analysis time compared to conventional methods. Deuterium abundances by FA-MS can currently be performed to an accuracy and precision of typical 1 %. Immediate applications that we have explored in clinical practice are the rapid measurement of total body water, studies of water dispersal kinetics in the body and the monitoring of water transport across the peritoneal membrane in patients being treated with peritoneal dialysis. We plan to use FA-MS to measure water loss during haemodialysis and the total body water of patients in intensive care units.

Acknowledgements

We are pleased to recognise the important contributions of our colleague Professor Simon Davies to the application of FA-MS to renal and body composition research.

References

1. Karasek F, Clement R. *Basic gas chromatography–mass spectrometry*. Amsterdam: Elsevier, 1988.
2. Begley I, Scrimgeour C. High-precision delta ^{2}H and delta ^{18}O measurement for water and volatile organic compounds by continuous-flow pyrolysis isotope ratio mass spectrometry. *Anal Chem* 1997; **69**: 1530–1535.

3. Horita J, Kendall C. Stable isotope analysis of water and aqueous solutions by conventional dual-inlet mass spectrometry. In: de Groot P ed. *Handbook of Stable Isotope Analytical Techniques* (Volume I), Amsterdam: Elsevier, 2004.

4. Smith D, Španěl P. Selected ion flow tube mass spectrometry, SIFT-MS, for on-line trace gas analysis of breath. In: Amann A, Smith D, eds. *Breath Analysis for Clinical Diagnosis and Therapeutic Monitoring,* Singapore: World Scientific, 2005.

5. Španěl P, Smith D. Selected Ion Flow Tube Mass Spectrometry (SIFT-MS) and Flowing Afterglow Mass Spectrometry (FA-MS) for the Determination of the Deuterium Abundance in Water Vapour. In: de Groot P ed. *Handbook of Stable Isotope Analytical Techniques* (Volume I), Amsterdam: Elsevier, 2004.

6. van Hook W. Vapor pressure isotope effect in aqueous systems. III. The Vapor pressure of HOD (-60 to 200 $^\circ$C). *J Phys Chem* 1972; **76**: 3040–3043.

7. Jancso G, van Hook W. Condensed Phase Isotope Effects. *Chem Rev* 1974; **74**: 689–710.

8. Španěl P, Smith D. Selected ion flow tube mass spectrometry analyses of stable isotopes in water: Isotopic composition of H_3O^+ and $H_3O^+(H_2O)_3$ ions in exchange reactions with water vapor. *J Am Soc Mass Spectrom* 2000; **11**: 866–875.

9. Smith D, Španěl P. On-line determination of the deuterium abundance in breath water vapour by flowing afterglow mass spectrometry, FA-MS, with applications to measurements of total body water. *Rapid Comm Mass Spectrom* 2001; **15**: 25–32.

10. Adams N, Smith D, Henchman M. Isotope exchange in the reactions $H_3O^+ + D_2O$, $NH_4^+ + ND_3$, $CH_5^+ + CD_4$ and their mirror isotope reactions at thermal energies. *Int J Mass Spectrom Ion Phys* 1982; **42**: 11–23.

11. Španěl P, Smith D. Accuracy and precision of flowing afterglow mass spectrometry for the determination of the deuterium abundance in the headspace of aqueous liquids and exhaled breath water. *Rapid Comm Mass Spectrom* 2001; **15**: 867–872.

12. Fahey A. Measurements of dead time and characterization of ion counting systems for mass spectrometry. *Rev Sci Instruments* 1998; **69**: 1282–1288.

13. Li W, Ni B, Jin D, Zhang T. Measurement of the absolute abundance of ^{17}O in VSMOW. *Chinese Sci Bulletin* 1988; **33**: 1610–1613.

14. Baertschi P. Absolute ^{18}O content of standard mean ocean water. *Earth Planetary Sci Lett* 1976; **31**: 341–351.

15. Wilson P, Freeman C, McEwan M, Milligan D, Allardyce R, Shaw G. Alcohol in breath and blood: a selected ion flow tube mass spectrometric study. *Rapid Comm Mass Spectrom* 2001; **15**: 413–417.

16. Davies S, Španěl P, Smith D. Rapid measurement of deuterium content of breath following oral ingestion to determine body water. *Physiol Meas* 2001; **22**: 651–659.

17. Crawford DH, Shepherd RW, Halliday JW, Cooksley GW, Golding SD, Cheng WS, Powell LW. Body composition in nonalcoholic cirrhosis: the effect

of disease etiology and severity on nutritional compartments. *Gastroenterology* 1994; **106**: 1611–1617.

18. Abraham WT, Schrier RW. Edematous disorders: pathophysiology of renal sodium and water retention and treatment with diuretics. *Curr Opin Nephrol Hypertens* 1993; **2**: 798–805.

19. Woodrow G, Oldroyd B, Turney JH, Davies PS, Day JM, Smith MA. Measurement of total body water and urea kinetic modelling in peritoneal dialysis. *Clin Nephrol* 1997; **47**: 52–57.

20. Matthie J, Zarowitz B, De Lorenzo A, Andreoli A, Katzarski K, Pan G, Withers P. Analytic assessment of the various bioimpedance methods used to estimate body water. *J Appl Physiol* 1998; **84**: 1801–1816.

21. Piccoli A, Pillon L, Favaro E. Asymmetry of the total body water prediction bias using the impedance index. *Nutrition* 1997; **13**: 438–441.

22. Cooper BA, Aslani A, Ryan M, Zhu FY, Ibels LS, Allen BJ, Pollock CA. Comparing different methods of assessing body composition in end-stage renal failure. *Kidney Int* 2000; **58**: 408–416.

23. Schoeller DA, van Santen E, Peterson DW, Dietz W, Jaspan J, Klein PD. Total body water measurement in humans with ^{18}O and ^{2}H labeled water. *Am J Clin Nutr* 1980; **33**: 2686–2693.

24. Watson PE, Watson ID, Batt RD. Total body water volumes for adult males and females estimated from simple anthropometric measurements. *Am J Clin Nutr* 1980; **33**: 27–39.

25. Jones PJ, Leatherdale ST. Stable isotopes in clinical research: safety reaffirmed. *Clin Sci (Lond)* 1991; **80**: 277–280.

26. Smith D, Engel B, Diskin AM, Španěl P, Davies SJ. Comparative measurements of total body water in healthy volunteers by online breath deuterium measurement and other near-subject methods. *Am J Clin Nutr* 2002; **76**: 1295–1301.

27. Chumlea WC, Guo SS, Zeller CM, Reo NV, Baumgartner RN, Garry PJ, Wang J, Pierson RN, Jr., Heymsfield SB, Siervogel RM. Total body water reference values and prediction equations for adults. *Kidney Int* 2001; **59**: 2250–2258.

28. Asghar RB, Diskin AM, Španěl P, Smith D, Davies SJ. Measuring transport of water across the peritoneal membrane. *Kidney Int* 2003; **64**: 1911–1915.

29. Asghar R, Diskin A, Španěl P, Smith D, Davies S. Influence of convection on the diffusive transport and sieving of water and small solutes across the peritoneal membrane. *J Am Soc Nephrol* 2005; 16: 437–443.

30. Flessner MF. The peritoneal dialysis system: importance of each component. *Perit Dial Int* 1997; **17** Suppl 2: S91–97.

^{13}C BREATH TESTS: TRANSITION FROM RESEARCH TO CLINICAL PRACTICE

A. S. MODAK

Cambridge Isotope Laboratories Inc.,
50 Frontage Road, Andover, MA 01810, USA

1. Introduction

Stable isotope ^{13}C labeled compounds have been widely used as diagnostic probes in research laboratories for over 30 years. In 1973, ^{13}C-glucose was the substrate in the first report on the use of a naturally occurring ^{13}C compound for a metabolic study in humans.[1] Prior to this report, similar investigations were conducted using the radioactive isotope ^{14}C instead of the stable isotope ^{13}C. Subsequent to the wide availability of low cost ^{13}C-substrates and the development of nondispersive isotope selective IR spectrometry (NDIRS), research groups from around the world have increasingly used these tracers in nutritional, medicinal, and veterinary research. These diagnostic ^{13}C stable isotope probes are now being expanded in their scope, to provide precise evaluations of the presence or absence of etiologically significant changes in metabolism due to a specific disease or the lack of a specific enzyme. This concept exploits the use of the ^{13}C-label that is incorporated at the appropriate site into a selected substrate specifically designed for the targeted enzyme (foreign or inherent) in a discrete metabolic pathway. The enzyme-substrate interaction, results in the release of ^{13}CO$_2$ in the expired breath. The subsequent quantification of ^{13}CO$_2$ allows for the indirect determination of pharmacokinetics and the evaluation of enzyme activity. A number of ^{13}C-substrates have been used for monitoring a certain physiological function or evaluating enzyme activity as shown in Table 1.

To date only three breath tests have been approved in the U.S. by the FDA and have made the transition to clinical practice, only one with a ^{13}C-substrate:

Table 1. ^{13}C-tracer probes and their diagnostic metabolic implications

Bacterial Overgrowth: D-sorbitol (1-^{13}C) D-xylose (1,2-^{13}C$_2$) **Identifying Hypercapnia:** sodium bicarbonate (^{13}C) **Ulcer and *H. pylori* Infection:** urea (^{13}C) (FDA-approved breath test)	**Liver Function:** aminopyrine (N,N-dimethyl-^{13}C) caffeine (3-methyl-^{13}C) erythromycin (N,N-dimethyl-^{14}C$_2$) D-fructose (1-^{13}C) D-galactose (1-^{13}C) D-glucose (1-^{13}C) D-ketoisocaproic acid (1-^{13}C), sodium salt	L-leucine (1-^{13}C) L-leucine (1,2-^{13}C$_2$) L-methionine (1-^{13}C) methacetin (methoxy-^{13}C) L-phenylalanine (1-^{13}C) D-sorbitol (1-^{13}C) sodium propionate (1-^{13}C)
Gastric Emptying: octanoic acid (1-^{13}C) sodium acetate (1-^{13}C) sodium octanoate (1-^{13}C) lactose-ureide (^{13}C) breath test glycine (1-^{13}C)	**Fat Malabsorption and Pancreatic Function:** mixed triglyceride (^{13}C) trioctanoin (1,1,1-^{13}C$_3$) triolein (1,1,1-^{13}C$_3$) tripalmitin (1,1,1-^{13}C$_3$) D-fructose (1-^{13}C) hiolein (1-^{13}C)	**DPD Enzyme Deficiency:** uracil (2-^{13}C) **Oro-Caecal Transit Time:** lactose-ureide (^{13}C) **Nutritional studies:** L-leucine (1-^{13}C)

1. ^{13}C-Urea breath test for the detection of *H. pylori*[2]
2. NO breath test for monitoring asthma[3]
3. Alkanes breath test for heart transplant rejection[4]

The feasibility of administering an oral dose of a ^{13}C-substrate and procuring metabolic or diagnostic information from its metabolism and conversion to $^{13}CO_2$ is attractive due to its noninvasive nature. The salient features of the ^{13}C-breath test are that they are noninvasive, non-radioactive, safe, simple, and effective. Breath tests have the potential to be useful screening methods that can be applied at the point of care (*e.g.*, hospitals and physicians' offices) and do not require patients to wait for hours or days for results. The noninvasive method is especially attractive for infants, children, pregnant and lactating women, seniors in poor health and subjects averse to the use of needles.

The simplicity of the ^{13}C-breath test makes it very applicable in a clinical setting: the physician can obtain valuable diagnostic information by distinguishing between two groups or populations on the basis of the recovery of $^{13}CO_2$ from the ingested ^{13}C-substrate. However, for the breath test to have significant clinical utility, it has to be compared to a gold standard test or an established method of diagnosis and more importantly, the accuracy of the breath test must be proven.

2. Breath Test Accuracy

The accuracy of a breath test versus the current gold standard test is evaluated by the simultaneous application of both these tests in the two groups: normal and those with a medical problem. These two groups should preferably be the same size. However, if the gold standard method is an invasive procedure (biopsy or endoscopy), the recruitment of normal volunteers becomes a problem. Statistically, at least 100 individuals must be studied in both categories and compared to the gold standard test. Four possible outcomes are possible from these comparisons: the breath test might correctly identify the true positive (TP) and true negative (TN) individuals.[b] The breath test might also falsely identify individuals as false positive (FP) or as false negative (FN). It is possible to calculate the following parameters of the breath test following the clinical trial:

$$\text{Sensitivity} = \frac{\text{TP}}{\text{TP} + \text{FN}} \qquad \text{Positive predictive value} = \frac{\text{TP}}{\text{TP} + \text{FP}}$$

$$\text{Specificity} = \frac{\text{TN}}{\text{TN} + \text{FP}} \qquad \text{Negative predictive value} = \frac{\text{TN}}{\text{TN} + \text{FN}}$$

$$\text{Accuracy} = \frac{\text{TP} + \text{TN}}{\text{total}}$$

The data can also be evaluated by generating a receiver operator characteristic curve in which sensitivity is plotted against (1-specificity). In these
plots, the rectilinear curve signifies a test with good discriminative ability.
For a breath test to have great clinical utility, the specificity and sensitivity
needs to be relatively high (higher than 90%).

3. How to Transform Research Tracer Probes to Clinical Tests

The successful FDA approval of the ^{13}C-urea breath test in 1996 provides
a strategy for the launch of a breath test from a research probe to an
established clinical test. Four different criteria are involved:

1. establish the accuracy of the test,
2. assess the market for the test and how it will reduce the cost of health
   care delivery
3. obtain regulatory approval of the test and obtain a reimbursement code
4. provide the financial resources required to market the test to the healthcare providers, physicians, and the consumer.

3.1. *Establishment of Accuracy*

In the pre-clinical development or proof of principle phase, normally carried
out at university research laboratories, a number of breath test parameters
need to be optimized to establish the accuracy of the test prior to Phase
I, II and III clinical trials in conjunction with the FDA. This ensures the
success of clinical trials, which are complex and expensive to organize and
execute especially when conducted at multiple sites. Although the goal of
clinical trials is to obtain data on the safety and accuracy of the breath
test, the overriding consideration in these studies is the safety of those in
the trials. The Center for Drug Evaluation and Research (CDER) monitors
the study design and conduct of clinical trials to ensure that people in the
trials are not exposed to unnecessary risks. In order to obtain meaningful
results, the trial must be conducted in accordance with the ground rules
of good clinical practice (GCP) set forth by the FDA. The accuracy of the
breath test has to be equivalent or superior to the gold standard test in
terms of sensitivity and specificity.

3.2. *Financial Cost Benefits of Test Use and Impact on Health Care Delivery Costs*

The cost per subject in clinical trials can vary from $\$1,000$ to $\$5,000$ depending on the breath test and the gold standard tests to be performed for comparisons. Even for an efficiently organized trial, the cost is likely to be $\$500,000$ to a million. Pharmaceutical companies must evaluate the market for such a test to ensure that it has a profitable proposition before proceeding to conduct clinical trials. FDA approval of a diagnostic procedure does not ensure its adoption by the medical community as is widely seen in the reluctance of physicians to use the urea-^{13}C breath test instead of invasive endoscopy for *H. pylori* detection. It is essential to evaluate the cost benefits of the breath test with respect to the currently used diagnostic test. The commercial success of the breath test depends on the cost savings and benefits to the insurance companies or healthcare providers covering the expense of the procedure. Overall cost of patient care and safety issues alone should compel physicians to adopt the novel breath tests in routine practice instead of the existing highly invasive tests and patients should demand these noninvasive breath tests.

3.3. *Regulatory Approval of the Test and a Reimbursement Code*

In the US, approval of a noninvasive device, such as a breath test, submitted as a new drug application (NDA) or as a 510K application, primarily hinges on its accuracy and its safety. Since most of the substrates or tracer probes for the breath tests are either approved drugs or chemical substances on FDA's Generally Recognized As Safe (GRAS) list (`vm.cfsan.fda.gov/~dms/eafus.html`), most of these substances do not have safety issues. However, in addition, the substrate must be produced in accordance with chemical, manufacturing and control processes that follow good manufacturing practices (GMP). The manufacturer is required to prepare a certificate of analysis, which documents the chemical and isotopic purity of the product, using previously validated analytical methods, and is required to document the stability of the bulk substance under conventional and accelerated aging conditions. A Drug Master File (DMF) has to be submitted to the FDA with all the manufacturing and analytical methods of the substrate. Theoretically, the entire approval process for a diagnostic test is completed within one year. Subsequently, an application for the reimbursement or current procedural terminology (CPT) code must be filed. Once a CPT code has been assigned, a reimbursement fee can be determined for the breath test so that physicians may charge insurance companies or health care providers.

3.4. *Financial Resources*

The real challenge for a pharmaceutical/biotechnology company after the breath test gets FDA approval is to provide the financial resources for the extensive infrastructure required to manufacture, package, and market the breath test kits with the tracer probes. Thereafter, the test has to be skillfully marketed and advertised to physicians, consumers (patients), and healthcare providers/insurance companies.

4. Hurdles and Pitfalls in Transition of Breath Test from Research to Clinical Practice

In the research arena, ^{13}C-substrates have been extensively used in a number of metabolic studies with clinical applications. The results of these studies are the subject of numerous presentations and posters at scientific meetings as well as over 1500 publications. The metabolic study protocols at universities/research hospitals merely require the blessing of the local Institutional Review Board (IRB) and minimal precautions in substrate manufacture and administration. The protocols are usually funded by research grants from the NIH. There are numerous reasons for the paucity of FDA approved breath tests using ^{13}C substrates, other than the urea-^{13}C breath test for the detection of *H. pylori*:

- Pharmaceutical/biotechnology companies have been reluctant to invest in breath test protocols with potential clinical utility because they need to conduct clinical trials to get them approved by the FDA as a NDA or as a 510K application (see websites `www.fda.gov/cder/`; `www.fda.gov/cdrh/`; `www.fda.gov/cdrh/devadvice/` of the FDA). Subsequently, they need to obtain a reimbursement or CPT code for the tracer probe test. As with all medical product research and design these can be prohibitive costs. Unless pharmaceutical companies see a large profit margin selling the test kits or physicians and patients demand the use of noninvasive tests in routine medical practice, the transition of these tests from research to the clinic will be limited.
- In the past the analytical instruments for measurements of ^{13}C/^{12}C ratios in breath samples, the isotope ratio mass spectrometers (IRMS),

were very expensive, required skilled operation and maintenance and were available only in academic research institutions. The introduction of the Automatic Breath Carbon Analyzer, a gas isotope ratio mass spectrometer, from Europa Scientific Ltd (`www.europa-uk.com/Products/ABCA4/ABCAmain.html`), significantly simplified and broadened breath gas measurements. However, the mass spectroscopic instrument still costs between $100K to $200K and is not affordable at primary care clinics. With the advent of bench top, inexpensive optical spectrophotometers (IR[6,7] and laser[8]) the breath tests can now be routinely performed in a clinic setting.

- ^{13}C-Substrates were relatively expensive until recently. A number of companies have started to manufacture the tracer probes thereby getting prices down and affordable.

- A fasting requirement for up to 12 h prior to the test and not participating in physical activity for at least 2 h prior to the test makes it especially difficult for pediatric use. Breath test results can be compromised with noncompliance.

- The ^{13}C-breath tests are too time-consuming if the breath samples need to be collected at regular intervals for 60–90 minutes. A single time point breath sample collection test capable of distinguishing between two groups or populations, with a high degree of sensitivity and specificity, would be ideal.

- Poor sensitivity and specificity of breath tests compared to the usually invasive gold standard tests due to the oral administration of ^{13}C-substrates. The target organ for most of these tests is the liver and variable interindividual gastrointestinal absorption and transport to the liver results in poor sensitivity and specificity. Concurrent medications or diseases like diabetes (delayed gastric emptying) or gastrointestinal diseases (GERD, IBD) can cause variability in absorption of ^{13}C-substrates. One way to overcome variable gastrointestinal absorption and transport is to administer the ^{13}C-substrates by the intravenous (*iv*) route. This is a very radical idea, moving away from the conventional "noninvasive breath test" paradigm. However, the ^{13}C-substrates administered by the *iv* route will go directly to the target organ and get metabolized by the relevant enzyme into $^{13}CO_2$, thereby increasing the specificity and sensitivity of the test as well as reducing the duration of the test. Non-compliance by subjects on the fasting requirement for the oral breath tests can also be overcome by the *iv* dosing of the ^{13}C-tracer probe.

- A gap exists in interaction between scientists at specialized stable isotope centers around the world and potentially interested clinicians. A closer working relationship needs to be developed.
- Lack of standardization of diagnostic protocols. The two methods of analysis of $^{13}CO_2$ breath samples, IRMS and bench top IR spectrophotometers, have proven to be equivalent in a number of studies. However, clinical trials use either method according to availability at the research center. Unfortunately, standardization will be very costly and time-consuming to accomplish since the number of breath test parameters that can be used to establish the efficacy of the test are varied depending on each test.

5. ^{13}C-Tracer Probe Breath Tests with Clinical Significance

5.1. *H. Pylori Detection by the ^{13}C-Urea Breath Test*

The first use of ^{13}C-urea in a breath test to detect the presence of *H. pylori* was described by Graham *et al.*[2] in 1987 and was widely reproduced by others in over 750 subsequent publications. In this test, a baseline breath sample is collected before ingesting 75 mg of ^{13}C-urea. One breath sample is collected 20 minutes after substrate ingestion. If *H. pylori* are present in the stomach, the organisms will hydrolyze the urea with consequent liberation of $^{13}CO_2$ that will be detected in expired air as an increase over the baseline abundance. A change as small as $2.4\,\%_{00}$, or approximately 26 parts per million of $^{13}CO_2$, is evidence of active *H. pylori* infection. The test is easy to perform and approved by the FDA with a reimbursement CPT code. The use of the test has reduced endoscopy costs in clinical trials. A commercial breath test diagnostic kit for the diagnosis of *H. pylori* appeared on the market in January 1997 (Meretek, `meretek.com/ubit.html`, introduced this breath test kit).

5.2. *Bacterial Overgrowth*

Bacterial overgrowth of the small intestine can be a hidden, unsuspected cause of chronic bowel problems such as indigestion, bloating, abdominal pain, gas, and irregularity. The most common causes of bacterial overgrowth of the small intestine usually relate to a decrease in gastric acidity or digestive enzymes, which create a non-sterile environment for the small intestine. Other possible causes of bacterial overgrowth of the small intestine include intestinal obstructions caused by Crohn's disease, adhesions, radiation damage and lymphoma. Treating bacterial overgrowth of the small intestine has been shown to significantly alleviate chronic symptoms, such as diarrhea and abdominal pain in patients with Irritable Bowel Syndrome.

Methane and hydrogen are two main gases produced due to bacterial overgrowth and measurement of these two is considered more sensitive for detecting small bowel bacterial overgrowth. However, the ^{13}C-xylose,[9] the ^{13}C-D-sorbitol,[10] and the ^{13}C-glycocholic acid[11] breath tests offer a diagnostic alternative to the microbiological analysis of jejunal fluid for the diagnosis of small bowel bacterial overgrowth. These tests offer a practical way of monitoring a condition that is often persistent throughout life.[9-11]

5.3. *Gastric Emptying*

Breath tests with ^{13}C-tracers offer an alternative to gold standard scintigraphic (radioactive substrates) techniques for measuring gastric emptying. The rate of emptying can be evaluated with ^{13}C-octanoic acid or ^{13}C-sodium octanoate for solid foods in human[12-15] as well as dogs[16] and ^{13}C-sodium acetate for semi-solid and liquid meals.[17-20] The safety of the ^{13}C-breath test and the ability to use it repeatedly has made it particularly desirable for the assessment of the efficacy of new motility drugs. ^{13}C-sodium octanoate breath tests can be used to evaluate delayed gastric emptying in patients with type I diabetes,[21-23], dyspepsia,[24] renal failure,[25] and cystic fibrosis.[26]

5.4. *Liver Function*

There are numerous ^{13}C-breath tests that can provide quantitative information on hepatic dysfunction. More ^{13}C-tracer probes have been used as substrates to quantify liver diseases or ailments than for any other diagnostic medical problem. Historically, blood tests and scoring indexes have been employed to identify and monitor patients with liver disease. These tests reflect a static end point of hepatocellular damage, but do not evaluate functional hepatic reserve. Therefore, while advanced liver disease can be diagnosed with confidence, early or marginal hepatic disease is poorly defined. A number of specific liver function breath tests targeted at exploring the functionality of cytosolic (Phe-1-^{13}C),[27-31] microsomal (cytochrome P450 enzymes with ^{13}C-aminopyrine,[32,33] P450 3A4 with ^{14}C-erythromycin,[34-37] 1A2 with ^{13}C-caffeine,[38,39] and ^{13}C-methacetin[40,41]) and mitochondrial (^{13}C-methionine[42,43] and ^{13}C-KIC[44-46]) enzyme systems within the hepatocyte have been developed and optimized over the last 20 years. Other ^{13}C-substrates used for evaluating liver functional reserve are ^{13}C-galactose[47] and ^{13}C-fructose.[48] These breath tests provide information on:

- monitoring the regeneration of the liver and its functional capacity[49–55] following living donor and orthotopic liver transplantations (OLT),
- decision in optimum transplant timing by monitoring disease severity,[56,57]
- prediction of long term liver disease prognosis,[33,58–60]
- monitoring the progression of liver disease,[49,61–64]
- determining the efficacy of a therapeutic regimen or surgical intervention,[65]
- deficiencies in certain enzymes produced in the liver leading to diseases such as PKU (phenylalanine hydroxylase deficiency), maple syrup disease[66,67] and propionic acidemia.[68]

5.5. *Oro-Caecal Transit Time*

^{13}C-lactose-ureide is not metabolized by the human intestinal or brush border enzymes and is not metabolized until reaching the colonic bacteria. The tracer stays intact down to the caecum at the beginning of the large intestine after oral ingestion. There it is split to lactose and urea and further metabolized by the bacteria resulting in ^{13}CO$_2$ in the expired breath and NH$_3$. ^{13}C-lactose-ureide has thus proven to be a reliable marker to follow oro-caecal transit time[69–73] instead of scintigraphy.

5.6. *Fat Malabsorption and Pancreatic Insufficiency*

Fat malabsorption results either from an absence of bile acids or pancreatic lipase or from inadequate intestinal mucosa. The use of ^{13}C-labeled lipids to detect fat malabsorption in children is of particular advantage in a pediatric population because of the simplicity of the breath test. The collection of fecal samples is inconvenient for outpatients and stool analysis is unpleasant to laboratory technicians. Pancreatic exocrine insufficiency is assessed by means of faecal elastase 1 determination. The use of breath tests (BT) with ^{13}C-labeled lipids (cholesteryloctanoate, mixed triglyceride, trioctanoin, triolein, and palmitic acid) for the diagnosis of pancreatic exocrine insufficiency[74–82] is on the rise. ^{13}C-lipid breath tests are also an accurate, noninvasive way of repeatedly measuring fat digestion[83–89] especially in a pediatric setting. These tests are especially useful in monitoring the progress of children on enzyme supplementation therapy.

5.7. Nutritional Studies

Tracer techniques are attractive for the *in vivo* study of different aspects of nutrient assimilation and metabolism. A number of ^{13}C-labeled amino acids have been used in nutritional studies to understand *in vivo* amino acid kinetics with subsequent estimation of whole body protein turnover. Constant infusions of labelled amino acids such as L-[1-^{13}C]-leucine[90–92] are generally used. ^{13}C-tracer amino acids, carbohydrates and lipids could be used in the future for optimizing the nutritional requirements for athletes and sportsmen to enable them to perform at peak levels during competitions.

5.8. Dihydropyrimidine Dehydrogenase Enzyme Deficiency

5-Fluorouracil (5-FU) is one of the most frequently prescribed antineoplastic agents for the treatment of solid tumours. However, unanticipated severe 5 FU toxicity and death may occur in a small but significant subpopulation of patients, thereby hindering optimum therapy. About 80% to 90% of 5-FU is inactivated via catabolism, where dihydropyrimidine dehydrogenase (DPD) is the rate-limiting enzyme. There is extensive evidence linking the pharmacogenetic syndrome known as "DPD deficiency" with severe 5-FU toxicity. Population studies have shown the prevalence of partial and profound DPD deficiency to be 3–5 % and 0.1 % in the general population, respectively in Caucasians,[93–95] and about 10 % of African Americans. Until recently, it has been impossible to rapidly screen for DPD deficiency, in particular prior to administration of fluoropyrimidine chemotherapy in the clinic. A novel ^{13}C-uracil breath test (UraBT)[96–98] has recently been developed, capable of rapidly phenotyping DPD activity in a healthy volunteer population.

5.9. Miscellaneous Breath Tests

Sodium bicarbonate-^{13}C has been used as a tracer probe in numerous clinical applications — gastric emptying time,[99] total parenteral nutrition,[100] energy expenditure,[101–103] and predicting hypercapnia.[104]

6. Future of ^{13}C-Tracer Probes in Clinical Practice

An ideal drug is one that effectively treats or prevents disease with a minimum of undesired adverse events. Heterogeneity within a treated population precludes all members of the population being safely and effectively treated with the "same dose" of medication. One important consequence of interindividual variability in drug disposition and response is the risk of adverse drug reactions (ADRs), a major problem in clinical medicine and drug development. A widely cited (and criticized) meta-analysis suggested that severe ADRs occurred in 6.7% of hospitalized patients affecting an estimated 2 million individuals, ranking ADRs as between the fourth and sixth leading cause of death in the United States.[105] A recent literature review identified 27 medications that were frequently cited in studies of ADR.[106] Of these, 59% were subject to biotransformation by enzymes that display functional polymorphism.

The cytochromes P450 (CYPs) are quantitatively the most important Phase I drug biotransformation enzymes and genetic variation of several members of this gene superfamily has been extensively examined. Stable isotope tracer probes can be ideal tools for the noninvasive kinetic assessment of the *in vivo* metabolism of drugs especially in the pediatric population. In the future, stable isotope labeled xenobiotics can be used to evaluate the clearance of drugs in the liver by CYP (cytochrome P450) enzymes. A majority of the drugs approved by the FDA are metabolized by the P450 enzymes. Approximately 40% of human P450-dependent drug metabolism is carried out by polymorphic enzymes, which can cause abolished, quantitatively or qualitatively altered or enhanced drug metabolism. The latter situation is due to stable duplication, multiduplication or amplification of active genes, most likely in response to dietary components that have resulted in a selection of alleles with multiple noninducible genes. Genetic polymorphisms are known to contribute considerably to interindividual variations in the metabolism of numerous drugs and xenobiotics. The phase I enzymes of the cytochrome P450 family (CYP450) are the most important enzymes in drug and xenobiotics metabolism. The CYP2A6, CYP2D6, CYP2C9, and CYP2C19 enzymes exhibit functional polymorphism that alters or abolishes enzyme activity. Normal, impaired, and enhanced enzyme activity result in the extensive, poor, and ultra-rapid drug metabolizing phenotypes, respectively. Subjects with impaired or absent enzyme activity will have supra-therapeutic plasma concentrations of drugs that are primarily metabolized by the affected enzyme when given conventional doses of the drug resulting in ADR's and/or toxicity. In contrast, sub-therapeutic plasma concentrations and therapeutic failure may occur when patients are treated with conventional doses of drugs metabolized through enzyme pathways that exhibit enhanced activity. Stable isotope tracers will be able to evaluate, *in vivo*, the characteristics of these polymorphic enzyme systems in the body and identify their response to stress or infection or foods or co-administered inhibitor drugs as well as to treatment regimes. The outcome will allow for safer and more efficient drug therapies. In the future, breath tests with stable isotope ^{13}C-tracers can be used for effective personalized medicine.

7. Conclusions

A number of reviews on the clinical applications and visions on the future for breath tests have appeared in the scientific literature over the last 5 years.[107–114] Despite over 50 diverse, accurate diagnostic ^{13}C-breath tests over a wide range of clinical applications, physicians have not been routinely utilizing them in clinical practice. The onus is now on pharmaceutical companies to come forward with the necessary funding for clinical trials in order to get noninvasive breath tests approved by the FDA and obtain reimbursement codes. This will enable physicians and patients to benefit from rapid, novel and noninvasive ways to detect enzyme deficiencies, to monitor the progress of disease severity, to trace acquired and/or congenital metabolic defects, to study *in vivo* the pharmacokinetics of xenobiotics, and to optimize individually tailored treatment therapies.

Acknowledgements

The author wishes to thank Dr. Anton Amann, Medical University of Innsbruck, for the opportunity to write this review article. He wishes to dedicate this work to his beloved deceased mother.

References

1. Lacroix M, Mosora F, Pontus M, Lefebvre P, Luyckz A, Lopez-Habib G. Glucose naturally labeled with carbon-13: use for metabolic studies in man. *Science* 1973; **181**: 445–446.
2. Graham DY, Klein PD, Evans DJ, Jr., Evans DG, Alpert LC, Opekun AR, Boutton TW. Campylobacter pylori detected noninvasively by the ^{13}C-urea breath test. *Lancet* 1987; **320**: 1174–1177.
3. Alving K, Weitzberg E, Lundberg JM. Increased amount of nitric oxide in exhaled air of asthmatics. *Eur Respir J* 1993; **6**: 1368–1370.

4. Phillips M, Boehmer JP, Cataneo RN, Cheema T, Eisen HJ, Fallon JT, Fisher PE, Gass A, Greenberg J, Kobashigawa J, Mancini D, Rayburn B, Zucker MJ. Heart allograft rejection: detection with breath alkanes in low levels (the HARDBALL study). *J Heart Lung Transplant* 2004; **23**: 701–708.

5. Nau H, Rating D, Koch S, Hauser I, Helge H. Valproic acid and its metabolites: placental transfer, neonatal pharmacokinetics, transfer via mother's milk and clinical status in neonates of epileptic mothers. *J Pharmacol Exp Ther* 1981; **219**: 768–777.

6. Koletzko S, Haisch M, Seeboth I, Braden B, Hengels K, Koletzko B, Hering P. Isotope-selective non-dispersive infrared spectrometry for detection of Helicobacter pylori infection with ^{13}C-urea breath test. *Lancet* 1995; **345**: 961–962.

7. Kato M, Asaka M, Saito M. Evaluation of a new ^{13}CO$_2$ infrared analyzer (UBiT-IR300) for ^{13}C-urea breath test. *Nippon Shokakibyo Gakkai Zasshi* 2001; **98**: 853.

8. Crosson ER, Ricci KN, Richman BA, Chilese FC, Owano TG, Provencal RA, Todd MW, Glasser J, Kachanov AA, Paldus BA, Spence TG, Zare RN. Stable isotope ratios using cavity ring-down spectroscopy: determination of ^{13}C/^{12}C for carbon dioxide in human breath. *Anal Chem* 2002; **74**: 2003–2007.

9. Dellert SF, Nowicki MJ, Farrell MK, Delente J, Heubi JE. The ^{13}C-xylose breath test for the diagnosis of small bowel bacterial overgrowth in children. *J Pediatr Gastroenterol Nutr* 1997; **25**: 153–158.

10. Somogyi L, Amann S, Wagner D, Toskes P. Preliminary evaluation of ^{13}C-sorbitol breath test in diagnosis of small bowel bacterial overgrowth. *Gastroenterology* 1998; **114**: A417.

11. Solomons NW, Schoeller DA, Wagonfeld JB, Ott D, Rosenberg IH, Klein PD. Application of a stable isotope ^{13}C-labeled glycocholate breath test to diagnosis of bacterial overgrowth and ileal dysfunction. *J Lab Clin Med* 1977; **90**: 431–439.

12. Ghoos Y, Geypens B. Gastric emptying test-kit and method of testing gastric emptying of solid meal. PCN 2001-10-04 2001072342/WO-A1.

13. Aygen S. Method for determining gastric evacuation using a ^{13}C-labelled test meal. PCN 2004-05-06 2004037298/WO-A1.

14. Sanaka M, Yamamoto T, Kuyama Y, Shimomura Y, Hattori K, Anjiki H. The ratio of ^{13}CO$_2$ exhalation at 120 min to ^{13}CO$_2$ exhalation at 60 min as a simpler gastric emptying parameter in the ^{13}C-octanoic acid breath test: a preliminary study. *J Gastroenterol* 2003; **38**: 298–299.

15. Chen CP, Chen CY, Lu CL, Chang FY, Lee SD, Chu LS, Liu RS, Wu HC. Infrared spectrometry based ^{13}C-octanoic acid breath test in measuring human solid gastric emptying. *J Gastroenterol Hepatol* 2003; **18**: 41–46.

16. Wyse CA, Preston T, Love S, Morrison DJ, Cooper JM, Yam PS. Use of the ^{13}C-octanoic acid breath test for assessment of solid-phase gastric emptying in dogs. *Am J Vet Res* 2001; **62**: 1939–1944.

17. Braden B, Adams S, Duan LP, Orth KH, Maul FD, Lembcke B, Hor G, Caspary WF. The ^{13}C-acetate breath test accurately reflects gastric emp-

tying of liquids in both liquid and semisolid test meals. *Gastroenterology* 1995; **108**: 1048–1055.

18. Shimamoto C, Hirata I, Hiraike Y, Takeuchi N, Nomura T, Katsu K. Evaluation of gastric motor activity in the elderly by electrogastrography and the ^{13}C-acetate breath test. *Gerontology* 2002; **48**: 381–386.

19. Pfluger T, Antos D, Demmelmair J, Hahn K, Koletzko S. Comparison of ^{13}C-acetate breath test and Tc-99m gastric emptying scintigraphy in children with impaired gastrointestinal motility. *Journal of Nuclear Medicine* 2004; **44**: 348P–349P.

20. Braden B, Peterknecht A, Piepho T, Schneider A, Caspary WF, Hamscho N, Ahrens P. Measuring gastric emptying of semisolids in children using the ^{13}C-acetate breath test: a validation study. *Dig Liver Dis* 2004; **36**: 260–264.

21. Lee JS, Camilleri M, Zinsmeister AR, Burton DD, Choi MG, Nair KS, Verlinden M. Toward office-based measurement of gastric emptying in symptomatic diabetics using ^{13}C-octanoic acid breath test. *Am J Gastroenterol* 2000; **95**: 2751–2761.

22. Folwaczny C, Wawarta R, Otto B, Friedrich S, Landgraf R, Riepl RL. Gastric emptying of solid and liquid meals in healthy controls compared with long-term type-1 diabetes mellitus under optimal glucose control. *Exp Clin Endocrinol Diabetes* 2003; **111**: 223–229.

23. Zahn A, Langhans CD, Hoffner S, Haberkorn U, Rating D, Haass M, Enck P, Stremmel W, Ruhl A. Measurement of gastric emptying by ^{13}C-octanoic acid breath test versus scintigraphy in diabetics. *Z Gastroenterol* 2003; **41**: 383–390.

24. Aoki S, Haruma K, Kusunoki H, Hata J, Hara M, Yoshida S, Tanaka S, Chayama K. Evaluation of gastric emptying measured with the ^{13}C-octanoic acid breath test in patients with functional dyspepsia: comparison with ultrasonography. *Scand J Gastroenterol* 2002; **37**: 662–666.

25. Van Vlem B, Schoonjans R, Vanholder R, Vandamme W, De Vos M, Lameire N. Dyspepsia and gastric emptying in chronic renal failure patients. *Clin Nephrol* 2001; **56**: 302–307.

26. Symonds EL, Omari TI, Webster JM, Davidson GP, Butle RN. Relation between pancreatic lipase activity and gastric emptying rate in children with cystic fibrosis. *J Pediatr* 2003; **143**: 772–775

27. Ishii T, Takatori K, Iida K, Higuchi T, Ohshima A, Naruse H, Kajiwara M. Optimum conditions for the ^{13}C-phenylalanine breath test. *Chem Pharm Bull (Tokyo)* 1998; **46**: 1330–1332.

28. Tugtekin I, Radermacher P, Wachter U, Barth E, Weidenbach H, Adler G, Georgieff M, Vogt J. Comparison between the oral and intravenous L-[1-^{13}C]-phenylalanine breath test for the assessment of liver function. *Isotopes Environ Health Stud* 1999; **35**: 147–156.

29. Kobayashi T, Kubota K, Imamura H, Hasegawa K, Inoue Y, Takayama T, Makuuchi M. Hepatic phenylalanine metabolism measured by the ^{13}C-phenylalanine breath test. *Eur J Clin Invest* 2001; **31**: 356–361.

30. Perri F, Marras RM, Ricciardi R, Quitadamo M, Andriulli A. ^{13}C-breath tests in hepatology (cytosolic liver function). *Eur Rev Med Pharmacol Sci* 2004; **8**: 47–49.

31. Wagner D, Baker M, Burke P, Forse R, Palombo J, Bistrian B. Liver function breath test using aromatic amino acids. PCN 1994-12-22 1994028941/WO-A1.

32. Bastien MC, Leblond F, Pichette V, Villeneuve JP. Differential alteration of cytochrome P450 isoenzymes in two experimental models of cirrhosis. *Can J Physiol Pharmacol* 2000; **78**: 912–919.

33. Fasoli A, Giannini E, Botta F, Romagnoli P, Risso D, Celle G, Testa R. ^{13}CO$_2$ excretion in breath of normal subjects and cirrhotic patients after ^{13}C-aminopyrine oral load. Comparison with MEGX test in functional differentiation between chronic hepatitis and liver cirrhosis. *Hepatogastroenterology* 2000; **47**: 234–238.

34. Schmidt LE, Olsen AK, Stentoft K, Rasmussen A, Kirkegaard P, Dalhoff K. Early postoperative erythromycin breath test correlates with hepatic cytochrome P4503A activity in liver transplant recipients. *Clin Pharmacol Ther* 2001; **70**: 446–454.

35. Dowling TC, Briglia AE, Fink JC, Hanes DS, Light PD, Stackiewicz L, Karyekar CS, Eddington ND, Weir MR, Henrich WL. Characterization of hepatic cytochrome p4503A activity in patients with end-stage renal disease. *Clin Pharmacol Ther* 2003; **73**: 427–434.

36. Salvat C, Mouly S, Rizzo-Padoin N, Knellwolf AL, Simoneau G, Duet M, Nataf V, Bailliart O, Bergmann JF. The [^{14}C-*N*-methyl]-erythromycin breath test dosimetry complies with the French regulations for radiation safety. *Fundam Clin Pharmacol* 2003; **17**: 349–353.

37. Lemahieu WP, Maes BD, Ghoos Y, Rutgeerts P, Verbeke K, Vanrenterghem Y. Measurement of hepatic and intestinal CYP3A4 and PGP activity by combined po + iv [^{14}C]-erythromycin breath and urine test. *Am J Physiol Gastrointest Liver Physiol* 2003; **285**: G470–482.

38. Park GJ, Katelaris PH, Jones DB, Seow F, Le Couteur DG, Ngu MC. Validity of the ^{13}C-caffeine breath test as a noninvasive, quantitative test of liver function. *Hepatology* 2003; **38**: 1227–1236.

39. Webster E, McIntyre J, Choonara I, Preston T. The Caffeine Breath Test and CYP1A2 Activity in Children. *Paediatric and Perinatal Drug Therapy* 2002; **5**: 28–33.

40. Pfaffenbach B, Gotze O, Szymanski C, Hagemann D, Adamek RJ. The ^{13}C-methacetin breath test for quantitative noninvasive liver function analysis with an isotope-specific nondispersive infrared spectrometer in liver cirrhosis. *Dtsch Med Wochenschr* 1998; **123**: 1467–1471.

41. Ciccocioppo R, Candelli M, Di Francesco D, Ciocca F, Taglieri G, Armuzzi A, Gasbarrini G, Gasbarrini A. Study of liver function in healthy elderly subjects using the ^{13}C-methacetin breath test. *Aliment Pharmacol Ther* 2003; **17**: 271–277.

42. Armuzzi A, Marcoccia S, Zocco MA, De Lorenzo A, Grieco A, Tondi P, Pola P, Gasbarrini G, Gasbarrini A. Non-Invasive assessment of human hep-

atic mitochondrial function through the ^{13}C-methionine breath test. *Scand J Gastroenterol* 2000; **35**: 650–653.

43. Spahr L, Negro F, Leandro G, Marinescu O, Goodman KJ, Rubbia-Brandt L, Jordan M, Hadengue A. Impaired hepatic mitochondrial oxidation using the ^{13}C-methionine breath test in patients with macrovesicular steatosis and patients with cirrhosis. *Med Sci Monit* 2003; **9**: CR6–11.

44. Mion F, Rousseau M, Brazier JL, Minaire Y. Human hepatic macrovesicular steatosis: a noninvasive study of mitochondrial ketoisocaproic acid decarboxylation. *Metabolism* 1995; **44**: 699–700.

45. Gabe S, Williams R, Silk D. The ketoisocaproic acid breath test is a dynamic in vivo test of mitochondrial energy production. *Gastroenterology* 1997; **112**: A1268.

46. Candelli M, Armuzzi A, Nista E, Zocco M, Grieco A, Miele L, Pola P, Gasbarrini G, Gasbarrini A. Gender affects ^{13}C-ketoisocaproic breath test for liver mithocondrial function. *Journal of Hepatology* 2001; **34**: 198.

47. Becker M. ^{13}C breath test for measurement of liver function. *Gut* 1998; **43** Suppl 3: S25–27.

48. Suzuki S, Ishii Y, Asai S, Kohno T, Mazaki T, Takahashi Y, Iwai S, Ishikawa K. [1-^{13}C] breath test of galactose and fructose for quantitative liver function. *J Surg Res* 2001; **96**: 90–95.

49. Ishii Y, Asai S, Kohno T, Takahashi Y, Nagata T, Suzuki S, Iwai S, Ishikawa K. Evaluation of liver regeneration using the L-[1-^{13}C]-methionine breath test. *J Surg Res* 2001; **95**: 195–199.

50. Ishii Y, Asai S, Kohno T, Ito A, Iwai S, Ishikawa K. Recovery of liver function in two-third partial hepatectomized rats evaluated by L-[1-^{13}C]-phenylalanine breath test. *Surgery* 2002; **132**: 849–856.

51. Di Campli C, Angelini G, Armuzzi A, Nardo B, Zocco MA, Candelli M, Santoliquido A, Cavallari A, Bernardi M, Gasbarrini A. Quantitative evaluation of liver function by the methionine and aminopyrine breath tests in the early stages of liver transplantation. *Eur J Gastroenterol Hepatol* 2003; **15**: 727–732.

52. Petrolati A, Festi D, De Berardinis G, Colaiocco-Ferrante L, Di Paolo D, Tisone G, Angelico M. ^{13}C-methacetin breath test for monitoring hepatic function in cirrhotic patients before and after liver transplantation. *Aliment Pharmacol Ther* 2003; **18**: 785–790.

53. Candelli M, Armuzzi A, Nista EC, Fini L, Gasbarrini G, Gasbarrini A. ^{13}C-methacetin breath test for monitoring hepatic function in cirrhotic patients before and after liver transplantation. *Aliment Pharmacol Ther* 2004; **19**: 243.

54. Ishii Y, Asai S, Ishikawa K, Iwai S, Katoh K, Kohno T, Masuda H, Mazaki T, Suzuki S. Evaluation of regenerated liver using 1-^{13}C-phenylalanine breath test. *Gastroenterology* 2000; **118**: AGA A559.

55. Freeman R, Dixon M, Horth B, Palladino M, Melanson A, Cooper J, Rohror R, Modak A. Hepatic oxidation of orally delivered amino acids remains impaired for weeks after living liver donation. *Am J Transplantation* 2004; **4** (Suppl 8): P1051.

56. Zambonin L, Sottili S, Roda E, Roda A, Mazzella G, Jaboli M, Fabbri C, Cipolla A. ^{13}C-phenylalanine and ^{13}C-aminopyrine breath tests for the assessment of hepatic disease severity. *Journal of Hepatology* 1999; **30**: 263.

57. Romano F, Papponetti M, Marcuccitti J, Festi D, Ferrante L, Colaiocco Di Ilio C, Di Carlo M, Cuccurullo F, Bonitatibus A, Mazzella G, Sergiacomo L, Simoni P, Tullio G. ^{13}C-phenylalanine and ^{13}C-methacetin breath tests for the evaluation of functional liver capacity and disease severity in chronic liver diseases. *Journal of Hepatology* 1999; **30**: 274.

58. Mion F, Queneau PE, Rousseau M, Brazier JL, Paliard P, Minaire Y. Aminopyrine breath test: development of a ^{13}C-breath test for quantitative assessment of liver function in humans. *Hepatogastroenterology* 1995; **42**: 931–938.

59. Klatt S, Taut C, Mayer D, Adler G, Beckh K. Evaluation of the ^{13}C-methacetin breath test for quantitative liver function testing. *Z Gastroenterol* 1997; **35**: 609–614.

60. Ishii Y, Suzuki S, Kohno T, Aoki M, Ito A, Takayama T, Asai S. L-[1-^{13}C]-phenylalanine breath test reflects histological changes in the liver. *J Surg Res* 2003; **114**: 120–125.

61. Mion F, Rousseau M, Scoazec JY, Berger F, Minaire Y. [^{13}C]-galactose breath test: correlation with liver fibrosis in chronic hepatitis C. *Eur J Clin Invest* 1999; **29**: 624–629.

62. Lara Baruque S, Razquin M, Jimenez I, Vazquez A, Gisbert JP, Pajares JM. ^{13}C-phenylalanine and ^{13}C-methacetin breath test to evaluate functional capacity of hepatocyte in chronic liver disease. *Dig Liver Dis* 2000; **32**: 226–232.

63. Tugtekin I, Wachter U, Barth E, Weidenbach H, Wagner DA, Adler G, Georgieff M, Radermacher P, Vogt JA. Phenylalanine kinetics in healthy volunteers and liver cirrhotics: implications for the phenylalanine breath test. *Am J Physiol Endocrinol Metab* 2002; **283**: E1223–1231.

64. Ishii Y, Suzuki S, Kohno T, Aoki M, Goto I, Ito A, Asai S. Patients with severe liver cirrhosis followed up by L-[1-^{13}C]-phenylalanine breath test. *J Gastroenterol* 2003; **38**: 1086–1090.

65. Schmidt LE, Rasmussen A, Kirkegaard P, Dalhoff K. Relationship between postoperative erythromycin breath test and early morbidity in liver transplant recipients. *Transplantation* 2003; **76**: 358–363.

66. Okano Y, Hase Y, Kawajiri M, Nishi Y, Inui K, Sakai N, Tanaka Y, Takatori K, Kajiwara M, Yamano T. In vivo studies of phenylalanine hydroxylase by phenylalanine breath test: diagnosis of tetrahydrobiopterin-responsive phenylalanine hydroxylase deficiency. *Pediatr Res* 2004; **56**: 714–719.

67. Thompson GN, Bresson JL, Pacy PJ, Bonnefont JP, Walter JH, Leonard JV, Saudubray JM, Halliday D. Protein and leucine metabolism in maple syrup urine disease. *Am J Physiol* 1990; **258**: E654–660.

68. Barshop BA, Yoshida I, Ajami A, Sweetman L, Wolff JA, Sweetman FR, Prodanos C, Smith M, Nyhan WL. Metabolism of 1-^{13}C-propionate in vivo in patients with disorders of propionate metabolism. *Pediatr Res* 1991; **30**: 15–22.

69. Morrison DJ, Zavoshy R, Edwards CA, Dodson B, Preston T, Weaver LT. Lactose [^{13}C]-ureide as a marker for colonic fermentation and the deconvolution of a complex $^{13}CO_2$ breath test curve. *Biochem Soc Trans* 1998; **26**: S184.

70. Morrison DJ, Dodson B, Preston T. Measurement of urinary total ^{13}C and ^{13}C urea by isotope ratio mass spectrometry after administration of lactose [^{13}C]-ureide. *Rapid Commun Mass Spectrom* 1999; **13**: 1252–1256.

71. Christian M, Morrison D, Dodson B, Preston T, Amarri S, Franchini F, Edwards C, Weaver L. Measurement of oro-cecal transit time in young children using lactose [^{13}C]-ureide requires further validation. *J Pediatr Gastroenterol Nutr* 2002; **34**: 570–571; author reply 571.

72. Morrison DJ, Dodson B, Preston T, Weaver LT. Gastrointestinal handling of glycosyl [^{13}C]-ureides. *Eur J Clin Nutr* 2003; **57**: 1017–1024.

73. Coremans G, Geypens B, Vos R, Tack J, Margaritis V, Ghoos Y, Janssens J. Influence of continuous isobaric rectal distension on gastric emptying and small bowel transit in young healthy women. *Neurogastrocntcrol Motil* 2004; **16**: 107–111.

74. Kato H, Nakao A, Kishimoto W, Nonami T, Harada A, Hayakawa T, Takagi H ^{13}C-labeled trioctanoin breath test for exocrine pancreatic function test in patients after pancreatoduodenectomy. *Am J Gastroenterol* 1993; **88**: 64–69.

75. Lembcke B, Braden B, Caspary WF. Exocrine pancreatic insufficiency: accuracy and clinical value of the uniformly labelled ^{13}C-Hiolein breath test. *Gut* 1996; **39**: 668–674.

76. Braden B, Picard H, Caspary WF, Posselt HG, Lembcke B. Monitoring pancroatin supplomontation in cystic fibrosis patients with the ^{13}C-Hiolein breath test: evidence for normalized fat assimilation with high dose pancreatin therapy. *Z Gastroenterol* 1997; **35**: 123–129.

77. Amarri S, Harding M, Coward WA, Evans TJ, Weaver LT. ^{13}Carbon mixed triglyceride breath test and pancreatic enzyme supplementation in cystic fibrosis. *Arch Dis Child* 1997; **76**: 349–351.

78. Thomas A, Super M, Sood M, Hambleton G, Akbar A, Weller P. ^{13}C-Triolein breath test to assess the effect of pancreatic enzyme on intraluminal lipolysis during continues enteral feeds in cystic fibrosis. *Journal of Pediatric Gastroenterology and Nutrition* 1999; **28**: 594.

79. Ventrucci M, Cipolla A, Colaiocco L, Festi D, Middonno M, Papponetti M, Racchini C, Roda A, Russo C. Use of ^{13}C-breath tests in pancreatic exocrine insufficiency: A comparative study. *Gastroenterology* 2000; **118**: AGA A424.

80. van Dijk-van Aalst K, van den Driessche M, van der Schoor S, Schiffelers S, van't Westeinde T, Ghoos Y, Veereman-Wauters G. ^{13}C-mixed triglyceride breath test: A noninvasive method to assess lipase activity in children. *Journal of Pediatric Gastroenterology and Nutrition* 2001; **32**: 579–585.

81. Loser C, Brauer C, Aygen S, Hennemann O, Folsch UR. Comparative clinical evaluation of the ^{13}C-mixed triglyceride breath test as an indirect pancreatic function test. *Scand J Gastroenterol* 1998; **33** (3): 327–334.

82. Sun DY, Jiang YB, Rong L, Jin SJ, Xie WZ. Clinical application of ^{13}C-Hiolein breath test in assessing pancreatic exocrine insufficiency. *Hepatobiliary Pancreat Dis Int* 2003; **2**: 449–452.

83. Watkins JB, Klein PD, Schoeller DA, Kirschner BS, Park R, Perman JA. Diagnosis and differentiation of fat malabsorption in children using ^{13}C-labeled lipids: trioctanoin, triolein, and palmitic acid breath tests. *Gastroenterology* 1982; **82**: 911–917.

84. McClean P, Harding M, Coward WA, Green MR, Weaver LT. Measurement of fat digestion in early life using a stable isotope breath test. *Arch Dis Child* 1993; **69**: 366–370.

85. Bamba T, Chikamochi N, Fuse K, Fujiyama Y, Nakajo S, Hosoda S, Watanabe H, Morikawa J. The clinical usefulness of carbon-13 triolein breath test for the evaluation of malabsorption syndrome. *Radioisotopes* 1993; **42**: 409–412.

86. De Boeck K, Delbeke I, Eggermont E, Veereman-Wauters G, Ghoos Y. Lipid digestion in cystic fibrosis: comparison of conventional and high-lipase enzyme therapy using the mixed-triglyceride breath test. *J Pediatr Gastroenterol Nutr* 1998; **26**: 408–411.

87. Abbas KA, Bilal R, Sajjad MI, Latif Z, Mirza NH. Fat absorption in persistent diarrhoea using ^{13}C-labelled trioctanoin breath test. *J Trop Pediatr* 1999; **45**: 87–94.

88. Janghorbani M, Schuette S, Cohen M. Method for measuring fat digestion and absorption formulation to aid in measuring fat absorption. PAT 1999-12-28 06006754.

89. Ritz MA, Fraser RJ, Di Matteo AC, Greville H, Butler R, Cmielewski P, Davidson G. Evaluation of the ^{13}C-triolein breath test for fat malabsorption in adult patients with cystic fibrosis. *J Gastroenterol Hepatol* 2004; **19**: 448–453.

90. Beaufrere B, Putet G, Pachiaudi C, Salle B. Whole body protein turnover measured with ^{13}C-leucine and energy expenditure in preterm infants. *Pediatr Res* 1990; **28**: 147–152.

91. Ghoos Y, Rutgeerts P, Vantrappen G. [13]CO_2-breath tests in nutritional diagnosis: present applications and future possibilities. In: Dietze GJ, Grünert A, Kleinberger G, Wolfram G, eds. *Clinical Nutrition and Metabolic Research*, Basel: Karger, 1985: 192–207.

92. Garlick P, McNurlan A, Essen P, Wernerman J. Measurement of tissue protein synthesis rates in vivo: a critical analysis of contrasting methods. *Am J Physiol* 1994; **266**: E287–297.

93. Lu Z, Zhang R, Diasio RB. Dihydropyrimidine dehydrogenase activity in human peripheral blood mononuclear cells and liver: population characteristics, newly identified deficient patients, and clinical implication in 5-fluorouracil chemotherapy. *Cancer Res* 1993; **53**: 5433–5438.

94. Lu Z, Zhang R, Carpenter JT, Diasio RB. Decreased dihydropyrimidine dehydrogenase activity in a population of patients with breast cancer: implication for 5-fluorouracil-based chemotherapy. *Clin Cancer Res* 1998; **4**: 325–329.

95. Etienne MC, Lagrange JL, Dassonville O, Fleming R, Thyss A, Renee N, Schneider M, Demard F, Milano G. Population study of dihydropyrimidine dehydrogenase in cancer patients. *J Clin Oncol* 1994; **12**: 2248–2253.

96. Mattison LK, Ezzeldin H, Carpenter M, Modak A, Johnson MR, Diasio RB. Rapid identification of dihydropyrimidine dehydrogenase deficiency by using a novel 2-^{13}C-uracil breath test. *Clin Cancer Res* 2004; **10**: 2652–2658.

97. Ezzeldin H, Diasio R. Dihydropyrimidine dehydrogenase deficiency, a pharmacogenetic syndrome associated with potentially life-threatening toxicity following 5-fluorouracil administration. *Clin Colorectal Cancer* 2004; **4**: 181–189.

98. Mattison L, Johnson M, Saif W, Modak A, Hirao Y, Koga T, Shimizu T, Diasio R. Validation of a novel $[2$-$^{13}C]$-uracil breath test (UraBT) to detect dihydropyrimidine dehydrogenase (DPD) deficiency by LC-MS-MS analysis of $[2$-$^{13}C]$-uracil (URA) and $[2$-$^{13}C]$-dihydrouracil (DHU) plasma levels. *Journal of Clinical Oncology* 2004; **22** (14S): 2130.

99. Bjorkman DJ, Moore JG, Klein PD, Graham DY. ^{13}C-bicarbonate breath test as a measure of gastric emptying. *Am J Gastroenterol* 1991; **86**: 821–823.

100. Bresson JL, Mariotti A, Narcy P, Ricour C, Sachs C, Rey J. Recovery of $[^{13}C]$-bicarbonate as respiratory $^{13}CO_2$ in parenterally fed infants. *Eur J Clin Nutr* 1990; **44**: 3–9.

101. Leigh Richards M, Davies PS. Energy cost of activity assessed by indirect calorimetry and a $^{13}CO_2$ breath test. *Med Sci Sports Exerc* 2001; **33**: 834–838.

102. Shew SB, Beckett PR, Keshen TH, Jahoor F, Jaksic T. Validation of a $[^{13}C]$-bicarbonate tracer technique to measure neonatal energy expenditure. *Pediatr Res* 2000; **47**: 787–791.

103. Horswill C, Zipf W, Kien C. Measuring energy costs of leisure activity in adolescents using a $^{13}CO_2$ breath test. *Med SciSports Exerc* 1997; **29**: 1263–1268.

104. Benzo R, Modak A, Kurogi Y. A non-invasive bicarbonate breath test (BBT) to rapidly evaluate arterial paCO$_2$. *Eur Respiratory J* 2004; **24** (Suppl 48): P2081.

105. Lazarou J, Pomeranz BH, Corey PN. Incidence of adverse drug reactions in hospitalized patients: a meta analysis of prospective studies. *Jama* 1998; **279**: 1200–1205.

106. Phillips KA, Veenstra DL, Oren E, Lee JK, Sadee W. Potential role of pharmacogenomics in reducing adverse drug reactions: a systematic review. *Jama* 2001; **286**: 2270–2279.

107. Swart GR, van den Berg JW. ^{13}C breath test in gastroenterological practice. *Scand J Gastroenterol Suppl* 1998; **225**: 13–18.

108. de Meer K, Roof MJ, Kulik W, Jakobs C. In vivo research with stable isotopes in biochemistry, nutrition and clinical medicine: an overview. *Isotopes Environ Health Stud* 1999; **35**: 19–37.

109. Klein PD. ^{13}C breath tests: visions and realities. *J Nutr* 2001; **131**: 1637S–1642S.

110. Bodamer OA, Halliday D. Uses of stable isotopes in clinical diagnosis and research in the paediatric population. *Arch Dis Child* 2001; **84**: 444–448.

111. Kurpad AV, Ajami A, Young VR. ^{13}C breath tests in infections and beyond. *Food Nutr Bull* 2002; **23**: 21–29.

112. Fischer H, Wetzel K. The future of ^{13}C-breath tests. *Food Nutr Bull* 2002; **23**: 53–56.

113. Ghoos Y, Geypens B, Rutgeerts P. Stable isotopes and ^{13}CO$_2$ breath tests for investigating gastrointestinal functions. *Food Nutr Bull* 2002; **23**: 166–168.

114. Wyse CA, Preston T, Yam PS, Sutton DG, Christley RM, Hotchkiss JW, Mills CA, Glidle A, Cumming DR, Cooper JM, Love S. Current and future uses of breath analysis as a diagnostic tool. *Vet Rec* 2004; **154**: 353–360.

THE COMBINED USE OF SIFT-MS AND FA-MS TO INVESTIGATE FIRST-PASS METABOLISM OF ETHANOL

T. S. WANG

Institute of Science and Technology in Medicine,
Medical School, Keele University,
Thornburrow Drive, Hartshill, Stoke-on-Trent, ST4 7QB, UK

P. ŠPANĚL

V. Čermák Laboratory, J. Heyrovský Institute of Physical Chemistry,
Academy of Sciences of the Czech Republic,
Dolejškova 3, CZ-182 23 Prague 8, Czech Republic

D. SMITH

Institute of Science and Technology in Medicine,
Medical School, Keele University,
Thornburrow Drive, Hartshill, Stoke-on-Trent, ST4 7QB, UK

1. Introduction

A large amount of research has been carried out into the nature of ethanol in the human body, work driven to a large extent by clinical and legal implications. As is well known, when ethanol (alcohol) is ingested in excess and over the long term it is poisonous and is destructive to the liver. At any dosage, it can affect judgement and reaction time. Above a certain limit, ethanol can be detected in exhaled breath and this phenomenon is exploited by law enforcement agencies at the street side using so-called breathalysers.[1] Legal limits are set for acceptable levels of ethanol in the breath and blood of drivers; currently in the UK this limit in blood is set at 80 mg of ethanol in 100 ml of blood,[2] which is equivalent to a partial pressure in exhaled breath of 180 parts-per-million, ppm[3,4] (this is discussed further in Section 5). This is massively greater than the ethanol level in breath resulting from endogenous processes (principally produced by the action of gut bacteria on carbohydrates),[5] these being typically within the range of 0.01–1.0 ppm for healthy persons.[5,6] Quite sophisticated analytical devices are required to detect breath ethanol at these levels, such as our selected ion flow tube mass spectrometer, SIFT-MS, instrument which will briefly be described later.

Almost all the studies of ethanol metabolism have been carried out by monitoring venous blood levels with time following either oral or intravenous administration.[7] We have shown recently,[8] and we emphasise below, that using our SIFT-MS analytical method single breath exhalations can be analysed for ethanol, and indeed several other metabolites simultaneously, thus providing data from which accurate decay rates of breath ethanol can be determined. What is very clear from many studies is that (following oral ingestion) the speed of absorption of ethanol from the stomach and gut depends on time of day, drinking pattern, dosage and concentration of ethanol in the drink, and particularly the feeding or fasting state of the individual.[5] It is also clear that at high doses the rate of metabolism is zeroth-order, *i.e.* conforms to saturation kinetics, whereas at low doses this rate is first-order (unsaturated).[7]

There is much interest in so-called first-pass metabolism of ethanol (by the liver via the portal vein and partially also within the gastric system).[7] The contribution of this process is commonly estimated from the difference in the area under the ethanol blood concentration time curves obtained following oral and intravenous administration of ethanol, but it is not fully appreciated that this technique provides an accurate indicator of first-pass metabolism only when the clearance of the compound under consideration obeys first-order (unsaturated) kinetics throughout the range of blood concentrations observed.[7] Thus, following the comments in the previous paragraph, it follows that studies of first-pass metabolism should ideally be carried out at low ethanol concentrations. Better still, it is desirable that first-order kinetics should be seen to be occurring during the experiment. This can be checked using SIFT-MS breath analyses, as we show later. However, first-pass metabolism remains difficult to assess because of the dose and time factors mentioned above. Ethanol is transported by the bloodstream to all parts of the body and the rate of equilibration within the body is governed by the blood flow rate and the total body water (TBW) in which it readily dissolves; note that ethanol has low solubility in lipids and does not bind to plasma proteins.[9] It has been shown that TBW is very varied amongst individuals and is correlated with gender and age (greater in men than women; greater in the old).[10] These findings have been confirmed by experiments carried out using the recently developed flowing afterglow mass spectrometry, FA-MS, technique, which allows on-line, real time determination of TBW using non-invasive breath analysis[11,12] (see also Ref. 14, on page 439 of this book). If the TBW of a subject is known, this can only help to elucidate the course of ethanol metabolism. The bulk of ethanol ingested (more than 95 %) is metabolised (oxidised) and the remainder is excreted in breath, urine and sweat.[9] The rate-limiting step in oxidation is the conversion of ethanol into acetaldehyde by cytosolic alcohol dehydrogenase, which quickly becomes saturated at high ethanol doses. This enzyme also displays polymorphism, which accounts for racial and ethnic variations in ethanol pharmacokinetics.[9] Clearly, many factors influence the rate of ethanol metabolism and so the study design can seriously bias the results obtained.

In this short chapter, it is shown how the SIFT-MS and the FA-MS techniques are applied jointly to study the complex physiological problem that is ethanol metabolism, SIFT-MS providing high temporal resolution measurements of breath ethanol concentration and FA-MS providing measurements of TBW.

2. The SIFT-MS and FA-MS Techniques

These novel experimental techniques are described in details elsewhere in this book (see the chapters by Smith and Španěl[13] on page 3 and by Španěl and Smith[14] on page 439) and in several other key papers.[11,12,15−17] Thus, it is only necessary here to state the principles on which they are based.

2.1. *SIFT-MS*

Selected ion flow tube mass spectrometry involves the chemical ionisation, using selected precursor positive ions, of the trace gases in an air/breath sample that is introduced into a flow tube. The details of this technique and examples of its many applications in medicine and other areas are given in the SIFT-MS chapter[13] in this book on page 3 and the several references therein. In brief, in the present experiments, H_3O^+ ions were injected into fast flowing helium carrier gas in the flow tube. Then directly exhaled breath displaced the ambient air at the entrance to an open port and thus breath was sampled and entered the carrier gas/H_3O^+ ion swarm via a heated calibrated capillary. The essential point is that single breath exhalations are analysed, on-line and in real time, for several chosen trace gases simultaneously, obviating sample collection into bags or onto traps and all the potential problems such procedures can incur. Thus, accurate analyses can be carried out with exceptional time resolution, if necessary in successive exhalations of a few seconds. Also, the wide dynamic range of the SIFT-MS analytical method allows the variations of trace gas concentrations in air and breath to be followed over orders-of-magnitude, which allows physiological phenomenon to be studied with greater confidence.

2.2. *FA-MS*

Detailed discussions of this technique and its applications are given in the chapter on FA-MS[14] in this book on page 439 and the references therein, so here it is pertinent only to outline the fundamental principles involved. When water vapour, say that in a sample of exhaled breath, is introduced into helium carrier gas containing H_3O^+ precursor ions, the HDO molecules in the breath water and the predominant H_2O molecules undergo clustering reactions forming the isotopomer ions $H_3O^+(H_2O)_3$, $H_3O^+(H_2O)_2(HDO)$ and $H_3O^+(H_2O)_2(H_2{}^{18}O)$ at mass-to-charge ratios, m/z, of 73, 74 and 75, respectively. Hence, the signal levels of these ions can be used to determine the D/H ratio in the molecules of the water vapour sample. The essential point here is that using FA-MS the deuterium content of breath water vapour can be obtained following the ingestion of a known quantity of D_2O (which rapidly becomes HDO in an excess of water), again in real time in single breath exhalations with excellent temporal resolution. Thus, the dispersal of water (HDO) throughout the body compartments can be tracked in time. Then, following the principle of isotope dilution, the deuterium content of breath after the HDO is fully equilibrated with the blood/body water provides a value of the TBW. The blood deuterium abundances, $R_{1\,\mathrm{liq}}$, can be obtained directly from the deuterium abundance levels measured in the breath water vapour, R_{vap} using the known partition coefficient of HDO above H_2O at the appropriate temperature.[18]

3. Experimental Protocol for These Studies

Healthy volunteers were recruited for these studies.[19] Their body weights were routinely obtained and the body mass indices were calculated (BMI = (weight in kg)/(height in m)^2).

Small amounts of ethanol were ingested in proportion to body weight, typically at a dose equivalent to about 60 mg/kg body weight. The ethanol dose was diluted in about 300 mL of water before drinking. Exhaled breath ethanol was measured in single breath exhalations using SIFT-MS in real time every two-to-three minutes, typically over a period of about two hours. Additionally, some chosen breath metabolites were measured simultaneously, including acetaldehyde, ammonia and acetone, the last two compounds being indicators of nutritional status.[20]

A standard approach was also taken to the FA-MS measurements in that measured quantities of D_2O in proportion to the body weight, typically at a dose level of 0.3 g/kg body weight, were diluted in about 200 mL of drinking water before drinking. The deuterium content of the breath water vapour in single breath exhalations was determined using FA-MS, again over a period of some two hours. In both the SIFT-MS and FA-MS experiments, a few measurements were taken just before the ingestion of the ethanol and the D_2O, establishing the so-called base line or predose levels of ethanol and HDO.

4. Sample Results

In this short report chapter we present the results obtained for a single individual (male, body weight 60 kg, BMI 22) simply to demonstrate how a coordinated SIFT-MS and FA-MS study of ethanol dispersal/metabolism and water dispersal throughout the body allows the fraction of the ingested ethanol that is first-pass metabolised to be obtained.

4.1. *Ethanol Dispersal and Metabolism*

The typical time variations of the breath ethanol, acetaldehyde and ammonia after ingestion of 5 mL of ethanol are shown in Fig. 1. Also shown are the predose breath levels of these species. The breath ethanol level is relatively high immediately after ingestion due to unavoidable mouth/saliva contamination during drinking. This contamination then diminishes and a clear minimum in the breath ethanol is reached following which it increase towards a maxima value as the ethanol passes from the stomach, into the small intestine and then into the blood stream when it is immediately seen in the exhaled breath. Finally, the blood/ breath ethanol decreases due to the combination of dispersal and dilution into the TBW and metabolism. Actually, these processes occur together as the breath ethanol maximum is approached and is passed, but at later times metabolism dominates the loss of ethanol from the blood/breath and a near-exponential decay results with a time constant, τ, of 20.7 minutes in this example (see Fig. 1). This indicates that first-order (unsaturated) kinetics dominates, which means that first pass metabolism can be properly investigated at these low ethanol doses. This phenomenon will be examined later after the TBW (FA-MS) data have been discussed. Note that the previous SIFT-MS experiments[8] showed at an ethanol dose some 3 times greater that ethanol loss is better described by zero-order (saturated) kinetics. (At an ethanol dose about 3 times smaller, the ethanol was very rapidly removed, which we now understand — following the present study — is due to first-pass metabolism effectively removing the entire amount of ethanol). It can be seen in Fig. 1 that the physiological (pre-ingestion) ethanol level is re-established after about 2 hours. Note, also, that the acetaldehyde level tracks the ethanol level, as expected, with a short time lag.[21,22]

A further observation that demonstrates the extraordinary value of the SIFT-MS technique is the simultaneous observation of breath ammonia, as is also shown in Fig. 1. Ammonia is present in the breath of all healthy individuals, typically in the partial pressure range from 200 to 2000 ppb.[6] SIFT-MS experiments have shown that breath ammonia levels "dip" immediately after the ingestion of protein and carbohydrate meals following overnight starvation.[20] This phenomenon also occurs when the ethanol aqueous solution used in these experiments is ingested, as can be seen in Fig. 1. This is surely due to the stimulation of the portal blood flow and the enhanced removal of ammonia by the liver. Note that the minimum in the

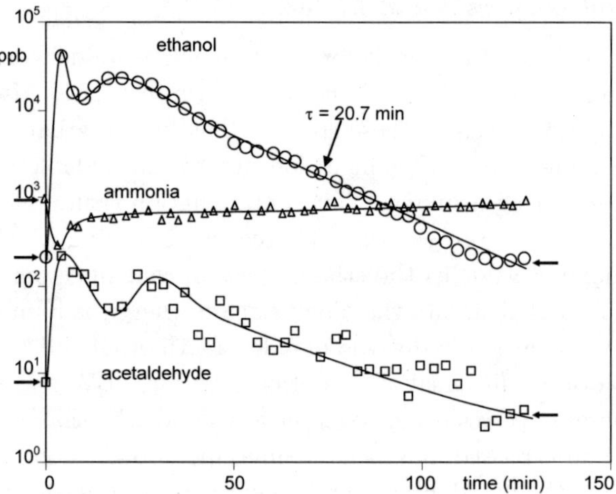

Fig. 1.   Time variations of the breath levels in parts-per-billion, ppb, of ethanol, acetaldehyde and ammonia after ingestion of the ethanol/water solution. The amount of ethanol ingested was 5 mL (0.067g/kg body weight). The time constant for the rate of ethanol metabolism, τ, at the later times is 20.7 min. The physiological (predose ethanol) levels of these compounds are indicated by the continuous arrows both at the start and end of the measurement period.

ammonia level occurs measurably earlier than that for the ethanol. This is probably because the stimulation of the portal blood flow is a rapid reflex reaction following which ammonia clearance is rapidly enhanced, whereas clearance of ethanol from the mouth relies on the slower process of saliva recycling. The ammonia level then relaxes back to the initial state when the portal blood flow normalises and a steady state is re-established in ammonia production and loss. A detailed discussion of the early metabolism of ingested material, including ethanol, must surely take this phenomenon into consideration.

4.2. *HDO Dispersal and TBW*

A plot of the time variations of the increase of blood deuterium abundances above the pre-dose value, $\Delta R_{1\,\mathrm{liq}}$ (as measured from the breath values, $\Delta R_{1\,\mathrm{vap}}$) after drinking the D_2O/water mixture containing 17 mL of D_2O is shown in Fig. 2 for the same subject. The initial high value of the breath deuterium is again due to the inevitable mouth contamination. A distinct minimum then occurs followed by a maximum and then an asymptotically decrease towards an equilibrium value as the HDO equilibrates with the TBW. The time required to reach the equilibrium value is about 90 minutes, since the time constant for the exponential approach to the asymptotic level is typically 20 minutes.[12]

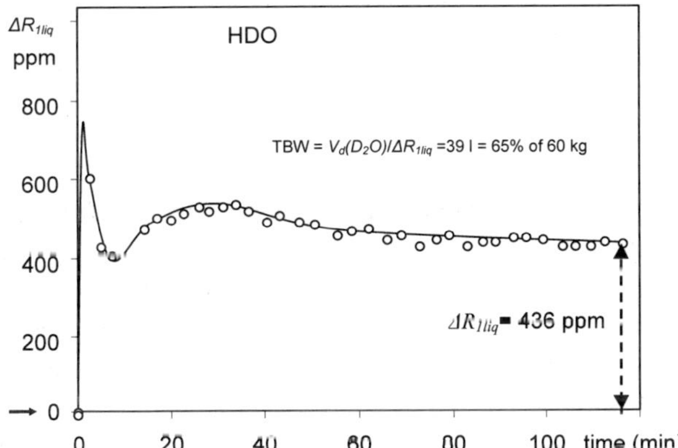

Fig. 2. Time variation of the increase of the blood deuterium abundances above the initial baseline, $\Delta R_{1\,\mathrm{liq}}$, in parts-per-million, ppm, determined after ingestion of 17 mL D_2O (about 0.283 g/kg body weight) by breath analysis using FA-MS. The equilibrium level reached at late times, $\Delta R_{1\,\mathrm{liq}}$, is used to derive the total body water, TBW, as indicated (see the text also).

The equilibrium value of $\Delta R_{1\,\mathrm{liq}}$, coupled with the known dose of D_2O, $V_\mathrm{d}(D_2O)$ [mL], provides a value for the TBW [mL] $= (V_\mathrm{d}(D_2O)/\Delta R_{1\,\mathrm{liq}})$, which is given in Fig. 2. The ratio of the derived TBW (39 litres) to the body mass (60 kg) indicates that the percentage of the body that is water for this individual is 65%. This value is within the range that has been derived by previous isotope dilution experiments[23] and our previous FA-MS experiments[12] for a male individual with a low BMI.

5. Discussion

The combined SIFT-MS and FA-MS data can be used to separately estimate the degree of ethanol metabolism, firstly during its first-pass transport from the stomach into the body fluids and, secondly, during its circulation in the blood stream and the dispersion into the body water.

In order to facilitate discussion of dispersion of the orally-ingested substances into the TBW, it is important to relate the measured breath levels to blood levels. This is a routine calculation for HDO.[10,11,18] For ethanol, an appropriate partition ratio relating the blood concentration to the breath concentration has to be applied.[3,4] This ratio is well established for ethanol due to its forensic importance and has been discussed in numerous publications.[2-4] Thus, a concentration of 177 ppm of ethanol in exhaled breath corresponds to a blood concentration of 1 mL per litre.[3] The time-dependent blood levels, $R(t)$, expressed as dimensionless volume mixing ratios are related to the breath levels as:

$$R(t) = \frac{C(t)}{K} \tag{1}$$

The $C(t)$ are the measured time-dependent breath concentrations, (in ppm for HDO and ppb for ethanol), K are the dimensionless partition coefficients between blood and breath (10^6 ppm for HDO and 1.77×10^8 ppb for ethanol). The breath concentrations are corrected for their respective baseline (predose) values, C_b, to obtain $\Delta R(t)$, which are normalised to the notional equilibrium concentration $R_\mathrm{d} = V_\mathrm{d}/V_\mathrm{TBW}$ that would be observed in breath if the volume of the ingested dose, V_d, was ideally diluted in the total body water of volume V_TBW (39 litres for the present subject) without any metabolism taking place, as:

$$\frac{\Delta R(t)}{R_\mathrm{d}} = \frac{C(t) - C_\mathrm{b}}{K} \cdot \frac{V_\mathrm{TBW}}{V_\mathrm{d}} \tag{2}$$

Equation (2) represents a simple linear transformation of the data, which does not change the shape of the time dependencies but allows direct comparison of dimensionless quantities for the two different ingested substances.

The $\Delta R(t)/R_\mathrm{d}$ values for the present subject for HDO and ethanol are shown as semi-logarithmic plots in Fig. 3. Note that the $\Delta R(t)/R_\mathrm{d}$ values of HDO acquire peak values above 1.0 and then asymptotically converge to 1.0 as the entire ingested dose is distributed throughout the TBW. However, the $\Delta R(t)/R_\mathrm{d}$ value for ethanol never exceeds 1.0. The ratios of the HDO and ethanol values at each time $(\Delta R_{\mathrm{ethanol}}(t)/R_{\mathrm{d\,ethanol}})/(\Delta R_{\mathrm{HDO}}(t)/R_{\mathrm{d\,HDO}})$, as read from the semi-logarithmic plot) correspond to the fraction of ethanol that has been metabolised at that time. This is based on the assumption that the ethanol dispersal rate into the blood/TBW is the same as or very similar to that of HDO,[5] an assumption that is reasonable only for times later than 10 minutes after ingestion, because at very early times the effects of mouth contamination from the ingested ethanol and D_2O are dominant and there will be some variation in the speeds of the gastric emptying processes.[1,24]

The $(\Delta R_{\mathrm{ethanol}}(t)/R_{\mathrm{d\,ethanol}})/(\Delta R_{\mathrm{HDO}}(t)/R_{\mathrm{d\,HDO}})$ value calculated for the time t corresponding to the maximum in the breath ethanol (see Fig. 3) thus provides the fraction of ethanol that is metabolised during the first-pass metabolism.[7]. This ratio is 0.7 for the present subject and so 30 % of the ingested ethanol (5 mL) has been metabolized during the first 20 min, *i.e.* before it has fully mixed with the blood circulation. Note it is very likely that if much larger doses of ethanol were used, the fractions metabolised

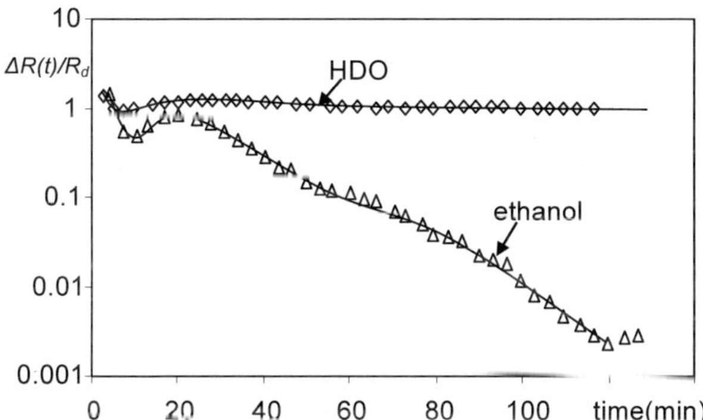

Fig. 3.   Semi-logarithmic plots of the dependence of $\Delta R(t)/R_\mathrm{d}$, the normalised blood levels of HDO and ethanol, as a function of time (see text and Eq. (2))

by the first-pass metabolism in the gut and liver would be smaller due to enzyme saturation.[7]

6. Concluding Remarks

The unique combination of SIFT-MS and FA-MS to study, via non-invasive breath analysis, the dispersal of ethanol and its metabolism and the dispersal of water throughout the body is providing more accurate data on these physiological phenomena. On-line breath analysis provides accurate data with good time resolution. Total body water can be measured easily by FA-MS, and knowing this important parameter the first-pass metabolism of ethanol can be reliably investigated using SIFT-MS following ethanol ingestion. The later time breath measurements indicate an exponential loss of ethanol from the body at a time constant that is well defined due to the multiple point decay curve that can easily be obtained by breath analysis and the wide range of concentrations that can be accessed using SIFT-MS. There is a clear need for multi-compartment models to thoroughly describe the dispersal and metabolism of ethanol. Breath analysis using the SIFT-MS and FA-MS techniques, individually and in combination, is ideally suitable to provide sufficiently accurate data for such modelling. The provision of such data relating to normal and abnormal physiology (diseased states), might improve clinical assessment and lead to more appropriate treatment.

Acknowledgements

We are grateful to Edward Hall for his help with the experimental work. We gratefully acknowledge financial support by the North Staffordshire Medical Institute.

References

1. Holt S, Stewart MJ, Adam RD, Heading RC. Alcohol absorption, gastric emptying and a breathalyser. *Br J Clin Pharmacol* 1980; **9**: 205–208.
2. National Highway Traffic Safety Administration. *Setting limits, saving lives — the case for .08 BAC laws.* DOT HS 809 241. Washington DC, U.S. Department of Transportation, 2001.
3. Španěl P, Diskin A, Abbott S, Wang TS, Smith D. Quantification of volatile compounds in the headspace of aqueous liquids using selected ion flow tube mass spectrometry. *Rapid Commun Mass Spectrom* 2002; **16**: 2148–2153.
4. Wilson PF, Freeman CG, McEwan MJ, Milligan DB, Allardyce RA, Shaw GM. Alcohol in breath and blood: a selected ion flow tube mass spectrometric study. *Rapid Commun Mass Spectrom* 2001; **15**: 413–417.

5. Owades J. Alcoholic Beverages and Human Responses. In: Francis F, ed. *Wiley Encyclopedia of Food Science and Technology* (2nd Edition), New York: John Wiley & Sons, 2000.

6. Diskin AM, Španěl P, Smith D. Time variation of ammonia, acetone, isoprene and ethanol in breath: a quantitative SIFT-MS study over 30 days. *Physiol Meas* 2003; **24**: 107–119.

7. Levitt MD, Levitt DG. Appropriate use and misuse of blood concentration measurements to quantitate first-pass metabolism. *J Lab Clin Med* 2000; **136**: 275–280.

8. Smith D, Wang TS, Španěl P. On-line, simultaneous quantification of ethanol, some metabolites and water vapour in breath following the ingestion of alcohol. *Physiol Meas* 2002; **23**: 477–489.

9. Norberg A, Jones AW, Hahn RG, Gabrielsson JL. Role of variability in explaining ethanol pharmacokinetics: research and forensic applications. *Clin Pharmacokinet* 2003; **42**: 1–31.

10. Chumlea WC, Guo SS, Zeller CM, Reo NV, Baumgartner RN, Garry PJ, Wang J, Pierson RN, Jr., Heymsfield SB, Siervogel RM. Total body water reference values and prediction equations for adults. *Kidney Int* 2001; **59**: 2250–2258.

11. Smith D, Španěl P. On-line determination of the deuterium abundance in breath water vapour by flowing afterglow mass spectrometry with applications to measurements of total body water. *Rapid Commun Mass Spectrom* 2001; **15**: 25–32.

12. Davies S, Španěl P, Smith D. Rapid measurement of deuterium content of breath following oral ingestion to determine body water. *Physiol Meas* 2001; **22**: 651–659.

13. Smith D, Španěl P. Selected ion flow tube mass spectrometry, SIFT-MS, for on-line trace gas analysis of breath. In: Amann A, Smith D, eds. *Breath Analysis for Clinical Diagnosis and Therapeutic Monitoring,* Singapore: World Scientific, 2005.

14. Španěl P, Smith D. Flowing afterglow mass spectrometry (FA-MS) for the determination of the deuterium abundance in breath water vapour and aqueous liquid headspace. In: Amann A, Smith D, eds. *Breath Analysis for Clinical Diagnosis and Therapeutic Monitoring,* Singapore: World Scientific, 2005.

15. Španěl P, Smith D. Selected ion flow tube mass spectrometry: detection and real-time monitoring of flavours released by food products. *Rapid Commun Mass Spectrom* 1999; **13**: 585–597.

16. Smith D, Španěl P, Thompson J, Rajan B, Cocker J, Rolfe P. The selected ion flow tube method for workplace analysis of trace gases in air and breath: its scope validation and applications. *Appl Occup Environ Hygiene* 1998; **13**: 817–823.

17. Španěl P, Smith D. Quantitative selected ion flow tube mass spectrometry: the influence of ionic diffusion and mass discrimination. *J Am Mass Spectrom Soc* 2001; **12**: 863–872.

18. Španěl P, Smith D. Selected Ion Flow Tube Mass Spectrometry (SIFT-MS) and Flowing Afterglow Mass Spectrometry (FA-MS) for the Determination of

the Deuterium Abundance in Water Vapour. In: de Groot P, ed. *Handbook of Stable Isotope Analytical Techniques* (Volume I), Amsterdam: Elsevier, 2004.

19. Španěl P, Wang TS, Smith D. Coordinated FA-MS and SIFT-MS analyses of breath following ingestion of D_2O and ethanol; total body water, dispersal kinetics and ethanol metabolism. *Physiol Meas* 2005: in press.

20. Smith D, Španěl P, Davies S. Trace gases in breath of healthy volunteers when fasting and after a protein-calorie meal: a preliminary study. *J Appl Physiol* 1999; **87**: 1584–1588.

21. Lieber CS. Alcohol, liver, and nutrition. *J Am Coll Nutr* 1991; **10**: 602–632.

22. Jones AW. Measuring and reporting the concentration of acetaldehyde in human breath. *Alcohol Alcohol* 1995; **30**: 271–285.

23. Schoeller DA, van Santen E, Peterson DW, Dietz W, Jaspan J, Klein PD. Total body water measurement in humans with ^{18}O and ^2H labeled water. *Am J Clin Nutr* 1980; **33**: 2686–2693.

24. Jones AW, Jonsson KA, Neri A. Peak blood-ethanol concentration and the time of its occurrence after rapid drinking on an empty stomach. *J Forensic Sci* 1991; **36**: 376-385.

PART F

ANIMAL STUDIES

BREATH ANALYSIS: TAKING THE NEEDLE OUT OF VETERINARY DIAGNOSTICS?

C. A. WYSE

Division of Companion Animal Science, Institute of Comparative Medicine,
University of Glasgow, Glasgow, G61 1QH, UK

K. D. SKELDON

Department of Physics and Astronomy,
University of Glasgow, Glasgow, G12 8QQ, UK

A. J. CATHCART

School of Sport and Exercise Sciences,
University of Leeds, Leeds, LS2 9JT, UK

R. SUTHERLAND

Centre for Exercise Science and Medicine, Institute of Biomedical and Life Sciences,
University of Glasgow, Glasgow, G12 8QQ, UK

S. A. WARD

School of Sport and Exercise Sciences,
University of Leeds, Leeds, LS2 9JT, UK

G. GIBSON

Department of Physics and Astronomy,
University of Glasgow, Glasgow, G12 8QQ, UK

L. C. MCMILLAN

Division of Community Health Sciences,
University of Dundee, Dundee, DD2 4BF, UK

M. J. PADGETT

Department of Physics and Astronomy,
University of Glasgow, Glasgow, G12 8QQ, UK

T. PRESTON

Scottish Universities Environmental Research Centre,
East Kilbride, G75 0QF, UK

P. S. YAM AND S. LOVE

Division of Companion Animal Science, Institute of Comparative Medicine,
University of Glasgow, Glasgow, G61 1QH, UK

1. Introduction

The non-invasive nature of the breath test makes this a particularly attractive investigative method for application in veterinary medicine and research. Veterinary research in this area has focused on development of breath tests for assessment of (i) gastrointestinal function, (ii) respiratory inflammation and (iii) oxidative stress in animals. Breath tests are very well accepted by animals and by their owners or trainers, and are ideal methods for screening or monitoring of disease. Because the collection of breath is non-invasive, research studies can often be performed on volunteer animals, without requiring the use of experimental animals. This is an important advantage of breath analysis, as reduction of the number of animals required for experimentation is a goal towards which the scientific community is striving.

Orthodox veterinary investigative methods often induce stress in animals, and activation of the hypothalamic-pituitary-adrenal axis with consequent production of catecholamines and cortisol, may affect the physiological parameters under investigation. In contrast, breath tests are asso-

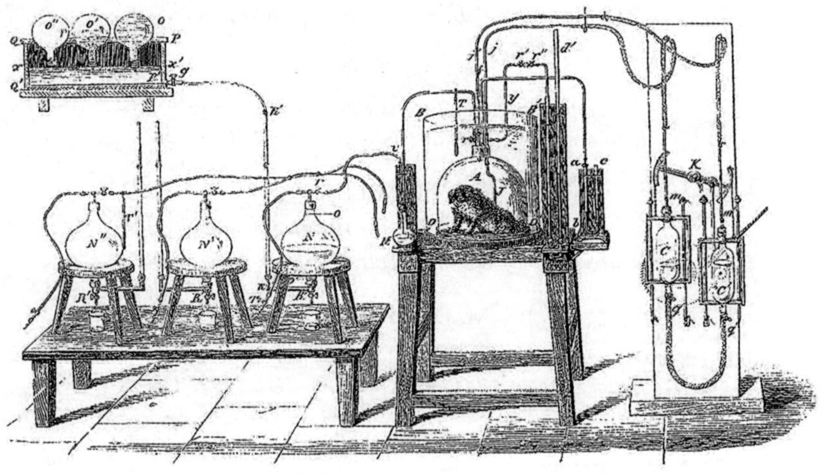

Fig. 1. Breath collection from a dog in the 19th century. This apparatus was developed by French scientists Henri Victor Regnault and Jules Reiset, for studies of respiration in animals. (Picture from Élie de Cyon, *Atlas zur Methodik der physiologischen Experimente und Vivisectionen*, Giessen, St. Petersburg: Carl Ricker, 1876. Reproduced with permission from digitised format at `vlp.mpiwg-berlin.mpg.de`)

ciated with minimal stress and thus facilitate assessment of physiological parameters under basal conditions.

Breath analysis is a rapidly expanding area of veterinary diagnostics, and there are now around 100 peer-reviewed publications in this area. The aim of this brief review is to summarise the work that has been carried out to date and to identify areas requiring further research.

2. Breath Collection Methods in Animals

The first description of breath analysis in a domestic animal can probably be attributed to the French scientists Henri Victor Regnault and Jules Reiset, in their studies of respiration in the late 19th century (Figure 1). Today, breath samples are generally collected from horses and dogs using a face-mask attached to a non-rebreathing valve and a breath collection bag (Figure 2). Breath samples can be collected from smaller animals, such as cats, rodents and birds, by placing the animal in a sealed breath collection chamber until the concentrations of the specific analyte of interest reach detectable levels. Breath is easily collected from anaesthetised animals directly through the endotrachael tube. Issues concerning the effect of respiratory rate or the portion of the exhaled breath collected have been largely ignored in veterinary medicine. Manipulation of the respiratory pattern is more difficult in animals than in cooperative human subjects; nevertheless, methods for collection of specific portions of the exhaled breath in animals require development. Methods for collection of exhaled breath condensate (EBC) have been described in horses,[1,2] dogs[3,4] and calves.[5] The relatively

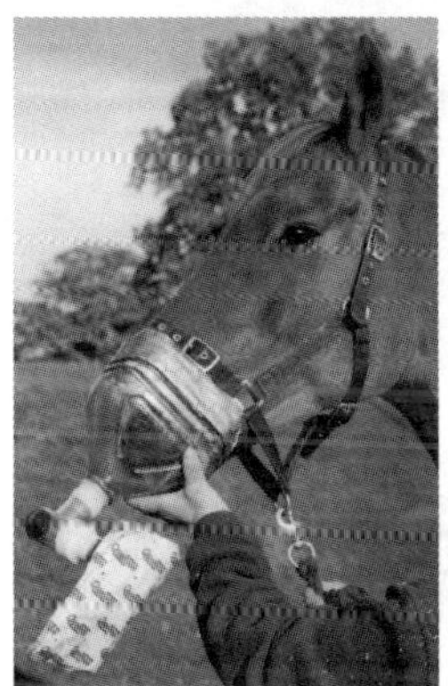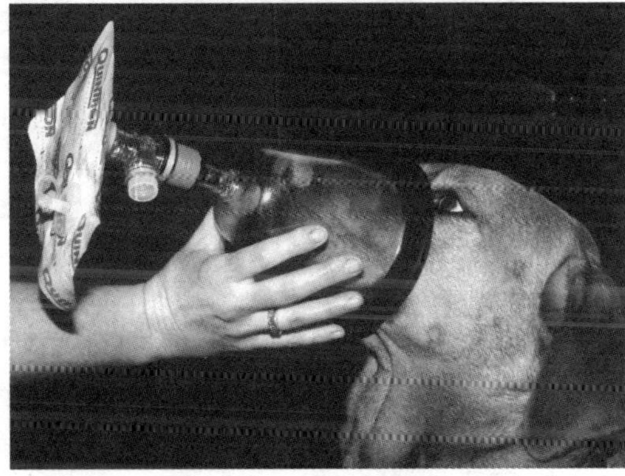

Fig. 2.   Collection of breath samples from a horse and a dog

large ventilation of the horse (approx. 65 litres/min) means that large volumes of condensate can be collected in short periods of time. The horse is an obligate nose breather, and upper respiratory tract secretions are likely to contribute significantly to the concentration of analytes in EBC. For this reason, the application of EBC tests in horses and in dogs may not be directly comparable to human medicine, where EBC is generally collected during mouth breathing.

3. Breath Analysis Techniques

Gas chromatography and mass spectrometry techniques are perhaps most commonly applied for analysis of animal breath, although electrochemical detection systems have been applied for analysis of exhaled carbon monoxide and hydrogen. The recent availability of highly sensitive laser spectroscopy methods has permitted real-time and rapid detection of ethane in exhaled breath (Figure 3). Sensor microarrays or "electronic nose" technology has also been applied for analysis of exhaled breath in cattle.[6] Advances in gas analysis technology will facilitate real-time and rapid analysis of exhaled breath, and consequently increased clinical application of breath tests in veterinary medicine. Sensitive analytical techniques are required for detection of the low concentrations of analytes in EBC in animals. The application of spectrophotometric techniques[1,2] and immunological assays[3,5] has been described.

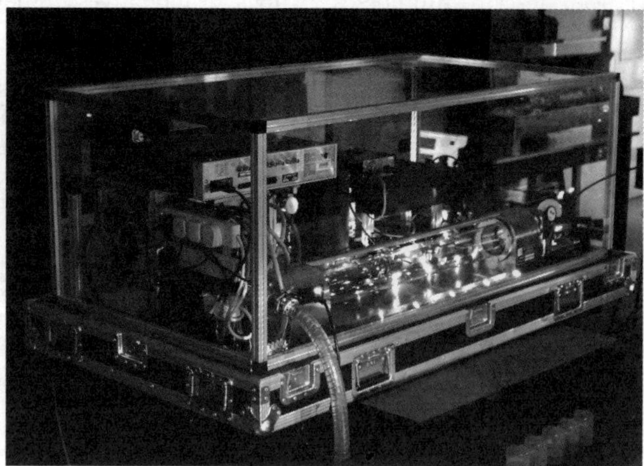

Fig. 3.   Laser spectroscopy facilitates rapid and sensitive detection of analytes in breath.

3.1. *Stable Isotope Breath Tests*

The stable isotope breath tests involve monitoring breath $^{13}CO_2$ following administration of a specific ^{13}C-labelled substrate. The rate and pattern of $^{13}CO_2$ recovery in breath represents substrate metabolism and can be used to probe various gastrointestinal and metabolic functions. The ^{13}C-octanoic acid breath test is used to assess gastric emptying and has been applied in several animal species including horses,[7–11] dogs,[12] cats[13] and rodents.[14] This test allows gastric emptying to be assessed non-invasively and without requiring restraint or sedation (Figure 4). Gastric emptying is usually assessed in animals using imaging techniques such as radiography or radioscintigraphy. These procedures require sedation or restraint of the animals, which can potently affect gastrointestinal motility, and preclude accurate assessment of the effects of disease or drugs on the rate of gastric emptying. The non-invasive assessment of gastric emptying using the ^{13}C-octanoic acid breath test has permitted the rate of gastric emptying in animals to be assessed under basal conditions.

Liver disease is commonly encountered in veterinary clinical practice, and stable isotope breath tests for non-invasive assessment of liver function would be useful clinical tools. The ^{13}C-aminopyrine breath test has been applied in dogs,[15] but the potential toxicity of aminopyrine presents an obstacle to the clinical use of this test. Various non-toxic ^{13}C-substrates have been described in human medicine for assessment of liver function and the application of these tests in veterinary medicine is anticipated.

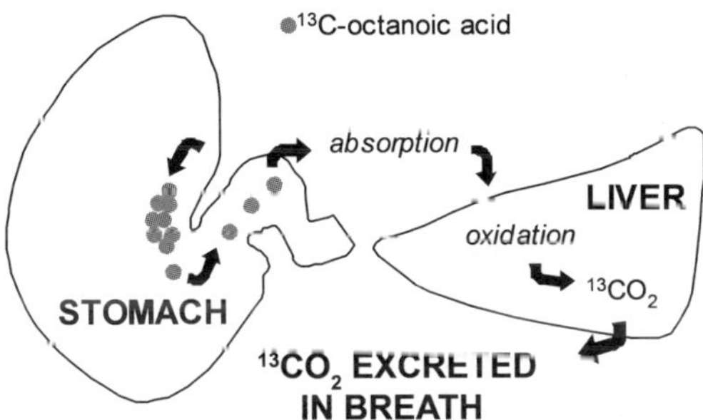

Fig. 4. The ^{13}C-octanoic acid breath test is used to measure gastric emptying. The animal ingests ^{13}C-octanoic acid which is rapidly absorbed in the duodenum and metabolised in the liver to $^{13}CO_2$. The rate of recovery of $^{13}CO_2$ in breath is then directly related to the rate of gastric emptying.

3.2. *Alkane Breath Tests*

Exhaled ethane and pentane have long been recognised as markers of *in vivo* oxidative stress.[16] There has been a recent surge in interest in the application of antioxidant therapeutics in human and in veterinary medicine, and research is required to elucidate the significance of oxidative stress in disease. The measurement of exhaled pentane in the horse has been described,[17] but high rates of endogenous metabolism of pentane make this an unsuitable marker of oxidative stress. In contrast, exhaled ethane is an excellent marker of oxidative stress, as samples can be collected non-invasively, and unlike other markers of oxidative stress, ethane is not subject to *ex vivo* oxidation, is poorly metabolised and poorly soluble in body tissues. Exhaled ethane has been applied for assessment of airway oxidative stress in numerous studies in human medicine[18,19] and similarly in horses; exhaled ethane was increased in horses with chronic respiratory disease (recurrent airway obstruction).[1] Respiratory disease is a significant problem in equine veterinary medicine and a non-invasive method for monitoring airway inflammation would be a useful clinical tool. However, further studies to correlate the ethane breath test against standard methods for assessment of equine airway inflammation are required.

Maximal exercise is a potent inducer of oxidative stress, and studies in racing dogs and horses have shown that exhaled ethane increased following exercise at gallop.[20] Antioxidant supplements are widely used in equine and canine sports, although the effects of oxidative stress on performance or on recovery from exercise are unclear. Further research is necessary to establish the implications of oxidative stress and antioxidant supplementation, for nutrition, exercise and disease in animals. Ethane can be measured rapidly and accurately using laser spectroscopy and this method will facilitate the detailed epidemiological studies that are required to establish the significance of oxidative stress in disease and in maintenance of health.

3.3. *Hydrogen Breath Test*

The hydrogen breath test is based on the detection of a hydrogen signal produced by microbial fermentation of non-digestible carbohydrates, either in the colon (for assessment of oro-caecal transit time) or in the small intestine (for detection of intestinal malabsorption). An oral dose of non-digestible carbohydrate (typically lactulose or xylose) is administered and breath hydrogen monitored for up to 24 hours. The hydrogen breath test has been applied for measurement of oro-caecal transit time in horses,[21] dogs[22] and cats[23,24] and for the detection of small intestinal malabsorbtion in dogs[25] and cats.[24]

The advantages of the hydrogen breath test are that inexpensive breath H_2 analysers are available commercially, and that the substrates are also freely available and inexpensive. However, H_2 is erratically produced in horse,[21] making the assessment of oro-caecal transit using this method difficult. It may also be difficult to differentiate between animals with small intestinal bacterial overgrowth and disordered small intestinal motility using this method, since both disorders could affect H_2 production.

3.4. *Carbon Monoxide and Nitric Oxide Breath Test*

Carbon monoxide (CO) is produced *in vivo* during the degradation of haem to bilirubin, by the enzyme haem oxygenase.[26] Nitric oxide (NO) is produced by the action of the enzyme nitric oxide synthase on the amino acid L-arginine.[27] Both nitric oxide synthase and haem oxygenase are up-regulated by inflammation, and the exhalation of CO and NO is thought to reflect respiratory inflammation.[28,29] However, in horses, exhalation of CO was only weakly associated with airway inflammation.[1,28,29] As with many other exhaled analytes, the detection of NO and CO in horses may be affected significantly by emissions from the upper airway, and this may preclude detection of inflammation of the lower airways in this species. The assessment of NO or CO in dogs or in cats has not yet been reported, although this is currently an active area investigation.

4. Exhaled Breath Condensate

Collection and analysis of EBC has been reported in the horse,[1,2,28,29] dog[3,4] and calf.[5] Recently, Deaton *et al.*[2] reported a significant association between percentage of inflammatory cells (neutrophils) in airway lining fluid and H_2O_2 in EBC in horses with respiratory inflammation. This finding indicates that analysis of EBC may have considerable potential for monitoring of airway inflammation in horses, so further research is warranted. In calves, the inflammatory mediator leukotriene B_4 was significantly increased in EBC following experimentally induced respiratory infection.[5] Collection of EBC in the dog is difficult because the low ventilation of this species mean that EBC collection requires at least 15–20 minutes of breathing through the condensation apparatus. In small dogs, this collection period is considerably longer, so this method is likely to be poorly tolerated by dogs and clinicians.

5. Conclusions

Non-invasive detection and monitoring of disease using breath tests could play an important role in the veterinary medicine of the future. At present, breath analysis is largely confined to the research laboratory where there are important issues to be addressed, including validation against standard investigative methods, standardisation of collection methods and establishment of reference ranges.

Acknowledgements

The authors are grateful for the support of the Faculty of Veterinary Medicine at the University of Glasgow and Hill's Pet Nutrition, and for the continued enthusiastic support of Professor Max Murray.

References

1. Wyse C, Skeldon K, Hotchkiss J, Gibson G, Christley R, Preston T, Cumming D, Padgett M, Cooper J, Love S. Effect of environmental modification on exhaled ethane, carbon monoxide and hydrogen peroxide in horses with respiratory inflammation. *Vet Rec* 2004: in press.
2. Deaton CM, Marlin DJ, Smith NC, Smith KC, Newton RJ, Gower SM, Cade SM, Roberts CA, Harris PA, Schroter RC, Kelly FJ. Breath condensate hydrogen peroxide correlates with both airway cytology and epithelial lining fluid ascorbic acid concentration in the horse. *Free Radic Res* 2004; **38**: 201–208.
3. Pietra M, Diana A, Forni M, Jochler M, Cinotti S. Evaluation of leukotriene B4 in the canine exhaled breath: standardization of a technique of sample collection. *Vet Res Commun* 2003; **27** Suppl 1: 425–428.
4. Wyse C, Hammond J, Arteaga A, Cumming D, Cooper J, Yam P. Collection and analysis of exhaled breath condensate H_2O_2 in conscious, healthy, dogs. *Vet Rec* 2004; **4**: 744–746.
5. Reinhold P, Becher G, Rothe M. Evaluation of the measurement of leukotriene B4 concentrations in exhaled condensate as a noninvasive method for assessing mediators of inflammation in the lungs of calves. *Am J Vet Res* 2000; **61**: 742–749.
6. Elliott-Martin R, Mottram T, Gardner J, Hobbs P, Barlett P. Preliminary investigation of breath sampling as a monitor of health in dairy cattle. *J Agric Eng Res* 1997; **67**: 267–275.
7. Wyse CA, Murphy DM, Preston T, Morrison DJ, Love S. Assessment of the rate of solid-phase gastric emptying in ponies by means of the ^{13}C-octanoic acid breath test: a preliminary study. *Equine Vet J* 2001; **33**: 197–203.
8. Wyse CA, Murphy DM, Preston T, Sutton DG, Morrison DJ, Christley RM, Love S. The ^{13}C-octanoic acid breath test for detection of effects of meal composition on the rate of solid-phase gastric emptying in ponies. *Res Vet Sci* 2001; **71**: 81–83.

9. Sutton DG, Bahr A, Preston T, Christley RM, Love S, Roussel AJ. Validation of the ^{13}C-octanoic acid breath test for measurement of equine gastric emptying rate of solids using radioscintigraphy. *Equine Vet J* 2003; **35**: 27–33.

10. Sutton DG, Bahr A, Preston T, Cohen ND, Love S, Roussel AJ. Quantitative detection of atropine-delayed gastric emptying in the horse by the ^{13}C-octanoic acid breath test. *Equine Vet J* 2002; **34**: 479–485.

11. Sutton DG, Preston T, Christley RM, Cohen ND, Love S, Roussel AJ. The effects of xylazine, detomidine, acepromazine and butorphanol on equine solid phase gastric emptying rate. *Equine Vet J* 2002; **34**: 486–492.

12. Wyse CA, Preston T, Love S, Morrison DJ, Cooper JM, Yam PS. Use of the ^{13}C-octanoic acid breath test for assessment of solid-phase gastric emptying in dogs. *Am J Vet Res* 2001; **62**: 1939–1944.

13. Peachey SE, Dawson JM, Harper EJ. Gastrointestinal transit times in young and old cats. *Comp Biochem Physiol A Mol Integr Physiol* 2000; **126**: 85–90.

14. Symonds EL, Butler RN, Omari TI. Assessment of gastric emptying in the mouse using the [13C]-octanoic acid breath test. *Clin Exp Pharmacol Physiol* 2000; **27**: 671–675.

15. Bieri HU, Bircher J. L-methionine ordinarily does not interfere with the aminopyrine breath test: studies in dogs and rats. *Biochem Pharmacol* 1981; **30**: 1421–1424.

16. Riely CA, Cohen G, Lieberman M. Ethane evolution: a new index of lipid peroxidation. *Science* 1974; **183**: 208–210.

17. Wyse CA, Love S, Christley RM, Yam PS, Cooper JM, Cumming DR, Preston T. Validation of a method for collection and assay of pentane in the exhaled breath of the horse. *Res Vet Sci* 2004; **76**: 109–112.

18. Paredi P, Kharitonov SA, Barnes PJ. Elevation of exhaled ethane concentration in asthma. *Am J Respir Crit Care Med* 2000; **162**: 1450–1454.

19. Paredi P, Kharitonov SA, Leak D, Ward S, Cramer D, Barnes PJ. Exhaled ethane, a marker of lipid peroxidation, is elevated in chronic obstructive pulmonary disease. *Am J Respir Crit Care Med* 2000; **162**: 369–373.

20. Cathcart A, Wyse C, Sutherland R, Ward S, Gibson G, Padgett M, Skeldon K. Effect of maximal dynamic exercise on exhaled ethane and carbon monoxide levels in human, equine and canine athletes. Abstract at the conference *Breath Gas Analysis in Medical Diagnostics*, September 23–26, 2004, Dornbirn (Austria).

21. Murphy D, Reid SW, Love S. Breath hydrogen measurement in ponies: a preliminary study. *Res Vet Sci* 1998; **65**: 47–51.

22. Papasouliotis K, Gruffydd-Jones TJ, Sparkes AH, Cripps PJ. A comparison of orocaecal transit times assessed by the breath hydrogen test and the sulphasalazine/sulphapyridine method in healthy beagle dogs. *Res Vet Sci* 1995; **58**: 263–267.

23. Papasouliotis K, Muir P, Gruffydd Jones TJ, Galloway P, Smerdon T, Cripps PJ. Decreased orocaecal transit time, as measured by the exhalation of hydrogen, in hyperthyroid cats. *Res Vet Sci* 1993; **55**: 115–118.

24. Muir P, Papassouliotis K, Gruffydd-Jones TJ, Cripps PJ, Harbour DA. Evaluation of carbohydrate malassimilation and intestinal transit time in cats

by measurement of breath hydrogen excretion. *Am J Vet Res* 1991; **52**: 1104–1109.

25. Washabau RJ, Strombeck DR, Buffington CA, Harrold D. Evaluation of intestinal carbohydrate malabsorption in the dog by pulmonary hydrogen gas excretion. *Am J Vet Res* 1986; **47**: 1402–1406.

26. Tenhunen R, Marver HS, Schmid R. Microsomal heme oxygenase. Characterization of the enzyme. *J Biol Chem* 1969; **244**: 6388–6394.

27. Palmer RM, Ashton DS, Moncada S. Vascular endothelial cells synthesize nitric oxide from L-arginine. *Nature* 1988; **333**: 664–666.

28. Horvath I, Donnelly LE, Kiss A, Paredi P, Kharitonov SA, Barnes PJ. Raised levels of exhaled carbon monoxide are associated with an increased expression of heme oxygenase-1 in airway macrophages in asthma: a new marker of oxidative stress. *Thorax* 1998; **53**: 668–672.

29. Kharitonov SA, Yates D, Robbins RA, Logan-Sinclair R, Shinebourne EA, Barnes PJ. Increased nitric oxide in exhaled air of asthmatic patients. *Lancet* 1994; **343**: 133–135.

POTENTIAL FOR AND LIMITATIONS OF EXHALED BREATH ANALYSIS IN ANIMAL MODELS

P. REINHOLD

Friedrich-Loeffler-Institut (FLI),
Institute of Molecular Pathogenesis,
Federal Research Institute for Animal Health,
Naumburger Straße 96a, D-07743 Jena, Germany

C. DEATON AND D. MARLIN

Animal Health Trust,
Kentford, Newmarket, Suffolk CB8 7UU, UK

1. Introduction

Because exhalate is the product of alveolar gas exchange and airway water loss, it most likely contains metabolites from the lungs or substances originating from biochemical reactions in the airway mucosa. With respect to respiratory physiology and the metabolic functions of the lung, various gaseous and non-gaseous components have already been detected in the exhaled breath of humans[1,2] and animals.[3-11] This paper summarises methodological and biological aspects of exhaled breath gas analysis and exhaled breath condensate sampling in order to assess non-invasively the respiratory system in animals.

2. Analysis of Exhaled Breath Gases in Animals

Measurements of volatile substances in exhaled breath have a long history; measurement of ammonia in exhaled breath was first reported approximately one hundred years ago. In modern human medicine, exhaled nitric oxide (NO),[1,12] but also carbon monoxide (CO) and other gases, including breath alkanes (*e.g.* ethane, pentane) are measured in exhaled breath and viewed as markers of airway inflammation.[13] In animals, measurements of NO in exhaled breath have been reported in elephants, horses, cattle, pigs, sheep, dogs and cats, as well as in anaesthetised and ventilated laboratory animals, including mice, rats, guinea pigs and rabbits.[3,6,11,14-16]

2.1. *Methodological Aspects of Exhaled Breath Gas Analysis in Animals*

NO has been the most widely studied exhaled marker both in humans and animals.[1,3,6,7,11–18] Concentrations of NO in exhaled breath can be determined by sampling the exhaled airstream directly (on-line measurement) or by analysing the concentration of NO in mixed exhaled air collected in a reservoir bag (off-line measurement). Since the measured values of exhaled NO depend on tidal volume and flow, a standardised breathing pattern (single breath manoeuvre) is considered ideal for NO measurements in conscious patients, in human medicine. This is not possible in children or in animals, in which collections of gas or on-line measurements can only be made during tidal breathing. In awake large animals (elephants, horses), three modified methods have been employed: (1) sampling exhaled gas with a syringe,[6] (2) continuously aspirating respiratory gas via a thin plastic tube and analysing NO concentrations on-line,[16], and (3) collecting exhaled NO into a reservoir bag and measuring the NO concentration off-line.[19]

In humans and several animal species, nasal NO concentrations were found to be much higher than tracheal concentrations of NO.[12,20] This is due to very high NO production in the epithelium of the nose and especially in the paranasal sinuses. Interestingly, nasal NO production is highly variable amongst different species and is much lower in mammals without paranasal sinuses (for example baboons) compared to species with paranasal sinuses.[7] In healthy horses, nasal occlusion does not result in a measured increase in the concentration of NO[19] and exhaled NO is not reduced when collected via an endo-tracheal tube as compared to that sampled from the nostrils under halothane anaesthesia,[16] suggesting that the nasal passages do not contribute significantly to exhaled NO in this species. However, halothane anaesthesia has been shown to markedly reduce exhaled NO in horses.[18] When exhaled NO was measured in horses anaesthetised with an intravenous regimen, the nasal NO concentration was found to be approximately double that exiting the endotracheal tube (see Fig. 1). However, as the volume and flow rate of the air exiting the lung is far in excess of that of the nasopharynx, the contribution to total exhaled NO is likely to be small.

From the current knowledge concerning exhaled NO analysis in human medicine, a number of limitations arise in applying exhaled breath analysis to spontaneously breathing animals:

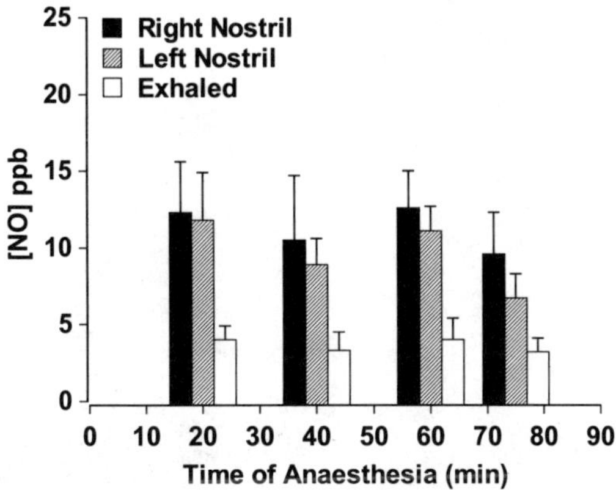

Fig. 1.   Nasal and exhaled NO concentrations (ppb) measured in eight intubated, anaesthetised horses during total intravenous anaesthesia (Marlin, Young and McMurphy, unpublished data)

- The concentration of NO in exhaled breath is dependent on the expired flow rate, which cannot easily be regulated in conscious animals.
- Due to the very high NO production in nose and paranasal sinuses, nasal NO should be eliminated from NO measurements in exhaled breath in order to assess the peripheral respiratory system and airway inflammation. However, nasal breathing is the predominant route of ventilation in most animals and is obligatory in the horse.
- Larger animals such as the horse and cow also have a significantly greater proportion of tidal volume that is dead space (somewhere between 50 % and 75 %), which is primarily due to a larger anatomical dead space.
- Inspired air must not contain any NO.
- The N_2-balance of the total organism may influence exhaled NO levels (carnivores are different from herbivores; the protein content of the diet could affect exhaled NO).
- NO analysers are mainly based on chemiluminescence (and are still relatively expensive).

2.2. *Analyses of NO and CO in Cats and Horses*

Despite these biological and technical limitations the concentration of NO in exhaled breath has been successfully determined in both cats (Fig. 2)

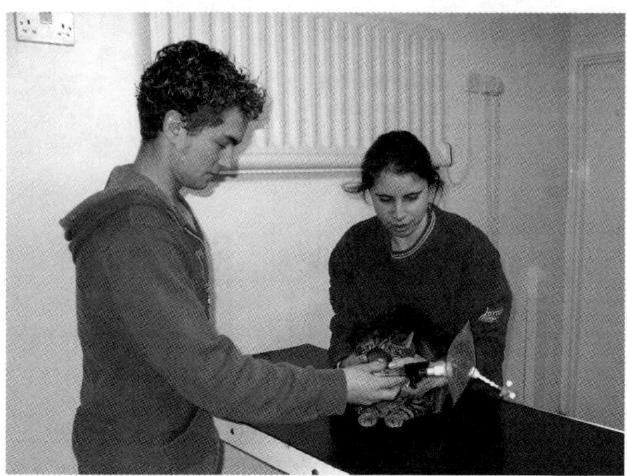

Fig. 2.   Exhaled breath collection in a non-sedated cat (photo: Marlin)

and horses.[19,21] In both species, exhaled air was collected into a Tedlar reservoir bag by use of a sealed facemask and non-rebreathing valve. The measurement of the NO concentration was reproducible within and between reservoir bags. There was no diurnal variation in exhaled NO concentrations in horses and the NO was not affected by feeding. In cats, NO concentrations in exhaled breath were higher in the afternoon than in the morning. In horses, mild neutrophilic airway inflammation did not result in an elevation in exhaled NO concentration. In contrast, cats with lower respiratory tract disease had significantly higher exhaled NO concentrations than healthy cats. The impact of ambient NO on the concentration of exhaled NO has also been investigated in horses. There was good agreement between concentrations of NO in exhaled breath when breathing NO-free air compared to ambient air when the concentration of NO in ambient air was less than one part-per-billion (ppb).[19]

There are far fewer studies of the concentration of CO in exhaled breath compared to NO in either human subjects or animals. However, a number of studies have demonstrated that exhaled CO concentration is greater in human patients with asthma, chronic obstructive pulmonary disease or cystic fibrosis compared to healthy controls (reviewed in Ref. 13). CO has been demonstrated to be undetectable in the exhaled breath of both healthy horses and cats (less than 0.1 parts-per-million, ppm) when measured off-line,[19,21] in contrast to the concentrations in exhaled breath from healthy human subjects (2.0 ± 0.2 ppm).[22]

3. Analysis of Exhaled Breath Condensate in Animals

As an alternative to the measurement of volatile markers in exhaled breath, a variety of compounds can be measured in condensed exhalate.[2,4,9,10,23–26] There is increasing interest in this technique, because the method of condensate collection is simple, completely non-invasive, repeatable and does not necessarily require patient cooperation (just spontaneous breathing). According to the recommendations of a joint Task Force of the European Respiratory and the American Thoracic Societies, "exhaled breath condensate" (EBC) is the preferred term to describe the sample collected by cooling the exhaled breath.

The rationale for making measurements in EBC is based on the hypothesis that water and aerosols (which are present in the exhaled breath) contain a range of compounds which reflect the concentrations within the extracellular epithelial lining fluid in the peripheral airways. To date, EBC samples have been collected in horses, calves, pigs, dogs and cats using different collection methods.[4,5,8,10,23–25,27,28]

3.1. *Methodological Aspects of Collection of Exhaled Breath Condensate in Different Species*

3.1.1. *Sampling devices*

A variety of custom made systems have been described to collect EBC from conscious, non-sedated animals as follows: Using a facemask with non-rebreathing valves (NRBV) and a cooled double-jacketed sample collection tube made of polytetrafluorethylene, EBC was collected from non-sedated calves in an early study.[24] EBC has also been collected from dogs using a facemask and NRBV with the expirate being passed through a cooled stainless steel collecting tube.[5] In conscious cats, EBC has been collected from a sealed chamber with a bias flow, with all the air leaving the chamber directed through a stainless steel tube cooled in iced water.[23,28] In conscious horses, two different custom made systems for collection of EBC have been described:[4,27] (*i*) Due to the use of an un-cuffed endotracheal tube, an undefined fraction of the total ventilation during the period of collection was directed through a condensing system.[27] (*ii*) In the system described by Deaton *et al.*,[4] the expiratory port of the facemask was connected to the stainless steel condensing tube (volume 5 litres) in iced water by a flexible PVC tube (volume 5 litres) maintained at approximately 35 °C by a heated outer tube.

The only commercially available system that has been used in animals is the ECoScreen (Viasys Healthcare, Hoechberg, Germany) and its use has been limited to calves and pigs in combination with a facemask using a non-rebreathing valve (Figs. 3 and 4). This system would not be suitable for animals larger than man due to unacceptably high resistance. Although the methodology of collecting EBC in spontaneously breathing animals is comparable to that used in humans when using the same technique, anatomical differences exist (*e.g.* nasal breathing) and equipment differences in using a facemask (instead of a mouthpiece) to adapt the collection system to the animal's head. Therefore, the equipment dead space in the collection systems will be greater in animals than in humans where there is direct connection to the mouth or nasal passages.

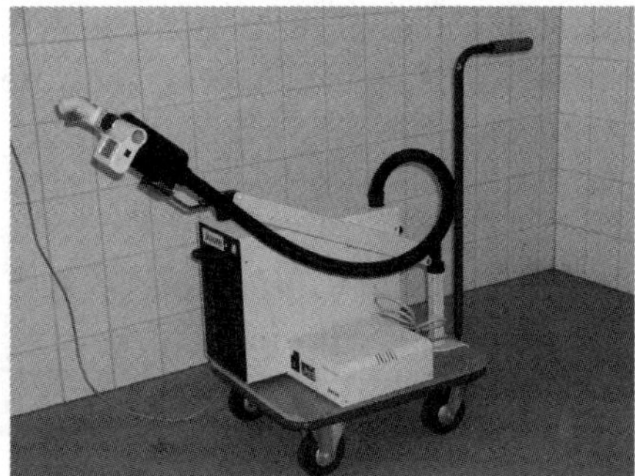

Fig. 3.   The collection system "ECoScreen" (Viasys Healthcare) — originally designed for human medicine — to be used in animals (photo: Reinhold)

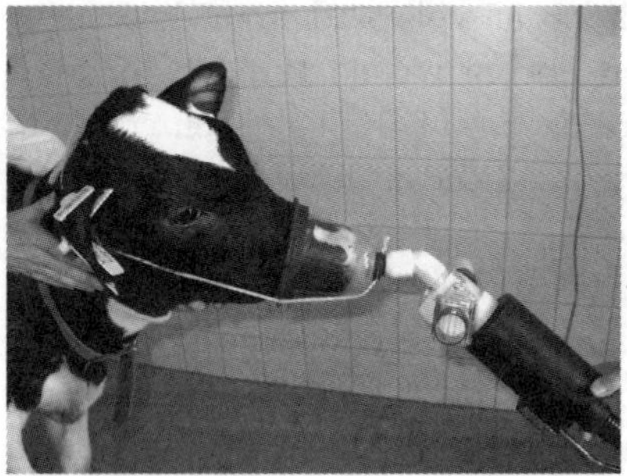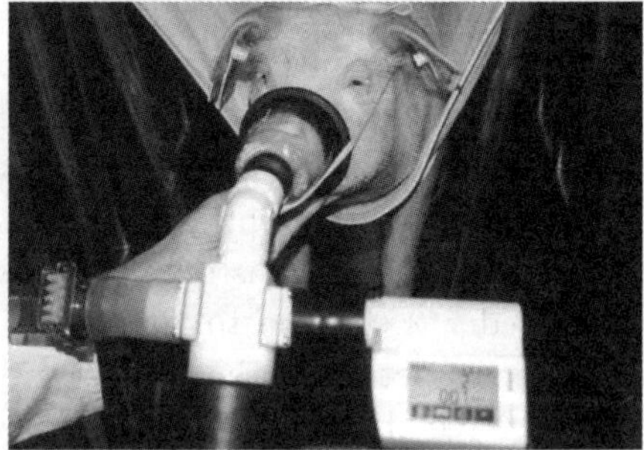

Fig. 4.   Collection of exhaled breath condensate using the system "ECoScreen" in a conscious calf and a sedated pig. On the system used to collect EBC from pigs, the electronic spirometer "ECoVent" can be seen attached to the expiratory port of the system on the right (photos: Reinhold).

3.1.2. *Lung function and ambient conditions*

Collection of EBC does not affect lung function in spontaneously breathing subjects,[29] however the volume collected is influenced by variables of lung function. As in humans, the volume of EBC collected per unit time depends mainly on individual minute ventilation.[24,30] Therefore, in small species, a longer period of collection is required to obtain the same volume of EBC as in a larger species. This may have the disadvantage that more labile components of the condensate may become degraded during prolonged collection periods. Despite minute ventilation being the most important factor affecting the collection of EBC, expiratory airflow rates and the ratio between dead space volume and tidal volume may also influence EBC-collection and the origin of exhaled breath condensate (Reinhold *et al.*, unpublished data).

Using the technique of collection described by Sparkes *et al.*[28] and Kirschvink *et al.*[23] EBC collection was combined with simultaneous measurements of lung function using whole body barometric plethysmography in cats. No effect of bias flow rate (2–6 L/min) or collection duration (20–40 min) on EBC collection was found. The volume of EBC collected was found to be positively linearly related to both ambient temperature and relative humidity.

Care should be taken to standardise the collection procedure as far as possible. Because species-specific conditions for EBC-collection must be accepted, the collection process should be standardised at least within each species in order to minimise unknown or variable factors that result from the collection process but may influence the composition of EBC. In order to allow comparison of different studies, not only the conditions of collection (temperature, duration of condensation, etc) but also the breathing pattern during EBC-collection should be reported.

3.2. *Substances Measured in EBC of Animals*

Different *non-volatile* substances or molecules have been examined in EBC with respect to airway inflammation and respiratory disease in large animal studies.

3.2.1. *Hydrogen peroxide*

Hydrogen peroxide (H_2O_2) has been measured in the EBC of horses, dogs and cats[4,5,23] and has been found to be elevated in inflammatory airway diseases.[4,23]

Horses with chronic airway inflammation had higher H_2O_2 concentrations in EBC (2.0 ± 0.5 μmol/L, mean $\pm$ SD) than healthy horses (0.4 ± 0.2 μmol/L).[4] The concentration of H_2O_2 in EBC was correlated positively with the neutrophil count and inversely with the ascorbic acid concentration in bronchoalveolar lavage fluid (BALF). In contrast, an acute neutrophilic inflammatory response did not result in an elevation in EBC H_2O_2 concentration.[31]

Kirschvink et al.[23] measured H_2O_2 in EBC samples collected in both healthy cats and in cats sensitised to Ascaris suum. In healthy cats there was a positive correlation between BALF neutrophil percentage and EBC H_2O_2 concentration. In Ascaris suum sensitised cats challenged with Ascaris suum aerosol, EBC H_2O_2 was increased, whilst there was no change in control cats following challenge. In addition, the EBC H_2O_2 concentration was positively correlated with BALF eosinophil percentage when both healthy and sensitised cats were combined. This suggests that in cats at least, increases in EBC H_2O_2 concentration may occur as a result of either neutrophilic or eosinophilic airway inflammation or both.

3.2.2. Leukotriene B4

Leukotriene B4 (LTB_4) has been mainly evaluated in the EBC of calves up to the age of 2 months.[9,24] In healthy calves, the measurements of LTB_4 were normally distributed, ranging from 32 to 225 pg/mL (116 ± 55 pg/mL, mean$\pm$SD).[24] Intra-individual variation in LTB_4 is much less than the inter-individual variability (Fig. 5) and indicates that it is more appropriate for comparing changes within individuals over time rather than between different animals.[9] EBC LTB_4 also correlates strongly with BALF neutrophil number. In the presence of both experimental bacterial and viral infections, EBC LTB_4 was increased.[24] In bacterial bronchopneumonia, there was a significant negative correlation between lung compliance and LTB_4. In viral disease high EBC LTB_4 appeared to be related to increased non-specific bronchial reactivity.[24]

3.2.3. Urea and ammonia

Since EBC contains large quantities of ammonia, which interfere with commercially available urea assays, urea alone cannot be accurately measured in EBC samples. Thus, the ammonia already present in the EBC must be measured separately and subtracted from the total "urea" measured. Both urea and ammonia have been measured in EBC samples from pigs and calves. Under physiological conditions, influences of food intake and

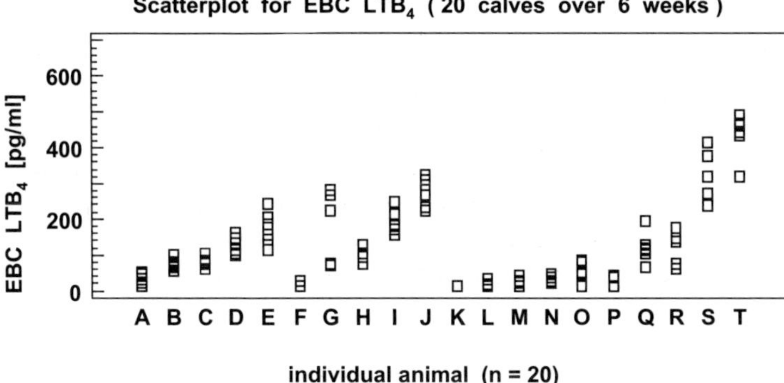

Fig. 5. Concentration of leukotriene B4 (LTB$_4$) in exhaled breath condensate samples collected from 20 calves (A...T) over 6 weeks (one EBC collection per animal weekly; $n = 6$ per animal). Individual LTB$_4$ ranges differed markedly between animals (mean range between animals: 372 pg/mL). Using variance component analysis, 21 % of total variance was related to intra-subject variability while 79 % of total variance was due to inter-subject variability (Reinhold, unpublished data).

ventilation must be taken into account on the concentration of urea and/or ammonia.[10,25] Under conditions of acute bacterial infection and/or pneumonia (induced by gram negative bacteria in a calf-model), urea increased significantly in the EBC as well as in the peripheral blood leading to the conclusion that the increase in EBC urea may be a result of a change in permeability of the lung-capillary barrier. In contrast, ammonia increased in the EBC (but not in the peripheral blood) indicating a local production of ammonia in the pneumonic lung.[26]

3.2.4. *pH*

In fresh (non-degassed) EBC samples of healthy calves and pigs, "physiological" pH measured immediately after collection was normally distributed, varying between 5.6 and 6.2, and was not significantly different between species.[8] This finding is in general agreement with results reported in humans, showing that fluid condensed from the breath of healthy volunteers is originally acidic. After degassing for 10 min with argon, the pH of EBC from healthy horses, dogs and cats was found to be above 7.0 (Marlin, Deaton and Kingston, unpublished data). The current consensus of opinion in the literature is that prior to EBC pH measurement, samples should always be degassed; however, un-degassed samples may more closely reflect the pH on the airway surface.

4. Conclusions

Exhaled breath analysis in animals has direct application in animal studies and veterinary medicine, but may also contribute to the understanding of the pathophysiology of human pulmonary disease and dysfunction. Animal models offer the opportunity to undertake studies that may not be possible in human subjects. Direct correlation of tissue histopathology at *post mortem* with *in vivo* measurements of markers or mediators of lung disease or dysfunction in cohorts of animals under controlled conditions is also possible.

References

1. Kharitonov SA, Barnes PJ. Clinical aspects of exhaled nitric oxide. *Eur Respir J* 2000; **16**: 781–792.
2. Scheideler L, Manke HG, Schwulera U, Inacker O, Hämmerle H. Detection of nonvolatile macromolecules in breath. A possible diagnostic tool? *Am Rev Respir Dis* 1993; **148**: 778–784.
3. Bernareggi M, Rossoni G, Clini E, Pasini E, Bachetti T, Cremona G, Ambrosino N, Berti F. Detection of nitric oxide in exhaled air of different animal species using a clinical chemiluminescence analyser. *Pharmacol Res* 1999; **39**: 221–224.
4. Deaton CM, Marlin DJ, Smith NC, Smith KC, Newton RJ, Gower SM, Cade SM, Roberts CA, Harris PA, Schroter RC, Kelly FJ. Breath condensate hydrogen peroxide correlates with both airway cytology and epithelial lining fluid ascorbic acid concentration in the horse. *Free Radic Res* 2004; **38**: 201–208.
5. Hirt R, Gütl A, Delvaux F, Gustin P, Marlin D, Kirschvink N. Hydrogen peroxide and pH analysis in exhaled breath condensate of healthy dogs (abstract). *J Vet Int Med* 2003; **17**: 746.
6. Lewandowski K, Busch T, Lewandowski M, Keske U, Gerlach H, Falke KJ. Evidence of nitric oxide in the exhaled gas of Asian elephants (*Elephas maximus*). *Respir Physiol* 1996; **106**: 91–98.
7. Lewandowski K, Busch T, Lohbrunner H, Rensing S, Keske U, Gerlach H, Falke KJ. Low nitric oxide concentrations in exhaled gas and nasal airways of mammals without paranasal sinuses. *J Appl Physiol* 1998; **85**: 405–410.
8. Reinhold P, Jäger J, Langenberg A, Födisch G, Marlin D. Physiological values for pH and pCO2 in exhaled breath condensate samples from pigs and calves. In: *Proceedings of the 21st Symposium of the Veterinary and Comparative Respiratory Society, San Antonio, Texas (USA)*, October 2–5, 2003: 43.
9. Reinhold P, Langenberg A, Becher G, Rothe M. Intra- and inter-subject variability of LTB4 in exhaled breath condensate samples of healthy subjects (calves). *Eur Respir J* 2003; **22** (Suppl 45): P364.
10. Reinhold P, Langenberg A, Rothe M, and Becher G. The influence of feeding on the concentration of urea and ammonium in exhaled breath condensate

and peripheral blood. In: *Proceedings of the 22nd Symposium of the Veterinary and Comparative Respiratory Society, Montreal (Canada)*, October 1–3, 2004: 79.

11. Schedin U, Röken BO, Nyman G, Frostell C, Gustafsson LE. Endogenous nitric oxide in the airways of different animal species. *Acta Anaesthesiol Scand* 1997; **41**: 1133–1141.

12. Gustafsson LE. Exhaled nitric oxide as a marker in asthma. *Eur Respir J Suppl* 1998; **26**: 49S–52S.

13. Kharitonov SA, Barnes PJ. Exhaled markers of pulmonary disease. *Am J Respir Crit Care Med* 2001; **163**: 1693–1722.

14. Cook S, Duplain H, Egli M, Nicod P, Scherrer U. Exhaled nitric oxide does not provide a marker of endothelial function. *Eur Respir J* 2000; **16** (Suppl 31): P1915.

15. Fujii Y, Goldberg P, Hussain SN. Intrathoracic and extrathoracic sources of exhaled nitric oxide in porcine endotoxemic shock. *Chest* 1998; **114**: 569–576.

16. Mills PC, Marlin DJ, Demoncheaux E, Scott C, Casas I, Smith NC, Higenbottam T. Nitric oxide and exercise in the horse. *J Physiol* 1996; **495** (Pt 3): 863–874.

17. Gustafsson LE, Leone AM, Persson MG, Wiklund NP, Moncada S. Endogenous nitric oxide is present in the exhaled air of rabbits, guinea pigs and humans. *Biochem Biophys Res Commun* 1991; **181**: 852–857.

18. Marlin DJ, Young LE, McMurphy R, Walsh K, Dixon P. Effect of two anaesthetic regimens on airway nitric oxide production in horses. *Br J Anaesth* 2001; **86**: 127–130.

19. Deaton C, Maxted C, Fehmi A, Marlin D. Measurement of exhaled nitric oxide and carbon monoxide in the horse. In: *Proceedings of the 22nd Symposium of the Veterinary and Comparative Respiratory Society, Montreal (Canada)*, October 1–3, 2004: 19.

20. Kirsten AM, Jörres RA, Kirsten D, Magnussen H. Comparison of nasal and bronchial production of nitric oxide in healthy probands and patients with asthma [in German]. *Pneumologie* 1997; **51**: 359–364.

21. Marlin D, Fehmi A, Sparkes A, Mardell E, Deaton C, Adams V. A preliminary investigation of exhaled NO and CO in healthy cats and cats with airway inflammation. In: *Proceedings of the 22nd Symposium of the Veterinary and Comparative Respiratory Society, Montreal (Canada)*, October 1–3, 2004: 56.

22. Zanconato S, Scollo M, Zaramella C, Landi L, Zacchello F, Baraldi E. Exhaled carbon monoxide levels after a course of oral prednisone in children with asthma exacerbation. *J Allergy Clin Immunol* 2002; **109**: 440–445.

23. Kirschvink N, Delvaux F, Leemans J, Clercx C, Marlin D, Sparkes A, Gustin P. Collection of exhaled breath condensate and analysis of hydrogen peroxide as potential marker of lower airway inflammation in cats. *The Veterinary J* 2005: in press.

24. Reinhold P, Becher G, Rothe M. Evaluation of the measurement of leukotriene B4 concentrations in exhaled condensate as a noninvasive method for assessing mediators of inflammation in the lungs of calves. *Am J Vet Res* 2000; **61**: 742–749.

25. Reinhold P, Langenberg A, Födisch G, Rothe M. The influence of variables of ventilation on the concentration of urea and ammonia in the exhaled breath condensate. *Eur Respir J* 2004; **24** (Suppl 48): P2486.

26. Reinhold P, Langenberg A, Seifert J, Rothe M, Becher G. Ammonia and urea in the exhaled breath condensate (EBC) and in corresponding blood samples. *Eur Respir J* 2002; **20** (Suppl 38): P3034.

27. Schack S, Fey K, Sasse HHL. Collection of breath condensate in horses. *Pferdeheilkunde* 2002; **18**: 612–616.

28. Sparkes A, Mardell E, Deaton C, Kirschvink N, Marlin D. Exhaled breath condensate (EBC) collection in cats-description of a non-invasive technique to investigate airway disease. *J Feline Med Surg* 2004; **6**: 335–338.

29. Reinhold P, Langenberg A, Födisch G, Jäger J. Die Gewinnung von Atemkondensat hat keinen negativen Einfluss auf die Lungenfunktion. *Pneumologie* 2003; **57**: 769.

30. Gessner C, Kuhn H, Seyfarth HJ, Pankau H, Winkler J, Schauer J, Wirtz H. Factors influencing breath condensate volume. *Pneumologie* 2001; **55**: 414–419.

31. Deaton C, Marlin D, Smith N, Harris P, Schroter R, Kelly F. Acute neutrophilic airway inflammation is associated with a decrease in pulmonary ascorbic acid concentration but not an elevation of exhaled hydrogen peroxide. *Eur Respir J* 2004; **24** (Suppl 48): 3651.

INDEX